BARTLETT'S MEDICAL
MANAGEMENT OF HIV
INFECTION

Bartlett's Medical Management of HIV Infection

17TH EDITION

John G. Bartlett,
Robert R. Redfield,
and Paul A. Pham

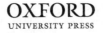

OXFORD
UNIVERSITY PRESS

OXFORD
UNIVERSITY PRESS

Oxford University Press is a department of the University of Oxford. It furthers
the University's objective of excellence in research, scholarship, and education
by publishing worldwide. Oxford is a registered trade mark of Oxford University
Press in the UK and certain other countries.

Published in the United States of America by Oxford University Press
198 Madison Avenue, New York, NY 10016, United States of America.

Library of Congress Cataloging-in-Publication Data
Names: Bartlett, John G., author. | Redfield, Robert R., author. | Pham, Paul A., author.
Title: Bartlett's medical management of HIV infection / John G. Bartlett,
Robert R. Redfield, Paul A. Pham.
Other titles: Medical management of HIV infection
Description: Oxford; New York : Oxford University Press, [2019] |
Includes bibliographical references and index.
Identifiers: LCCN 2018038498 | ISBN 9780190924775 (pbk. : alk. paper)
Subjects: | MESH: HIV Infections—therapy
Classification: LCC RC606.6 | NLM WC 503.2 | DDC 616.97/92—dc23
LC record available at https://lccn.loc.gov/2018038498

9 8 7 6 5 4 3

Printed by Sheridan Books, Inc., United States of America

CONTENTS

Pioneered by Dr. John Bartlett, and published every few years over the past 22 years, the *Medical Management of HIV Infection* has been the leading HIV diagnosis and treatment resource globally for physicians and healthcare professionals who provide care to patients with HIV. *Bartlett's Medical Management of HIV Infection— 17th Edition* maintains the tradition of excellence established by the previous editions and summarizes available data and knowledge from the medical literature, as well as from every relevant major conference, distills best practices, and presents guidance for hands-on patient management in a clear, authoritative, and reader-friendly format.

As was the case with the previous editions, *Bartlett's Medical Management of HIV Infection—17th Edition* will prove to be a trusted companion to all HIV clinicians, and will provide practical and up-to-date knowledge that can be directly applied to the care of persons living with HIV worldwide. This will lead to improvement in the health and well-being of individual patients, as well as contribute to ongoing efforts to eliminate HIV as a public health threat as we expand services to achieve universal health coverage.

—Eric P. Goosby, MD
UN Secretary-General's Special Envoy on Tuberculosis
MacArthur Foundation Chair in Global Health Sciences
Professor of Medicine
Director, Global Health Delivery and Diplomacy,
Global Health Sciences
University of California, San Francisco

CONTENTS

Foreword

With more than 30 million people living with HIV, nearly 2 million new HIV infections, and 1 million deaths in 2017 globally, the HIV epidemic continues to exert a considerable deleterious impact on the health of individuals, communities, and the economic growth of nations. However, remarkable advances have also been achieved: improvements in our scientific understanding of the biology of HIV, how it causes disease, and its prevention and treatment, coupled with unprecedented multisectoral global efforts, have resulted in rendering HIV infection essentially a manageable chronic disease.

These advances notwithstanding, considerable challenges remain: a substantial proportion of persons with HIV infections do not know that they are infected; of those who are diagnosed with HIV infection, a substantial proportion are not linked to care for antiretroviral therapy and other services; retention in care continues to be problematic; and the rate of viral suppression remains unacceptably low. The issues and challenges are not all problematic: there is a continued need for clinicians proficient in the medical management of HIV infection, from screening and testing for HIV infection, to prompt initiation of antiretroviral therapy for prevention and treatment, instituting prophylaxis against opportunistic infections where appropriate and managing complications of HIV and its treatment as well as associated co-morbidities.

Pioneered by Dr. John Bartlett, and published every few years over the past 22 years, the *Medical Management of HIV Infection* has been the leading HIV diagnosis and treatment resource globally for physicians and healthcare professionals who provide care to patients with HIV. *Bartlett's Medical Management of HIV Infection—17th Edition* maintains the tradition of excellence established by the previous editions and summarizes available data and knowledge from the medical literature, as well as from every relevant major conference, distills best practices, and presents guidance for hands-on patient management in a clear, authoritative, and reader-friendly format.

As was the case with the previous editions, *Bartlett's Medical Management of HIV Infection—17th Edition* will prove to be a trusted companion to all HIV clinicians, and will provide practical and up-to-date knowledge that can be directly applied to the care of persons living with HIV worldwide. This will lead to improvement in the health and well-being of individual patients, as well as contribute to ongoing efforts to eliminate HIV as a public health threat as we expand services to achieve universal health coverage.

—Eric P. Goosby, MD
UN Secretary-General's Special Envoy on Tuberculosis
MacArthur Foundation Chair in Global Health Sciences
Professor of Medicine
Director, Global Health Delivery and Diplomacy,
Global Health Sciences
University of California, San Francisco

Acknowledgments

We thank our colleagues for their contributions, consultation, and content review:

Okan Akay, MD
Shanna Berry, DO
Inderjeet Brar, MD
Aditya Chandorkar, MBBS
Alex Chen, MD
Joel Chua, MD
Cassidy Claassen, MD, MPH
Niel T. Constantine, PhD
Rhonda Dillon, MD
James Doub, MD
Shara Epstein, MD
Bruce Gilliam, MD
Thomasine Guberski, CRNP, PhD
Lottie Hachaambwa, MBChB
Niyati Jakharia, MBBS
Eurides Lopes, MD
Anjali Majumdar, MD
Poonam Mathur, DO
Sandra Medina Moreno, MS
Afua Ntem-Mensah, MBChB
Ibukun Oni, MBBS

Devang Patel, MD
Husain Poonawala, MBBS
Rekha Rapaka, MD, PhD
David Riedel, MD, MPH
Brenna Roth, MD, MPH
Patrick Ryscavage, MD
Kapil Saharia, MD, MPH
Paul Saleeb, MD
Sarah Schmalzle, MD
Kamini Shah, MD
Madeeha Shams, MBBS
Maryana Shenderov, MD
Lydia Tang, MBChB
Patricia Tellez-Watson, MD
Calvin Williams, MD, PhD
Eleanor Wilson, MD, MPH
Richard Y. Zhao, MS, PhD

Project Director: Kathy Cyryca

This publication was made possible through funding from Gilead to the University of Maryland, Baltimore Foundation.

Disclaimers and Disclosures

This book is provided as a resource for physicians and other healthcare professionals providing care and treatment to patients with HIV/AIDS. Every effort is made to ensure the accuracy and reliability of material presented in this book; however, recommendations for care and treatment change rapidly, and opinion can be controversial. Therefore, physicians and other healthcare professionals are encouraged to consult other sources and confirm the information contained within this book. The authors, reviewers, contributors, and production staff will not be held liable for errors, omissions, or inaccuracies in information or for any perceived harm to users of this book. It is up to the individual physician or healthcare professional to use his or her best medical judgment in determining appropriate patient care or treatment because no single reference or service can take the place of medical training, education, and experience.

Neither the Johns Hopkins University; the Johns Hopkins Health System Corporation; the University of Maryland, Baltimore; the University of Maryland Medical System; nor the authors, contributors, and reviewers are responsible for deletions or inaccuracies in information or for claims of injury resulting from any such deletions or inaccuracies. Mention of specific drugs or products within this book does not constitute endorsement by the authors; the Johns Hopkins University Division of Infectious

Diseases; the Johns Hopkins University School of Medicine; the University of Maryland, Baltimore Division of Infectious Diseases; the University of Maryland Baltimore, Institute of Human Virology; or the University of Maryland Baltimore, School of Medicine. With regard to specific drugs or products, physicians are advised to consult their normal resources before prescribing to their patients.

Dr. John G. Bartlett has no conflicts of interest to report.
Dr. Robert R. Redfield has no conflicts of interest to report.
Dr. Paul A. Pham has no conflicts of interest to report.

1

Natural History and Classification

Stages

The natural history of untreated HIV infection is divided into the following stages:

Viral transmission —— 2–3 weeks ——▶ Acute retroviral syndrome —— 2–3 weeks ——▶

Recovery & seroconversion —— 2–4 weeks ——▶ Asymptomatic chronic HIV infection

—— Avg 8 yrs ——▶ Symptomatic HIV infection/AIDS —— Avg 1.3 yrs ——▶ Death

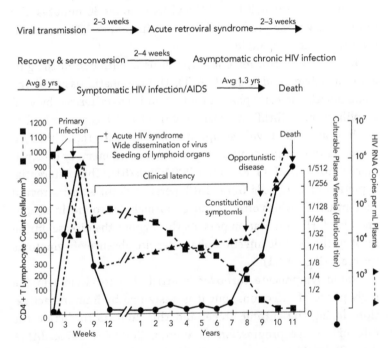

FIGURE 1.1 Natural history of HIV infection in an average patient without antiretroviral therapy from the time of HIV transmission of death at 10–11 years.

Life Cycle and Natural History of HIV

The external glycoprotein gp120 attaches to the CD4 cell receptor. This allows binding of gp120 to co-receptors (CCR5 and CXCR4) on the cell surface. Binding is followed by insertion of gp41 into the CD4 cell, resulting in membrane fusion and fusion within pores followed by release of viral core into the CD4 cell cytoplasm (Lancet 2006; 368:489). The HIV genome is then reverse transcribed to DNA by reverse transcriptase. Viral DNA is then carried into the nucleus and inserted into host DNA by the viral integrase enzyme. Finally, translated viral proteins are processed by viral proteases, allowing assembly of new virions, which are released from the cell to infect other targets, completing the viral life cycle. The half-life of the virus is about 30 minutes, the number of virions produced daily is estimated at 10^{10}, and lymphocyte turnover is rapid.

Immediately after infection, the virus is harbored in the gut-associated lymphoid tissue (GALT), the lymphatic tissue of the small bowel. The early phase of infection is characterized by viral amplification in GALT and peak viremia (10^6–10^7 copies/mL) that is often associated with symptoms of the "acute retroviral syndrome" and massive depletion of activated and memory cells primarily from GALT (J Exp Med 2004;200:761). The preferential depletion of CD4 cells from GALT persists despite antiretroviral therapy (ART), which often produces normal CD4 counts in peripheral blood. HIV replication persists throughout the disease during most of the chronic infection phase despite absence of symptoms for years (Figure 1.1).

Rapid lymphocyte turnover is attributed to viremia in the early phase of infections, but it is sustained by immune activation during the chronic stage, and this appears to dictate the rate of disease progression (J Immun 2003;170:2479; JAMA 2006;296:1498). The population of HIV is relatively homogeneous initially, but the virus is error-prone and multiple quasi-species are produced that facilitate evasion of viral control by immune mechanisms and antiretroviral agents. Common observations in

TABLE 1.1 Natural history of HIV infection

	Acute Wk 0-6	Chronic Year 1-10	Late Year >10
Symptoms	Variable	Asymptomatic	Opportunistic infections Table 1-2
Viral load (c/mL)	10^6-10^7 (c/mL)	10^5-10^6 (c/mL)	10^5-10^7 (c/mL)
Transmission	++++	++	+++
Cytotoxic T cells and antibody	0	++	++
CD4 count (cells/mm^3)	>600	300-500	<200
GALT depletion	Severe	Severe	Severe
Viral diversity	None	Modest	Great

From Lancet 2006;368:489.

the average patient in high-resource areas such as the U.S. and Europe are shown in Table 1.1.

Definitions of HIV Stages

Classification of the natural history of untreated HIV infection into discrete disease stages helped to optimize the treatment approach to those infected with HIV. However, due to the advancements in antiretroviral treatment and current treatment recommendations some of the subdivisions of chronic HIV infection are now seemingly more of historical than clinical value but are listed for the historical context. The clinically important stages are discussed in further detail. It is important to note that although ART has completely changed the disease course of HIV and altered the relevance of some of the disease stages there remains a gap in the life expectancy of treated HIV-infected individuals compared to uninfected controls in the general population. This is believed to be largely driven by immune activation and inflammation, which not only play a significant role in untreated patients with HIV but also in virally suppressed patients. It is now known that these factors have a significant impact on the contributions to morbidity and mortality of a panoply of comorbidities including cardiovascular disease, metabolic syndrome, osteopenia/osteoporosis, renal disease, liver disease, neurocognitive function, cancer, and frailty in addition to contributing to accentuated or accelerated aging in HIV (Curr HIV/AIDS Rep 2017;14:93–1100; Curr Opin HIV AIDS 2016;11:242–249). (See Table 1.2.) Addressing these factors is critical to managing comorbidities in HIV, narrowing the life expectancy gap between HIV-infected individuals and the general population and working toward a cure (Lancet 2013, Jun 15;381(9883):2109–2117).

TABLE 1.2 Correlation of complications with CD4 cell counts

CD4 Cell Count[a]	Infectious Complications	Noninfectious[b] Complications
>500 cells/mm^3	Acute retroviral syndrome Candidal vaginitis	Persistent generalized lymphadenopathy (PGL) Guillain-Barré syndrome Myopathy Aseptic meningitis
200–500 cells/mm^3	Pneumococcal and other bacterial pneumonia Pulmonary tuberculosis Herpes zoster Oropharyngeal candidiasis (thrush) Cryptosporidiosis, self-limited Kaposi's sarcoma Oral hairy leukoplakia	Cervical and anal cancer B-cell lymphoma Anemia Mononeuronal multiplex Idiopathic thrombocytopenic purpura Hodgkin lymphoma Lymphocytic interstitial pneumonitis

TABLE 1.2 Continued

CD4 Cell Count[a]	Infectious Complications	Noninfectious[b] Complications
<200 cells/ mm³	Pneumocystis pneumonia Disseminated histoplasmosis and coccidioidomycosis Miliary/ extrapulmonary TB Progressive multifocal leuko-encephalopathy (PML)	Wasting Peripheral neuropathy HIV-associated dementia Cardiomyopathy Vacuolar myelopathy Progressive polyradiculopathy Non-Hodgkin's lymphoma
<100 cells/ mm³	Disseminated herpes simplex Toxoplasmosis Cryptococcosis Cryptosporidiosis, chronic Microsporidiosis Candidal esophagitis	
<50 cells/mm³	Disseminated cytomegalovirus (CMV) Disseminated mycobacterium avium complex	Primary central nervous system lymphoma (PCNSL)

[a]Most complications occur with increasing frequency at lower CD4 cell counts.

[b]Some conditions listed as "noninfectious" are associated with transmissible microbes. Examples include lymphoma (Epstein-Barr virus [EBV]) and anal and cervical cancers (human papillomavirus [HPV]).

From Arch Intern Med 1995;155:1537.

Disease Stages

Primary HIV Infection

Evidence of HIV (HIV RNA or p24 antigen) prior to seroconversion (see below).

Chronic HIV Infection

CHRONIC PROGRESSOR: "Typical" disease progression as illustrated in Figure 1.1, usually with VL >10,000 c/mL and CD4 decline of 50–100 cells/mm³/yr.

CHRONIC NONPROGRESSORS (OR LONG-TERM NONPROGRESSORS): HIV infection without opportunistic infections and a CD4 count >500 cells/mm³ for greater than 10 years. This includes subsets of "slow progressors" who have slow CD4 loss, usually with a VL of 1,000–10,000 c/mL (PLoS Med 2009;97:2709) and "elite controllers" defined by a VL of <50 c/mL in the absence of therapy. However, not all elite controllers are nonprogressors; a small proportion experience progression, as defined by a decline in CD4 cell count.

AIDS: Defined by an AIDS-defining diagnosis or a CD4 count of <200 cells/mm³ (Tables 1.3, 1.4 and 1.5).

Primary HIV Infection

Primary HIV Infection refers to the initial events that occur in the weeks after HIV transmission. This early period is defined as (1) the period of HIV transmission to antibody detection, (2) the time between detectable HIV RNA until antibody detection, and (3) the brief period of symptomatic HIV with high viral titer (JID 2012:205:521). This has been studied most extensively with sexual transmission in humans and primates. Acute HIV has assumed increased importance for HIV management as it represents the stage of highest risk of HIV transmission and highlights the particular importance of preventive efforts (JID 2010;201:Suppl1:S1). A growing body of evidence suggests that this may be an optimal

TABLE 1.3 Stages of HIV

Stage	Days[a]	Test
Eclipse	0–10	None
I	10–17	HIV RNA (Viral load) detectable; latency established
II	17–22	p24 antigen detectable and inflammatory cytokines
III	22–25	ELISA detectable; peak viremia
IV	25–30	gp41 antibody present with decrease in HIV viral load
V	30–100	Western blot positive, p31 Ag negative
VI	100+	Infection established; viral load, p24 antigen, p31 antigen and Western blot positive

[a]Approximate with substantial individual variation.

TABLE 1.4 Indicator conditions in case definition of AIDS (Adults)—1997*

Indicator Conditions

Candidiasis of esophagus, trachea, bronchi, or lungs – 3,846 (16%)[a] [12.6 → 5.2][b]

Cervical cancer, invasive[c d] – 144 (0.6%)[a] [3.5 → 3.5][b]

Coccidioidomycosis, extrapulmonary[c] – 74 (0.3%)[a] [——]

Cryptococcosis, extrapulmonary – 1,168 (5%)[a] [2.6 → 0.8][b]

Cryptosporidiosis with diarrhea >1 mo – 314 (1.3%)[a] [7.3 → 0.8][b]

CMV of the eye or any organ other than liver, spleen, or lymph nodes; eye – 1,638 (7%)[a] [33.0 → 1.8][b]

Herpes simplex with mucocutaneous ulcer >1 mo; or bronchitis, pneumonitis, esophagitis – 1,250 (5%)[a] [1.6 → 1.0][b]

Histoplasmosis, extrapulmonary[c] – 208 (0.9%)[a] [——]

(continued)

TABLE 1.4 Continued

HIV-associated dementia[c]: Disabling cognitive and/or other dysfunction interfering with occupation or activities of daily living – 1,196 (5%)[a] [5.4 → 1.4][b]

HIV-associated wasting[c]: Involuntary weight loss >10% of baseline plus chronic diarrhea (≥2 loose stools/day lasting ≥30 days) or chronic weakness and documented enigmatic fever ≥30 days – 4,212 (18%)[a] [——]

Isosporiasis with diarrhea >1 mo[c] – 22 (0.1%)[a] [——]

Kaposi's sarcoma[c] – 1,500 (7%)[a] [16.4 → 1,2][b]

Lymphoma, Burkitt's – 162 (0.7%), immunoblastic – 518 (2.3%), primary CNS – 170 (0.7%)[a] [5.5 → 1.6][b]

Mycobacterium avium complex or M. kansasii—disseminated or extrapulmonary disease – 1,124 (5%)[a] [26.9 → 2.5][b]

Mycobacterium tuberculosis: pulmonary – 1,621 (7%); extrapulmonary – 491 (2%)[a] [5.0 → 0.8][b]

Pneumocystis pneumonia – 9,145 (38%)[a] [29.9 → 3.9][b]

Pneumonia, recurrent bacterial (≥ 2 episodes in 12 mos)[c d] – 1,347 (5%)[a] [——]

Progressive multifocal leukoencephalopathy – 213 (1%)[a] [2.7 → 0.7][b]

Salmonella septicemia (nontyphoid), recurrent[c] – 68 (0.3%)[a] [——]

Toxoplasmosis of internal organ – 1,073 (4%)[a] [4.1 → 0.7][b]

[a]Indicates frequency as the AIDS-indicator condition among 23,527 reported cases in adults for 1997. The AIDS diagnosis was based on CD4 count in an additional 36,643 or 61% of the 60,161 total cases. Numbers indicate sum of definitive and presumptive diagnoses for stated condition. The number in parentheses is the percentage of all patients reported with an AIDS-defining diagnosis; these do not total 100% because some had a dual diagnosis. This is the last year the CDC systematically collected these data and reflects the pre-HAART experience.

[b]Data are from the HIV Outpatient Study (HOPS), which is a prospective cohort study of 7,155 patients in 10 US Clinics. The numbers show the rate (/1,000 person–years for AIDS-defining conditions for 1994-97 (pre-HAART) – 2003-07 (post-HAART).

[--] indicates data not provided (AIDS 2008;22:1345).

[c]Requires positive HIV serology.

[d]Added in the revised case definition, 1993.

TABLE 1.5 CDC revised case definition for HIV in adults[a]

Stage	CD4 Data		Clinical
	Count	%	
1	≥500	≥29	No AIDS-defining dx
2	200–499	14–28	No AIDS-defining dx
3	<200	14	*or* Documentation of AIDS-defining dx
Unknown	No information		No information

[a]HIV infection (>13 yrs).
From MMWR 2008;RR10:1–8.

time for aggressive ART intervention to reduce viral replication (and transmissibility), preserve immune function against damage/depletion, limit the size of viral reservoirs, confine viral diversity, promote immune restoration, and possibly achieve long-term viral control.

In the VISCONTI study, 14 patients were treated before seroconversion for >1 year (median 3 years) and then had ART stopped. They maintained HIV VL levels of <50 copies/mL for the follow-up duration of at least 3 years and had HIV-1 DNA levels similar to spontaneous HIV controllers in PBMC (Saez-Cirion et al., PLoS Path 2013 Mar;9(3):e1003211). Similarly, 15 Thai patients with acute infection demonstrated reduced viral DNA in the blood and gut after 24 wks of ART; 3 patients had undetectable DNA levels in the blood after 24 wks (Ananworanich et al., PLoS One 2012;7(3):333948). These observations on prevention and early treatment are accompanied by the introduction of fourth-generation HIV tests that detect HIV antigen prior to seroconversion, thus facilitating early detection (JID 2012;201:528).

The clinical features of acute HIV are variable, and many patients are asymptomatic or have limited symptoms that do not prompt seeking medical attention. A review of a large number of patients with acute HIV showed the following symptoms (Ann Intern Med 2002;137:3811): fever 96%, adenopathy 74%, pharyngitis 70%, rash 70%, myalgias 54%, diarrhea 32%, headache 32%, nausea and vomiting 27%, hepatosplenomegaly 14%, weight loss 12%, thrush 12%, and neurological symptoms 12%. The rashes were described as erythematous and maculopapular on the face and trunk, sometimes on extremities, including palms and soles. Some patients had ulcerative lesions involving the mouth, esophagus, and/or genitals. The neurologic symptoms included aseptic meningitis, peripheral neuropathy, facial palsy, Guillain-Barré syndrome, brachial neuropathy, cognitive defects, and psychosis.

Results of the laboratory testing in early stage HIV depend on the test and the stage (NEJM 2011;364:1943; AIDS 2003;17:1871–1879), as summarized in Table 1.3.

Natural Viral Suppression/Elite Controller

HIV VL <50 COPIES/ML WITHOUT ART (JAMA 2010;302:194; AIDS 2008;22:541): Elite controllers make up <0.5–1.5% of persons with HIV infection (CID 2005;41:1053; JID 1999;180:526; Trop HIV Med 2007;15:134; J Acquir Immune Defic Syndr 2009 Apr 1;50(4):403–408; CID 2010;50:1187). Differences between elite controllers and "slow progressors" are that the latter usually have VLs of 1,000–10,000 c/mL, CD4 depletion over time, and eventual development of opportunistic conditions (Blood 1997;90:1133; Immunity 2008;29:1009). A review of 14 elite controllers with known HIV infection for a median of 13 years showed a median CD4 count of 812 cells/mm^3, and all had a VL of <50 copies/mL. Nine (64%) had a VL of <1 copies/mL, and the median VL in the other 6 was 26 copies/mL (CID 2008;47:102). The variation in VL is significantly greater than in patients receiving ART with viral suppression. The virus in elite controllers is replication competent, and there may be viral evolution with sequential testing (CID 2009;49:1763). Virologic control in elite controllers may be immunologically mediated, as suggested by the fact that the HLA-B*57 allele is highly overrepresented (PNAS 2000;97:2709). Of interest is the observation that ART in elite controllers with stable low VLs and high CD4 counts further reduces markers of immune activation (CID 2009;49:1763).

Diagnosis and Staging

Diagnosis and staging of HIV disease has been useful not only for clinical purposes but also for research.

Diagnosis

LABORATORY CRITERIA: (1) Positive screening test (enzyme immunoassay; EIA) confirmed by (a) Western blot, (b) indirect immunofluorescent test, or (c) supplemental HIV Ab test; or (2) detectable quantity within established laboratory limits for (a) HIV RNA or DNA, (b) HIV p24 antigen test with neutralization assay, or (c) HIV culture (PNAS 2008;105:75552; JID 2010;202 Suppl 2:S270).

It is important to make the diagnosis in the acute stage because it is associated with high rates of HIV transmission (JID 2004;189:1785; JID 2007;195:951), is a time when standard serologic tests for HIV antibody are deceptively negative, and diagnosis may explain an otherwise enigmatic illness. The ability to detect this stage of disease is facilitated by the availability of fourth-generation HIV tests that detect both antigen and antibody (Chapter 2) (JAIDS 2009;52:121; JCM 2009;47:2639).

Staging

Staging has proved useful in clinical care, public health, and research. Multiple staging systems have been developed, but the three most useful include the Centers for Disease Control (CDC), World Health Organization (WHO), and Walter Reed Staging Systems. The WHO and CDC systems are similar in their use of systems and CD4 cell count to stage disease, but the CDC system is most commonly used in the United States both for clinical care, research, and public health. The Walter Reed Staging System incorporates additional clinical factors, including delayed hypersensitivity to further refine clinical staging of patients, as well as including individuals who are uninfected but have had high-risk exposure. This is particularly important today with the availability of highly effective combination ART, when it is important to not only treat early, but also to promote earlier diagnosis of HIV in all at-risk populations, not all of whom are recognized to be at risk.

2

Laboratory Tests

Introduction

Since the development of the first HIV test in 1985 by Gallo and colleagues (Sarngadharan, Science, Vol 224, p 506–508, 1984), test methods and testing strategies for HIV have evolved to offer a large number and variety of choices to meet the needs of the various testing venues (Constantine et al., 2005); as new tests become available in the future, testing strategies will undoubtedly change. In 2016, major changes occurred in the availability of some tests and the introduction of additional assays; hence, recommended testing strategies have been forced to change. The selection of methods is determined on the basis of the objective for testing (i.e., screening blood for transfusion, diagnosis, monitoring infection, and viral resistance assessment) but may be determined on the basis of laboratory capabilities and limitations (e.g., no stable electricity in resource-limited countries). Methods are classified as (1) serologic assays for detecting antibodies or antigens of HIV, (2) molecular-based assays to determine RNA or DNA (qualitatively or quantitatively for the measurement of viral load [VL]) to diagnose or stage infection or to determine the genotype/phenotype to disclose resistance mutations for treatment management, and (3) CD4 cell phenotyping and quantification to monitor the immune system (Lancet 1996;348:176). In addition, test selection may be dependent on the nature of the virus (i.e., HIV-1, HIV-2, or the different groups of HIV). Accordingly, a short description of the HIV viruses follows.

The HIV Viruses

HIV-1

HIV types include HIV-1 and HIV-2, which show 40–60% amino acid homology. Within the HIV-1 types are the Groups M, N, and O, and within the M Group are a number of subtypes (also called clades) including A, B, C, D, F, G, H, J, and K; further, there are at least 15 circulating recombinant forms (CFRs) (AIDS 2000;14:S31; DL Robertson Science 2000—hiv.lanl.gov). HIV-1 accounts for the majority of cases throughout the world; HIV-2 is predominately found in West Africa, although there have been near to 200 HIV-2 cases identified in the United States (Centers for Disease Control [CDC] https://www.ncbi.nlm.nih.gov/pubmed/24717910). Group O shows 55–70% homology with the M subtypes, and, although not uncommon in Cameroon, not many cases have been found outside of Africa (only a few in the United States). Another group of viruses, Group N, was first reported in 1998 (Nat Med 1998;4:1032; Science 2000;287:607), but few cases have been reported. The O and N Groups are thought to represent divergent evolution or distinctive cross-species transmission. It should be noted that of the HIV viruses, HIV-2 and HIV-1 Group O sometimes produce diagnostic dilemmas both serologically and with molecular assays.

Most HIV infections are by the subtypes A, B, C, and D, and the CRFs—CRF01_AE and CRF02_AG (Table 2.1). More than 98% of HIV-1 infections in the United States are caused by subtype B; most non-B subtypes in the United States were acquired in other countries (JID 2000;181:470; JAIDS 2010, 3:297). In a review of subtypes from 196 immigrants in New York City in 2005, subtype B accounted for 111 (55%), subtype A for 54 (27%), and subtype C for 8 (4%) (JID 2006;41:399).

HIV-2

HIV-2 is primarily found in West Africa, where it is endemic in Benin, Burkina Faso, Cape Verde, Cote d'lvoire, Gambia, Ghana,

TABLE 2.1 Global distribution of HIV-1 by subtypes

Geographic Location	Number of Infections	HIV-1 Subtypes
North America	1,200,000	B
Caribbean	300,000	B
Latin America	1,800,000	B, BF
Western Europe	720,000	B
North Africa, Mid East	510,000	B, C
Sub-Saharan Africa	25,800,000	A, C, D, F, G, H, J, K, CRF
East Europe, central Asia	1,600,000	A, B
East Asia	870,000	B, C, BC, CRF 01
Southeast Asia	7,400,000	B, AE

From Lancet 2006;368:489.

Guinea, Guinea-Bissau, Liberia, Mali, Mauritania, Niger, Nigeria, São Tome, Senegal, Sierra Leone, and Togo and other African countries, such as Angola and Mozambique (MMWR 1992;4[RR-12]:1). Compared with HIV-1, HIV-2 infections are characterized by low VL, slow rates of clinical progression, low rates of transmission (vertically or sexually), and have unique treatment recommendations due to intrinsic resistance to non-nucleoside reverse transcriptase inhibitors (NNRTIs) (JAIDS 2004;37:1543; Retrovirology 2010;7:46; AIDS 2003;17:2591; AIDS Res Ther 2008;5:18; AIDS 2008;22:2069; Lancet 1994;344:1380; AIDS 1994;8 [suppl 1]:585; JID 1999;180:1116; JAIDS 2000;24:257; Arch Intern Med 2000;160:3286; AIDS 2000;14:441; JID 2002;185:905; AIDS 2008;22:211; CID 2010;51:2010:1334). Despite slow rates of progression, mortality rates for HIV-1 and HIV-2 infection are similar when adjusted for VL (JAIDS 2005;38:335). HIV-2 has less homology with HIV-1 than HIV-1 subtypes (Nature 1987;328:543), and serology can be negative in 20–30% depending on which assay is used. Because of this, HIV tests have been designed to also detect

HIV-2 by including specific HIV-2 antigens, and all are effective. A review of 40,300 cases of HIV infection in New York City for 2000–2008 showed 62 (0.15%) were caused by HIV-2. Sixty of the 62 were foreign-born (Africa, 58; Central America, 2), one was white, 11 (18%) had CDC-defined AIDS, 33 (62%) had a CD4 count <500 cells/mm^3, 40 (65%) were initially diagnosed as HIV-1 infection, and none had dual infection (CID 2010;51:1334). HIV-2 should be suspected if (1) patients are of West African origin, (2) patients have undetectable virus without therapy, (3) patients are epidemiologically linked to HIV-2 infection, and (4) in cases where an HIV-1 supplemental assay is negative, indeterminate, or atypical. In such cases, it is essential that the initial test detects both HIV-1 and HIV-2. HIV-2 infection is associated with immune activation that is comparable to that seen with HIV-1 infection when adjusted for VL (JID 2010;201:114). There are no treatment guidelines for HIV-2 infection based on comparative trials, but PI-based ART treatment is generally recommended (AIDS 2009;23:1171; BMC Infect Dis 2008;8:21). Several issues affect the management of HIV-2-infected patients because:

1. Many patients are co-infected with HIV-1 (AIDS 2001; 16:1775).
2. The doubling time is sixfold longer than for HIV-1, leading to a low VL, decreased transmission, and a long period of asymptomatic infection (JAMA 1993;270:2083).
3. Laboratory confirmation of infection may be difficult (see later discussion).
4. There are no commercially available VL assays or resistance testing for HIV-2, although these tests can be performed by some specialty laboratories (J Virol Methods 2000;88:81; CID 2004;38:1771; JAIDS 2000;24:257).

Serologic tests to detect HIV-2 include those combination assays that detect both HIV-1 and HIV-2 and specific tests that identify only HIV-2 infection. Test formats can be enzyme-linked immunosorbent assay (ELISA), chemiluminescence, rapid, or Western blots

(WB). In the United States, rapid tests and WBs for only HIV-2 are not available (the Multispot has been discontinued, although several internationally available tests can differentiate HIV-1 and HIV-2). The usual algorithm is to test samples initially with a HIV-1/2 screening assay that will identify infection by either virus, followed by a specific differentiating assay such as an HIV-2 ELISA or supplemental assay approved by the US Food and Drug Administration (FDA) (Bio-Rad Geenius™ HIV 1/2 Confirmatory Assay, see later discussion) that will identify the infection as HIV-1 or HIV-2. The HIV-2 ELISAs and the Geenius incorporate the gp36 antigen derived from HIV-2, and this antigen is specific for HIV-2. RNA tests for HIV infection may be negative with HIV-2 infection.

Viral Variants (Group O and Group N)

Viral variants are viruses other than HIV-1 of the M Group and HIV-2, and they are most often due to HIV-1 Group O and HIV-1 Group N viruses. Serologic detection of these variants may be less than perfect because it has been shown that a number failed to detect the O subtype, and none detected N subtypes (Lancet1994;343:1393; Lancet 1994;344:1333; MMWR 1996;45:561; JCM 2006;44:1856; JCM 2006;44:662; JCM 2008;6:2453; CID 2008;46:1936; JCM 2009;47:2906). Although only several patients with subtype O HIV infection were identified in the United States (MMWR 1996;45:561; Emerg Infect Dis 1996;2:209; AIDS 2002;18:269), the FDA mandated the requirement for all new tests to include Group O antigens for efficient detection; hence, most current FDA-approved tests can detect HIV-1 Group O. The N group can also cause false-negative screening test results but may be positive by WB (Nat Med 1998;4:1032). There have been no recognized infections with Group N in the United States through March 2000 (JID 2000;181:470). There is little evidence that Group M subtypes cannot be detected with HIV-1 assays. Nevertheless, it is important to consider the geographic origin of persons who are tested but produce nonconfirmed or unusual test results, especially if unusual results are obtained.

Immune Responses to HIV and Detection Markers

Immune responses are predictable in HIV infection, and the markers that occur are used to diagnose and, to some extent, stage infection. Although variations do occur depending on host factors, viral factors, and the tests used to detect these markers, the kinetics of marker appearance is nearly identical in all individuals. The most common markers that can be detected in blood following infection are (1) specific antibody to HIV (seropositivity), (2) p24 antigen (antigenemia), and 3) viral nucleic acid (viremia or VL). The CD4 lymphocyte number, a marker of immune competence, also follows a typical course during infection, although this marker is not used to diagnose infection because CD4 levels are not predictive of whether a person is infected. The phases and appearance of markers are listed in Table 2.2.

Infection by HIV can be defined as the time at which the virus becomes established in the host after exposure, and the kinetics of the appearance of markers is depicted in Figure 2.1. As shown, the first marker that can be detected in blood after infection is viral RNA. RNA can be detected at about 10–12 days postinfection, whereas p24 antigen detection requires 4–10 days after RNA appearance (J Int AIDS Soc. 2017;20(1):2165, Published online 2017 Jun 26. doi: 10.7448/IAS.20.1.21652).

Although both RNA and antigen appearance represent viral establishment and replication, RNA is detected earlier only because of the method used for detection (i.e., amplification method for RNA). This is exemplified when using research methods such as p24 Immuno-PCR where using amplification methods to detect p24 antigen can be shown to be as sensitive as, or than RNA detection (Barletta et al., Am J Clin Path 2004;122:20–27; Barletta et al., J Virol Meth 2009;157:122–132). Nevertheless, during the first 2 weeks after infection, viremia appears to increase exponentially as the virus replicates until the antibody and cell-mediated immune responses provide resistance to viral replication, at which time RNA levels reach a stable "set point."

TABLE 2.2 Phases and marker detection following HIV-1 infection

Time in Days (Post-Infection)	Phase	Marker Appearance	Marker Duration
0–10	Eclipse	None	
10–12	Acute infection	RNA	Throughout infection
15–17	Acute infection and antigenemia	Antigen (p24)	Antigen detection duration of 2–4 wks and later in disease
10–25	Window period	Seronegative	Seronegative until antibody appears
17–25	Seropositive	Antibody	Antibody appears during this time and lasts throughout infection
17–25 throughout infection	Established infection	IgG antibody sufficient to indicate confirmed infection rise and peak	Antibody and RNA persist throughout infection

The period after infection but before any marker (e.g., RNA, p24 antigen, antibody) can be detected (10–12 days) is known as the *eclipse phase*. During this time, the level of circulating virus is rising to about 10,000 RNA copies/mL (ramping up) with doubling rates of 21.5 hrs each day and finally peaking to levels of about 1 million RNA copies/mL within 1–2 mos (J AIDS 2005;39:133; Transfusion 2013;53:2384). Subsequently, a decrease in VL typically occurs to the set point of approximately 10,000 copies/mL and

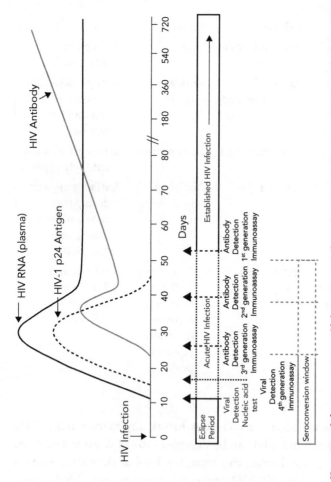

FIGURE 2.1 Kinetics of the appearance of laboratory markers for HIV-1 infection, different phases of infection, and detection by different generations of tests.

Note. Units for vertical axis are not noted because their magnitude differs for RNA, p24 antigen, and antibody. Modified from MP Busch, GA Satten (1997) with updated data from Fiebig (2003) Owen (2008) and Masciotra (2011, 2013).

later rises slowly throughout the remainder of infection. The efficient control of virus replication shortly after primary infection to a low set point is a paramount predictor of a long-term asymptomatic course of infection. Acute HIV infection is defined as the time from HIV infection to seroconversion. Detection of infection during this early stage is a priority because (1) it may be accompanied by symptoms of an otherwise unexplained illness, (2) treatment may be important at this stage to reduce symptoms and possibly to slow the subsequent course of disease (although this is unproven), and (3) undiagnosed individuals with acute infection are at high risk of further transmitting the virus because of high levels of viremia combined with ongoing high-risk behavior (JID 2005;191:1403; JID 2004;189:1785). The period after the eclipse period until antibody is detected is known as the *window period* (seronegative period). During this period, the appearance of p24 antigen in the serum (antigenemia) usually occurs within 2–3 wks after infection and 5–7 days after RNA detection and is the second earliest marker that can be detected. When using serologic assays, antigen detection signals infection earlier than antibody detection, and, because levels of antigen subsequently decrease at the time antibody appears, antigenemia is a determinate of acute infection (as is RNA detection) (Constantine, Kabat, Zhao 2005, Clin Lab Sci, 18:263; Cell Res 2005;15:870). Antigen detection can reduce the seronegative period by about 1 wk and therefore has been incorporated into many screening assays (fourth-generation tests, see below) to increase sensitivity. Seroconversion occurs with the detection of specific antibody to HIV, thus signaling the end of the window period, and the individual is now labeled as seropositive. Although IgM antibodies are expressed first, which can be detected by third- and fourth-generation immunoassays, assays to detect IgM are not widely accepted. However, assays that can detect IgM antibodies in addition to IgG (including rapid assays) have been shown to have a higher sensitivity over only IgG detection methods (Manuscript 22582v2, 2018, in press). IgG antibodies to HIV can be detected 3–5 days after p24 antigen or 10–13 days after the appearance of viral RNA (J Int AIDS Soc. 2017;20(1):21652, Published online 2017 Jun

26. doi: 10.7448/IAS.20.1.21652). However, the exact time when antibody can be detected is dependent on several factors, including the test used, individual host responses, and viral characteristics. In general, current assays for antibody allow detection within 3–4 wks following infection (Kucirka et al., Am J Transpl. 2011;11:1176). However, some individuals do not seroconvert for up to 12 wks or more (J Med Virol 2000;60:43; NEJM 1997;336:919). Once IgG antibody appears and meets the criterion for a confirmed infection, infection is considered as established, and this lasts throughout infection until a compromised immune system fails and antibody levels fall as antigen and RNA levels rise.

Antibodies to the major *gag* proteins (p17, p24, p40, p55) usually appear early during infection and are probably responsible for the decrease in p24 (core) antigen as the antibody response slows viral replication; that is, antibodies combine with circulating antigen and the complexes are removed. Subsequently, a decrease in p24 antibody occurs as the immune system becomes less responsive later in disease (AIDS) and viral antigens and RNA increase. Most individuals respond in a highly characteristic manner, with antibody production occurring within several weeks to all major HIV core (p15, p17, p24, p40, p55), polymerase (p31, p51, p66), and envelope (gp41, gp120, gp160) antigens. Rarely, seroreversion has been observed, suggesting exposure to nonviable virus or antigens (without infection) or from possible clearance of infection. It should also be noted that individuals who have received candidate vaccines will produce antibody responses to those specific antigens without being infected; thus, this could cause false-positive results.

It has been well-described that a number of individuals infected with HIV-2 produce negative or indeterminate results when tested by HIV-1 assays and vice versa. Similarly, a number of serological assays, designed to detect antibodies to HIV-1 and HIV-2, have been shown to produce false-negative results when testing individuals infected with HIV-1 Group O (CDC, https://www.cdc.gov/mmwr/preview/mmwrhtml/00042810.htm). However, most assays in use today are designed detect HIV-1 Group O.

It should be noted that the immune response to HIV is affected by successful highly active antiretroviral therapy (HAART) treatment, resulting in interruption of seroconversion or causing seroreversion. Thus, with treatment, serologic assays can produce varying or false-negative results. In one study, 46% of individuals initiating ART at Fiebig I–IV tested negative by the WB, and 67% were negative by a screening test at week 24. (Manak et al., 19th Annual International Meeting of the Institute of Human Virology at the University of Maryland, School of Medicine, October 23–26, 2017). This is explained by a decrease in viremia below the threshold levels required to continually sustain immune responses (i.e., a lesser antigenic stimulus) when on treatment.

In summary, in an infected individual, plasma viremia is the earliest detectable marker and can identify infection within 2 wks after infection. Viral p24 antigen appears within several days after viremia, and levels peak in the absence of antibody. When antibody appears, usually within several days to 2 wks after antigenemia, p24 levels decrease, whereas antibody levels increase and remain detectable throughout the infection.

HIV Serologic Tests

The initial tests, also referred to as screening tests, to identify HIV infection are always performed using serologic tests to detect antibodies to HIV. Because these tests may yield a small percentage (≤1%) of false-positive results, a repeatedly reactive result must be verified using a confirmatory assay (also known as a supplemental test) to maximize the chances that the reactivity is produced from antibodies that are truly directed against HIV (and not from cross-reacting antibodies or interfering blood components). These tests and the testing strategies are discussed here.

Initial Tests to Detect HIV Antibody

The current repertoire of initial tests (screening tests) for HIV include enzyme-linked immunoassays (EIA), chemiluminescence immunoassays (CIA), indirect immunofluorescent assays (IFA), and rapid tests. For high-volume and automated testing, the EIAs or CIAs are used, while rapid tests and IFA are more appropriate for smaller testing venues and/or point of care (POC) testing. Although whole-blood, fingerstick blood, and oral fluids can be used with some tests and offer advantages, especially in POC venues (PLoS One 2010:19:e11581; J AIDS 2012;15:588), serum and plasma are the most common media used for testing. The principles, performance characteristics, and limitations of EIAs, CIAs, the IFA, and rapid tests can be found elsewhere (Constantine et al., 2005), although some basic information is provided here. A list of all FDA-approved tests (for screening and confirmation) can be found at: http://www.fda.gov/BiologicsBloodVaccines/ BloodBloodProducts/ApprovedProducts/LicensedProductsBLAs/ BloodDonorScreening/InfectiousDisease/UCM080466#anti_ HIV1_Assays).

Following the introduction of third-generation screening tests that used an antigen sandwich configuration to include IgM detection to increase sensitivity, fourth-generation tests became available in which both antibodies to HIV and HIV p24 antigen are detected simultaneously in one assay. Because antigenemia precedes antibody production kinetically (by several days), these fourth-generation tests reduce the antibody window period and thus have increased sensitivity; they have been shown to detect 80% of acute HIV infections (Expert Rev Anti-Infect Ther 2010;8:63) and have been shown to be effective when used as initial tests. Recently, a fifth-generation test (BioPlex 2200 HIV Ag-Ab, Bio-Rad Laboratories) has been approved by the FDA that allows not only detection of antigen and antibody simultaneously, but also "differentiation" of antigen from antibody; thus, it not only identifies both acute and established infection, but it also indicates if the infection is acute. Identifying acute infection is important for treatment management and effective contact-tracing. The IFA test, which can be used for screening or confirming infection (but not both on the same specimen) is more difficult to perform and subjective; it is briefly described later.

EIAs and CIAs are most appropriate for high-volume screening, while rapid screening tests to detect HIV infection have advantages over automated methods, including (1) storage at temperatures up to 30°C, (2) use of alternative testing media (fingerstick and oral fluid), (3) fast results (1–25 minutes), and (4) simplicity (e.g., Clinical Laboratory Improvement Amendment of 1988 [CLIA]-waived, allowing POC testing by nonlaboratory persons; Constantine et al., 2005). Of particular importance, rapid tests are especially useful where rapid results are important, as with occupational exposure, in pregnant women who present in labor without prior testing, in outreach settings (MMWR 2006;55:673), and in settings where patients are unlikely to return for test results, including emergency rooms and STD clinics. There are at least 10 rapid HIV tests approved by the FDA (http://www.fda.gov/BiologicsBloodVaccines/BloodBloodProducts/ApprovedProducts/LicensedProductsBLAs/BloodDonorScreening/InfectiousDisease/UCM080466#anti_HIV1_Assays), although one (Multispot HIV) has been recently removed from the market (June 2016); there are two additional rapid tests approved for home use. Two of these approved rapid tests allow the use of oral fluids, most allow the use of fingerstick blood, most are CLIA-waived, and all can be performed within 25 minutes; one test produces results in 1 minute. None of the FDA approved rapid tests currently on the market has the ability to differentiate HIV-1 from HIV-2 infection. One rapid test is a fourth-generation assay (Determine HIV) that can detect and differentiate p24 antigen and antibody to HIV, thereby being able to identify acute infection; however, reports have shown that the sensitivity for p24 antigen is less than that of the automated fourth-generation tests (Masciotra et al., J Clin Viro;2013;58S:e54–e58). Nevertheless, the sensitivity for detecting HIV infection (antigen or antibody) is higher than antibody-only detection rapid tests. The sensitivity of rapid tests for antibody detection as compared to that of EIAs and CIAs is sometimes questioned, but most studies show comparable test indices, especially with the newer rapid tests. Finally, the cost of rapid tests is 2–3 times higher that of EIA and CIA, but their use is cost-effective in venues where a small number of tests are performed or where automated instruments are not available or can't be supported.

Confirmatory Tests to Detect Antibody, Antigen, or RNA

In contrast to initial screening tests, HIV confirmatory assays (or supplemental assays) for antibody detection are designed to indicate the presence of specific antibodies to HIV (i.e., are more specific). Another way to consider their purpose is that confirmatory tests rule out false-positive results that are sometimes produced by initial assays, thereby verifying true infection. However, not all confirmatory assays are 100% specific, and false-positive results by WB assays have been documented (J Clin Virol 2013;58:240). Nevertheless, they are more specific than initial assays, and, in nearly all cases of established infection, they are effective to confirm infection. Importantly, confirmatory assays should not be used as screening tests because they are less sensitive, and negative or indeterminate results can be misleading. For example, during early infection, a screening test result can be positive while the confirmatory test is negative at that time (but will become positive at a later date); thus, providing a negative result to an individual can be inaccurate. In the United States, confirmatory tests for HIV do not have to be licensed by the FDA if they are used for purposes other than the testing of blood donors; however, it is recommended to have FDA-approved confirmatory tests. Many state laboratories use in-house prepared WBs or IFA methods. There are several methods for confirming HIV infection: (1) WBs, (2) recombinant immunoblots (RIBAs), (3) LIAs, (4) RIPAs, (5) p24 antigen tests, (6) rapid confirmatory tests, (7) indirect fluorescence assays (IFAs), (8) viral culture, (9) the Geenius, and (10) molecular methods (nucleic acid tests [NATs]). In the United States, there are only four FDA-approved methods available for confirming HIV infection: (1) the Geenius, (2) IFA, (3) the p24 antigen test, and (4) one molecular method. Although FDA-licensed WBs are no longer available in the United States (as of June 2016), this test is described here because some state laboratories still use it for diagnostic confirmation.

1. *WESTERN BLOT*: The HIV-1 WB was the major confirmatory assay in the United States since 1986, but it has recently been removed from the market; thus, an FDA-approved WB is not available. It has been replaced by the Geenius HIV 1/2 Supplemental Assay (BioRad). The WB gains its specificity by allowing for the identification of antibodies to specific antigens of the virus, including the core antigens p15, p17, p24, p40, and p55; the integrase proteins p31, p51, p66; and the envelope glycoproteins gp41, gp120, and gp160. A negative result is the absence of reactivity to all antigens, while an indeterminate result is defined as reactivity to one or more antigens that does not meet the criterion for positive. Although the specific profile can sometimes suggest early infection (e.g., reactivity to a core antigen only during early infection), it is not possible to differentiate early infection from nonspecific reactivity if the profile does not meet the criterion for positive. A positive result is reactivity to at least 2 of the following antigens: p24, gp41, and gp120/160 (gp120 or gp160). Negative and indeterminate results require follow-up serology in 2–6 wks to assess seroprogression (MMWR 2001;50 RR-19:1), or confirmation by another method (e.g., RNA testing, IFA). For poorly understood reasons, many noninfected individuals continue to exhibit indeterminate results by WB for years but are not infected. If an individual does progress serologically (seroprogression) or converts to positive (seroconversion) during retesting, the individual was probably infected at the time of the first test (early infection). One reason that confirmatory tests such as the WB are not selected for use as screening assays is because nearly 15% of noninfected persons may show some reactivity to a component (nonspecific reactions), necessitating the classification of indeterminate. Another reason for inconclusive results on confirmatory assays is the occurrence of infection by HIV viral variants, most notably HIV-2 and HIV-1 group O Journal of Human Virology, 1: 46–52, 1997; Constantine et al., 2005).

As expected, infection by HIV viruses that are slightly different from the most common HIV-1 group M may produce incomplete positive profiles or weak reactions to certain antigens, particularly the envelope antigens (gp41, gp120, and gp160) that are less conserved between viral variants when the tests use antigens derived from group M viruses. False-positive results by WB have been documented (Kleinman, 1998). Although uncommon, these false-positive WB results occur mostly in individuals who produce a WB profile that meets the criterion for positivity but show a lack of reactivity to p31 (integrase). Therefore, a vigilant laboratory should alert a caregiver when such a profile is produced.

GEENIUS: The Geenius HIV 1/2 Supplemental Assay (BioRad) is a qualitative, immunochromagraphic assay for the confirmation and differentiation of individual antibodies to HIV-1 and HIV-2 in whole blood, serum, or plasma. It differentiates between six distinct HIV antibodies: HIV-1 gp160, gp41, p31, and p24; and HIV-2 gp140 and gp36. It can be used for diagnosis in individuals beginning at age 2 ys. Results are generated are interpreted by software that is read by an instrument as positive, negative, or indeterminate for each HIV-1 and HIV-2; thus, this test is both a confirmatory assay and a viral type-differentiating assay. This automated method does not allow the user to make subjective interpretation; results are complete in 30 minutes, and it has been evaluated (Hawthorne et al., Clin Vac Immuno 2014;21:1192; Montesinos et al. J Clin Viro 2014;60:399).

IFA: In the IFA technique, cells (usually lymphocytes) that have been infected with HIV are fixed to a microscope slide. Serum containing HIV antibodies is added, and the anti-HIV antibodies react with the intracellular HIV before being detected with a conjugate that produces fluorescence. This technique has the advantage of sometimes providing definitive diagnosis of samples that have yielded indeterminate results by WB analysis but has the disadvantages of requiring an expensive and well-maintained microscope and requiring a subjective interpretation; therefore, the method requires well-trained individuals (Internat J Infect Dis 2010;14:e10930). Unless autoantibodies are present in the sample, the result is not difficult to interpret by well-trained individuals; it does require more time to read the results if large numbers of specimens are tested at one time. Also, if a patient has received a therapy such as fluorescence angiograms, false-positive results may occur. The sensitivity and specificity of the IFA are equivalent to the WB. Currently, the IFA is widely used in Europe, and it is used in a number of laboratories in the United States, including blood banks. There is only one FDA-approved IFA test—Fluorognost HIV-1 Indirect Immunofluorescence Assay (Sanochemia).

P24 ANTIGEN ASSAY: Although an EIA to detect p24 antigen alone was used for confirmation of infection in the past, its use as a confirmatory test has been replaced by the tests for nucleic acids (e.g., RNA) because of the high sensitivity of NATs. Currently, the detection of p24 antigen is incorporated into the fourth- and fifth-generation assays to decrease the antibody window period. In laboratories that cannot support nucleic acid testing (e.g., in resource-limited countries), antigen testing may be used for confirmation if there is stable electricity and the capability to perform EIAs. Now that there is a rapid fourth-generation rapid test (that detects and differentiates antibody and antigen) (Masciotra et al., J Clin Viro 2013;58S:e54–e58), antigen-only testing by EIA will most likely be discontinued. Details of the p24 antigen test, including the requirement for confirming antigenemia by a neutralization step, can be found elsewhere (Constantine et al., 2005).

MOLECULAR ASSAYS: Qualitative tests for HIV RNA have been used to confirm infection for many years but, until recently, were not included in most acceptable confirmatory strategies primarily because of their high cost. Until now, their use was mostly to resolve inconclusive serologic results. With the discontinuation of Multispot rapid test that was recommended by the CDC as a second test in a two-test confirmatory strategy, an RNA test will most likely be recommended in the near future for laboratories that do not wish to use the WB, Geenius, or IFA (see algorithm section). Details and characteristics of molecular tests and their use are presented under the section on "Molecular Assays." Only one FDA-licensed RNA test is available for diagnosis of HIV (see below).

False-Negative and False-Positive Results

1. False-negative results by serologic screening tests usually occur because of testing during the window period before the antibody response has fully developed in an infected person or late in disease when the immune system has failed. The rate of false negatives ranges from 0.3% in a high-prevalence population (JID 1993;168:327) to <0.001% in low-prevalence populations (NEJM 1991;325:593). The largest review of unexplained persistently seronegative HIV infection includes 25 patients (median age 30 yrs) who generally presented with late-stage disease with CD4 counts of <200 cells/mm^3 (20 patients), an AIDS-defining condition at presentation, high VL (median 600,000 c/mL), and clade B virus infection (11/17) (AIDS 2010;1407). Other reasons for false-negative results include infection with a viral variant or HIV-2, technical or clerical errors (Constantine et al., 2015), unusual causes (Ann Intern Med 2008;149:71; JCM 2003;41:2153), and persons on treatment (Manak et al., 19th Annual International Meeting of the Institute of Human Virology at the University of Maryland School of Medicine, October 23–26, 2017). False-negative results can also occur because of the lesser degree of analytical sensitivity (level of detection) of some tests. For example, it is documented that certain tests cannot detect infection as early as others, as shown when testing seroconversion panels where sequential bleeds after infection of an infected person are tested Acquired Immunodeficiency Syndrome, 8: 1715–1720, 1994; J Clin Virol, 2013 e54-e58.

And a fourth-generation rapid test is less sensitive for detection of antigen as compared with automated fourth-generation tests (Stekler; Gillis, HIV Conference). Although there are minor differences in the sensitivity of some assays by 1–2 wks, the differences do not represent a substantial concern because a very small percentage of persons would be within this time interval when tested. Nevertheless, this might be significant if a high-incidence population is being tested, where a larger number of persons are becoming infected and might be within the window period. Of note, it has been shown that the tests that use oral fluids for testing have a lesser sensitivity as compared with the testing of blood. False-negative results also occur with confirmatory assays and are most likely the result of the same reasons as for screening tests but primarily because the serologic response has not fully evolved to produce high titers of antibody to all HIV antigens. A not-uncommon reason for false-negative results is human error or technical error (JAMA 1993;269:2876, Arch Intern Med 2003;163:1857), but, in many cases, the cause of false negative serology is largely unexplained (AIDS 1995;9:95; MMWR 1996;45:181; CID 1997;25:98; JID 1997;175:955; AIDS 1999;13:89; CID 2008;46:785). Finally, failure to mount an immunologic response can occur in patients with agammaglobulinemia (NEJM 2005;353:1074), but this is not always the explanation (JID 1999;180:1033).

False-positive results occur in about 1% of tests (test specificity of 99%). In low-risk populations, the rate is lower based on a report from the American Red Cross where 20 false positives occurred among 5.02 million donations from 1991 to 1995 or 1/251,000 (JAMA 1998;280:1081). The lower percentage in a low-prevalence population may be due to a lesser degree of other infectious diseases that are known to cause interference (e.g., syphilis). Although the causes of false-positive results are not definitively known in many cases, likely causes include (1) autoantibodies (NEJM 1993;328:1281); (2) infections such as malaria, influenza, malaria, dengue, trypanosomiasis, and schistosomiasis, possibly due to polyclonal B cell activation (JCM 2010;48:2836; JCM 2010;48;1570; JCM 2006;44:3024; CID 2007;45:139; CID 2000;30:819; JAIDS 2010;54:641); (3) hypergammaglobulinemia; (4) vaccines such as HIV (JAMA 2010;304:275; Am J Epidemiol 1995;141:1089; NEJM 2006;354:1422; Cell 1997;89:263); (5) test-dependent issues (the OraQuick test using oral fluids has shown sporadic reports of higher false-positive results, sometimes in substantial numbers) (PLoS One 2007;2:e185; MMWR 2008;57:660; Ann Intern Med 2008;149:153; AIDS 2006;20:1661); (6) cross-reacting nonspecific antibodies, as seen with collagen-vascular disease, autoimmune diseases, lymphoma, liver disease, injection drug use, multiple sclerosis, parity, or recent immunization (Am J Kidney Dis 1999;34:146; Pediatr Nephrol 2004;19:547); and (7) in pregnancy (positive-screening EIA tests with negative or indeterminate WB appear overrepresented in pregnancy, but those with indeterminate tests usually revert to negative after delivery, suggesting that pregnancy per se may cause these results [Am J Perinatol 2011;28:467]).

Testing Strategies and Algorithms

A testing strategy refers to the selection of the best type of test or more than one test type to use for identifying and confirming HIV infection in a particular testing situation. Usually, the strategy involves a logical sequence of performing two or more tests in tandem (one after the other) to arrive at a conclusion on the HIV status of the person being tested. Sometimes, regulatory agencies or national programs dictate a testing strategy, whereas in other situations a particular facility may decide on the strategy.

A testing *algorithm* refers to the selection of specific tests that are used to fulfill the testing strategy. For example, if a testing strategy requires one test for screening and one for confirmation of infection, a particular ELISA followed by a differentiating supplemental test (e.g., Geenius) may be used. Similarly, if two tests that are usually classified as screening tests constitute the testing strategy, a given ELISA followed by a given rapid test may constitute the testing algorithm. Therefore, a testing algorithm that is selected using particular tests is decided upon depending on the testing strategy. The CDC has published recommendations for HIV testing algorithms and interpretations, updated in January 2018 (https://stacks.cdc.gov/view/cdc/50872).

Testing strategies and testing algorithms almost always involve at least two tests but can include as many as five tests before a final and conclusive result is accomplished. For example, if an infection is caused by HIV-1 group O virus and a specific diagnosis is required, antibody screening and confirmatory tests may initially identify

HIV infection, but specific antibody tests for HIV-2, for HIV-1 group O, and even NATs may be required before the infection is confirmed to be of HIV-1 group O. A number of different testing strategies (and many algorithms) are available for determining the HIV status of individuals. Furthermore, different strategies may be required depending on (1) surveillance versus blood screening, (2) the need for cost-savings strategies when resources are limited or certain tests are unavailable (e.g., resource-limited countries), and (3) to increase the ability to identify different HIV variants depending on the geographic location of testing. Specific testing strategies have been devised and endorsed by a number of agencies, including the World Health Organization, and have been shown to be effective for a wide range of purposes (http://www.who.int/diagnostics_laboratory/documents/guidance/pm_module4.pdf).

Although each laboratory must determine its own testing strategies and algorithms based on the purpose of testing, the available tests, and regulations, there are some general guidelines which should be followed. A highly sensitive screening test is first used to identify samples that contain antibody to HIV (i.e., to detect all positives). The first screening test should be selected based on high sensitivity and high negative predictive values. Samples with initially reactive results are repeated in duplicate to rule out technical error (although some test manufacturers do not require repeat testing). If repeatedly reactive (at least two of the three results are reactive), the sample is then tested by a supplemental or confirmatory test that preferably has the ability to differentiate HIV-1 from HIV-2 infection (differentiating test); these tests are highly specific, have a high positive predictive value, and will usually clarify the status. Thus, the use of one screening assay followed by a supplemental test is nearly always the strategy (except in resource-limited countries). For confirmation of infection, the CDC states that an individual must be positive by *both* a screening test and a confirmatory test; therefore, a positive result by just one of these is not sufficient to label a person as confirmed positive.

In the recent past, the CDC recommended an algorithm that included a rapid differentiation test as a means to confirm infection and

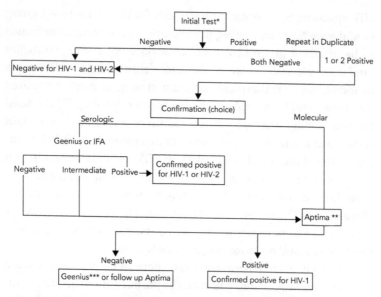

FIGURE 2.2 Testing strategy/algorithm for HIV-1 and HIV-2.
Geenius, Geenius HIV 1/2 Supplemental Assay (BioRad); Aptima, Aptima HIV-1 RNA Qualitative Assay (Hologic); IFA, Fluorognost HIV-1 Indirect Immunofluorescence Assay (Sanochemia).
* A fourth-generation test (Ag/Ab) is recommended, but the initial test can be an EIA, CIA, a rapid test, or the IFA.
** Aptima is the only molecular assay approved by the FDA for diagnosis.
*** If the Geenius is positive after a negative Aptima, an Elite Suppressor is likely.

to specifically identify HIV-2 infection. With the discontinuation of that second test (Multispot HIV-1/2) in June 2016, algorithms have been forced to change. Figure 2.2 depicts a suitable testing strategy and allows for a choice for confirmation. Other strategies exist in different countries, and studies are planned to evaluate alternative strategies for the United States.

As noted, the serologic supplemental tests (Geenius and IFA) and RNA detection are definitive for HIV infection if they are positive. However, negative or indeterminate results by these tests require further analysis or follow-up to verify infection. Noteworthy, elite suppressors (Sajadi et al., JAIDS 2009;50:403–408) may be confirmed positive serologically but negative by RNA and VL assays, thus necessitating further testing and follow-up. A proportion of individuals will not serologically convert upon follow-up and thus are subsequently found to be noninfected (i.e., were false-positive screening test results).

If the IFA method is used as the serologic confirmatory test, it may not confirm infection by HIV-2; in such cases, a negative or indeterminate result by the IFA should signal further testing by the Geenius or a specific HIV-2 test. For cases in which a WB is used as the confirmatory test and is indeterminate or negative, an IFA can be performed, and if the IFA is positive, the result is definitive. When the IFA is negative, some IFA algorithms allow a final result to be reported as HIV-negative; however, others recommend that such patients be followed by retesting (or performing RNA testing).

Alternative Testing Strategies for Resource-Limited Countries

Alternatives to classical algorithms have been in use since the late 1980s, primarily as a means to save on costs and provide simplicity for facilities that have limited resources. The goal is to maximize the chance of verifying HIV infection with accuracy but without the need for incorporating confirmatory assays that are costly and rigorous to perform. Therefore, alternative strategies offer a response for laboratories that do not have the capability to use tests that required instrumentation or stable electricity or that require expertise for interpretation of results. Results from a number of studies have consistently shown that the use of selected tests in alternative testing strategies can result in a 70–82% cost savings over classical ELISA/WB testing strategies (http://www.who.int/diagnostics_laboratory/documents/guidance/pm_module4.pdf). The degree of cost savings depends on the prevalence of HIV infection in the population being tested. Alternative strategies are also of value in those testing situations where a small number of tests are performed and in outreach or peripheral laboratories (decentralized testing). Consequently, a number of testing facilities, particularly in resource-limited countries, have adopted these alternative strategies.

These types of alternative strategies and algorithms are usually based on performing two screening tests in tandem, with the second test acting as a confirmation for samples that were positive by the first screening test. Thus, a negative result using a highly sensitive rapid or EIA screening test is considered as negative with no need to perform a second test (similar to most other algorithms). A positive result by the first test requires a second screening test. If positive, the result is considered to be from a truly infected person. If the sample that was positive by the first test is negative by the second test, further testing is required for resolution; this can be accomplished by a third screening test (tie-breaker) or another means (confirmatory test). Information on alternative testing strategies from USAID and WHO can be found at: http://www.who.int/hiv/pub/posters/Testingstrategies_policy_poster.pdf?ua=1.

Home Tests and Tests that Use Oral Fluids

Oral fluids consist of crevicular fluid from the tooth–gum margin as a transudate of blood and fluid from the salivary glands; details of the constitution of oral fluids has been described (Tamashiro & Constantine; editorial review, Bull World Health Org. 1994;72:35–143; Constantine et al., 2005). For HIV oral fluid testing, specific devices are incorporated to preferentially collect crevicular fluid which contains IgG antibodies (unlike IgA from the salivary glands). HIV tests that use oral fluid (saliva) as a sample medium offer a number of advantages, including (1) being more acceptable to persons being tested (Peralta et al., Arch Pediatr Adolesc Med. 2001;155:838–843), (2) a reduced risk of occupational exposure from needlesticks, (3) availability in places that do not have phlebotomy services, and (4) extreme simplicity for users from sample collection to test results. Currently, there are two rapid tests that are FDA-approved for using oral fluids, including the OraQuick HIV-1/2 (OraSure Technologies www.orasure.com) and the Chembio DPP HIV 1/2 Assay (Chembio Diagnostics Systems). Both use an FDA-approved device for collecting the sample and concentrating IgG for application to detect HIV antibody. The OraQuick test is the only truly "home test" that can be performed at home by the public. It is available for purchase at OraQuick.com or at retailers. The test consists of a specially treated pad used to swab the gums; the swab is then inserted into a vial for 20 minutes and read at 20 minutes. As compared with blood tests, including the OraQuick with blood, a few reports indicate a lesser sensitivity as compared with blood tests (Lancet Infect Dis. 2012 May;12(5):373–80. There are several other reports of a higher false-positive rate as compared to blood tests when using the OraQuick with blood samples. Nevertheless, the test is suitable for use and is valuable for getting more persons tested. The Chembio DPP HIV 1/2 Assay detects antibodies to HIV-1 and HIV-2 in oral fluid and all blood matrices. A video showing collection and testing can be found at http://chembio.com/products/human-diagnostics/dpp-hiv-12-assayx/).

Molecular Tests to Detect and Monitor HIV Infection

NATs for HIV are used to directly detect nucleic acids (RNA or DNA). The verification of viral nucleic acid confirms infection, and monitoring VL or levels of viral copies is used to stage infection and guide therapy. Importantly, detection of viral nucleic acids is used to identify acute HIV because detection through amplification techniques can be accomplished up to 1 wk prior to antigen detection and 1–2 wks prior to antibody detection (Figure 2.1) (AIDS 2003;17:1871). RNA detection is most commonly used, but DNA detection may have advantages in certain situations (J Antimicrob Chemother 2015;12:3311; J Clin Microbiol 2002;40:675). RNA detection is most often used for diagnosis and monitoring infection using qualitative and quantitative methods, respectively. There are at least 10 NATs that have been approved by the FDA, but many have been discontinued; these can be found at http://www.fda.gov/ BiologicsBloodVaccines/BloodBloodProducts/ApprovedProducts/ LicensedProductsBLAs/BloodDonorScreening/InfectiousDisease/ UCM080466#anti_HIV1_Assays. Internationally, there are many more NATs available, and some are available for research only. Table 2.3 presents some popular RNA VL tests and indicates characteristics of each.

All of the HIV-1 VL tests listed in Table 2.3 detect the major (M) group of viruses (A–D and F–H). Thus, all these tests detect HIV-1 B subtype, which is the predominant form in industrialized countries such as the United StatesEurope and Australia (J Med Virol 2006;78:883). However, non-B subtypes are seen increasingly in the United States (AIDS Res Hum Retroviruses 2016 Apr 22; Infect Genet Evol 2014;28:358; J AIDS 2010;54:297), and in Europe (AIDS 2014;28:773; Clin Infect Dis 2013;56:880). There is significant performance variation with the detection of non-subtype B viruses such as Group O and Group N, as well as the circulating recombinant forms (CRFs) with different types of RNA assays (Virol J 2011;8:10; J Acq Imm Def Synd 1999;29:330). The Roche COBAS AmpliPrep/ COBAS TaqMan HIV-1, v2.0 and the Abbott m2000 RealTime HIV-1 assays are quite comparable in their detection of B and non-B subtypes (J Clin Virol 2011;52:181; J Antivirals Antiretrovirals 2010;2:42). However, at the low end of VL, these two assays behave quite differently (J Med Virol 2016;88:724), suggesting that a single assay should be used to monitor disease progression. There is no commercially available quantitative NAT for HIV-2.

Kinetics of Viral Nucleic Acid Production

The time from infection when RNA tests can detect infection after exposure is estimated to be between 10–12 days (eclipse phase, Figure 2.1). During this period, all markers of infection, including RNA, are negative, but the person is infectious. There are approximately 4–5 days when RNA and p24 antigen levels may be detectable but HIV antibody tests are negative (seronegative

TABLE 2.3 Examples of HIV-1 viral load tests that are currently available

Company	Roche	Siemens	Abbott	bioMérieux
Trade name(s)	1) Amplicor HIV Monitor 1.5 2) COBAS TaqMan HIV-1 Test, v2.0,3 COBAS 6800/8800 HIV-1 VL test	VERSANT HIV-1 RNA 1.5 Assay (kPCR)	RealTime HIV-1	NucliSENS EasyQ HIV-1 v2.0
Technique	TaqMan Real-time RT-PCR	kPCR	Real-time PCR	NASBA
Dynamic range	20–100,000 20–10,000,000 20–10,000,000	37–11,000,000	40–10,000,000	10–10,000,000
Subtype amplified	A–H A–H and O A–H, CRF and O	A–H, CRF and O	A–H, O and N	A–H
Sample type	Plasma	Plasma	Plasma	Plasma and Dry blood spot (DBS)
Collection tube	EDTA	EDTA, ACD-A, PPT	EDTA, ACD-A	EDTA
Specimen volume	0.5 mL 1 mL 0.5mL	0.5 mL	0.2, 0.5, 0.6, and 1.0 mL	0.1, 0.5, and 1.0 mL

(continued)

TABLE 2.3 Continued

Company	Roche	Siemens	Abbott	bioMérieux
Requirement	Separate plasma <6 hrs and freeze prior to shipping at −20°C or −70°C.	Separate plasma <4 hrs and freeze prior to shipping at −20°C or −70°C.	Freshly drawn specimens (whole blood) may be held at 15–30°C for up to 6 hrs or at 2–8°C for up to 24 hrs, prior to centrifugation.	Separate serum or plasma <4 hrs and freeze prior to shipping at −20°C or −70°C.
Instrument	COBAS AMPLICOR Analyzer COBAS AmpliPrep/COBAS TaqMan System COBAS 6800/8800 Systems	VERSANT kPCR Molecular System	M2000 RealTime System	NucliSentral solution
Contact	800-526-1247	800-434-2447	800-553-7042	800-682-2666

period). During the time when RNA can be detected, but all other markers are negative, the VL is usually between 100 and 10,000 copies/mL; this is sometimes called the "ramping up period" and represents HIV doubling rates of 21.5 hrs each day (J AIDS 2005;39:133; Transfusion 2013;53:2384). Once p24 antigen becomes detectable at about 16 days, RNA levels are always greater than 10,000 copies/mL. Peak viremia usually occurs within 2–4 mos after infection, thereby occurring after the time of seroconversion.

Without treatment during early infection, viral RNA levels rise exponentially during the first 5–6 wks, peak within about 50 days to 1 million copies/mL or higher, drop 2–3 logs (to about 10,000 copies) with some fluctuation, and subsequently reach the "set point" by about 6 mos after infection. Subsequently, the VL remains at fairly constant levels (low to moderate) for up to 10 yrs before rising when AIDS occurs. Although the constant levels of VL for long periods of time suggest low viral replication, it is known that viral production is exceedingly high, with about 1 billion virions produced each day regardless of the stage of infection (STEP Perspect 1995;7:10). The physiological factors that determine the set point remain unknown, but they probably relate to the effectiveness of the host antiviral immune responses, the degree of immune activation, and/or the characteristics of the virus. HIV-infected individuals generally have set points of 1,000–10,000 copies/mL in plasma and, once established, the set points remain fairly constant for months to years in most infected individuals (AIDS 1997;15:1799; Retrovirol 2007;4:65). Those persons whose clinical course of disease is short (fast progression toward AIDS) are commonly referred to as *rapid progressors*. They have higher set points, whereas *slow progressors* usually have lower set points. In established infections, set point levels range from 200 copies/mL in those who are nonprogressors to approximately 1 million copies/mL in persons who have advanced disease. Although the levels of viral RNA differ between individuals, the kinetics are similar in most persons.

Qualitative RNA Tests

As of the time of writing, there is only one HIV RNA test that is FDA-approved for diagnosis. This test, the Aptima HIV-1 RNA Qualitative Assay (Hologic), is a qualitative molecular assay that detects HIV-1 RNA in plasma. It is most often used for diagnosis, and it can be used to detect acute HIV before antigen or antibody appears. In addition, it is valuable as a means to resolve negative or indeterminate serologic results produced by confirmatory assays (see Figure 2.2). The method, transcription-mediated amplification (TMA), involves several enzymes and a complex series of reactions that all take place simultaneously at the same temperature (isothermal). The advantages of TMA include its very rapid kinetics and the lack of requirement for a thermocycler. Reaction in a single tube with a rapidly degradable product (RNA) helps minimize contamination risks. RNA isolation and DNase pretreatment are not required. Plasma specimens are lysed, and RNA is stabilized and captured on magnetic particles containing poly (dT) oligonucleotides and oligonucleotides complementary to the viral RNA. The manufacturer claims a sensitivity of 33 copies/mL with 100% reliability when a diluted WHO standard is used (Product Insert). However, quantitative RNA tests that measure VL are often used for diagnosis, and this might be justified if the Aptima test is not available.

Quantitative RNA (Viral Load) Tests

Although the choice of a particular test may be by preference or may be dictated by which test is available at healthcare-associated reference laboratories, all are essentially comparable in performance. Even though some RNA tests may claim a slightly higher sensitivity (copy number detection), a lesser cost, or a more simplified procedure, all produce results that are sufficient to guide therapy (JCM 1996;34:3016; J Med Virol 1996;50:293; JCM 1996;34:1058; JCM 1998;36:3392; J Antivirals Antiretrovirals 2010;2:42). However, it is important that the same method be used for sequential assessments in order to minimize differences due to the methodologies (JCM 2011;49:292; J Med Virol 2016;88:724).

All of the assays listed in Table 2.3 have very similar linear dynamic ranges, from log10(1) to log10(7) with the exception of the Amplicor (Roche) assay version 1.5, which ranges from log10(1) to log10(5); all have similar lower limits of detection. It is arguable if a lower limit of detection of 10 versus 40 copies/mL is clinically relevant for monitoring infection. Some of the HIV-1 VL tests listed in the previous edition of this book are no longer available, such as the branched chain DNA (bDNA) assay (Versant 3.0). The three Roche assays differ by their amplification targets and instrument platforms, but all detect multiple subtypes, and only several can detect HIV-1 Group O. The Amplicor HIV-1 Monitor Test detects a conserved region in HIV-1 gag and uses the COBAS Amplicor Analyzer with the conventional RT-PCR method. The COBAS TagMan HIV-1 test v2.0 is performed using the COBAS AmpliPrep/COBAS TaqMan System and adapts a dual-target strategy that includes the long terminal repeat region (5′ LTR, U5), as well as gag (J Clin Virol 2010;49:41). A concern with this assay is an apparent reduced accuracy with persistently detectable levels (>50 c/mL) reported in patients who do not have evidence of failure with sequential testing and have <50 c/mL with duplicate Amplicor monitor tests (HIV Clin Trials 2008;9:283; J Clin Virol 2012;53:354). This has prompted concern for the need to repeat the test or change treatment with low-level viremia using that assay. The COBAS 6800/8800 HIV-1 VL test was approved by the FDA in 2015. It uses the same dual-target strategy, but the test is carried out on the completely automated COBAS 6800/8800 Systems with faster turnaround times. The NucliSENS EasyQ HIV-1 v2.0 test is the only one that can test dried blood spot (DBS). However, many HIV-1 VL testing laboratories may also test other samples types such as seminal fluid, cerebrospinal fluid, breast milk, saliva, and vaginal fluid (JCM 2000;38:1414) as long as their tests have been fully validated internally as a laboratory developed test (LDT). In general, the newer versions of the HIV-1 VL tests, such as Abbott's RealTime HIV-1, Siemen's Versant HIV-1 RNA 1.5 (kPCR), and Roche's TaqMan HIV-1 test, are more suitable to detect non-B subtypes. These quantitative RNA VL assays are based on different principles, including polymerase chain reaction (PCR) for the Roche, Siemens, and Abbott assays, and nucleic acid sequence-based amplification (NASBA) for the bioMerieus assay. The VERSANT HIV-1 RNA 1.5 Assay (kPCR) is performed on the VERSANT kPCR Molecular System and is combined with Siemen's nucleic acid extraction technology.

HIV-1 DNA Assessment

The detection of integrated and nonintegrated forms of proviral DNA sequences in CD4 lymphocytes or whole blood by PCR continues to be an important means of diagnosing HIV infection in some situations and in research. It is sometimes used to confirm HIV-1 infection, particularly in (1) cases of conflicting serology and molecular test results, (2) in long-term survivors with undetectable RNA VLs in plasma, (3) in the diagnosis of HIV infection in the newborn, and (4) in patients receiving effective antiretroviral therapy where RNA levels in plasma are undetectable (Int J Infect Dis 2000;4:187). Clinically, the detection of HIV-1 proviral DNA is usually sufficient to provide a diagnosis of infection, although it requires blood cells for analysis and a more rigorous procedure. HIV-1 DNA detection is a highly sensitive method to identify HIV-1 infection, being able to detect 1–10 copies of HIV-1 proviral DNA (J Clin Microbiol 2002;40:675). Recently, the use of RNA tests, rather than tests for DNA, have been suggested for assessment of infection in the newborn because of an increased sensitivity and a more routine methodology. Qualitative DNA PCR is used to detect cell-associated proviral DNA, including HIV-1 reservoirs in peripheral CD4 cells in patients responding to ART with a sensitivity of about 5 copies/10^6 cells (J Virol Methods 2005;124:157). This is not considered sufficiently accurate for diagnosis without confirmation, and these tests are not FDA-approved (Ann Intern Med 1996;124:803).

The Uses of Viral Load Tests

In addition to the ability to resolve the infection status of those who have inconclusive serologic confirmatory results, the VL is accepted as the most important barometer of therapeutic response, although CD4 count best predicts clinical progression (NEJM 1996;335:1091; Ann Intern Med 1996;124:984; JID 2002;185:178). The most important long-term goal of treatment is achieving a VL of <50 c/mL because some authorities note that clonal sequence analyses show no viral evolution with resistance mutations at that level (JID 2004;189:1452; JID 2004;189:1444), and some studies show that VL of <1 copy/mL is common (AIDS 2011;25:341). The implication is that there is no viral replication and little likelihood of developing resistance or disease progression. Nevertheless, some blips are associated with lapses in adherence, which could lead to drug failure and resistance (JID 2007;193:1773). Given the variability in VL assays and results with long-term outcome, most authorities endorse a therapeutic goal of maintaining the VL at <50 copies/mL (JAMA 2005;293:817), although clinicians would like to see as low a VL as possible. A minority of patients are long-term nonprogressors with persistently high CD4 cell counts. The "elite controllers" or "elite suppressors" are defined as those having a VL of <50 copies/mL (or nondetectable) without therapy but while being fully seropositive (Sajadi et al., JAIDS 2009;50:403–408).

Tests should be performed at baseline and followed by routine testing at 3- to 6-mo intervals (CID 2001;33:1060). With new therapy and changes in therapy, assays should be performed at 2–4 wks, then at 4- to 8-wk intervals until a VL of <50 copies/mL is achieved. An expected response to therapy is a decrease of 0.75–1.0 log10 copies/mL at 1 wk (Lancet 2001;358:1760; JAIDS 2002;30:167), a decrease of 1.5–2.0 log10- copies/mLat 4 wks (JAIDS 2000;25:36; AIDS 1999;13:1873; JAIDS 2004;37:1155), <500 copies/mL at 8–16 wks (Ann Intern Med 2001;135:945; JAIDS 2000;24:433), and <50 copies/mL at 24–48 wks. The 2003 Swiss guidelines define treatment failure as a failure to decrease the VL by 1.5 log10 copies/mL within 4 wks or to achieve undetectable virus by 4 mos (Scand JID 2003;35:155). The time to VL nadir is dependent on the pre-treatment VL as well as on the potency of the regimen, adherence, pharmacology, and resistance. Patients with high baseline VL take longer to achieve maximum suppression. Failure to reduce the VL by 1 log10 copies/mL (90%) at 4 wks suggests virologic failure due to nonadherence, preexisting resistance, or inadequate drug exposure. The expectation is to reduce the VL to <50 copies/mL by 16–24 wks (JAMA 2006;296:827; JCI 2000;105:777). The VL should then be measured in patients on treatment every 3–6 mos to assure that a VL of <50 copies/mL is maintained (JID 1999;180:1347). Blips are usually inconsequential but can also indicate nonadherence (JID 2007;196:1773), and sustained levels of >50 copies/mL indicate virologic failure (JAMA 2005;293:817; JAC2008;61:699). Virologic failure is now defined by the 2011 DHHS Guidelines panel as a con-firmed VL of >200 copies/mL. Changes of ≥50% (0.3 log10 copies/mL) are considered significant.

The VL can predict the time until AIDS and the degree of trans-missibility. VLs of >100,000 are a good predictor of rapid progres-sion to AIDS. For example, in persons with baseline VL levels of <500 copies/mL, 5% of persons progressed to AIDS within 6 yrs, as compared with 80% progressing if the VL level is >30,000 (Proc Natl Acad Sci USA 2007;30:17441). Infected persons whose HIV RNA VL levels exceed 100,000 copies/mL at 6 mos of infection are 10-fold more likely to progress to AIDS within 5 yrs than those with levels of <100,000 copies/mL. Persons with a baseline set point of >100,000 copies/mL have a median survival of only 3.5 yrs. In infected individuals with VL levels >10,200 copies/mL and CD4 cell counts >500 cells/μL, more than 70% will progress to AIDS and will die within 10 yrs, as compared with less than 30% of patients who have <10,200 copies/mL. The association between viral set point and progression has been described (Ann Intern Med 1995;122:573; Science 1996;272:1167; JID 1996;174:696; JID 1996;174:704; AIDS 1999;13:1305; NEJM 2001;349,720; AIDS 2002;16:2455; Lancet 2003;362:679; JAIDS 2005;38:289). In the treatment era, outcome is determined primarily by therapy and is less dependent on baseline VL (AIDS 2006;20:1197; CID 2006;42:136; JID 2004;190:280).

VL and DNA tests are also used in a research capacity to identify latent reservoirs of HIV that reside in some anatomical sites that may be differentially affected by antiretroviral drugs and may be the source of archived strains resistant to those drugs. The most important and best characterized reservoirs are resting CD4 cells; others are cells in the central nervous system (CNS), gut-associated lymphoid tissue (GALT), macrophages (Curr Opin Infect Dis 2013 26:561), and genital tract (AIDS 2002;16:39; JCM 2000;38:1414; Ann Intern Med 2007;146:591; Top HIV Med 2010;18:104; PNAS 2008;105:3879; Ann Rev Med 2008;59:487). Discussions on measuring viral nucleic acid for identifying and characterizing viral reservoirs have been published (J Virol Methods 2005;124:157).

Rapid Molecular Tests

Recent advances have offered NATs that can be performed more simply and faster. These are especially important if they can be performed as POC tests in nonlaboratory settings and in resource-limited countries where facilities may be limited and cost-savings methods are important. Some tests listed here are rapid and simpler than conventional nucleic acid assays but still require moderate laboratory resources and facilities that can support instrumentation (e.g., stable electricity). Because HIV-1 VL testing is recommended by the WHO for monitoring patients on treatment, alternatives to more rigorous assays are important.

One alternative to routine PCR methods is the Whole Blood Alere Q NAT Point-of-Care RNA Assay (Alere Technologies) (http://www.alere.com/en/home/product-details/alere-q-hiv-12-detect.html). The method incorporates a PCR chamber, uses 25 µL of whole blood (venous or capillary), detects HIV-1 and HIV-2, and produces results in 52 minutes. When the VL is above 10,000 copies/mL, results generated were shown to be very similar to those as generated by the Roche COBAS AmpliPrep/COBAS TaqMan v assay (JCM 2016; Jun 1, doi: 10.1128/JCM.00362-16 JCM.00362-16).

However, below this cutoff, much higher and variable results were obtained. This high variability limits its use in monitoring ART failure. Nevertheless, it is a POC molecular method that offers an alternative to routine PCR, but it still must be performed in a laboratory setting that can support instrumentation.

Another alternative is the Xpert HIV-1 Qual (qualitative) test (Cepheid) that received WHO prequalification in June 2016. The test can detect HIV-1 in whole blood and dried blood spots from individuals suspected of HIV infection, including infants. Inclusion in the prequalification list signifies that Xpert HIV-1 Qual meets WHO's stringent performance, quality, safety, and reliability standards and fulfills a performance measure established for many developing countries and global health participants. The method is run on the GeneXpert System and detects viral RNA and proviral DNA in one fully integrated cartridge. It requires 100 µL of whole blood or dried blood spot material; there is no requirement for PCR room settings, it requires just 1 minute of hands-on time, and produces results in 90 minutes. Although this assay is not available in the United States, it has important applications in resource-limited countries for detecting HIV in the newborn up to 18 mos of age (when infant antibody becomes identifiable). As with other rapid NATs, a certain degree of laboratory infrastructure is required. Information can be found at http://www.cepheid.com/en/cepheid-solutions-uk/clinical-ivd-tests/virology/xpert-hiv-1-qual and www.cepheidinternational.com.

In contrast to PCR-based NATs, the HIV-1 RT-LAMP method is an alternative (PLoS One 2015;10:e0126609). This method detects acute HIV infection by an isothermal amplification technique (reverse-transcription loop-mediated isothermal amplification); it is quick, easy to perform, and does not require complex, dedicated equipment and laboratory space; it may be performed using low-tech, portable heating devices. It can detect both viral DNA and RNA in a single reaction, and it incorporates two primer sets directed against highly conserved regions within the reverse transcriptase (RT) and integrase (IN) genes. Using well-characterized seroconversion panels from recent seroconverters, it was demonstrated that the HIV-1 RT-LAMP assay was able to detect samples from acutely infected individuals up to 24 days prior to a representative rapid antibody test and up to 2 wks earlier than a lab-based antigen/antibody (Ag/Ab) combo enzyme immunoassay. But it was not as sensitive as a laboratory-based qualitative RNA assay (the APTIMA detected infection up to 5 days earlier). The HIV-1 RT-LAMP assay is estimated to cost 15–40 times less per test compared to the APTIMA depending on the individual laboratory's cost for purchasing the APTIMA kit. When used in conjunction with current rapid antibody tests, it has the potential to increase the number of individuals who receive an accurate, timely, and definitive HIV result at POC or in select laboratory settings, where cost and time restraints prohibit the use of standard NAT platforms.

Resistance Testing

Purpose and Scope

Resistance testing is aimed at providing information to facilitate the selection of antiretroviral agents in patients with HIV infection. There are two commercially available strategies, genotype and phenotype resistance tests, both of which provide information relevant to the selection of nucleoside analogue reverse transcriptase inhibitors (NRTIs), non-nucleoside reverse transcriptase inhibitors (NNRTIs) and protease inhibitors (PIs); testing for resistance to enfurvitide (ENF), chemokine receptor 5 (CCR5) antagonists, and integrase inhibitors is also available but requires separate tests. There is a genotype assay of the V-3 coding region to detect CCR5 antagonist resistance, but the Trofile phenotypic assay (see below) is preferred due to better sensitivity (2011 DHHS Guidelines). Resources that are recommended for information relevant to genotypic, phenotypic, and integrase inhibitor resistance include the International Antiviral Society (http://iasusa.org) and the Stanford University HIV database (http://hivdb.stanford.edu).

Most guidelines recommend resistance testing at the time of diagnosis for either acute or chronic HIV infection regardless of intent to start ART. Resistance testing is also recommended in patients with virologic failure (JAMA 2010;304:321, 2011 DHHS Guidelines; Top HIV Med 2009;18:132). Implementation can be considered as follows:

ACUTE HIV INFECTION: A genotypic resistance test is recommended in all patients at the time of diagnosis; testing should be performed at the time of diagnosis, regardless of the duration of infection and whether therapy will be initiated immediately (JAIDS 2006;41:573; JAIDS 2004;37:1665; 2011 DHHS Guidelines). This is the suggested time to test because resistant mutants may later become undetectable, particularly minority strains that subsequently emerge due to selective pressure (J Virol 2008;82:5510; JID 2010;65:548). If ART is to be initiated during acute infection, the regimen may need to be chosen and initiated before test results are available. In this case, the regimen should be based on anticipated resistance patterns for treatment-naïve patients, local resistance patterns, or data from the transmission source if this information is available. In most cases, the use of a ritonavir-boosted PI-based regimen is preferred in this setting since transmitted NNRTI resistance is more common than transmitted PI resistance.

CHRONIC HIV INFECTION: The baseline genotype should be considered when selecting the initial ART regimen (CID 2005;40:468; JID 2010;65:548; PLoS Med 2008;5:e158; JID 2009;199:693). Waiting to test until the decision has been made to start ART may decrease the yield of testing due to time-dependent reversion to wild-type virus. Despite this limitation, baseline genotypic resistance testing is also recommended at the time ART is initiated based on studies showing better virologic responses when the results are considered (NEJM 2002;347:385; JID 2008;197:867; HIV Clin Trials 2002;3:1; AIDS 2006;20:21; JAIDS 2010;53:633). Baseline genotypic resistance testing is now considered the standard of care because mutations in transmitted strains tend to persist. Resistance testing may fail to detect mutations present at low levels, which is most likely to be a problem in patients with acquired resistance from failed ART rather than in those with transmitted resistance.

In either case, this testing is best for defining what drugs not to use. Detection of minority variants is not currently possible with commercially available assays. The more complete baseline data require testing for resistance in the "minority pool," which is technically possible but not commercially available (J Clin Micro 2006 44:2612; JAMA 2011;305:1327).

VIROLOGIC FAILURE: Genotypic resistance testing is recommended with virologic failure, assuming there is a sufficient VL (>500–1000 c/mL). Suboptimal response is also considered an indication, as defined by the failure to achieve a decrease in VL of (1) 0.5–0.7 $\log_{10}$ c/mL by 4 wks, (2) a reduction by 1 $\log_{10}$ c/mL (10-fold reduction) by 8 wks, and (3) a VL >1,000 c/mL at 16–24 wks. Possibly the most important studies of the value of resistance testing with therapeutic failure were TORO-1 and TORO-2 (NEJM 2003;348:2175) and other salvage trials that found a strong correlation between the number of active drugs in the background regimen (by genotype or phenotype analysis) and virologic response. Multiple salvage trials have confirmed this observation. Table 2.4 shows resistance test results for several studies.

Resistance Test Methods

GENOTYPIC ASSAYS: Genotype analysis identifies mutations associated with phenotypic resistance. Testing may be performed using commercial kits or "home brews" that have been validated. Assays vary in cost and the method of reporting, but there was 98% concordance when two commercial kits were tested by the same laboratory (Antiviral Ther 2000;5 suppl 4:60; Antiviral Ther 2000;suppl 3:53). A study found a 0.3% frequency of false-positive results and a 6.4% frequency of false-negative results (Antiviral Ther 2001;6 suppl 1:1). The methodology involves (1) amplification of the RT and PR genes by RT-PCR, (2) DNA sequencing of amplicons generated for the dominant species (mutations are limited to those present in >20% of plasma virions), and (3) reporting of mutations for each gene using a letter-number-letter standard, in which the first

TABLE 2.4 Resistance test results in patients with acute or recent HIV infection

CPCRA-US[1]	1999–01	491	11.6%	7.8%	3.0%	0.7%
Europe Commission[2]	2002–05	2793	8.4%	4.7%	2.3%	2.9%
Canada[3]	2000–01	494	6.1%	3.1%	1.2%	1.2%
10 North American cities[4]	1995–01	377	11.6%	7.8%	3.0%	0.7%
United Kingdom[5]	2002–03	171	19.2%	12.4%	8.1%	6.6%
CDC survey[6]	2003–06	3130	10.4%	3.6%	6.9%	2.4%
UK CHIC[7]	1997–07	7994	9.0%	5.3%	2.9%	1.5%
France[8]	2006–07	530	9.5%	5.8%	2.8%	4.7%

1. CID 2005;40:468 5. BMJ 2005;331:1368

2. JID 2009;200:1503 6. Topics HIV Med 2007;15:150

3. JAIDS 2006;42:86 7. AIDS 2010;24:1917

4. NEJM 2002;347:385 8. JAC 2010;65:2620

TABLE 2.5 Letter designations for amino acids

A	Alanine	I	Isoleucine	R	Arginine
C	Cysteine	K	Lysine	S	Serine
D	Aspartate	L	Leucine	T	Threonine
E	Glutamate	M	Methionine	V	Valine
F	Phenylalanine	N	Asparagine	W	Tryptophan
G	Glycine	P	Proline	Y	Tyrosine
H	Histidine	Q	Glutamine		

Single-letter codes are used in describing genotypes.

letter indicates the wild-type amino acid at the designated codon, the number is the codon position, and the second letter indicates the amino acid substituted in the mutation. Thus, the RT mutation K103N indicates that asparagine (N) has replaced lysine (K) on codon 103. Table 2.5 shows the amino acids and corresponding letter codes used to describe mutations in genotype analyses.

Mutations associated with HIV resistance to RT or PR inhibitors are summarized in Table 2.6 – Table 2.12.

Interpretation is based on lists of drug resistance mutations or computerized rules-based algorithms. Interpretation of genotype resistance patterns in drug selection may be improved by consultation with an expert (AIDS 2002;16:209; Curr Opin HIV AIDS 2009;4:474) and by use of genotypic interpretation scores (GIS) that are available from the Stanford University HIV database (http://hivdb.stanford.edu) or the International Antiviral Society USA (http://iasusa.org). Genotypic susceptibility scores (GSS) are derived from GIS and used to predict virologic response (NEJM 2008;359:355; NEJM 2008;359:1442; AIDS 2007;21:2033). Genotypic resistance tests are generally preferred for baseline (pretreatment) testing, with early failures of initial regimens in which multiple mutations are not expected, and in patients who have discontinued therapy. Arguments for this approach are that genotypes are easy to interpret at early stages of failure and are more sensitive

TABLE 2.6 Resistance mutations adapted from IAS-USA

Drug	Mutations[a] Selected	Comments

Nucleoside Reverse Transcriptase Inhibitors (NRTIs): RT gene mutations

Drug	Mutations Selected	Comments
AZT	41L, 67N, 70R, 210W, 215Y/F, 219Q/E	Thymidine analog mutations (TAMs): reduce susceptibility to all NRTIs (see TAMs below). Most frequent TAMs are 41L, 210W, 215Y, which have greatest impact on NRTI susceptibility. 184V increases AZT susceptibility and reduces the emergence of TAMs. 44D and 118I further decrease susceptibility when present with TAMs. Some NRTI mutations may mutate to produce hypersensitivity to NNRTIs. The 118Y, 208Y and 215Y mutations are examples and have shown improved response with EFV or NVP treatment (AIDS 2002;16:F33; JID 2004;189:F33; HIV Clin Trials 2008;9:11). TAMs infrequently coexist with 65R.
d4T	41L, 65R, 67N, 70R, 210W, 215Y/F, 219Q/E	Most d4T resistance is due to TAMs (AZT). 65R causes low-level resistance, occasionally selected by d4T. 75T/M/A seen infrequently.
3TC	65R,184V	184V/I: high-level 3TC and FTC resistance, with increase in activity of AZT, d4T, and TDF, and partial reduction of resistance due to TAMs; also delays emergence of TAMs. Reduces susceptibility to ddI, ABC, though not clinically significant with 184V alone. 44D and 118I not selected by 3TC, but they confer moderate 3TC resistance. 65R not selected by 3TC, but can cause intermediate resistance to 3TC.

TABLE 2.6 Continued

Drug	Mutations[a] Selected	Comments
FTC	65R,184V	See 3TC.
ddI	65R, 74V	ddI resistance is seen with any three of the following: 41L, 67N, 210 W, 215Y/F, 219Q/E (AAC 2005;49:1739; the 70R and 184V mutations alone did not reduce viral response (JID 2005;191:840). 74V or 65R mutations alone or combined with 184V are associated with ddI resistance and cross-resistance to ABC (74V, 65R) and TDF (65R).
ABC	65R, 74V, 115F, 184V	Resistance with 65R or 74V, increased if 184V/I also present. 74V more commonly selected by ABC then 65R. TAM-mediated resistance depends on number of TAMs and TAM-pathway. 184V alone does not confer clinically significant resistance but further decreases in vivo response when in combination with TAMs or ABC mutations (JID 2000;181:912; Antivir Ther 2004;9:37).
TDF	65R, 70E	Reduced activity with 65R or with ≥3 TAMs that include 41L and 210W. 184V/I increases TDF activity, partially compensating for 65R or TAMs. 70E is uncommon, but reduces TDF susceptibility.

[a]The distinction between primary and secondary mutations has been eliminated for non-nucleoside reverse transcriptase inhibitors (NRTIs/NNRTs) by the IAS-USA Expert Committee; this distinction has been retained for protease inhibitors (PIs), but the terms have been replaced by "major" or "minor" mutations.

From Top HIV Med 2010;18:156.

TABLE 2.7 Multi-nucleoside resistance

Drug	Mutations[a] Selected	Comments
Multi-Nucleoside Resistance		
Multi- nucleoside resistance: Q151M complex	151M plus 62V, 75I, 77L, 116Y, 151M	Uncommon with 3TC- or FTC-containing regimens. Occurs with or without TAMs. The 151M complex confers high-level resistance to AZT,d4T, ABC, ddI, intermediate resistance to TDF, and low-level resistance to 3TC, FTC. TDF has activity against Q151M mutant strains (JID 2004;189:837).
Multi- nucleoside resistance: T69 insertion	69 insertion 41L, 62V, 70R, 210W, 215Y/F, 219Q/E	The 69 insertion complex confers resistance to all NRTIs when combined with a TAM at codons 41, 210 or 215.
Multi nucleoside resistance: multiple TAMs	41L, 67N, 70R, 210W, 215Y/F, 219Q/E	TAMs reduce in vitro susceptibility of all NRTIs, but the clinical significance of the in vitro findings is unclear (CID 2010;51:620; JID 2010;201:1054). Most common cause of multinucleoside resistance. Only AZT and d4T select for TAMs. 44D and 118I further decrease NRTI susceptibility.

TABLE 2.7 Continued

Drug	Mutations[a] Selected	Comments

Non-Nucleoside Reverse Transcriptase Inhibitors (NNRTIs): RT gene mutations

Drug	Mutations[a] Selected	Comments
NVP	100I:101P, 103N, 106A/M, 108I, 181C/I, 188C/L/H, 190A	181C is the favored mutation with NVP unless combined with AZT, in which case 103N is favored. 103N, 106M, 188L/C cause high-level NVP resistance. 188H causes low-level NVP resistance.
DLV	103N, 106M, 181C, 188L, 236L	Some NNRTI mutations (190A/S, 225) decrease susceptibility to NVP and EFV but cause DLV hypersusceptibility; clinical significance unknown.
EFV	100I, 101P, 103N, 106M, 108I, 181CI, 188L, 190S/A, 225H	103N is the favored mutation with EFV, causing high-level NNRTI resistance. 188L and 106M also cause high-level EFV resistance. Although 181C (and some other NNRTI mutations) cause only low-level EFV resistance phenotypically, response to EFV is generally poor, and other NNRTI mutations may be present in sub-populations.

(continued)

TABLE 2.7 Continued

Drug	Mutations[a] Selected	Comments
ETR	90I, 98G, 100I, 181V/I, 101P, 106I, 138AGK, 179DFT, 181C/I/V, 106I, 138AGK, 179DFT	Weighted resistance score Score 3: 181/V/I 2.5: 101P, 100I, 181C, 230L 1.5: 138A, 106I, 190S, 179F 1.0: 90I, 179D, 101E, 101H, 98G, 190A, 179T Failure 0–2: 38%; 2.5–3.5: 52%; ≥4: 74%. The IAS-USA December 2010 update on drug resistance mutations did not provide a weighted ETR resistance ETR resistance score but noted that the most important mutations are 181C/I/C, 101P and 100L.

TABLE 2.8 Protease Inhibitors (PIs): Protease gene mutations

Drug	Major[a] Mutations	Minor[b] Mutations	Comments
Protease Inhibitors (PIs): Protease gene mutations			
IDV and IDV/r	46I/L, 82A/F/T, 84V	10I/R/V, 20M/R, 24I, 32I, 36I, 54V, 71V/T, 73S/A, 76V, 77I, 90M	At least 3 mutations required for resistance to unboosted IDV (>4-fold decrease in susceptibility).

TABLE 2.8 Continued

Drug	Major[a] Mutations	Minor[b] Mutations	Comments
NFV	30N, 90M	10F/I, 36I, 46I/L, 71V/T, 77I, 82A/F/T/S, 84V, 88D/S	30N is the most common mutation, causing no PI cross-resistance. 90M occurs in some (especially non-B subtypes), causing greater PI cross-resistance.
SQV and SQV/r	48V, 90M	10I/R/V, 24I, 54L/V, 62V, 71V/T, 73S, 77I, 82A/F/T/S, 84V	With unboosted SQV, 90M is typically the first mutation, then 48V. 48V is unique to SQV, but 90M causes PI cross-resistance. Selection of PI mutations is unlikely with SQV/r in PI-naïve patients.
FPV and FPV/r	50V, 84V	10F/I/R/V, 32I, 46I/L, 47V, 54L/V/M, 73S, 76V, 82A/F/T/S, 90M	50V is associated with cross-resistance to LPV. 50V, 84V, 32I, 54L/M, 47V decrease DRV susceptibility. 10V, 47V, 54M, 84V decrease TPV susceptibility. PI mutations are unlikely to be selected by FPV/r in PI-naïve patients.

(continued)

TABLE 2.8 Continued

Drug	Major[a] Mutations	Minor[b] Mutations	Comments
LPV/r	32I, 47V/A, 76V, 82A/F/T/S	10F/I/R/V, 20M/R, 24I, 33F, 46I/L, 50V, 53L, 54V/L/A/M/T/S, 63P, 71V/T, 73S, 84V, 90M	Most PI-naïve patients failing LPV/r as the first PI have no PI mutations. 47A, 32I and possible 47V confer intermediate-to-high level LPV resistance. It is usually thought that >6 mutations are required for LPV resistance (package insert; AAC 2002;46:2926; J Virol 2001;75:7462), but more recent data suggests 147 V, 32I and possibly 147V produce high-level resistance and the combination of 76V and 3PI resistances LPV resistance (J Virol 2005;79:333;Protein Sci 2005;15:1870).

TABLE 2.8 Continued

Drug	Major[a] Mutations	Minor[b] Mutations	Comments
TPV/r	47V, 74P, 82L/T, 83D, 84V	10V, 33F, 36I/L/V, 46L, 54A/M/V, 69K/R, 89I/M/V	The best response is seen with 0–1 TPV mutations; an intermediate response with 2–7 mutations, and minimal response with 8 or more mutations. However, the validity of these scores in terms of clinical correlates is not well established with limited clinical experience. (TOP HIV Med 2010;18:156).
DRV/r	47V, 50V, 54M/L, 84V	11I, 32I, 33F, 74P,76V, 89V	Reduced response with increasing DRV mutations; poor response with ≥3 mutations.

[a]Major mutations emerge first or are associated with decreased drug binding or reduced viral activity; these effect phenotype resistance.

[b]Minor mutations appear later and, by themselves, do not significantly change phenotypic resistance, but they may further decrease susceptibility in combination with major mutations or help to compensate for loss of fitness caused by major mutations.

TABLE 2.9 Protease Inhibitors (PIs): Protease gene mutations

Drug	Major Mutations	Minor Mutations	Comments
Protease Inhibitors (PIs): Protease gene mutations (continued)			
ATV and ATV/r	50L, 84V, 88S	10I/F/V/C, 16E, 20R/M/I/T/V, 24I, 32I, 33I/F/V, 34Q, 36I/L/V, 46I/L, 48V, 53L/Y, 54L/V/M/T/A, 60E, 62V, 64L/M/V, 71V/I/T/L, 73C/S/T/A, 82A/T/F/I, 85V, 90M, 93L/M	50L causes no PI cross-resistance, and possible hypersusceptibility to other PIs. Reduced in vivo activity is associated with ≥3 of the following: 10F/V/I, 16E, 33F/I/V, 46I/L, 60E, 84V, 85V. Boosted ATV increases the number of mutations necessary to reduce activity. Selection of PI mutations is uncommon with ATV/r in PI-naïve patients. One report showed 75% or 0% response with 2 or > 3 of the following: 10V/I/C, 32I, 34Q, 46I/L, 53L, 54 A/M/V, 82A/F/I/T and 184V. Mutations 46I + 76V may increase the activity of ATV.
Fusion inhibitors: gp41 mutations			
ENF		36D/S, 37V, 38A/M/E, 39R, 40H, 42T, 43D	Mutations in other viral envelope regions may affect sensitivity. Resistance correlates with mutations at the HR1 region of gp41. Mutations in other parts of the envelope gene may be associated with reduced activity (PNAS 2002;99:16249; AAC 2005;49:113).

CCR5 antagonists: gp120 mutations

MVC   92Q,
       143R/H/C,
       148
       H/K/R,
       155H

Activity is limited to patients with purely R5- tropic virus. Resistance is most common with selection of X4 or D/M virus. Mutations in gp120 that allow viral binding of the drug-bound form have been reported with virologic failure despite R5 virus. Most mutations are in the V3 loop, which is the major determinant of HIV tropism. There is no consensus on the specific mutations associated with MVC resistance.

Resistance has also been noted with gp41 mutations without involving the V3 loop (Top HIV Med 2010;18:156).

Integrase Inhibitors: Integrase gene mutations

RAL   92Q,
       143R/H/C,
       148H/K/R,
       155H

There are 3 genetic resistance pathways with a signature mutation at 148 H/K/R, 155H or 143R/H/C, each combined with minor mutations.

The combination of 148H and 140S is the most Common, and causes the greatest loss of activity.

Other significant mutations with 148H/K/R include 74M + 138A, 138K or 140S. Significant mutations in the 155H pathway are 74M, 92Q, 97A and 92Q + 97A and 92Q = 97A, 143H, 163 K/R, 151I or 232N (Antiviral Ther 2007;12:S10). The 143 R/H/C pathway is rare.

TABLE 2.10 Mutations

Mutation Category	Mutation	Comments
Thymidine analog mutations (TAMs)	M41L, D67N/G, K70R, L210W, T215F/Y, K219E/Q/N	Selected by thymidine analogs (AZT, d4T) but cause resistance to all NRTIs. The M41L, L210W, and T215F/Y patterns are more common in subtype B virus and cause higher-level NRTI resistance than D67N/G, K70R, or K219E/Q/N. T215C/D/E/S/I/V are "revertants" that typically indicate "back mutation" after initial infection with NRTI-resistant virus. Revertants do not cause resistance themselves, but may indicate the presence of archived resistant virus.
Accessory mutations	E44D, VI118I	Contribute to NRTI resistance when accompanied by multiple TAMs.
Non-TAM nucleoside analog mutation	K65R	Selected by TDF, ABC, ddI. Causes variable decrease in susceptibility to those drugs and to d4T, 3TC, and FTC, but hypersusceptibility to AZT. Rarely occurs in patients on AZT-containing regimens or in the setting of TAMs. Can also be selected by d4T. Selection appears less common with TDF/FTC than with TDF/3TC.
Non-TAM nucleoside analog mutation	L74V	Selected by ABC, ddI (more common than K65R with ABC/3TC-containing regimens). Causes variable decrease in susceptibility to ABC and ddI, but hypersusceptibility to AZT, TDF. Rarely occurs in patients on AZT-containing regimens or in setting of TAMs.

3TC/FTC resistance mutation	M184V/I	Selected by 3TC, FTC. Causes high-level resistance to both drugs and modest decrease in susceptibility to ABC and ddI (not clinically significant when present alone). Increases susceptibility to AZT, d4T, TDF. Delays emergence of TAMs in thymidine analog-containing regimens.
Multi-nucleoside resistance mutations	T69 insertion	Selected by thymidine analogs, but rare in the HAART era, especially with 3TC-or FTC-containing regimens. Causes high-level resistance to all NRTIs and TDF.
Multi-nucleoside resistance mutations	Q151M complex	Selected by thymidine analogs, but rare in the HAART era, especially with 3TC-or FTC-containing regimens. Causes high-level resistance to all NRTIs when combined V75I, F77L, F116Y. TDF may retain activity.
d4T mutation	V75T/M/A	Selected by d4T in vitro and results in decreased d4T susceptibility, but uncommon with clinical use of d4T.
ABC mutation	Y115F	Selected by ABC, resulting in ~3-fold decrease in ABC susceptibility.

TABLE 2.11 Non-nucleoside reverse transcriptase inhibitor (NNRTI) resistant mutations

Mutation	Comments
V90I	Associated with decrease ETR susceptibility in combination with other ETR mutations
A98G	Selected by NVP (uncommon), resulting in minimal decrease in NVP susceptibility. Associated with decreased ETR susceptibility in combination with other ETR mutations.
L100I	Causes intermediate resistance to DLV, NVP, and EFV. Usually occurs with K103N, resulting in further loss of NNRTI susceptibility especially to EFV and DLV. Associated with decreased ETR susceptibility in combination with other ETR mutations. Increases susceptibility to AZT and possibly d4T.
K101E/H/P	**K101E:** Selected by NVP and EFV (uncommon), resulting in intermediate- level resistance to NVP and DLV, and low-level resistance to EFV. **K101P:** Associated with intermediate resistance to DLV, NVP, and EFV, but usually occurs in combination with K103N, resulting in high-level resistance. **K103E/H/P** is associated with decreased ETR susceptibility in combination with other ETR mutations.
K103N/S/R	**K103N:** Commonly selected by all NNRTIs, resulting in high-level resistance to DLV, NVP, and EFV. Does not affect ETR susceptibility. **K103S:** less common, resulting in lower degree of resistance to DLV and EFV, but moderate resistance to NVP. **K103R:** Polymorphism with minimal effect on NNRTI susceptibility, unless combined with V179D.

TABLE 2.11 Continued

Mutation	Comments
V106M/A	**V106M**: Selected by NVP (common with subtype C), resulting in high-level resistance to DLV, NVP, and EFV. Does not affect ETR susceptibility. **V106A**: Selected by NVP (uncommon), resulting in high-level NVP resistance, intermediate DLV resistance, and low-level EFV resistance. **V106I** was considered a polymorphism that does not cause NNRTI resistance; however, in the DUET studies it was associated with decreased ETR susceptibility in combination with other ETR mutations.
V108I	Selected by NVP and EFV (uncommon), resulting in minimal decrease in DLV, NVP and EFV susceptibility. Does not affect ETR susceptibility.
E138A/G/K	Included in Monogram (**A/G**) and Tibotec (**A**) scoring systems as ETR mutations, reducing ETR susceptibility in combination with other mutations. **E138K** selected by RPV, and causes cross-resistance to ETR.
V179 D/E/F/M/T	**V179D**: Selected by NNRTIs (uncommon), resulting in low-level resistance to DLV, NVP, and EFV. Greater resistance with V179D + K103R. Associated with decreased ETR susceptibility in combination with other ETR mutations. **V179E**: Low-level resistance to DLV, NVP, and EFV. **V179F**: Associated with intermediate resistance to NVP and DLV, low- level resistance to EFV, and decreased ETR susceptibility in combination with other ETR mutations. Usually occurs in combination with Y181C, resulting in high-level ETR resistance. **V179D**: Decreases susceptibility to ETR in combination with other ETR mutations.

(continued)

TABLE 2.11 Continued

Mutation	Comments
Y181C/I/V	Selected by NVP and DLV, causing resistance to both. Causes only low- level resistance to EFV, but clinical response to EFV is unlikely, possibly because of the presence of viral subpopulations with other resistance mutations. Increases susceptibility to AZT. Associated with decreased ETR susceptibility in combination with other ETR mutations. Alone, it causes 5–10 fold decrease in ETR susceptibility.
Y188 L/H/C	**Y188L:** Selected by NVP, DLV, and EFV (uncommon) resulting in high- level resistance to NVP And EFV and low-level resistance to DLV. Decreased ETR susceptibility in combination with Other mutations. **Y188C:** Selected by NVP; causes high-level NVP resistance and low-level EFV and DLV resistance. **Y188H:** Low-level NNRTI resistance. **Y188H/C:** Effects on ETR susceptibility unknown.
G190 S/A/E/Q	**G190A:** Selected by NVP and EFV, causing high-level resistance to NVP and intermediate resistance To EFV. Associated with decreased ETR susceptibility in combination with other ETR mutations. Increases DLV susceptibility (clinical relevance unknown). **G190S:** cause high-level resistance to NVP and EFV and hypersusceptibility to DLV. Associated With decreased ETR susceptibility in combination with other ETR mutations. **G190E/Q:** Causes high-level resistance to EFV and NVP, low-level resistance to DLV. Associated With decreased ETR susceptibility in combination with other ETR mutations.

TABLE 2.11 Continued

Mutation	Comments
P225H	Usually occurs with K103N, resulting in further loss of EFV susceptibility. Decreased ETR susceptibility in combination with other mutations.
F227L	Sometimes seen in combination with V106A, resulting in further loss of NVP susceptibility.
M230L	Selected by NNRTIs (uncommon), resulting in high-level resistance to DLV and NVP and intermediate resistance to EFV. Decreased ETR susceptibility in combination with other mutations.
P236L	Selected by DLV (uncommon), resulting in high-level DLV resistance.
K238T/N	Selected by NNRTIs (uncommon), usually in combination with K103N or other NNRTI mutations. Causes intermediate resistance to DLV and NVP and low-level resistance to EFV.
Y318F	Selected by NNRTIs (uncommon), resulting in intermediate-to-high-level DLV resistance and low-to-intermediate NVP resistance.

TABLE 2.12 Protease inhibitor (PI) resistance mutations

Mutation	Comment
L10 I/V/F/R/V	Accessory mutations that can contribute to reduced susceptibility in the presence of other PI mutations. L10V: Contributes to TPV resistance in the presence of other TPV mutations.
V11I	Contributes to DRV resistance in the presence of other DRV mutations.

TABLE 2.12 Continued

Mutation	Comment
I13V	Contributes to TPV resistance in the presence of other TPV mutations.
K20 R/I/M/T/V	Accessory mutations/polymorphisms that may contribute to reduced susceptibility in the presence of other PI mutations. K20M/R/V: Contribute to TPV resistance in presence of other TPV mutations.
L23I	Uncommon mutation; low-level NFV resistance.
L24I/F	L24I: PI resistance, especially to IDV, when combined with other PI mutations. L24F: Rare mutation with unknown effect on PI susceptibility.
D30N	Primary PI mutation selected only by NFV, especially with subtype B virus; intermediate NFV resistance; further loss of susceptibility with N88D/S.
V32I	Accessory mutation that confers low-level resistance to IDV, RTV, APV, LPV. Contributes to DRV resistance in the presence of other DRV mutations.
L33F/I/V	L33F: decreases susceptibility to RTV, APV, LPV, ATV, TPV, and DRV in the presence of other PI mutations. L33I/V: Polymorphisms not known to be associated with drug resistance.
E35G	Contributes to TPV resistance in the presence of other TPV mutations.
M36I/V/L	M36I/V: Accessory mutations that contribute to reduced PI susceptibility in the presence of other PI mutations. M36I: Contributes to TPV resistance in the presence of other TPV mutations. M36L: Unknown effect on PI susceptibility.

TABLE 2.12 Continued

Mutation	Comment
K43T	Contributes to TPV resistance in the presence of other TPV mutations.
M46I/L/V	M46I/L: Accessory mutation that contributes to reduced PI susceptibility in the presence of other PI mutations. M46L: Contributes to TPV resistance in presence of other TPV mutations. M46V: Uncommon mutation with unknown effect on PI susceptibility.
I47A/V	I47V: Reduced susceptibility to APV, IDV, RTV, LPV, TPV, and DRV in combination with other PI mutations. I47A: Moderate to high-level LPV resistance.
G48V/M	G48V: Selected by SQV; intermediate SQV resistance; low-level resistance to other PIs. G48M: Effect on PI susceptibility unknown.
I50V/L	I50V: Selected by APV in PI-naïve patients; intermediate APV resistance; low to intermediate resistance to RTV, LPV. Contributes to DRV resistance in the presence of other DRV mutations. I50L: Selected by ATV in PI-naïve patients; moderate to high-level ATV resistance; susceptibility to other PIs maintained or increased.
F53L	Associated with PI resistance when combined with other PI mutations.
I54V/M/L/T/S/A	I54V: Increases resistance to PIs when combined with other PI mutations. I54M/L: Selected by APV or FPV, causing low to intermediate resistance. Contributes to DRV resistance in presence of other DRV mutations. I54T/S/A: Effect on PI susceptibility unknown. I54A/M/V: Contribute to TPV resistance in the presence of other TPV mutations.

(continued)

TABLE 2.12 Continued

Mutation	Comment
Q58E	Contributes to TPV resistance in presence of other TPV mutations.
L63A/C/E/H/P/Q/R/S/T/V/I	L63P: Common polymorphism that increases PI resistance when combined with other PI mutations. Others: Effect on PI susceptibility unclear.
H69K	Contributes to TPV resistance in presence of other TPV mutations.
A71V/T/I	A71V/T: Decreases susceptibility to all PIs when combined with other mutations. A71I: Effect on PI susceptibility unknown.
G73S/C/T/A	G73S/C/T: Resistance to NFV, IDV, SQV, ATV in combination with other PI mutations. G73A: Uncommon variant.
T74P	Contributes to TPV and DRV resistance in the presence of other mutations.
L76V	Decreases LPV susceptibility to unknown degree. Contributes to DRV resistance in the presence of other DRV mutations.
V77I	Polymorphism associated with slight decrease in NFV susceptibility.
V82A/T/F/S/ I/G/L	V82A/T/F/S: Primary PI mutation that reduces susceptibility to LPV, IDV, RTV, and also to NFV, SQV, APV, ATV when combined with other PI mutations. V82I: Polymorphism with minimal effect on PI susceptibility. V82M: Seen with subtype G infection; reduces IDV susceptibility. V82L/T: Contributes to TPV resistance in the presence of other TPV mutations.
N83D	Contributes to TPV resistance in the presence of other TPV mutations.

TABLE 2.12 Continued

Mutation	Comment
I84V/A/C	I84V: Decreases susceptibility to all PIs: greatest effect on APV, NFV, SQV, and lowest on LPV. Contributes to TPV and DRV resistance in the presence of other mutations. I84A/C: Effects similar to I84V, but rare.
N88S/D	N88D: Intermediate resistance to NFV; low-level resistance to SQV, ATV. N88S: Intermediate resistance to NFV, ATV; low-level resistance to IDV; hypersusceptibility to APV.
L89V	Contributes to DRV resistance in the presence of other DRV mutations.
L90M	By itself, causes intermediate resistance to SQV and NFV and low-level resistance to other PIs. Contributes to TPV resistance in the presence of other TPV mutations.
I93L/M	I93L: Common polymorphism that increases PI resistance when combined with other PI mutations. I93M: PI mutation with unknown effect on PI susceptibility.

for detecting wild-type/mutant mixtures, which may be present in treatment-naïve patients or in patients who have discontinued therapy. In addition, clinical trials demonstrated better outcomes in this setting when compared to the standard of care (GART [AIDS 2000;14:F83], VIRADAPT [Lancet 1999;353:2195]; HAVANA [AIDS 2002;16:209]) or when compared to phenotypic testing (REALVIRFEN [Antiviral Ther 2003;8:577]; NARVAL [Antiviral Ther 2003;8:427]). Genotypic testing is less expensive and appears cost-effective when used for first or second regimen failures (Ann Intern Med 2001;134:440; JAIDS 2000;24:227).

PHENOTYPIC ASSAYS: Phenotype analysis measures the ability of HIV to replicate at different concentrations of tested drugs. The test involves insertion of the RT and PR genes from the patient's strain into a backbone laboratory clone by molecular cloning or recombination. Replication is monitored at various drug concentrations and compared with a reference wild-type virus. This strategy is comparable with conventional in vitro tests of antimicrobial sensitivity in which the microbe is grown in serial dilutions of antimicrobial agents. Results are reported as the IC_{50} for the test strain relative to that of a reference, or wild-type strain. The interpretation uses either biologic thresholds based on the normal distribution of wild-type virus from untreated patients or, for most drugs, clinical thresholds based on data from clinical trials. Two cutoffs are provided for most drugs: a lower cutoff that indicates the fold-change for declining activity, and an upper cutoff that indicates the threshold for total loss of activity as reported by two commercial suppliers, Monogram (PhenoSense) and Virco (Antivirogram) (see Table 2.13). A "virtual phenotype" (VircoTYPE) is also provided by Virco and uses the genotype to predict phenotype based on a large database with genotype–phenotype pairs. It is unclear whether this provides additional advantage beyond standard genotype testing (JID 2003;126:194; Curr Opinion HIV AIDS 2009;4:474). Phenotype resistance may supplement genotypic test results in patients with more extensive resistance after multiple regimen failures (CID 2004;38:723) and TORO (NEJM 2003;348:2175). Phenotypes provide quantitative results, allowing comparison of relative susceptibility and resistance. They assess interactions among mutations and may be preferable for the assessment of susceptibility to new drugs for which genotypic correlates of resistance have not been completely determined. In the POWER studies, phenotypic susceptibility to Darunavir (DRV) was the best predictor of response to therapy (Antiviral Ther 2006;11:S83).

Table 2.14 shows a comparison of genotypic and phenotypic assays, with the advantages and disadvantages of each (JAC 2004;53:555; Top HIV Med 2008;16:89).

TABLE 2.13 Fold-change cut-offs for phenotype and VircoTYPE assays

Drug		Monogram PhenoSense				Virco Antivirogram		
		LCO	UCO	SCO	B/C	LCO	UCO	BCO
Abacavir	ABC	4.5	6.5		C	3.2	7.5	2.2
Didanosine	ddI	1.3	2.2		C			2.2
Emtricitabine	FTC			3.5	B			3.5
Lamivudine	3TC			3.5	C			2.4
Stavudine	d4T			1.7	C			2.3
Tenofovir DF	TDF	1.4	4.0		C			2.1
Zidovudine	AZT			1.9	B			2.7
Delavirdine	DLV			6.2	B			
Efavirenz	EFV			3.0	B			3.4
Etravirine	ETR							
Nevirapine	NVP			4.5	B			5.5
Amprenavir	APV							2.2
Amprenavir/Ritonavir	APV/r							
Atazanavir	ATV			2.2	C			2.4

(continued)

TABLE 2.13 Continued

Drug		Monogram PhenoSense				Virco Antivirogram		
		LCO	UCO	SCO	B/C	LCO	UCO	BCO
Atazanavir/Ritonavir	ATV/r			5.2	C			
Darunavir/Ritonavir	DRV/r	10.0	90.0		C	10	40.0	2.4
Fosamprenavir	FPV			2.0	B			
Fosamprenavir/Ritonavir	FPV/r	4.0	11.0		C			
Indinavir	IDV			2.1	B			2.4
Indinavir/Ritonavir	IDV/r			10	C			
Lopinavir/Ritonavir	LPV/r	9.0	55.0		C	10	40.0	1.7
Nelfinavir	NFV			3.6	B			2.2
Ritonavir	RTV			2.5	B			
Saquinavir	SQV			1.7	B			1.8
Saquinavir/Ritonavir	SQV/r	2.3	12.0		C			
Tipranavir/Ritonavir	TPV/r	2.0	8.0		C	3.0	10.0	1.8

LCO, lower cutoff; UCO, upper cutoff; SCO, single cutoff; B, biological; C, clinical; CCO1, lower clinical cutoff; CCO2, upper clinical cutoff; BCO, biological cutoff.

TABLE 2.14 Comparison of genotypic and phenotypic assays

Genotypic Assays

Advantages

Less expensive ($300–480/test).
Short turnaround of 1–2 wks.
Well standardized
Good reproducibility
Possibility of virtual phenotype[a]
More sensitive for detection of
    mixtures that can occur with
    emerging or disappearing
    resistance
Favored in comparative studies
    with failure of first or second
    regimens.

Disadvantages

Detect resistance only in
    dominant species (>20%).
Interpretation requires expertise
    or use of algorithms that
    vary in their ability to predict
    susceptibility.
Algorithms may be incomplete,
    especially for new drugs.
Require VL >500–1000 c/mL.
Limited data on non-clade
    B virus
Separate test required for
    integrase or fusion inhibitor
    resistance

Phenotypic Assays

Advantages

Interpretation is more
    straightforward and familiar.
Assess total effect, including
    mutational interactions.
Do not require data on genotypic
    correlates of resistance
    (advantageous with newer
    agents).
Reproducibility is good.
Advantage over genotype when
    there are complex mutation
    patterns, especially with PIs.
Provide quantitative assessment
    of susceptibility

Disadvantages

More expensive (usually $800–
    1000). High cost may affect
    reimbursement.
Report takes longer than for
    genotypic assay.
Clinically determined thresholds
    are not available for all drugs.
Detect resistance only in
    dominant species (>20%).
Require VL >500–1000 c/mL.
Separate test required for
    integrase inhibitor or fusion
    inhibitor resistance

[a]VircoTYPE, a genotype that estimates phenotype, is rapid, easily performed, and less expensive than phenotypic assays; the disadvantage is that its ability to predict phenotype is dependent on the accuracy of the algorithms derived from the database.

Other Assays

Tropism assays are used to determine whether patients are candidates for therapy with CCR5 antagonists that are indicated only in patients with exclusively R5-tropic virus. HIV binds to the host CD4 cell by attachment of gp120 to a CD4 receptor. This results in a conformational change in gp120 that allows binding to one of two chemokine co-receptors on the CD4 cell surface, namely CCR5 or CXCR4. There are four categories of tropism:

1. *R5-tropism*: Viruses that bind only to the CCR5 co-receptor
2. *X4-tropism*: Viruses that bind only to the CXCR4 co-receptor
3. *Dual-tropism*: Viruses that bind to either co-receptor
4. *Mixed-tropism*: Mixed populations that include both R5-tropic and X4-tropic viruses

Tropism assays cannot distinguish between dual- and mixed-tropic virus; therefore, these viruses are collectively referred to as dual/ mixed (D/M)-tropic virus. Sequential data show that transmitted virus is almost always R5 virus even when the source has D/M-tropic virus (Ann Rev Immunol 2003;21:265). Therefore, patients with early HIV infection typically have R5 virus exclusively. With progressive disease, a shift to D/M-tropic virus can occur (CID 2007;44:591). Patients with extensive treatment experience or rapid progression have a higher frequency of X4 virus, but pure X4 populations are rare (JID 2005;191:806; CID 2007;44:591; JID 2006;194:926). The presence of X4 virus is associated with more rapid clinical progression, but this does not alter the response to standard therapy (CID 2008;46:1617). Table 2.15 shows the prevalence of different viruses.

There are two high-throughput phenotypic assays: Phenoscript (VIRalliance, Paris, France) and Trofile (Monogram Biosciences, Inc., San Francisco CA). The Trofile test requires a VL of ≥1000 c/ mL, the cost is $1,960/test, and the turnaround time is about 2 wks

TABLE 2.15 Prevalence of R5, D/M, and X4 viruses in patients with HIV infection

Source	Treatment	N	R5	D/M	X4
JID 2005; 192:466	Naïve	979	82%	18%	<1%
JID 2005; 191:866	Naïve	462	81%	18%	<1%
CID 2007; 44:591	Experienced	391	50%	46%	4%
Viral Entry 2007;3:10	Experienced	2,560	56%	41%	3%
NEJM 2008;359:1429	Experienced	3,244	61%	–	–

(www.trofileassay.com). The indication for the test is consideration of using a CCR5 antagonist because the drug should be used only in patients with exclusive R5 virus. In MOTIVATE-1 and -2, the Trofile test was used to screen treatment-experienced patients with three-class resistance; 61% of 3,244 potential participants had R5 virus. A subsequent report showed that some of the failures had D/M virus detected only with the more recent and more sensitive Trofile ES (enhanced sensitivity) that has the ability to detect X4 virus with 100% sensitivity when X4 or D/M virus accounted for >0.3% of the viral population (JCM 2009;47:2604). Disadvantages of the Trofile assay include cost, requirement for a VL of >1000 c/mL, occasional cases of "nonreportable" results, and the 2- to 3-wk turnaround time. An alternative to the Trofile test is the tropism co-receptor assay information or "TROCAI" assay based on the virologic response to short-term exposure to the CCR5 antagonist (MVC). Results of this tests have correlated well with the Trofile (JCM 2010;48:4453). There is also a genotypic assay of the HIV-1 env V3 loop to determine co-receptor tropism (AIDS 2010;24:2517). This assay is less expensive and does not require a VL of >1,000 c/mL (JCM 2010;48:4453), but it is less sensitive for detecting X4 virus (Antiviral Res 2011;89:182) and is consequently not recommended in the 2011 DHHS Guidelines. Trofile is preferred for cases with a VL of >1,000 c/mL.

Routine Laboratory Tests

The routine repertoire of screening laboratory tests advocated for patients with established HIV infection is summarized in Table 2.16 (Primary Care Guidelines IDSA, CID 2004;39:609).

Tests for Sexually Transmitted Infections

A *syphilis serology* (MMWR 2010;59:RR-12) screen with a nontreponemal test (VDRL or RPR) at baseline and annually thereafter is recommended in sexually active patients due to high rates of co-infection. The screening test is confirmed with a treponemal-specific test including the fluorescent treponemal antibody absorbed (FTA-ABS) test, the *T. pallidum* passive particle agglutination (TP-PA), or EIAs/chemiluminescence immunoassays (Kashyap et al., Sex Transm Dis 2015;36:162–165). Confirmation is important due to frequent false-positive screening tests often ascribed to autoimmune disease, advanced age, injection drug use, pregnancy, and HIV infection (CID 1994;19:1040; JID 1992;165:1124; JAIDS 1994;7:1134; Am J Med 1995;99:55). In one review of 300,000 VDRLs, the rate of biologic false positives was 2.1% in persons with HIV compared to 0.24% in those without HIV (Int J STD AIDS 2005;16:722). Nontreponemal tests give antibody titers that correlate with disease activity. Many patients will have positive treponemal tests for life, but the VDRL and RPR usually become negative or persist at low titer, especially with successful treatment. Some HIV-infected patients have "atypical serology" with unusually high, unusually low, or fluctuating titers, but "for most HIV-infected patients, serologic tests are accurate and reliable for the diagnosis of syphilis and for the response to therapy" (MMWR 2002;51[RR-6]:19; Myer et al., Sex Transm Infect 2003;79:208–213). Some laboratories and blood banks now screen for syphilis with a treponemal test, usually an EIA. These may also show false positives and need to be confirmed with a nontreponemal test with titer; such a "reverse algorithm" has been suggested primarily to increase the efficiency of screening (treponemal-specific tests are more

TABLE 2.16 Routine laboratory tests

Test	Cost[a]	Frequency and Comment
HIV Tests		
HIV confirmation	$40–100	HIV serology. Rapid HIV tests and EIAs need confirmation by the Geenius, WB, IFA or HIV RNA. If confirmatory test is negative or indeterminate, use a different confirmatory test or repeat in 1 mo on a new sample. As of 2017, FDA approved WB assays are not available in the US.
HIV VL or Amplicor for diagnosis	$150–300	Baseline and every 3–6 mos.
CD4 count and CD4%	$100–150	Baseline and every 3–6 mos. Monitoring at 6- to 12-mo intervals is appropriate in clinically stable patients with consistent HIV suppression.
HIV genotypic resistance test	$100–150	Baseline and with virologic failure.
HLA-B*5701	$100	Indicated if plan is to treat with ABC.
Tropism test	$1960	Indicated if plan is to use CCR5 antagonist (i.e., MVC) and with MVC failure.
Serologic Tests		
Hepatitis screen	$60–80	If acute hepatitis is suspected, screen for anti-HAV IgM, anti-HCV, and HBsAg, anti-HBc IgM.; HCV RNA testing can be considered.

(continued)

TABLE 2.16 Continued

Test	Cost[a]	Frequency and Comment
Total anti-HAV antibody[†]	$20–30	For chronic hepatitis and immune status, screen for anti-HAV, anti-HCV, HBsAg, anti-HBs, and anti-HBc.
anti-HBc or anti-HBs[†]	$10–15	Screen at baseline for HAV immunity to determine need for vaccination.
		HBV: Screen at baseline for immunity with anti-HBc, anti-HBs and HBsAg to determine need for vaccination. If prior HBV vaccination, then test anti-HBs. If anti-HBc present without anti-HBs or HBsAg, screen for chronic HBV with HBV DNA; if HBV DNA negative, give HBV vaccine. Repeat anti-HBs at 1–2 mos after 3d vaccine dose to determine "take."
HBsAg[†]	$20–25	Screen for chronic hepatitis B. Consider HBV DNA in HBsAg negatives with abnormal transaminases.
anti-HCV[†]	$25 HCV EIA	Screen with anti-HCV; confirm positives with quantitative HCV RNA at $150. Consider HCV RNA in HCV-seronegatives at high risk, with abnormal transaminases, or with CD4 counts <200.

Test	Cost	Comments
Syphilis: VDRL, RPR or treponema specific test	$5–16	Confirm positives with FTA-ABS, MHA-TP or TP-PA. Repeat test annually in at-risk sexually active patients. Non-treponemal and treponemal tests may not always correlate. May consider reverse-algorithm.
anti-Toxoplasma IgG[†]	$12–15	Screen all patients at baseline, and repeat in seronegatives if CD4 cell count is <100 cells/mm^3 and patient does not take TMP-SMX for PCP prophylaxis or has symptoms suggestive of toxoplasmosis encephalitis. Agglutination assays for IgG are preferred. IgM is not useful.
Varicella IgG	$10	If negative or unknown history for chickenpox or shingles to promote protection against exposure, varicella vaccination and/or post-exposure ZIG.
Chemistry		
Comprehensive Chemistry panel[†]	$10–15	Includes liver enzymes and renal function. Repeat every 6–12 mos or more frequently in patients with abnormal results and with administration of hepatotoxic or nephrotoxic drugs, including most ART regimens. FBS at entry to care and repeat annually.
G6PD	$14–20	Timing and need for this test depends on the host demographics and use of high risk drugs.

(*continued*)

TABLE 2.16 Continued

Test	Cost[a]	Frequency and Comment
Lipid profile and blood glucose (fasting)	$20–40	Test at baseline and at 4–8 wks after starting new ART regimen. Routine testing at 6- to 12-mo intervals; more frequently based on initial results and risks.[†]
Hematology		
Complete blood count (CBC)[†]	$6–8	Repeat every 3–6 mos, more frequently for low values and with marrow-toxic drugs.
Other		
Chest x-ray	$40–140	May be routine or restricted to those with past pulmonary disease, chronic pulmonary disease or a positive PPD or IFN-γ release assay.[a]
PAP smear[b]	$25–40	Repeat at 6 mos and then annually if results are normal. Results reported as "inadequate" should be repeated. Refer to a gynecologist for results showing atypia or greater on the Bethesda scale.
PPD test or interferon-γ release assay	$10/PPD test $40/IFN-$\gamma$ release assay	Test at baseline. Annual testing should be considered in previously PPD-negative patients who have risk for tuberculosis, and repeat testing should be considered if initial test was negative and the CD4 count has subsequently increased to >200 cells/mm^3 in response to ART.

Urine NAT: *C. trachomatis* in sexually active females ≤25 yrs[b]	$40–100	Recommended by CDC HIV prevention guidelines for sexually active females <25 yrs (MMWR 2010; 59:RR12). Advocated as marker of high risk behavior with need for enhanced counseling and for treatment and contact tracing. Repeat annually in sexually active patients, and more often in high-risk patients. The Primary Care HIV Guidelines recommend screening all men and women for gonorrhea and *C. trachomatis* (CID 2009;49:651).
Urinalysis	$10	Assessment is especially important in African Americans, those on TDF, and with comorbidities such as diabetes, hypertension or hepatitis C. If ≥1+ proteinuria, measure hourly urine protein/creatinine ratio.

[a] Cost to purchase; with labor and administrative costs, the cost could be 2–5 times higher. General estimation; varies between laboratories and countries.

[b] Recommendations of Primary HIV Care Guidelines of IDSA (CID 2004;39:609).

automated), but the CDC still recommends the classical algorithm of a nontreponemal screening test with a specific test if positive for confirmation (CDC MMWR Morb Mortal Wkly Rep 2011;60:133–137). Some laboratories use a second specific treponemal test if the first was negative. If the second treponemal test is negative, no further evaluation or treatment is needed (MMWR 2010;59:RR-12). Overall, the nontreponemal and treponemal-specific tests, used in tandem, are excellent for diagnosis.

N. gonorrhoeae and/or C. trachomatis are common sexually transmitted infections (STIs) in HIV-infected patients (AIDS 2000;14:297) and are often asymptomatic in both men and women (STD 2001;28:33; CID 2002:35:1010). Diagnosis of STIs is important because (1) they usually indicate ongoing high-risk behavior, (2) they may enhance transmission of HIV, and (3) detection and treatment can reduce the likelihood of transmission (Sex Transm Infect 1999;75:3; Lancet 1995;346:530). Urine-based NATs are available for N. gonorrhoeae and C. trachomatis screening of men and women with the attributes of good sensitivity, good specificity, and ease of specimen collection (MMWR 2010;59:RR-12). Rectal and pharyngeal C. trachomatis infections can be diagnosed by NATs; these tests may be more sensitive than culture (STD 2008;35:435 and 637; JCM 2010;48:1827; JCM 2009;47:902), but they are FDA-cleared only for diagnostic testing for urethral or endocervical infection. Alternative, less expensive tests include endocervical and urethral swabs to detect N. gonorrhoeae and/or C. trachomatis by culture, nucleic acid hybridization, direct fluorescent antibody (DFA), or EIA. The CDC recommends annual screening for C. trachomatis in all females <25 yrs who are sexually active. For women who are >25 yrs, this screening is recommended if there are specific risks such as a new sex partner or multiple sex partners. C. trachomatis screening of sexually active young men is recommended in settings of high C. trachomatis prevalence such as STD clinics and in some men who have sex with men (MSM) (MMWR 2010;59:RR-12). Routine screening of sexually active MSM is recommended at least annually for (1) HIV (if not known to be positive); (2) syphilis; (3) urinary NAT testing for N. gonorrhoeae and C. trachomatis, (4) rectal infection with *N. gonorrhoeae* and *C. trachomatis* in men who have had insertive intercourse in the prior year, preferably with a rectal swab for NAT testing; and (5) a pharyngeal test for *N. gonorrhoeae* in men who have had receptive oral intercourse in the prior year, preferably using NAT (testing for pharyngeal *C. trachomatis* is not recommended). The HIV Primary Care Guidelines (CID 2009;49:651) recommend screening all patients for syphilis (RPR or VDRL) and to "consider" first-voided urine NAT tests for *N. gonorrhoeae* and *C. trachomatis*. Women should have vaginal secretions examined for *Trichomonas*, and women <26 yrs and others at increased risk should have a cervical specimen for NAT for *Chlamydia* species. Patients reporting receptive anal sex should have rectal cultures for *N. gonorrhoeae* and *C. trachomatis*. The screening tests noted should be repeated annually in sexually active patients.

TUBERCULOSIS: Routine testing includes a chest X-ray and tuberculin skin test. Other tests, including interferon-γ release assays (IGRAs), lateral flow antigen tests, and molecular tests are used also.

CHEST X-RAY: A routine baseline chest x-ray is sometimes recommended for detection of asymptomatic tuberculosis and as a baseline for patients who are at high risk for pulmonary disease. Nevertheless, in a longitudinal study of 1,065 patients at various stages of HIV infection, it was shown that routine chest x-rays performed at 0, 3, 6, and 12 mos (Arch Intern Med 1996;156:191) detected an abnormality in only 123 (2%) of 5,263 x-rays. None of the asymptomatic PPD-negative patients had evidence of active tuberculosis, and only 1 of 82 with a positive PPD had an abnormality on x-ray. The authors concluded that routine chest x-rays in asymptomatic HIV-infected patients with negative PPD skin tests are not warranted.

TUBERCULIN SKIN TEST: The CDC recommends the Mantoux method tuberculin skin test (TST) or IGRAs for detection of latent TB. The TST test uses the intradermal injection of 5TU of PPD for HIV-infected patients who have not had a prior positive test. TST should be repeated annually if initial test(s) were negative or if the patient belongs to a population with a high risk of tuberculosis (such as residents of prisons or jails, injection drug users, and homeless individuals). The PPD should also be repeated following immune reconstitution when the CD4 count increases to >200 cells/mm^3. Induration of ≥5 mm at 48–72 hrs constitutes a positive test. Anergy testing is not recommended. A meta-analysis of TST showed good performance characteristics except in patients with a prior BCG (Ann Intern Med 2007;16:340).

IGRA TESTS: These are FDA-approved tests that measure the release of interferon-γ derived from *M. tuberculosis* and include the QuantiFERON-TB Gold test, QuantiFERON-TB Gold In-Tube test, and the T-Spot.TB test. All require fresh whole blood that is mixed with TB antigens and reported as positive, negative, or indeterminate (T-Spot.TB also has a "borderline" result). Advantages of these tests compared to PPD testing include (1) better specificity (92–97% vs. 55–95%), (2) only a single patient visit is required, (3) results are available in 24 hrs, (4) it does not boost with subsequent tests, and (5) there are no false-positive results with BCG vaccination. Disadvantages include (1) the need to process blood sample within 8–16 hrs; (2) there are limited data on the ability to predict who will get active TB; (3) limited data exist in selected populations such as in children <5 yrs, recent TB exposures, immunocompromised patients, and results with serial testing; and 4) high cost (Ann Intern Med 2007;146:340; PLoS One 2008;6:e2665; MMWR 2006;54 RR15:49; Proc Am Thorac Soc 2006;3:103). In the CDC-published guidelines in 2010 on the use of IGRAs (MMWR. 2010:59[No. RR-5]: 1–25), it was recommended for latent TB infection in all situations in which the tuberculin skin testing is used. The specificity of the IGRAs tends to be higher than that of the skin test (Check W., CAP Today, March 2013). The cost of IGRAs is more expensive; however, a false-positive with the skin test may require more chest x-rays and the possible need to offer more people medication. Therefore, there may be greater cost-effectiveness with IGRAs. The higher specificity of the IGRAs comes from their not giving a positive result for those who have received BCG vaccination. In addition, rheumatologists are screening arthritis patient for latent TB infection with IGRAs before instituting anti-TNF therapy, and gastroenterologists are screening prior to biological therapy for inflammatory bowel diseases. Furthermore, patients do not need to return to have their results read, as they do with skin testing, and the results are more objective than those of a skin test. Whether to continue to use TST or to adopt an IGRA may depend on the prevalence and incidence of TB in foreign-born persons and how common is BCG vaccination in the population. In a high-incidence area, it might be best to screen employees with an IGRA, as compared to in a low-risk general population where there would be a higher ratio of false-positive results. In patients who are immunocompromised, discordant results between the TST and the IGRA make the diagnosis less certain (Check, W.; CAP Today, March 2013). The T-Spot TB requires no special phlebotomy (one green top tube), no tube shaking, and no incubation (i.e., one visit and one tube). It claims a sensitivity and specificity exceeding 95% in clinical studies (www. tspot.com), and the sensitivity remains high in HIV patients regardless of CD4 counts and immunosuppression (Clark et al., Clin Exp Immunol. 2007;1501:238–244).

RAPID CHROMATOGRAPHIC LATERAL FLOW ASSAYS (LFA): These have been developed (marketed since early 2000) for the discrimination of the *Mycobacterium tuberculosis* complex (MTbC) from the nontuberculous mycobacteria (Vong et al., Diagnostic Micro and Infect Dis 2011;70:154–156; Ismail et al., 2009). Two LFA tests have been evaluated, including the SD Bioline Ag MPT64 Rapid assay and the MGIT TBc Identification Test. These tests provide rapid culture confirmation of MTbC in AFB-positive cultures from liquid and solid media, can provide results in about 2 minutes, and their cost is less than $5 per test (Vong et al., Diagnostic Micro and Infect Dis 2011;70:154–156). However, the tests cannot distinguish between species of the MTbC, and a weak inoculum below 10^5 CFU/mL can be negative (Park et al., 2009). Vong et al., concluded that in high TB endemic countries, these tests can efficiently replace the conventional methods. Another LFA is the Alere Determine-TB LAM Ag strip test that detects LAM antigen in urine (Peter et al., 2010; Curr

Opin Pulm Med 16:262–270), and it has been shown to offer the greatest benefit in hospitalized HIV co-infected patients with advanced immunosuppression (Peter et al., 2012; Official J European Society for Clinical Respiratory Physiology).

MOLECULAR METHODS: The MTB/RIF assay is a novel, automated molecular TB diagnostic that can detect the presence of both *M. tuberculosis* complex DNA and rifampicin drug-resistance in less than 2 hrs; it has been endorsed by the World Health Organization (WHO;2010 WHO, Geneva Switzerland; WHO; 2011, publication number WHO/HTM/TB2011.2). The assay has a sensitivity and specificity of 90% and 99%, respectively (Boehme et al., 2011; Lancet 377;1495–1505) and is an advance over smear microscopy for the diagnosis of pulmonary-TB (Peter et al., 2012; PLos ONE 7; e39966, www.plosone.org). A major drawback of this method is the need for sputum, which may be difficult in HIV-infected sputum-scarce patients, particularly in resource-limited venues when sputum induction methods and other tissues may not be available. Boehme et al. found that this method, when used on urine samples, may aid in the rapid diagnosis of TB in sputum-scarce HIV-infected patients with advanced immunosuppression; it can offer about 70% of HIV co-infected persons a TB diagnosis within 24 hrs of being admitted to a hospital and additionally provides information on rifampicin drug susceptibility.

PAP TESTS: The CDC recommends that a gynecological evaluation with pelvic exam and Pap smear be performed at baseline, repeated at 6 mos, and annually in women with HIV infection. The cervical screening is performed with conventional, or liquid-based cytologic tests (Paps test) and can include human papilloma virus (HPV)-DNA tests. Cytopathic findings are reported by the Bethesda classification: atypical squamous cells (ACS), low grade squamous epithelial lesions (LSIL), or high-grade squamous epithelial lesions (HSIL). The ACS category is subclassified as atypical squamous cells of undetermined origin (ASC-US), and atypical squamous cells cannot exclude HSIL (ACS-H). HIV-infected women with ASC-H, LSIL, or HSIL should undergo colposcopy. With ASC-US (indicating some abnormal areas on the cervix) the recommendations include (1) colposcopy, (2) repeat Pap test at 6- to 12-mo intervals until there are two consecutive negatives, or (3) a test for high-risk HPV DNA. Recommendations for women with an abnormal Pap test are based on the 2006 Consensus Guidelines for Management of Abnormal Cervical Cytology (www.mmhiv.com/link/2006-ASCCP-Abnormal). More aggressive testing in women with HIV is recommended because of prior reports indicating a several-fold increase in rates of squamous intraepithelial lesion (33–45% in HIV positive vs. 7–14% in HIV-negative) and a 0- to 9-fold increase in rates of cervical cancer in women with HIV (Arch Pediatr Adolesc Med 2000;154:127; Obstet Gynecol Clin N Am 1996;23,861; JAIDS 2003;32:527; JAIDS 2004;36:978). The severity and frequency of cervical dysplasia increase with progressive immune compromise, but this association is weak and there is some evidence that cervical cancer rates are not decreasing in the HAART era (Curr HIV Res 2010;8:493; JID 2010;201:681; JID 2010;201:650). There is a strong association between HIV infection and detectable and persistent HPV infection by the HPV types associated with cervical cancer (16, 18, 31, 33, and 35) (CID 1995;21[suppl 1]:S121; NEJM 1997;337:1343; JID 2001;184:682).

The anal PAP smear for anal cancer is similar to that for cervical cancer in many ways; both are caused by infection with one of several oncogenic HPV subtypes, low-grade lesions often progress to high-grade lesions, and a Pap smear may be an effective screening method (Am J Med 2000;108:674). The prevalence of HPV in MSM is 60–75% (JID 1998;177:361), and the frequency of anal carcinoma in MSM with HIV infection is 35/100,000 or about 80 times that of the general population (Lancet 1998;351:1833; Cancer 2010;116:5507; Int J Cancer 2010;127:875; AIDS 2010;24:535). The rate increases with persons who have CD4 counts of <500 cells/mm^3 (AIDS 1998;12:495).

It is important that the instructions for collection be followed. A review of seven reports on anal cytology showed sensitivities of 42–98% and specificities of 33–96% (AIDS 2010;24:463), with a specificity of 32–59% for anal Pap smears (CID 2006;43:223).

Abnormal anal Pap smears should lead to referral for high-resolution anoscopy (HRA) and biopsy (CID 2004;38:1490). HRA should be considered for patients with cytology results showing ASC-US, LSIL, or HSIL, which is comparable to cervical colposcopy and considered complementary to cytology in high-risk patients (Dis Colon Rectum 2009;52:1854; AIDS 2010;24:373). The American Society for Colposcopy and Cervical Pathology offers an annual workshop on HRA (www.mmhiv.com/link/ASCCP-HRA-Workshop). A cost analysis concluded that direct use of HRA was more cost effective than cytology or HPV testing (AIDS 2011;25:635). Some authorities recommend anal Pap smears in all patients with histories of receptive anal intercourse at 1–3 yr intervals, which is comparable to recommendations for cervical Pap smears (Am J Med 2000;108:634). Others are more selective based on the large variation in reported sensitivity and specificity and the uncertain relative value of Pap tests versus HRA (AIDS 2010;24:463). The 2010 STD Guidelines (MMWR 2010;59 RR-12:1) state, "Because the increased incidence of anal cancer in HIV-infected men screening for anal intraepithelial neoplasia by cytology can be considered." A cost-effective analysis (Canada) found that the best strategy was use of HRA without prescreening by anal PAP. A meta-analysis of 21 published studies from 1996 to 2005 (CID 2006;43:223) concluded that anal Pap smears are of "modest accuracy" that is similar to cervical Pap smears. A comparison of cervical PAP and anal PAP is shown in Table 2.17.

HUMAN PAPILLOMA VIRUS TESTING: HPV is the most common STI in the United States. More than 4 million new HPV infections are reported annually, and up to 10% of the sexually active US population is infected (McConnell, Lippincott Williams & Wilkins, 2007); there are more than 100 HPV types. High-risk oncogenic types (especially type 16 and 18) may cause cancer of the cervix, penis, vulva, vagina, anus, or oropharynx. Nononcogenic types (especially types 6 and 11) may cause genital warts or respiratory papillomatosis. The lifetime risk of HPV in sexually active persons is >50%, and persistence of the oncogenic type is the greatest risk

TABLE 2.17 Comparison of cervical and anal cancer

Issue	Cervical Cancer Decreasing	Anal Cancer Increasing
Prevalence in general population	8.1/100,000	1.6/100,000
Prevalence in HIV population	5.6/100,000	34.6/100,000
Median CD4 at diagnosis (cells/mm^3)	287	276
Duration of HIV (median)	8.2 yrs	12.4 yrs
HPV types	16–50%	16–66%
	18–20%	18–5%
National guidelines	Yes	No
Median age at diagnosis	48 yrs	60 yrs
Palpation useful	No	Yes
Cytology useful	Yes	Probably
HPV testing useful in screening	Yes	No
Management	Colposcopy	High resolution anoscopy
Availability of well-trained cytologists	Extensive	Limited
Treatment: High grade lesions	Laser, LEEP	Infrared coagulation, excision

Adapted from Darragh and Winkler, Cancer Cytopath 2011;119:5.

for cancer. HPV tests include the HCII High-Risk HPV test (Qiagen), HCII Low-Risk HPV test (Qiagen), Cervista 16/18 test, and the Cervista HPV High-Risk test (Hologics) (2010 CDC Guidelines for Sexually Transmitted Diseases; MMWR 2010;59 RR-12:1); the Pap smear is the gold standard for detecting abnormal cervical epithelial cells using microscopic analysis. A number of molecular diagnostic methods, including PCR, signal amplification technologies, and line immunoassays, are available to detect HPV DNA; a summary is provided by Arney et al., Lab Med 2010;41:524–530). HPV screening is less clinically effective for younger women because women under the age of 30 have a high incidence of HPV, but the majority will clear spontaneously and will never get cancer (Arney et al., Lab Med 2010;41:524–530). In 2006, the FDA approved a prophylactic HPV vaccine to help guard against four common types of HPV (6, 11, 16, and 18) that cause genital warts or are associated with up to 70% of cervical cancer cases (Smith et al., Int J Cancer 2007;121:621–632). In 2009, the FDA approved another vaccine (Cervarix) that prevents only HPV 16 and 18 and is indicated for prevention of cervical cancer in females 10–25 yrs of age (Cervarix, FDA; www. fda.gov/BiologiccsBlood   Vaccines/Vaccines/ApprovedProducts/ ucm186957.htm, March 18, 2010).

Screening Tests for Other Infectious Agents

HEPATITIS A SEROLOGY: HAV serology (total anti-HAV antibody) is performed to identify candidates for the HAV vaccine, which is indicated for susceptible persons with chronic HCV infection, injection drug use, MSM, persons with clotting disorders, persons with chronic liver disease, and travelers to HAV-endemic areas (MMWR 1996;45[RR-15]:1). Some authorities believe that all HIV-infected persons who are susceptible should be vaccinated. The prevalence of anti-HAV IgG is 40–70% in adults in the United States and most European countries (CID 1997;25:726; MMWR 1999;48:[RR-12]:1), indicating past infection or vaccination. To diagnose acute hepatitis, the preferred test is anti-HAV IgM, along with HBsAg and HCV RNA. For HAV, the serologic assays include total anti-HAV, anti-HAV IgM, and anti-HAV IgG; the kinetics of appearance of these markers have been published (Hollinger & Dreesman; Hepatitis viruses, In: Rose et al., *Manual of Clinical Laboratory Immunology*; ASM; p. 702; 1997). Anti-HAV IgM appears within 3–6 wks of infection, peaks at about 6 wks, and gradually decreases to undetectable levels by about 12 wks. The anti-HAV IgG becomes positive at 4–6 wks, peaks at about 10 wks, and remains positive apparently for life (unless there is immunosuppression). Therefore, the detection of anti-HAV IgM during the first 12 wks usually indicates a recent infection. Total anti-HAV (IgM and IgG) tests that do not differentiate antibody isotypes are used to determine susceptibility to infection, particularly for those traveling to high-risk areas, or to determine immune status for vaccination decisions. Although not commonly used, the presence of HAV RNA can be determined by molecular methods to elicit acute infection, but the most reliable method is for identifying anti-HAV IgM because it is invariably present when symptoms appear, and its appearance provides presumptive evidence of acute HAV infection (Hollinger and Dreesman; Hepatitis viruses, In: Rose et al., *Manual of Clinical Laboratory Immunology*; ASM; p. 702; 1997).

HEPATITIS B VIRUS (HBV) TESTS: HBV infection is most easily diagnosed using serologic means for the detection of antibody and antigen. There are several antigenic subtypes of HBV, but their occurrence does not seem to present a diagnostic dilemma. A number of serologic markers for HBV infection are available (Hollinger and Dreesman; Hepatitis viruses, In: Rose et al., *Manual of Clinical Laboratory Immunology*; ASM; p. 702; 1997), including:

HBsAg: The detection of HBV surface antigen evaluates individuals for acute and chronic infection with HBV. HBsAg appears 2–4 wks prior to liver abnormalities or 3–5 wks before clinical symptoms; it gradually declines to undetectable levels in 4–6 mos. Persons who are positive have acute infection, or, if HBsAg positive for at least 6 mos, are chronically infected. The presence may indicate the need to evaluate.

HBeAg positivity, HBV DNA, and/or for liver function tests: Persons who are HBsAg positive are infectious.

HBeAg: This marker is tested only in those individuals who are HBsAg-positive, and indicates infection that has a high rate of infectivity and of viral replication (i.e., those positive for HBeAg are highly infectious). This is particularly concerning with pregnant women.

Anti-HBe (HBeAb): May be present with chronic infection or immunity, and its presence usually indicates a lesser degree of infectivity (i.e., not highly infectious). The main use is in chronic infection for which HBV DNA indicates low viral titer and a low degree of infectivity.

Anti-HBc IgM and anti-HBcIgG: IgM antibody appears at about 2 mos and may last for up to 8 mos. It indicates recent infection (within 6–8 mos) and is generally used to resolve the window at 4–6 mos where HBsAg has disappeared and prior to the development of HBsAb; it usually disappears at 8 mos regardless if the infection resolves or becomes chronic. Anti-HBcAb IgG usually appears at 8 mos and persists for a long period of time.

HBsAb: Indicates immunity and provides protection against re-infection. HBsAb will be present in those who have resolved infection or those who have been vaccinated.

HBV DNA: HBV DNA tests are available as a marker for viral replication, but their utility has not been fully described.

All HIV-infected patients should be screened with HBsAg and anti-HBs. Routine testing for HBcAb is optional. For those who are anti-HBs and HBsAg negative, vaccination is recommended. For those that are anti-HBc positive, anti-HBs/HBsAg-negative, chronic HBV infection can be ruled out. Table 2.18 provides a summary for interpretation.

HEPATITIS C VIRUS (HCV) TESTS: Reviews on the seroprevalence and testing for HCV have been published (Smith et al., CID:53, p780, 1011; McGibbon et al., Am J Med 2013;126:718; MMWR 2013;62; Hollinger and Dreesman; Hepatitis viruses, In: Rose et al., *Manual of Clinical Laboratory Immunology*; ASM; p. 702; 1997). HCV is a serious public health issue, with about 3.2 million persons in the United States having chronic HCV infection; the prevalence is highest among intravenous drug injection (IVD) users, the homeless, and incarcerated individuals (Institute of Med [IOM], The National Academies Press; 2010). HCV screening is recommended for patients with risk factors, a history of IVD, a

TABLE 2.18 Hepatitis B serology

HBsAgg	Total Anti-HBc	Anti-HBcAb IgM	Anti-HBsAb	Interpretation
–	–	–	–	Never infected
+	–	–	–	Acute HBV
+	+	+	–	Acute HBV
–	+	+	–	Recent and resolving
–	+	–	+	Past infection—Immune
+	+	–	–	Chronic HBV
–	+	–	–	False positive (susceptible)
–	+	–	+	Immune if >10 lU/mL

Modified from MMWR 2010;59 RR-12.

receipt of a blood transfusion before 1992, and all persons born from 1945 to 1965 (Smith et al. MMWR Recomm Rep. 2012;61 (RR-4):1–32). Screening tests for HCV antibody, available since the early 1990s, include ELISA, chemiluminescent assays, rapid tests, and RNA tests; RNA tests were approved by the FDA in 2001 and became more widely used in 2003 (New York State Department of Health; Medicaid management DOH Medicaid Update: 2003;18[7]). In 2011, a rapid test for HCV antibody (OraQuick HCV Rapid Antibody Test (OraSure Technologies) became available; it is CLIA waived and allows fingerstick capillary blood and venipuncture whole blood; its sensitivity and specificity are similar to FDA-approved laboratory-based HCV antibody assays (Shivkumar et al., Ann Intern Med 2012;157:558–566), and results are available in 10–20 minutes.

Other rapid HCV assays have been evaluated, with sensitivities and specificities ranging from 79–97% and 83–100%, respectively (Smith et al., CID 2011:53;780–786). All screening tests produce some degree of false-positive results, so confirmatory or supplemental tests are required for a definitive diagnosis. However, many testing facilities rely only on the screening test results. Alternatively, the "intensity" of screening test results by ELISA-type assays can be used to increase the predictive value of a screening test result (high signal-to-cutoff [S/CO]) ratios, most likely indicating a true positive result); however, the use of this strategy should only be used with test kits for which the package insert indicates the usefulness (MMWR Vol. 62, May 7, 2013). Nevertheless, an RNA test is indicated when an HCV antibody test is reactive, regardless of S/CO. Another strategy cited is to use a second antibody screening test with a different format or antigenic source to verify the antibody-positive status (MMWR Vol. 62, May 7, 2013; Vermeersch et al., 2008; J Clin Virol:42;394–398). In the 2013 guidelines, the CDC recommended that all HCV antibody positive persons be further tested for HCV RNA; there are no supplemental confirmatory serologic assays available in the United States (the RIBA was discontinued). FDA-approved qualitative tests must be used (unless other tests have been validated by the laboratory); quantitative RNA tests should only be used for monitoring infection (not for diagnosis). Qualitative HCV RNA assays have a limit of detection of 7.5–100 IU/mL. If RNA positive, the interpretation is current or past infection, while a RNA-negative result indicates no current infection. Because 15–25% of persons who test HCV antibody positive have no detectable HCV RNA, they have either resolved infection or a false-positive antibody test occurred. RNA tests include typical PCR or more rapid RNA tests such as the HCV Xpert (http://www.prnewswire.com/news-releases/cepheid-announces-european-approval-of-xpert-hcv-viral-load-300066101.html, 2015). The Xpert HCV VL is a quantitative test that provides on-demand molecular testing for diagnosis and monitoring of HCV and is based on the GeneXpert technology that utilizes an automated RT-PCR using fluorescence to detect and quantify RNA for HCV genotypes 1–6 over the range of 10–100,000,000 IU/mL. In summary, the current recommendation is to perform an initial screening test, followed by an HCV RNA qualitative test if the screening test was positive. If RNA is negative, repeat RNA testing is suggested; a negative test does not exclude HCV because HCV RNA levels may periodically decline below limits of detection. Repeat testing at 3–6 mos is recommended to rule out chronic HCV infection.

All HIV-infected persons should be tested for HCV infection. The current third-generation EIAs have a sensitivity and specificity of >99% in immunocompetent patients, but there may be false negatives with severe immunosuppression (e.g., CD4 counts of <100 cells/mm^3) (JAIDS 2002;31:154) and some with acute HCV infections. The HCV VL (quantitative RNA tests) does not correlate with disease severity or rate of progression; its principal use is to monitor response to therapy. Hepatic transaminases should be measured in patients with chronic HCV infection, although there may be significant liver disease with persistently normal AST and ALT levels. An HCV genotype should be measured because the genotype is an important predictor of response to therapy. Genotype 1 accounts for about 75% of cases in the United States. Table 2.19 provides some basic information on HCV tests.

TOXOPLASMA SEROLOGY: Toxoplasma serology (anti-Toxoplasma IgG, or IgM) is recommended to assist in the differential diagnosis of complications involving the CNS, to identify candidates for toxoplasmosis prophylaxis (Ann Intern Med 1992;117:163), and to counsel patients on preventive measures if seronegative. The gold-standard Sabin-Feldman dye test is less frequently used, and most testing is performed using ELISA assays. As with most serologic viral assays, IgG antibodies signal past or present infection, while IgM antibodies are more associated with recent infection. If a person is IgG positive, an IgM test can be performed (IgM-capture ELISA) to further define the time of infection. A negative IgM test essentially excludes recent infection, but a positive IgM test is difficult to interpret because *Toxoplasma*-specific IgM antibodies may be detected for as long as 18 mos after acutely acquired infection. A major problem with *Toxoplasma*-specific IgM testing is a lack of specificity. A positive IgM result with a negative IgG result in the same specimen should be viewed with great suspicion; the patient's blood should be redrawn 2–4 wks after the first and tested together with the first specimen to assess seroprogression, where IgG should

TABLE 2.19 Tests for HCV

Test	Comment
Anti-HCV screening tests	Indicates past or present HCV infection. Sensitivity of the third-generation tests is >99%.
	Screening tests lack specificity and have a low predictive value in low-prevalence populations.
Qualitative HCV RNA (HCV RT-PCR)	Although very sensitive and specific, RT-PCR tests to detect HCV RNA may produce false-positives and false negatives.
	Threshold for detection is as low as 7.5 IU/mL. The recommended use is to confirm serologic results.
Quantitative HCV RNA tests (VL)	The HCV RNA level is not useful for determining prognosis; it is used to monitor response to therapy. The magnitude of HCV RNA level may predict response.
Genotype	Of the 6 major genotypes, genotype 1 predominates in US (70%). Genotyping was used to predict response to therapy in the past, but is less used now that current therapies are more effective.

become positive. If the IgG is negative and the IgM is positive in both specimens, the IgM result should be considered to be a false positive, and the patient should be considered to be not infected. If the patient is pregnant and IgG/IgM positive, an IgG avidity test could be performed. A high avidity result in the first 12–16 wks of pregnancy (time dependent upon the commercial test kit) essentially rules out an infection acquired during gestation. A low IgG avidity result should not be interpreted as indicating recent infection because some individuals have persistent low IgG avidity for many months after infection. The interpretation of IgG and IgM assay results is shown in Table 2.8, and additional information has been published (McAuley et al., In: Jorgensen et al., editors; *Manual of Clinical Microbiology*. 11th ed. Washington, D.C.: ASM; p. 2373–2386; 2015). Molecular techniques that can detect the parasite's DNA in the amniotic fluid can be useful in cases of possible mother-to-child (congenital) transmission.

The seroprevalence among healthy adults in the United States varies widely but can approach 60% (IBL, package insert), and the seroconversion rate is up to 1% per year. Most infections in AIDS patients represent relapse of latent infection, which is noted in 20–47% of those with the combination of CD4 counts of <100 cells/mm^3, positive *Toxoplasma* serology, and no prophylaxis (CID 1992;15:211; CID 2002;34:103). A negative *Toxoplasma* serology should be repeated after the CD4 cell count is ≤100 cells/mm^3, if the patient does not take atovaquone or TMP-SMX prophylaxis for PCP (2009 Guidelines for Prevention and Treatment of Opportunistic Infections in HIV-Infected Adults and Adolescents: www.mmhiv.com/link/2009-OI-NIH-CDC-IDSA), or whenever the diagnosis of toxoplasmosis encephalitis is being considered when prior tests were negative or not performed. Table 2.20 summarizes the interpretation of serologic results.

CMV SEROLOGY: Serologic tests for cytomegalovirus (CMV) are very similar in principle and interpretation to those for toxoplasmosis. The major potential benefit is that a negative test usually excludes CMV disease (Ann Intern Med 1993;118:12; Lancet 2004; Lancet 2004;363:2116). IgM antibodies are the first to be produced and are present in most individuals within a week or two after the initial exposure. IgM antibody production rises for a short time period and then declines to undetectable after several months. Additional IgM antibodies are produced when latent virus is reactivated (https://labtestsonline.org/understanding/analytes/cmv/tab/test/). IgG antibodies are produced several weeks after the initial CMV infection and provide protection for life; testing is routinely used to determine immunity for people prior to organ or bone marrow transplantation and for a person diagnosed with HIV/AIDS. Antibody testing and viral CMV detection may be used to help diagnose primary CMV infection in young adults, pregnant women,

TABLE 2.20 Interpretation of serologic results for Toxoplasmosis

IgG Result	IgM Result	Report/Interpretation for Humans[a]
Negative	Negative	No serological evidence of infection with *Toxoplasma*.
Negative	Equivocal	Possible early acute infection or false-positive IgM reaction. Obtain a new specimen for IgG and IgM testing. If results for the second specimen remain the same, the patient is probably not infected with *Toxoplasma*.
Negative	Positive	Possible acute infection or false-positive IgM result. Obtain a new specimen for IgG and IgM testing. If results for the second specimen remain the same, the IgM reaction is probably a false-positive.
Equivocal	Negative	Indeterminate result; obtain a new specimen for testing or retest this specimen for IgG using a different essay.
Equivocal	Equivocal	Indeterminate result: obtain a new specimen for both IgG and IgM testing.
Equivocal	Positive	Possible acute infection with Toxoplasma. Obtain a new specimen for IgG and IgM testing. If results for the second specimen remain the same or if the IgG becomes positive, both specimens could be sent to a reference laboratory with experience in diagnosis of toxoplasmosis for further testing.
Positive	Negative	Infected with *Toxoplasma* for six months or more.

TABLE 2.20 Continued

IgG Result	IgM Result	Report/Interpretation for Humans[a]
Positive	Equivocal	Infected with *Toxoplasma* for probably more than 1 yr or false-positive IgM reaction. Obtain a new specimen for IgM testing. If results with the second specimen remain the same, both specimens could be sent to a reference laboratory with experience in the diagnosis of toxoplasmosis for further testing.
Positive	Positive	Possible recent infection within the last 12 mos, or false-positive IgM reaction. Send the specimen to a reference laboratory with experience in the diagnosis of toxoplasmosis for further testing.

[a]Except infants.

Modified from CDC (https://www.cdc.gov/dpdx/toxoplasmosis/dx.html, 2015).

and immunocompromised persons with flu- or mononucleosis-like symptoms. A serologic test for CMV is not recommended for baseline screening in the 2009 Guidelines for Prevention and Treatment of Opportunistic Infections in HIV-Infected Adults and Adolescents (www.mmhiv.com/link/2009-OI-NIH-CDC-IDSA) due to limited clinical utility in most patients. However, it is recommended in the IDSA HIV Primary Care Guidelines for persons defined as having low risk for CMV infection (CID 2009;49:66). Viral DNA detection is used to diagnose congenital infection in newborns and may be used to detect and/or confirm active infections in others. PCR DNA testing can be qualitative or quantitative for measuring the amount of virus present in immune-compromised people with active CMV to monitor response to therapy. Other uses of serology include (1) identification of seronegative patients for counseling on CMV prevention (although the message is not different from the "safe sex message" for preventing HIV transmission); (2) assessment of the likelihood of CMV disease in late-stage HIV infection, although invasive CMV disease has become a rare complication in the HAART era; (3) identification of seronegative individuals who should receive CMV antibody-negative blood or leukocyte-reduced blood products for nonemergent transfusions (JAMA 2001;285:1592); and (4) CMV serology is the "C" in TORCH testing for neonates. The seroprevalence for adults in the United States is about 50%, although it can be greater than 80% in older adults and is >90% in MSM and injection drug users (JID 1985;152:243; Am J Med 1987;82:593). The 2009 Primary Care Guidelines for HIV Management from IDSA (CID 2009;49:651) recommend a baseline anti-CMV IgG in low-prevalence populations, but this has never proved useful in preventing or predicting CMV disease in HIV-infected persons (JCM 2000;38:563).

Recommended General Reading

https://stacks.cdc.gov/view/cdc/50872
https://www.cdc.gov/hiv/guidelines/testing.html
http://www.who.int/diagnostics_laboratory/documents/guidance/
    pm_module4.pdf
http://www.who.int/hiv/pub/posters/testing-strategies-uptake/en/
https://www.cdc.gov/hiv/testing/laboratorytests.html
www.who.int/hiv/pub/guidelines/hiv-testing-services/en/
Alexander TS. Human immunodeficiency virus diagnostic testing: 30 years of evolution. *Clin Vaccine Immunol* 2016;23(4):249–253.
Bruns DE, Burtis CA. *Fundamentals of molecular diagnostics*, ed. H.H. Kessler. New York: Elsevier Health Sciences, 2007: 267.
Clutter DS, et al. HIV-1 drug resistance and resistance testing. *Infect Genet Evol* 2016.;46:292–307.

Constantine N, Zhao R. Molecular-based laboratory testing and monitoring for human immunodeficiency virus infections. *Clin Lab Sci* 2005;18(4):263–270.

Constantine NT, Kabat W, Zhao RY. Update on the laboratory diagnosis and monitoring of HIV infection. *Cell Res* 2005;15(11–12):870–876.

Constantine NT, Saville RD, Dax EM. Retroviral testing and quality assurance: Essentials for laboratory diagnosis. ISBN 0-9785982-0-2; Malloy Printers, 1–696; 2005.

Delaney KP, Hanson DL, Masciotra S, et al. Time until emergence of HIV test reactivity following infection with HIV-1: Implications for interpreting test results and retesting after exposure. *Clin Infect Dis* 2017;64(1):53–59.

Highsmith J, Edward W. *Molecular diagnostics: 12 tests that changed everything*, ed. J. Highsmith, W. Edward. New York: Springer, 2013: 257.

Nkeze JN, Constantine NT, Zhao RY. Laboratory testing for HIV infection: Advances after 28 years. In *Molecular diagnostics: 12 tests that changed everything*, ed. J. Highsmith, W. Edward. New York: Springer, 2013: pp. 81–106.

Obermeier M, Symons J, Wensing AM. HIV population genotypic tropism testing and its clinical significance. *Curr Opin HIV AIDS* 2012;7(5):470–477.

Van Laethem K, Theys K, Vandamme AM. HIV-1 genotypic drug resistance testing: digging deep, reaching wide? *Curr Opin Virol* 2015;14:16–23.

Wittek M, et al. Molecular assays for monitoring HIV infection and antiretroviral therapy. *Expert Rev Mol Diagn* 2007;7(3):237–246.

3

Prevention of HIV and Prevention of Infection in PLWH

Prevention of HIV

Background

After HIV was identified as a sexually transmitted infection (STI), early HIV prevention efforts focused on barrier protection methods, specifically condom use. Studies ultimately confirmed condom use efficacy to be 70–95% when used consistently (Cochrane Database Syst Rev 2002;CD003255; Soc Sci Med 1997;44:1303; JAIDS 2015;68:337). Condom use has the added benefit of preventing transmission of other STIs. Unfortunately, consistent condom use appears to be uncommon and may be especially low among men who have sex with men (MSM) (JAIDS 2015;68:337). Studies have also confirmed modest additional HIV prevention efficacy through male circumcision (50–60%), STI treatment (38%), and needle exchange programs (44–68%) (PLoS Med 2005;2:e298; Lancet 2007;369:643; Lancet 2007;369:657; Lancet 1995 Aug 26; 346(8974):530; Sex Transm Infect 1999;75:3; Int J Epidemiol 2014;43:235). Taken together, these approaches offer an effective array of strategies that should be incorporated into any comprehensive HIV prevention package. However, there is now an emerged consensus on the singular efficacy of antiretroviral therapy (ART) as a prevention tool, both through decreasing transmissibility from HIV-infected patients and as a chemoprophylactic strategy in HIV-uninfected individuals.

Treatment as Prevention

Treatment as prevention (TasP) is defined as the reduction in risk of HIV transmission through HIV viral suppression. Early evidence for the concept was derived from studies evaluating strategies to prevent mother-to-child HIV transmission (MMWR 1994;43:285). A subsequent early observational study of HIV serodiscordant couples found no evidence of HIV transmission when the HIV-infected partner had a viral load (VL) of <1,500 cpm (NEJM 2000;342:921). The landmark HPTN 052 study was a large, randomized trial in 1,763 heterosexual HIV serodiscordant couples which initially demonstrated a 96% reduction (93% in final analysis) in linked transmissions among couples whose HIV-infected partner began ART "early" (prior to CD4 <250 cells/mm^3 or the development of an AIDS-associated illness) compared to those whose partner had delayed ART initiation, and zero transmissions among couples whose HIV-infected partner was virally suppressed (NEJM 2011;365:493; NEJM 2016;375:830). In recent years these results have been corroborated by large observational cohort studies among serodiscordant couples (both heterosexual and MSM) practicing condomless sex (PARTNERS Study, Opposites Attract), which have found no evidence of linked HIV transmissions when the HIV-infected partner is virally suppressed (JAMA 2016;316:171; 9th IAS Conference; 2017; Abstract TUAC0506LB). In 2017, an "Undetectable=Untransmittable (U=U)" consensus statement was published and widely endorsed (including by the CDC), stating that "people living with HIV on ART with an undetectable VL in their blood have a negligible risk of sexual transmission of HIV" (https://www.preventionaccess.org/consensus).

HIV Pre-exposure Prophylaxis

PrEP Clinical Trials

The concept of HIV *pre-exposure prophylaxis* (PrEP) was de-rived from the observation that studies examining the efficacy of PEP inferred maximal efficacy in the setting of therapeutic antiretroviral drug levels prior to HIV exposure (J Virol 2000 Oct;74(20):9771). This led to several randomized clinical trials examining the clinical efficacy of PrEP, the first of which was the Pre-exposure Prophylaxis Initiative (iPrEx) trial. This trial enrolled 2,499 initially HIV-negative MSM at high risk of HIV infection (averaging 18 sexual partners in the preceding 3 mos), across nine cities on four continents. Subjects were randomized to receive ei-ther tenofovir disoproxil fumarate plus emtricitabine (TDF/FTC, Truvada®) or placebo, and all subjects received standardized safe sex counseling, access to condoms, and STI testing and treat-ment. Overall efficacy in HIV prevention was 44%. A subsequent post-hoc analysis determined that efficacy among those with drug levels approximating 4 doses per week was 96% (Sci Transl Med 2012 Sep 12;4(151):151ra125). Following iPrEx, several ad-ditional clinical trials confirmed PrEP efficacy in serodiscordant heterosexual couples (62–75%), injection drug users (49%), and MSM (86%) (NEJM 2012;367:423; NEJM 2012;367:399; Lancet 2013;381:2083; Lancet 2015;387:53; NEJM 2015;373:2237). By contrast, two studies conducted only among women found poor efficacy of PrEP, though these findings may have correlated with poor ART adherence (NEJM 2012;367:411; NEJM 2015;372:509). In 2012, the US Food and Drug Administration (FDA) approved TDF/FTC for PrEP use, and the Centers for Disease Control (CDC) followed with published guidance for the provision of PrEP. From 2013 to 2015, TDF/FTC prescriptions for PrEP rose >500%, though much of this uptake was restricted to a handful of cities and remains underutilized among women and people of color (AIDS 2016 Durban, South Africa. Oral #TUAX0105LB).

Recommendations for PrEP Delivery

Indications

Patients with the following risks for acquiring HIV should be considered for PrEP:

1. *Men who have sex with men*:
   a. Ongoing sexual relationship with HIV-positive sexual partner within the previous 6 mos
   b. Recent bacterial STI within the previous 6 mos
   c. High number of sex partners
   d. History of inconsistent or no condom use within the previous 6 mos
   e. Commercial sex work
2. *Heterosexual men and women*:
   a. Ongoing sexual relationship with HIV-positive sexual partner
   b. Recent bacterial STI within the previous 6 mos
   c. High number of sex partners
   d. History of inconsistent or no condom use
   e. Commercial sex work
   f. In high prevalence area or network
3. *Injection drug users*:
   a. HIV-positive injecting partner
   b. Sharing injection equipment
   c. Recent drug treatment (but currently injecting) within the previous 6 mos
4. *HIV serodiscordant couples who wish to conceive*: PrEP can be considered in this setting, though this should be individualized. Other strategies in this setting include viral suppression of HIV-infected partner, intrauterine insemination (IUI) of the female partner, in vitro fertilization (IVF), and/or two-step sperm washing (MMWR 2017;66(21);554).

Other considerations for risk assessment include epidemiologic area of residence (including zip code) and ongoing alcohol abuse. Risk assessment calculators are available online and include https://ictrweb.johnshopkins.edu/ictr/utility/prep.cfm and http://www.cdc.gov/hiv/pdf/PrEPProviderSupplement2014.pdf

Initial Assessment for PrEP

1. Obtain and document negative serum HIV testing within 1 wk before starting PrEP medication. Baseline HIV screening should include a fourth-generation HIV antigen/antibody test.
2. If the patient has symptoms consistent with acute HIV infection, or if the patient has had a high-risk exposure (unprotected sexual intercourse with a partner with known HIV infection, IDU) within the previous 6 wks, obtain HIV VL in addition to a fourth-generation HIV antigen/antibody test.
3. Advise patients to remain abstinent until they have taken PrEP for at least 1 wk and ideally up to 20 days (tenofovir/emtricitabine achieves maximum intracellular levels in rectal tissue after 7 days; in blood after 20 days; and in cervico-vaginal tissue after 20 days).
4. Confirm that the patient's glomerular filtration rate is greater than or equal to 60 mL/minute (EPIC laboratory calculation is acceptable) and screen for proteinuria with urinalysis.
5. Screen for HAV, HBV, and HCV infection and vaccinate against HAV (for MSM) and/or HBV if susceptible.
6. Screen and treat (as needed) for STIs through:
   a. Nucleic acid amplification test (NAAT) for gonococcal and chlamydial infection via three-site screening (genital, rectal, pharyngeal)
   b. Treponemal and/or or nontreponemal testing for syphilis.
7. In women of reproductive age or transmen who have sex with men, screen for pregnancy with β-HCG testing and determine if patient is planning to become pregnant or if patient is breastfeeding.

8. Review any potential drug interactions.

9. Identify and address potential barriers to PrEP medication and clinic visit adherence, including mental health disease, substance use, socioeconomic barriers (housing instability, insurance, other).

10. Counsel patients that PrEP is only one part of an ongoing sexual risk reduction program which should include ongoing consistent condom use for HIV and STI prevention.

Contraindications to PrEP

1. Persons who are HIV infected or have not had an HIV test to rule out infection.

2. Persons who have signs or symptoms of acute HIV infection.

3. Persons seeking occupational or nonoccupational post-exposure prophylaxis

4. Women who are breastfeeding.

5. Persons who are not able or willing to strictly adhere to treatment protocol as prescribed.

6. Persons who are not available or not willing to adhere to recommended counseling service.

7. Persons who are not available or not willing to participate in frequent diagnostic monitoring.

Prescribing PrEP

1. Prescribe 1 tablet of TDF 300 mg plus FTC 200 mg (Truvada®) by mouth daily. In general, prescribe no more than a 90-day supply, renewable only after HIV testing confirms that a patient remains HIV-uninfected.

2. Provider and patient-oriented materials are available from the CDC at http://www.cdc.gov/hiv/pdf/PrEPProviderSupplement2014.pdf.

3. Inform patient of correlation between daily PrEP dosing and efficacy.

4. Educate the patient regarding potential side effects of TDF/FTC, including
   a. Occasional: Generally well tolerated. Diarrhea, dizziness, nausea, headache, fatigue, abnormal dreams, sleep problems, rash, depression
   b. Serious (rare): Lactic acidosis (weakness, unusual pain, trouble breathing, nausea, vomiting, fast heartbeat, feeling cold/dizzy/lightheaded), liver problems (jaundice, biliuria, light colored stools, lack of appetite, nausea, abdominal pain)
5. Inform the patient of patient assistance programs that may help the patient pay for medication if he or she is eligible, and provide information for same if patient is interested.
6. Educate the patient about acute HIV infection symptoms.

Monitoring During PrEP Use

1. All patients newly initiating PrEP should be seen for a 1-mo follow-up visit to review side effects and adherence.
2. After the 1-mo follow-up visit, the patient should be evaluated by the provider at least every 3 mos. Consider more frequent visits in adolescent and younger patients or anyone with expected adherence difficulties. These visits should include:
   a. Confirmation of HIV-negative status using a fourth-generation HIV Antibody test (and an HIV VL if concern for acute HIV infection).
   b. Evaluation of PrEP medication adherence.
   c. Assessment of risk behaviors and provision of risk-reduction counseling and condoms.
   d. Assessment of STI symptoms and, if present, testing and treatment for STIs, as needed (at least every 6 mos).
   e. Blood urea nitrogen (BUN), serum creatinine, and urinalysis should be checked 3 mos after PrEP initiation, then every 6 mos while on PrEP medication. More frequent assessment may be necessary per provider discretion.

f. Consider bone mineral density (BMD) testing if patient is expect to remain on TDF/FTC for ≥1 yr and has any predisposing risk factors for bone disease, including but not limited to perimenopausal women, long-term tobacco use, significant alcohol intake, history of fragility fractures, chronic glucocorticoid use.

g. In women of reproductive age and transmen, a pregnancy test should be administered at every visit and, if pregnant, discussion should occur regarding continued use of PrEP.

h. Consideration should be made at each visit regarding the ongoing necessity of PrEP for the individual patient. This decision will be based on risk assessment and discussion with the patient, who may move through "seasons of risk."

3. Reasons to discontinue PrEP:
   a. Patient request
   b. Safety concerns
   c. Medication nonadherence
   d. Clinic nonadherence
   e. Concern for drug diversion
   f. Patient becomes HIV-positive: If a patient discontinues PrEP due to seroconversion, he or she should receive immediate linkage to HIV care.
   g. Patient becomes pregnant: Patient should receive linkage to care for OBGYN services.
   h. Patient is no longer considered at high risk based on behavioral risk assessment

HIV Post-exposure Prophylaxis

Definitions

oPEP: "Occupational" PEP generally refers to PEP given to healthcare workers (HCW) for percutaneous or mucous membrane exposures sustained in the practice of their occupation. Janitorial/custodial staff in hospital and nonhospital settings are also at risk of being exposed to used needles through the trash. oPEP programs are often organized through healthcare system occupational health departments, sometimes with the aid of emergency department or infectious disease providers.

nPEP: Nonoccupational PEP refers to PEP given to people exposed through sexual encounters (consensual and nonconsensual) and shared needles (not limited to injection drug users [IDUs]; also possible through shared needles for nonprescribed hormone or silicone injections).

PEP Data

The basis for current-day PEP administration largely comes from two small prospective nonhuman primate studies. In the first, 24 macaques injected with 10× the LD_{50} of IV simian immunodeficiency virus (SIV) were immediately given a 3-, 10-, or 28-day course of TDF or placebo. Rates of infection were 100% for all placebo arms, 100% for 3 days, 50% for 10 days, and 0% for 28 days (J Virol 1998;72:4265). HIV-2 was intravaginally administered to 16 female macaques in the second study, followed by TDF or placebo starting at 12, 36, or 72 hrs, each for a 28-day course. Rates of infection were 75% in the placebo arms, 0% at 12 and 36 hrs, and 25% at 72 hrs (J Virol 2000;74:9771). Studies to more specifically define infection risk at alternate start times or treatment durations (e.g., 14 vs. 21 vs. 28 days or 48 vs. 72 vs. 84 hrs) are not available.

A retrospective case control study of 33 HCW who contracted HIV via needlestick and 679 controls who did not contract HIV following needlestick from a HIV-positive source identified a protective effect of PEP with AZT (aOR 0.19; NEJM 1997;337:1485). A meta-analysis of nonhuman primate PEP studies (180 receiving PEP, 103 placebo) similarly showed protective effect (OR 0.11; CID 2016;60:S165).

Of an estimated 600,000–800,000 annual percutaneous exposures in HCW, there have been 58 confirmed cases of HIV transmission between 1985 and 2013, the vast majority before the CDC began recommending oPEP in 1996 (MMWR 2015;63:1245).

This group includes 6 HCWs who received PEP using recommended regimens (in that era) that were initiated within 2 hrs of exposure. Sixty-nine percent of the 58 infected were nurses or clinical laboratory technicians.

Estimating Risk of Tranmission

Risk of HIV transmission is dependent on exposure type and severity and HIV status of the source. There is no defined numerical threshold for what is considered an exposure worthy of PEP.

For sexual exposures, additional details should be sought to help clinicians and patients best understand the level of risk. Genital ulcer disease, cervical ectopy, genital trauma or bleeding, use of sex toys, and ejaculation all increase risk of HIV transmission, while condom use and male circumcision (statistically significant for heterosexual uninfected male partners and uninfected homosexual male insertive partners) decrease the risk (AIDS 2014;28:1509). Consensual sex leads to vaginal lacerations in 5% of women, while 40% of sexual assault victims suffer vaginal lacerations (70% in nulliparous women). Prevalence of HIV was found to be 1% in convicted sex offenders, compared to 0.3% in the general population (HIV Clinician 2009;22:5). Data on sexual transmission with partner on ART from a meta-analysis of studies published through 2012 are included in Table 3.1; subsequent research suggests a negligible risk if the HIV-infected partner has a suppressed HIV VL (see TasP section). Similarly, risk is greatest during acute HIV infection— 0.008 transmissions/coital act were seen in 5 mos after conversion compared to 0.0007/coital act in 8 yrs with chronic infection (JID 2005;191:1403).

Needlestick injuries carry an average 0.23% risk of HIV transmission (AIDS 2014;28:1509). The risks for seroconversion following any individual occupational needlestick are dependent on the severity of the exposure, which is reflective of the relative inoculum size. Factors associated with higher risk include deep injury (aOR 15.0), visible blood on the device (aOR 6.2), needle in source vein or artery (aOR 4.3), and source with late-stage HIV infection

TABLE 3.1 Risk of HIV transmission with single exposure from an HIV-infected source

Exposure	Risk			
	Without Male Condom or ART Use	With Male Condom	With ART Use	With Male Condom and ART Use
Blood transfusion	90%	–	–	–
Receptive anal intercourse	1.38%	0.28%	0.06%	0.011%
Needle-sharing IDU	0.63%	–	–	–
Needle stick injury	0.23%	–	–	–
Insertive anal intercourse	0.11%	0.02%	0.004%	0.0009%
Receptive vaginal intercourse	0.08%	0.016%	0.0032%	0.0006%
Insertive vaginal intercourse	0.04%	0.008%	0.0016%	0.0003%
Receptive oral intercourse	Low	–	–	–
Insertive oral intercourse	Low	–	–	–
Mucous membrane exposure	0.09%	–	–	–
Intact skin exposure	negligible	–	–	–
Biting, spitting, throwing body fluids, sharing sex toys	negligible	–	–	–

From AIDS 2014;28:1509; Arch Intern Med 1993;153:1451.

(aOR 5.6; presumably reflective of high VL) (NEJM 1997;337:1485). A porcine tissue model of simulated needlesticks showed larger needles and deeper injury were associated with larger blood transfer volumes, with volume ranging from 0.47 +/− 0.26 µL (30-gauge needle, 0.5-cm depth) to 5.88 +/− 1.45 µL (18-gauge needle, 2.0-cm depth). Gloves reduced volume transferred by 46–86% (JID 1993;168:1589–1592).

The risk of transmission following HIV-positive body fluid splashes to broken skin or mucous membranes is estimated at 0.09%; 0 transmissions were seen in 2,712 exposures to intact skin (Arch Intern Med 1993;153:1451).

Timing of PEP Initiation

- A 72-hr cutoff or "window period" for PEP is used, based on reduction in transmission in nonhuman primate study (noted above) at 12, 36, and 72 hrs. Delays within this time period are likely important and relative, so PEP should always be initiated as quickly as possible and need not be delayed while waiting for additional testing or information. It is far better to stop PEP after a few doses if found to be unnecessary than to miss an opportunity to prevent transmission.
- HCW often present very soon following exposure. The median time from exposure to treatment in 432 HCWs with HIV exposure from October 1996 to December 1998 was 1.8 hrs (Infect Control Hosp Epidemiol 2000;21:780).
- Patients presenting after sexual exposure may present closer to the end of the "window period." It is unknown if there is still a degree of benefit past 72 hrs.

Laboratory Testing of Source Person: Baseline

- If the source patient is available, immediately obtain HIV Ag/Ab (or Ab alone, if Ag/Ab unavailable), HBV surface Ab, HBV core Ab, HBV surface Ag, and HCV Ab.

- In most cases of nPEP, the source person is not available and assumptions on HIV status should take local prevalence data into account.
- The source patient should be offered routine opt-out HIV testing if allowed per local laws to encourage testing. In some states, previously collected blood that is available in the laboratory can be used in this situation. Refer to local laws.
- If source patient HIV testing is negative and there is no clinical reason to suspect acute HIV, discontinue or do not offer HIV PEP to the exposed person.
  - If the source has had an illness compatible with acute retroviral syndrome or is at high risk of HIV acquisition, testing should include plasma HIV RNA levels. Be aware that false positives can occur with VL testing, and an approved screening test should also be used.
- If source patient is known to be HIV-positive, attempts should be made to obtain any available information on their CD4 count, VL, resistance history, cART regimen, and adherence, to guide assessment of transmission risk. If not available,
  - People living with HIV (PLHIV) with documented suppressed VL, and 100% adherence to medication regimen could be considered to be noninfectious based on TasP data. Currently available guidelines do not address this, and so each case should be judged independently and discussed directly with exposed person at risk.
  - Consult an HIV expert in cases of proved or suspected resistance. In a review of 52 patients who were the source of occupational exposures, 39% involved strains with major mutations conferring resistance (NEJM 2003;348:826).

Laboratory Testing of Exposed Person: Baseline and Follow-Up

Exposures from an unknown source, such as needle in trash, do not require testing above due to risk of additional injury, and lack of standardized testing or interpretation (Table 3.2).

TABLE 3.2 Laboratory testing of exposed person

	Baseline	4–6 Wks	3 Mo	6 Mo
	Laboratory testing for all persons considered for PEP			
HIV Ag/Ab[a]	+	+	+	prn[b]
HBV surface Ab	+	–	–	prn[c]
HBV core Ab	+	–	–	prn[c]
HBV surface Ag	+	–	–	prn[c]
HCV Ab	+	–	–	prn[c]
	Additional tests for persons exposed sexually			
STI testing[d]	+	+	–	prn
Pregnancy (women of reproductive age)[e]	+	+	prn	prn
	Additional tests for persons being prescribed PEP			
CBC, AST, ALT, BUN, Cr	+	+ (2 wks) – (4-6 wks)	–	–
Pregnancy (women of reproductive age)	+	prn	prn	prn

a. If HIV Ag/Ab is not available, use rapid HIV Ab test. If no rapid test is immediately available, do not delay initiation of PEP while waiting for baseline HIV test result. Do not obtain HIV RNA at baseline in exposed patient, due to risk of false positives (JID 2004;190:598). HIV RNA testing can be used anytime during follow-up that patient presents with symptoms that could be due to acute retroviral syndrome.

b. If exposed patient has incident HCV infection from original exposure, repeat HIV testing at 6 mos, as acute HCV infection can delay HIV seroconversion. If HIV Ab test is used, last follow-up test should be extended to 6 mos.

c. If susceptible to HBV or HCV at baseline, repeat respective testing at 6 mos.
d. STI testing to include *Neisseria gonorrhea* NAAT, *Chlamydia trachomatis* NAAT, *Treponema pallidum* serology. If syphilis infection is diagnosed, treat and retest 6 mos after treatment. If gonorrhea or chlamydia diagnosed, treat, and retest 3 mos after treatment. Note: In cases of sexual assault some programs choose to treat possible gonorrhea, chlamydia, and syphilis empirically. Testing may then be avoided, as positive baseline tests are representative of prior infection and may be used against the victim in court.
e. Pregnancy status should be established at baseline and repeated at 4–6 wks in women of childbearing age having one-time or ongoing unprotected vaginal intercourse. It can be repeated outside of these defined windows in those with suspicion or symptoms of pregnancy.

Exposed Persons Testing Positive for HIV

- Positive results of HIV test should preferably be given face-to-face.
- All patients testing positive should be linked to HIV care, and baseline HIV-related laboratory tests should be obtained according to guidelines (i.e. CD4, VL, genotype, etc.).
- If testing positive at baseline, do not prescribe PEP.
- If testing positive at follow-up, instances of occupationally acquired HIV and/or PEP failure should be reported to state health department HIV surveillance staff and the CDC coordinator for Cases of Public Health Importance at 404-639-2050.

Counseling at Time of PEP Evaluation

The exposed person should be counseled on these topics:

- *All exposed patients*:
  - Risk of transmission based on specific exposure sustained

- Efficacy of PEP
- Importance of follow-up HIV testing
- Symptoms of acute retroviral syndrome
- Precautions to prevention transmission, if HIV seroconversion occurs: (a) barrier protection for sexual interactions, (b) prevention of pregnancy, (c) discontinuation of breastfeeding, and (d) avoidance of any blood or tissue donations, shared needles, or other drug paraphernalia. These precautions should be observed until last recommended follow-up HIV test is confirmed to be negative.
- Discussion on PrEP in cases of ongoing elevated risk. This topic should be avoided in cases of sexual assault to avoid placing blame on victim.
- *Patients prescribed PEP*:
  - Necessity of adherence to full 28-day prescription
  - Review of insurance coverage of PEP; availability of Patient Assistance Programs to cover cost
  - Common side effects; when to seek emergency care
  - Possible drug interactions
  - Importance of follow-up evaluations while taking PEP
  - Clear follow-up plan with appointment and contact information
- *Legal and work-related issues*:
  - HCW evaluated for oPEP likely require close follow-up and documentation through their occupational health service.
  - Some HCW (or other professions with occupational exposure) may require worker's compensation evaluation.
  - Victims of sexual assault should be notified of applicable resources and may be eligible for reimbursement or up-front coverage of medical expenses depending on local laws.

Is PEP Indicated?

- If patient is judged to have potential benefit from PEP due to risk assessment and baseline laboratory testing in source and exposed patient, PEP should be offered. The exposed person

should be counseled on risk of transmission and risks and benefits of PEP and allowed to make an informed decision on receipt of PEP.
- For nPEP, the following algorithm should be used:
- *nPEP is recommended if there is:*
  - Substantial risk, based on:
    - Exposure of: Vagina, rectum, eye, mouth, other mucosal surface, nonintact skin or subcutaneous tissue, AND
    - Exposure with: Blood, semen, vaginal secretions, rectal secretions, breast milk, or any bloody fluid, AND
  - From: Source likely to be infected, AND
  - Time from exposure: <72 hrs
- *nPEP is not recommended if there is:*
  - Time from exposure: >72 hrs (if close, seek expert input), OR
  - Negligible risk, based on exposure with: Urine, nasal secretions, saliva, sweat, or tears, if not visibly contaminated with blood (regardless of HIV status of source)
- *nPEP may be recommended on a case-by-case basis if:*
  - Substantial risk exposure (defined above), AND
  - Time from exposure: <72 hs, AND
  - Source patient HIV status unknown

PEP Regimen

Choice of PEP Regimen

- If patient chooses to take PEP, their medical history, medication list, and current information on CrCl, HBV status, and pregnancy status should be taken into account when selecting regimen. Pill burden and tolerability of each PEP regimen and drug–drug interactions with patient's mediations should be considered.
- Recommendations from CDC's oPEP (2013) and nPEP (2016) guidelines are reflective of most potent and tolerable regimens at time of publication rather than efficacy of different regimens for oPEP or nPEP. Most recent guidelines are summarized in Table 3.3.

TABLE 3.3 Recommended nonoccupational post-exposure prophylaxis (nPEP) and occupational post-exposure prophylaxis (oPEP) regimens for adolescents ≥13 yrs and adults

Renal Function	Medication
CrCl ≥ 60	Preferred: (FDC of TDF300 mg/FTC200 mg/d) + (RAL 400 mg bid or DTG 50 mg/d) Alternative: (FDC of TDF300 mg/FTC200 mg/d) + (DRV 800 mg/d + RTV 100 mg/d)
CrCl <60	Preferred: (AZT + 3TC, renally dosed) + (RAL 400 mg bid or DTG 50 mg/d) Alternative: (AZT + 3TC, renally dosed) + (DRV 800 mg/d + RTV 100 mg/d)

Similar medications available since last guidelines:
1) FDC of TAF/FTC[a]
2) FDC of DRV/cobi

Not routinely recommended, or contraindicated:
1) ABC is contraindicated due to risk of fatal hypersensitivity reaction and inability to pre-test for HLA-B*5701 allele before PEP given.
2) NVP is contraindicated due to risk of fatal hepatotoxicity if CD4 >250 cells/mm^3 in women and >400 cells/mm^3 in men (which is expected in HIV-negative persons).
3) Other medications not routinely recommended due to tolerability issues: EFV, d4T, ddI, NFV, TPV, SQV, FPV, T20.

[a]TAF/FTC has not been evaluated for PEP and nPEP. Ongoing study for PrEP
See CDC guidelines for additional medications that can be used as alternatives.

Providing PEP Prescription

- PEP programs should take into account the quickest, easiest, and most cost-effective way for programs and patients to obtain PEP medications. Options include having first dose available to give immediately upon presentation, providing 3 or 7 day "starter packs" or "to-go packs," and providing assistance with obtaining medications through pharmaceutical sponsored patient assistance programs (PAP). A meta-analysis found higher PEP refusal rates for patients given a "starter pack," but evidence was rated as very low quality (CID 2015;60(S3):S182).

- Programs should also ensure that the patient's selected pharmacy has the necessary PEP medication in stock.
- Programs must ensure patient is able to attend a follow-up appointment before their initial PEP supply runs out. This 3- to 7-day follow-up can also allow for provider to obtain further details about exposure that patient has recalled and to further educate on PEP and HIV when patient may be in a calmer state.

Resources

- PEPline at the National HIV/AIDS Clinicians' Consultation Center in San Francisco for expert consultation on HIV, HBV, and HCV PEP (1-888-448-4911, 9 AM to 9 PM, 7 days/week).
- Local resources usually include occupational health, infectious disease/HIV experts, and emergency departments.
- Expert consultation is recommended for these situations: (a) delayed presentation beyond 72 hrs, (b) unknown source (e.g., needle in trash), (c) pregnancy or breastfeeding in exposed person, (d) known or suspected resistant HIV, (e) PEP toxicity, (f) significant comorbidities or drug–drug interactions.

Follow-Up and Monitoring or Source and Exposed Persons

Follow-Up of Baseline Labs from Source

- If laboratory tests were not available at time of initiation of PEP, but become available, they should be taken into account. This may require follow-up with occupational health departments that often coordinate source patient testing.

- If the source patient tests negative for HIV and there is no reason to suspect recent or acute infection, PEP can be discontinued.

PEP Tolerability and Adverse Drug Reactions

- For HCWs who receive PEP, data from older PEP regimens show that about 74% experience side effects; primarily nausea (58%), fatigue (37%), headache (16%), vomiting (16%), or diarrhea (14%). TDF-based regimens are better tolerated that AZT-based regimens, and TDF/FTC/RAL had only a 1.9% discontinuation rate in a more recent analysis (CID 2015;60(S3):S170).
- Patients should be evaluated for intolerability and adverse drug reactions while on PEP, including at any early (3- to 7-day) follow-up visits and at a 2-wk follow-up visit.
- For any side effects that threaten serious harm or discontinuation of therapy, an expert familiar with ARVs should be consulted to consider a change in PEP regimen.

Reporting

- Instances of occupationally acquired HIV and/or PEP failure should be reported to state health department HIV surveillance staff and the CDC coordinator for Cases of Public Health Importance at 404-639-2050.
- Unusual or severe toxicities from ARV drugs should be reported to the manufacturer or FDA (1-800-332-1088, http://www.accessdata.fda.gov/scripts/medwatch/medwatch-online.htm).
- If PEP is prescribed to a woman who is pregnant at the time of exposure or becomes pregnant while on PEP, healthcare providers should enter the patient's information (anonymously) into the Antiretroviral Pregnancy Registry (http://www.apregistry.com).

Hepatitis B and C PEP

- HCWs with sharps injuries also have the risk for HBV and HCV transmission. See recommendations for management of HBV exposure and HCV exposure.
- HCW living with HBV or HCV infection could potentially transmit these viral infections to patients. See Society for Healthcare Epidemiology of America (SHEA) guideline for further information (Infect Contr Hosp Epidemiol 2010;31).

Overlap of PEP and PrEP

- Any patients evaluated for either PEP or PrEP should be educated on the other and assessed for eligibility.
- As patients adherent to PrEP do not have a 100% protection rate, use of PrEP should not preclude use of PEP.

HCW Living with HIV

- Transmission from HIV-positive HCW to patients first became a concern in 1990 when a dentist in Florida was identified as the source of HIV infection in six patients through an unknown route of exposure (Ann Intern Med 1992;116:798 and 1994;121:886; J Virol 1998;116:798). This led to a series of "look-backs" in which serologic tests were performed on >22,000 patients who received care from 59 HCW with known HIV infection; no transmissions were identified (Ann Intern Med 1995;122:653). There have since been three additional proven cases, one traced to a total hip procedure and two others to C-sections (AIDS 2006;20:285; Ann Intern Med 1999;130:1).
- A federal US law in 1991 required states to establish guidelines for HIV-positive HCWs, many of which delineate high-risk procedures for transmission, VL cutoffs, and advisory boards to make case-by-case decisions. Some require disclosure of

status and written informed consent of the patient prior to surgical procedures where a HCW involved in the operation is known to be HIV-infected. Refer to individual state laws for more information.

- A 2010 SHEA guideline recommends HCW with HIV RNA of >500 copies/mL who performs Category 3 procedures (procedure where there is definite risk of blood-borne virus transmission, a.k.a. "exposure prone procedures," using previous language) be restricted from these procedures until HIV RNA is <500 copies/mL.

- Patients with HIV RNA <500 copies/mL do not have any procedural restrictions, provided that (a) there is no history of transmitted infections, (b) an expert review panel advises on continued practice, (c) there is routine follow-up with occupational medicine or public health official who confirm with twice-annual labs that HIV RNA remains <500 copies/mL, (d) there is routine follow-up with a personal physician treating the HIV who can confer with the panel, (e) there is consultation with an infection control expert and adherence to recommended practices (including double-gloving and frequent glove changes depending on category of procedure), and (f) HCW agrees and signs contract with the review panel.

- See SHEA guideline (Infect Contr Hosp Epidemiol 2010;31), local infection control policies, and state laws for further information.

- Patients possibly exposed to HIV through a HCW should be evaluated and treated the same as in all other PEP cases.

Prevention of Infection in PLWH

Recommendations are largely based on CDC, National Institutes of Health (NIH), and HIV Medical Association (HIVMA), and Infectious Diseases Society of America (IDSA) recommendations on opportunistic infections (OIs) in HIV-infected adults and adolescents and on

Guidelines by the Advisory Committee for Immunization Practices (Table 3.4). Other pertinent studies are noted also. Information on treatment and secondary prophylaxis for each OI is found in pertinent OI sections.

TABLE 3.4

Vaccine	CD4 <200 cells/mm³	CD4 >200 cells/mm³
Hepatitis A (HAV)	2 doses Havrix 1440 or VAQTA 50 or 3 doses Twinrix (see text)	
Hepatitis B (HBV)	3 doses Recombivax HB and Engerix B (see text for alternative dosing strategies)	
Herpes Zoster Virus (HZV, VZV)	Zostavax: Contraindicated Shingrix: No recommendation	Zostavax: Can be considered for pt >60 yrs old Shingrix: insufficient data
Inactivated or Recombinant Influenza (IIV, RIV)	One dose annually (see text)	
Live Influenza	Not recommended	
Haemophilus influenza type B (HiB)	Only recommended if other indications (asplenia, complement deficiencies) (see text)	
Human Papillomavirus (HPV)	2–3 doses through age 26 (see text)	
Measles, Mumps, and Rubella (MMR)	Contraindicated	If no evidence of immunity: 2 doses at least 28 days apart
Meningococcal serogroups A, C, W, Y (MenACWY)	2 doses, at least 8 wks apart, then booster every 5 yrs (see text)	

(*continued*)

TABLE 3.4 Continued

Vaccine	CD4 <200 cells/mm³	CD4 >200 cells/mm³
Meningococcal serogroup B (MenB)	Only recommended if other indications (asplenia, complement deficiencies, eculizumab use, other) (see text	
Pneumococcal	PPV-23: 1–3 doses depending on indication (see text) PPV-13: 1 dose (see text)	
TDAP	1 dose TDAP, then Td booster every 10 yrs	
Varicella	Contraindicated	If nonimmune: 2 doses, 4–8 wks apart

Travel-Related Vaccines		
Vaccine	CD4 <200 cells/mm³	CD4 >200 cells/mm³
Parenteral (inactivated) Typhoid	Single dose, protective for 2 yrs	
Oral (Live) Typhoid (Ty21a)	Contraindicated	No recommendation
Yellow Fever	Contraindicated	No recommendation
Rabies	Appropriate if indicated (dosing varies)	
Rotavirus	Contraindicated	
Live Cholera (CVD-103HgR)	Contraindicated	
Killed Cholera (WC/rBs)	Consider if travel to highly endemic area, 2 doses, 10–14 days apart	
Japanese Encephalitis	Consider if travel to highly endemic area	
Tick-Borne Encephalitis	Consider in appropriate setting, 3 doses: 0, 1–2, and 9–12 mos	

Infections Due to Fungi

Candidiasis, Mucocutaneous

RISK: Oropharyngeal candidiasis and esophageal candidiasis are associated with HIV-related immune suppression. The odds ratio (OR) for oropharyngeal candidiasis is 3.1 in those with CD4 <200 cell/mm^3 compared to >200 cell/mm^3 (J Oral Sci 2011;53:203). Vulvovaginal candidiasis is not increased in PLHIV.

PREVENTING EXPOSURE: Candida spp. are commensals on mucosal surfaces and cannot be avoided.

ANTIMICROBIAL PRIMARY PROPHYLAXIS: Not recommended due to low morbidity and mortality of active infection, effective treatment, and risk of drug–drug interactions and azole-resistant Candida spp. with use of prophylaxis. A study of 215 PLHIV in Texas showed 29% of colonizing Candida spp. were non-albicans, and 10% of all isolates were fluconazole-resistant (AIDS Res Treat 2012, doi 10.1155/2012/262471).

POST-EXPOSURE PROPHYLAXIS: Not indicated

VACCINATION: Not available.

Coccidioides immitis and posadasii

RISK: PLHIV with a CD4 count of <250 cells/mm^3 or AIDS diagnosis and resident in or traveling to endemic areas (Southwest US, including parts of AZ, CA, NM, NV, TX, UT) are at increased risk. People of African and Philippine descent and immunocompromised hosts have much higher rates of disseminated infection but no difference in risk of exposure or pulmonary/localized infection (Mayo Clin Proc 2011;86(1):63).

PREVENTING EXPOSURE: For those living in endemic areas, complete avoidance of exposure is not feasible. It is prudent to avoid extensive exposure to disturbed soil and dust storms, as possible.

ANTIMICROBIAL PRIMARY PROPHYLAXIS: Indications: Check serology (IgG and IgM, via enzyme-linked immunoassays [EIA] or immunodiffusion technique) every 6–12 mos in patients with CD4 counts of <250 cells/mm^3 and current or prior exposure or resident in an endemic area. Patients with newly positive serology should be evaluated clinically for active infection; if excluded, initiate prophylaxis. *Primary regimens*: Fluconazole 400 mg/d. *Discontinuation*: Discontinue when CD4 is >250 cells/mm^3 and VL is suppressed.

POST-EXPOSURE PROPHYLAXIS: Based on expert opinion, laboratory workers with occupational exposure can be given itraconazole or fluconazole, 400 mg po qd for 6 wks if previously unexposed. Exposures in individuals residing in endemic areas is controversial but can be considered, if they have risks for dissemination (CID 2009;49(6):919).

VACCINATION: Not available. Natural immunity following infection is expected.

Cryptococcus neoformans

RISK: PLHIV with a CD4 count of <100 cells/mm^3 are at highest risk. A recent analysis estimates global serum cryptococcal antigen (sCrAg) positivity at 6% in those with CD4 of <100 cells/mm^3. Those on ART without virological failure and without antigenemia have no risk of developing cryptococcosis (Lancet ID 2017;17:873). The majority of cases of cryptococcal meningitis (CM) occur in PLHIV not on ART or soon after initiating ART.

PREVENTING EXPOSURE: *C. neoformans* is found worldwide in soil contaminated by bird excreta (Mem Inst Oswaldo Cruz 2011;106:781). Clinical infection in PLHIV may be either due to reactivation or may follow exposure. Therefore it is likely prudent to avoid areas contaminated with bird excreta.

ANTIMICROBIAL PRIMARY PROPHYLAXIS: Azole prophylaxis does reduce the incidence of cryptococcosis, but does not confer a survival benefit. Due to low rates of antigenemia, cost-benefit analyses, potential development of resistance, azole side effects, drug interactions, and teratogenicity, primary prophylaxis is not recommended.

sCrAg SCREENING AND PRE-EMPTIVE THERAPY: Screening cART-naïve PLHIV with CD4 of <100 cells/mm^3, evaluating for CM if positive, and treating pre-emptively with oral fluconazole (200–400 mg daily for 2–4 wks) if CM is not present is cost effective in resource-limited settings where local antigenemia is >3% (CID 2010;51:448). Cost-effectiveness in other areas depends on local drug pricing, antigenemia rates, and type/cost of test used. This strategy is not yet recommended universally.

POST-EXPOSURE PROPHYLAXIS: Not indicated

VACCINATION: Not available

Histoplasma capsulatum

RISK: PLHIV with a CD4 count <100 cells/mm^3 and residence in, or travel to, endemic areas (central and south-central US, particularly Ohio and Mississippi river valleys, and Latin America) are at increased risk. Severely immunosuppressed people have higher rates of dissemination.

PREVENTING EXPOSURE: For those living in endemic areas, it is prudent to avoid dust from demolition, cleaning, or remodeling of older buildings; exploring in caves; and cleaning bird or bat droppings.

ANTIMICROBIAL PROPHYLAXIS: *Indications*: CD4 count of <150 cells/mm^3 and at high risk because of occupational exposure or residence in a community with a hyperendemic rate of histoplasmosis (>10 cases/100 person years). *Primary regimens*: Itraconazole 200 mg/d. *Discontinuation*: Discontinue when CD4 is >150 cells/mm^3 for 6 mos and on cART.

POST-EXPOSURE PROPHYLAXIS: Occupational PEP used in some healthcare institutions; PEP in PLHIV is not advised.

VACCINATION: Not available.

Talaromyces marneffei (formerly Penicillium marneffei)

RISK: PLHIV with a CD4 count of <100 cells/mm^3 and residence in endemic areas (southern China, Southeast Asia, especially northern Thailand and Vietnam, and possibly parts of India) are at increased risk.

PREVENTING EXPOSURE: No specific recommendation for those in endemic areas. Avoid travel to these areas in advanced HIV.

ANTIMICROBIAL PROPHYLAXIS: Indication: CD4 count of <100 cells/mm^3 and travel to or residence in endemic area. Primary regimen: Itraconazole 200 mg/d. Alternative regimen: Fluconazole 400 mg weekly. Discontinuation: On cART and CD4 count of >100 cells/mm^3 for 6 mos.

POST-EXPOSURE PROPHYLAXIS: Not described

VACCINATION: Not available

Pneumocystis jirovecii

RISK: PLHIV with CD4 of <200 cells/mm^3 or CD4% of <14 are at highest risk; 80–95% of cases occur with CD4 <200 cells/mm^3 (Arch Int Med 1995;155;1538; Am J Respir Crit Care Med 1997;155:60). Relative risk (RR) for pneumocystis pneumonia (PCP) with CD4 <200 cells/mm^3 is 4.9 (NEJM 1990;322:161), but this risk is somewhat abrogated if the VL is also suppressed (CID 2010;51:611). Other factors associated with increased risk during the pre-HAART era were prior PCP, oral thrush, recurrent bacterial pneumonia, unintentional weight loss, and high plasma VL. PCP prophylaxis reduces the rate of PCP ninefold and reduces mortality in those who develop PCP (Am J Respir Crit Care Med 1997;155:60).

PREVENTING EXPOSURE: P. jirovecii is ubiquitous, and two-thirds are exposed in early childhood. Nosocomial airborne transmission and outbreaks in susceptible hosts have been well documented (J Hosp Infect 2016;93:1), prompting consideration of isolation for patients with active infection. This is not currently recommended as standard practice, but can be considered.

ANTIMICROBIAL PROPHYLAXIS: Indication: CD4 of <200 cells/mm^3 or CD4% <14. Consider in patients unable to start cART and with CD4 count 200–250 cells/mm^3 where frequent monitoring (every 3 mos) not available and in others at risk (see preceding sections). In resource-limited settings, trimethoprim-sulfamethoxazole (TMP-SMX) prophylaxis is used universally in PLHIV to prevent PCP and several other infections. *PRIMARY REGIMENS*: TMP-SMX 1 DS qd (preferred) or 1 SS qd (may be better tolerated).

ALTERNATIVE REGIMENS:

- TMP-SMX 1 DS 3×/wk
- Dapsone 100 mg/d or 50 mg bid
- Dapsone 50 mg/d + pyrimethamine 50 mg/wk + leucovorin 25 mg/wk
- Dapsone 200 mg/wk + pyrimethamine 75 mg/wk + leucovorin 25 mg/wk
- Aerosolized pentamidine 300 mg monthly by Respirgard II nebulizer using 6 mL diluent delivered at 6 L/min from a 50-psi compressed air source until reservoir is dry (usually 45 minutes), with or without albuterol (2 whiffs) to reduce cough and bronchospasm
- Atovaquone 1,500 mg/d with food (can be cost prohibitive)
- Atovaquone 1,500 mg/d + pyrimethamine 25 mg/d + leucovorin 10 mg/d with food
- Aerosolized pentamidine via other nebulization devices, intermittent parenteral pentamidine, and oral clindamycin + primaquine do not have sufficient efficacy data to be recommended but are sometimes used if other options have been exhausted.
- Patients receiving pyrimethamine-sulfadiazine for toxoplasmosis do not require additional PCP prophylaxis.

ADVERSE DRUG REACTIONS: PLHIV have higher rates of drug hypersensitivity. Adverse reactions sufficiently severe to require discontinuation of the drug are noted in 25–50% with TMP-SMX, 25–40%

with dapsone, and 2–4% with aerosolized pentamidine (NEJM 1995:332:693). Patients who have a non–life-threatening reaction to TMP-SMX can continue use or be rechallenged, possibly using desensitization. Gradual initiation of TMP-SMX prophylaxis reduces the rate of rash and/or fever by about 50% (JAIDS 2000;24:337).

- *"Sulfa" allergy*: SMX is a sulfonamide antibiotic. Dapsone is a sulfone (low likelihood of cross-allergy with sulfonamide). Hypersensitivity to either can include fever, rash, hepatitis, lymphadenopathy, and hemolysis. A small study showed 21.7% with reaction to TMP/SMX also had cross-reactivity to dapsone; most reactions were mild or moderate, and 30.8% of people were able to continue dapsone (Pharmacotherapy 1998;18:831).
- *G6PD deficiency*: G6PD deficiency affects up to 25% of people, mostly male, who are of Asian, African, or Mediterranean descent. 10% of black males in the United States have moderate deficiency. It is a disorder with variable clinic presentation based on type of mutation and homo- versus heterozygosity. Exposure to SMX or dapsone in those with G6PD deficiency can provoke methemoglobinemia and hemolysis, usually beginning 24–72 hrs after exposure. Rates of hemolysis from SMX are low. Testing for G6PD deficiency prior to dapsone and primaquine use is recommended.

DISCONTINUATION: Generally, PCP primary prophylaxis should be discontinued when CD4 increases from <200 to >200 cells/mm^3 × 3 mos. A cohort study including >100,000 patient years of follow-up showed low rates of PCP in virally suppressed patients regardless of CD4 count or PCP prophylaxis and no significant benefit to prophylaxis for patients with CD4 101–200 cells/mm^3 (CID 2010;51:611). Stopping PCP prophylaxis in those with CD4 100–200 cells/mm^3 on cART and virally suppressed for at least 3–6 mos can be considered.

POST-EXPOSURE PROPHYLAXIS: Not indicated.

VACCINATION: Not available.

Infections Due to Protozoa

Cryptosporidiosis (Cryptosporidium parvum, C. hominis, C. meleagridis)

RISK: CD4 count of <200 cells/mm^3. Highest risk in those with CD4 <100 cells/mm^3

PREVENTING EXPOSURE: Sources are stool from infected people and animals and contaminated food and water. Patients with HIV should (1) avoid contact with stool from patients with possible cryptosporidiosis and stool from pets, especially dogs and cats <6 mos of age, and calves and lambs. If contact is unavoidable, gloves should be used; (2) strict handwashing after exposure to human feces (including after changing diapers in young children), after handling animals, after contact with soil; (3) avoid sex practices that involve oral contact with feces; (4) avoid drinking water from lakes or rivers; (5) avoid eating raw oysters; and 6) avoid drinking tap water when traveling to developing countries. During outbreaks involving municipal water supply, boil water for 3 minutes, put water through a 1 μm micrometer, or use bottled water (see www. bottledwater.org, or call 1-703-683-5213). Also note that bottled water is unregulated and many commercial supplies are no different from municipal water supplies, which are regulated.

ANTIMICROBIAL PRIMARY PROPHYLAXIS: Rifabutin and azithromycin may have a protective effect but there is insufficient evidence to recommend primary prophylaxis (JAMA 1998;279(5):384; AIDS 2000;14(18):2889).

POST-EXPOSURE PROPHYLAXIS: Not indicated.

VACCINATION: Not available.

Cystoisospora belli (Isospora belli)

RISK: Uncommon in the United States. Predominantly found in subtropical and tropical regions. No defined CD4 count is associated with increased risk of infection. Incidence has declined in the ART era except among those with CD4 counts of <50 cells/mm³ (HIV Med 2007;8:124).

PREVENTING EXPOSURE: Sources are thought to be largely contaminated water and food. Patients with HIV should (1) wash and peel fruits and vegetables, especially in endemic regions and (2) avoid drinking tap water when traveling to developing countries.

ANTIMICROBIAL PRIMARY PROPHYLAXIS: There is limited evidence that prophylaxis with TMP-SMX, sulfadiazine, or pyrimethamine lowers the risk of isosporiasis, but there is insufficient evidence to recommend primary prophylaxis (Am J Trop Med Hyg 1995;53:656; Lancet 1999;353:1463).

POST-EXPOSURE PROPHYLAXIS: Not indicated.

VACCINATION: Not available.

Microsporidiosis

RISK: CD4 count of <200 cells/mm³.

PREVENTING EXPOSURE: Sources are thought to be contaminated water, and/or animal exposure. Patients at risk should (1) avoid drinking water from lakes or rivers, (2) avoid contact with animals known to be infected with microsporidia (if contact is unavoidable gloves should be used), (3) avoid consumption of undercooked meat and/or seafood, and (4) avoid drinking tap water when traveling to developing countries.

ANTIMICROBIAL PRIMARY PROPHYLAXIS: There is no recommended chemoprophylaxis for microsporidiosis.

POST-EXPOSURE PROPHYLAXIS: Not indicated.

VACCINATION: Not available.

Leishmania spp.

RISK: Not found in the United States. Risk is highest in subtropical and tropical regions, as well as in southern Europe.

PREVENTING EXPOSURE: Disease is spread through the bite of infected sand fleas or through injection drug use (IDU) (Trans R Soc Trop Med Hyg 2002;96:S93; Lancet 2002;359:1124). HIV-infected travelers to endemic countries should (1) apply insect repellant and wear protective clothing, (2) avoid nocturnal activities outdoors as sand fly bites largely occur from dusk to dawn, (3) consider use of fine mesh insecticide-treated bed nets, and (4) for injection drug users, employ needle sterility at all times.

ANTIMICROBIAL PRIMARY PROPHYLAXIS: There is no recommended chemoprophylaxis for leishmaniasis.

POST-EXPOSURE PROPHYLAXIS: Not described.

VACCINATION: Not available.

Plasmodium spp. (Malaria)

RISK: Autochthonous transmission is extremely uncommon in the United States. Higher frequency and clinical severity is noted among those with CD4 counts of <350 cells/mm^3 (*AIDS* 2009;23:1997).

PREVENTING EXPOSURE: Disease is transmitted by the bite of an infected female *Anopheles* mosquito. Patients with HIV should utilize the same exposure prevention methods recommended for all travelers to endemic regions, including (1) avoid nocturnal activities outdoors as *Anopheles* mosquito bites largely occur from dusk to dawn; (2) apply insect repellant, specifically N,N-diethyl-m-toluamide (DEET) and/or picaridin (NEJM 2002;347:13); (3) wear protective clothing; and (4) use fine mesh insecticide-treated bed nets. Finally, patients with HIV should consider deferral of travel to endemic region if CD4 counts are <350 cells/mm^3.

ANTIMICROBIAL PRIMARY PROPHYLAXIS: Patients with HIV should utilize the same chemoprophylactic strategies recommended for all travelers to endemic regions (https://www.cdc.gov/malaria). In addition, cotrimoxazole prophylaxis has been found to decrease risk of malaria by 70%, though this method should not replace standard antimalarial chemoprophylaxis (Lancet 2006;367:1256). Check for ART drug–drug interactions with antimalarial agents.

POST-EXPOSURE PROPHYLAXIS: Not described.

VACCINATION: Not available.

Toxoplasma gondii

RISK: CD4 count of <100 cells/mm^3 plus positive anti-Toxoplasma IgG confers a risk of toxoplasmosis encephalitis of 33% per year in the absence of ART (JID 1996;173:91; CID 2001;33:1747).

PREVENTING EXPOSURE: Major sources are ingestion of uncooked meat (tissue cysts), contaminated stool from infected cats (oocysts), soil contact, and eating raw shellfish. Seronegative patients with HIV infection should (1) avoid undercooked pork, lamb, beef, venison, and shellfish including oysters, clams, and mussels; (2) wash hands after gardening, contact with raw meat or change of cat litter (consider gloves for the latter); (3) not feed cats undercooked meat; and (4) wash vegetables before eating them raw

ANTIMICROBIAL PRIMARY PROPHYLAXIS: *Indication*: Toxoplasma IgG positive plus CD4 <100 cells/mm^3. *Note*: Seronegative patients on PCP prophylaxis that does not cover *Toxoplasma* should have the serologic test repeated if the CD4 count decreases to <100 cells/mm^3.

    Preferred: TMP-SMX 1 DS qd
    Alternatives:
- TMP-SMX 1 SS qd
- TMP-SMX 1 DS 3×per week
- Dapsone 50 mg/d po + pyrimethamine 50 mg/wk + leucovorin

    25 mg/wk
- Dapsone 200 mg/wk po + pyrimethamine 75 mg/wk po + leucovorin

    25 mg/wk po
- Atovaquone 1,500 mg/d
- Atovaquone 1,500 mg/d + pyrimethamine 25 mg/d + leucovorin 10 mg/d

    Discontinuation: Discontinue prophylaxis with CD4 count >200 cells/mm^3 for >3 mos; restart when CD4 count is <100–200

cells/mm^3. Can consider discontinuing primary prophylaxis when patient is taking ART with CD4 counts of 100–200 cells/mm^3 and HIV plasma RNA is below the limits for detection for at least 3–6 mos (CROI; 2016; Boston, Massachusetts; Abstract 765).

Trypanosoma cruzi (Chagas disease)

RISK: Autochthonous transmission is extremely uncommon in the United States. Disease is found almost exclusively in Latin America, especially rural areas. However, given disease latency, an estimated 300,000 immigrants to the United States are infected with T. cruzi.

PREVENTING EXPOSURE: T. cruzi is transmitted through the bite of the triatomine vector. It has also been rarely associated with blood transfusion, organ transplantation, vertical transmission, and ingestion of contaminated water or food. HIV-infected travelers to endemic countries should (1) avoid sleeping in adobe brick, mud, or thatch buildings in rural areas; (2) avoid nocturnal activities outdoors as triatomine vectors are most active at night; and (3) use fine mesh insecticide-treated bed nets if sleeping outdoors.

ANTIMICROBIAL PRIMARY PROPHYLAXIS: There is no recommended primary chemoprophylaxis for T. cruzi.

POST-EXPOSURE PROPHYLAXIS: Indication: (1) Antibody to T. cruzi, (2) no prior therapy, and (3) infection likely to be <20 yrs' duration (and no evidence of advanced Chagas cardiomyopathy).

Preferred agent: Benznidazole 5–8 mg/kg/d po in two divided doses × 30–60 days

Alternative: Nifurtimox 8–10 mg/kg/d po in 3 divided doses × 90–120 days

Note: Neither benznidazole nor nifurtimox is available in United States: obtain from CDC drug service.

VACCINATION: Not available.

Infections Due to Mycobacteria

Mycobacterium avium complex (MAC)

RISK: PLHIV with CD4 count of <50 cells/mm^3 are at increased risk; incidence of MAC without cART or prophylaxis is 20–40% (JID 1997;176:126; CID 1993;17:7). Other factors contributing to risk are VL >100,000 copies/mL, previous OIs, colonization of respiratory or gastrointestinal (GI) tract, and reduced T-cell response to M. avium antigens.

PREVENTING EXPOSURE: Organisms in this complex are ubiquitous and cannot be avoided. Person-to-person transmission is unlikely.

ANTIMICROBIAL PRIMARY PROPHYLAXIS: Indication: CD4 count <50 cells/mm^3 after ruling out disseminated MAC infection through clinical assessment (may include mycobacterial blood culture).

> Primary regimens:
> - Azithromycin 1,200 mg po once weekly
> - Clarithromycin 500 mg po bid
> - Azithromycin 600 mg po twice weekly
>
> Alternative regimens: Rifabutin 300 mg po daily with dose adjustment for concurrent ARV agents. M. tuberculosis (MTB) infection should be ruled out prior to initiating rifabutin due to possible development of resistance.
>
> Discontinuation: Discontinue prophylaxis with CD4 count increases to >100 cells/mm^3 for >3 mos.

POST-EXPOSURE PROPHYLAXIS: Not indicated

VACCINATION: BCG vaccination may confer some protection against MAC, but is not used for this purpose.

Mycobacterium tuberculosis

RISK: Risk of exposure to MTB may be higher in PLHIV based on overlapping socioeconomic factors and residence in areas with concurrent epidemics. The RR of progression to active TB in PLHIV with latent TB infection (LTBI) is 9.4–9.9 compared to those with LTBI, but without HIV (NEJM 2004;350:2060). TB incidence doubles in the first year of HIV infection (aRR 2.1, JID 2005;191:150) and is related to degree of immunosuppression; TB-free survival is lower in patients with stage 3 or 4 disease compared to stage 1 or 2 in both low- and high-prevalence settings (JAIDS 2000;23:75). cART reduces rates of TB in PLHIV (Int J Tuberc Lung Dis 2000;4:1026; NEJM 2010;363:257; Lancet 2002;359:2059).

PREVENTING EXPOSURE: PLHIV should follow general guidance on avoidance of scenarios that increase risk of exposure. No extra precautions are needed. Due to increased risk of progression from LTBI to active TB, anyone traveling to endemic areas should have testing for LTBI upon return.

ANTIMICROBIAL PRIMARY PROPHYLAXIS: Isoniazid preventative therapy (IPT) is recommended by the World Health Organization (WHO) for high-prevalence areas, including in resource-limited settings that are unable to offer testing for LTBI.

TESTING FOR LTBI: All PLHIV should undergo testing for LTBI at time of HIV diagnosis and annually if at risk for exposure to MTB. If test was done when CD4 <200 cell/mm^3, it should be repeated when CD4 increases to >200 cell/mm^3. Testing can be done with a tuberculin skin test (TST; result >5 mm in PLHIV considered positive) or interferon-γ release assay (IGRA). Unfortunately, correlation between these tests and reproducibility of each can be poor. Use of both together is not recommended based on lack of predictive and cost-efficacy data. IGRAs have several practical advantages—they do not require two visits for administration and interpretation, do not cross react with BCG and most nontuberculous mycobacteria, and have higher specificity. Once a patient has a positive test for LTBI, there is no utility in repeating these tests to assess for repeat exposure.

TREATMENT OF LTBI:

Indications:
- Patients with LTBI should be evaluated for active TB by symptom screen +/– chest x-ray. If active TB is excluded, LTBI should be treated.

- PLHIV who are close contacts of active TB cases should be evaluated to exclude active TB and should receive treatment for LTBI regardless of TST/IGRA results.

Primary regimens:

- Isoniazid (INH) 300 mg po + pyridoxine 25–50 mg/d × 9 mo
- INH 900 mg po + pyridoxine 100 mg twice weekly with directly observed treatment (DOT) × 9 mo
- Exposure to drug-resistant TB: consult expert

Alternative regimens:

- Rifampin 10 mg/kg/d (max 600 mg) qd × 4 mo
- Rifabutin (dose adjusted based on cART regimen) × 4 mo
- Rifapentine (750 mg if weight 32.1–49.9 kg; 900 mg if weight >50 kg) + INH 15 mg/kg (900 mg max) + pyridoxine 50 mg qwk × 12 wk by DOT is safe in patients on EFV or RAL based regimens, but has not been studied in other regimens.
- Pyrazinamide + rifampin × 2 mos is no longer recommended due to unacceptably high rates of severe hepatotoxicity and death (MMWR 2002;51:998; MMWR 2002;51:998; Am Rev Respir Crit Care Med 2001;164:1319).

Pregnancy: In pregnancy, the risk of progression from LTBI to active TB should be weighed against the risk of INH hepatotoxicity, which may be increased during pregnancy. INH is the recommended regimen, but monitoring should be frequent.

Efficacy of LTBI treatment: A Cochrane review showed lower rate of progression to active TB in PLHIV with LTBI if treated with INH versus placebo (RR 0.38; confidence interval [CI] 0.25–0.57), but also showed a decrease regardless of baseline TST result (RR 0.68; CI 0.54–0.85). Mortality was reduced in those with LTBI treated with INH (RR 0.74, CI 0.55–1.00) (Cochrane Database Syst Rev 2010;20:CD000171).

Monitoring and discontinuation: For those taking INH, baseline bilirubin, ALT, or AST should be obtained and repeated during treatment if abnormal. Those with chronic viral hepatitis should be monitored closely. All patients should be clinically monitored monthly to detect hepatotoxicity or neuropathy, and should stop treatment and report their symptoms if any symptoms of hepatitis occur (jaundice, dark urine, nausea, vomiting, abdominal pain, and/or fever >3 days). INH should be discontinued with aminotransferase elevations to >5× ULN without symptoms, >3× ULN with symptoms, or 2× ULN in those with abnormal baseline values. Rates of serious adverse reactions are low. At monthly appointments providers should assess for adherence and any other side effects.

POST-EXPOSURE PROPHYLAXIS: In the event of exposure to known or suspected TB case (pulmonary or laryngeal TB with positive culture), test for LTBI should be obtained and treatment initiated if positive. All PLHIV and children <5 yrs who are exposed to TB should have an initial LTBI test and CXR. If both are negative treat for LTBI and repeat LTBI test 8–10 wks after exposure has ended—if still negative and there is not concern for anergy, LTBI treatment can be stopped. Those exposed to INH resistant TB should receive rifampin for 4 mos. Seek expert consultation for anyone exposed to MDR TB.

VACCINATION: BCG is recommended as routine part of routine neonatal vaccinations in areas of high endemnicity. It is generally not recommended in infants known to be HIV-infected, but if HIV testing is not available and the infant is asymptomatic, it can be considered. BCG is not recommended as part of the TB prevention strategy in the United States; it can be considered only in (a) infants and children in settings with high likelihood of transmission and infection who cannot be removed from the source of infection and (b) HCW in settings with high likelihood of transmission and infection with INH-/RIF-resistant strains, provided infection control measures have been implemented but are unsuccessful (MMWR 1996;45(RR-4):1).

VACCINE RESPONSE: BCG given to HIV-uninfected infants does not provide primary protection or prevent reactivation but decreases TB-related death, TB meningitis, and disseminated TB by 65–80%

(Lancet 2006;367:1173). Immunity wanes to nonsignificant levels after 10–20 yrs.

Infections Due to Bacteria

Bartonella quintina and hensalae

RISK: CD4 count of <100 cells/mm³.

PREVENTING EXPOSURE: Risk of B. *quintana* infection is associated with exposure to the body louse and is largely seen among the homeless (NEJM 1997;337:1876). Risk of B. *henselae* is associated with exposure to cats (through the cat flea). Patients with HIV and CD4 <100 cells/mm³ should (1) avoid and treat body lice infestations, (2) ensure pet cats have good veterinary care and are treated for flea infestation, (3) avoid cat scratches (if a cat scratch occurs the wound should washed immediately with soap and water), and (4) avoid contact with flea feces.

ANTIMICROBIAL PRIMARY PROPHYLAXIS: There is no recommended chemoprophylaxis for *Bartonella* spp. Of note, patients taking prophylactic macrolides and/or rifamycins may have some protection against bartonellosis (NEJM 1997;337:1876).

POST-EXPOSURE PROPHYLAXIS: Not described.

VACCINATION: Not available.

Enteric Bacteria

RISK: The risk of infection with enteric bacterial pathogens is significantly increased with HIV infection and immunosuppression (greatest with CD4 count of <200 cells/mm³. The risk is most striking for *Salmonella* (JID 1987;156:998; AIDS 1992;6:1495; CID 1995;21:S84), but also noted with *Shigella* (CID 2007;44:327) and *Campylobacter* (Ann Intern Med 1984;101:187). A CD4 count of <50 cells/mm³ may be an independent risk factor for C. *difficile* infection (AIDS 2013;27:2799).

PREVENTING EXPOSURE: These pathogens are generally transmitted by contaminated food or water and less commonly by oral–fecal contact. Patients with HIV should (1) apply good handwashing practices (soap and water preferred over alcohol-based cleansers for *C. difficile* spores), especially after contact with feces, soil, contact with animals, and before and after sex; (2) avoid undercooked eggs and other common food sources of *Salmonella*; (3) avoid undercooked meat; (4) avoid cross-contamination with cutting boards, knives, hands, and the like; (5) when traveling to developing countries, avoid undercooked meat, tap water or ice from tap water, unpasteurized milk, and raw vegetables; and (6) avoid sex practices that involve oral contact with feces and consider use of dental dams if such exposure is anticipated.

ANTIMICROBIAL PRIMARY PROPHYLAXIS: Chemoprophylaxis is generally not recommended, even among travelers. Consideration for fluoroquinolone or rifaximin prophylaxis may be considered on a case-by-case basis. TMP-SMX may have some protective effect for traveler's diarrhea.

POST-EXPOSURE PROPHYLAXIS: Not described.

VACCINATION: Not available.

Haemophilus influenzae

RISK: The risk to adults with HIV infection is low for *H. influenzae* type B. Most infections are due to non-type B strains that are not covered by the vaccine.

PREVENTING EXPOSURE: There are no evident means to decrease risk of exposure to *H. influenza* besides routine handwashing and vaccination.

ANTIMICROBIAL PRIMARY PROPHYLAXIS: There is no recommended primary chemoprophylaxis for *H. influenza*.

POST-EXPOSURE PROPHYLAXIS: As per guidance for the general population, consider chemoprophylaxis for close contacts of patients with confirmed *H. influenzae* type B infections, in appropriate circumstances (MMWR Recomm Rep 2014;63:1).

VACCINATION: The *H. influenzae* type B vaccine is not recommended unless there is coexisting asplenia.

Neisseria meningitides

RISK: Compared with HIV-uninfected individuals, patients with HIV are at an elevated risk of meningococcal disease, and this risk may correlate with CD4 counts of <200 cells/mm^3 and high HIV VLs (Ann Intern Med 2014;160:30; Open Forum Infect Dis 2016;3:226). Among the general population, the highest risk is in travelers to developing countries, living in crowded conditions, and having close contact to those with meningococcal disease.

PREVENTING EXPOSURE: There are no evident means to decrease risk of exposure to *N. meningitidis* besides routine handwashing and vaccination.

ANTIMICROBIAL PRIMARY PROPHYLAXIS: HIV-infected individuals should (1) if feasible, avoid close contact with those known to be infected with meningococcal disease until at least 24 hrs after meningococcal treatment has commenced (MMWR Recomm Rep 2013;62:1), and (2) observe strict handwashing practices.

POST-EXPOSURE PROPHYLAXIS: Recommendations for antibiotic prophylaxis for close contacts of those with meningococcal disease are the same in HIV-infected individuals as for the general population (MMWR 2016 65;1189).

VACCINATION: Routine vaccination is now recommended for all HIV-infected individuals >2 mos of age with meningococcal conjugate vaccine, two doses of MenACWY-D or MenACWY-CRM administered 8 wks apart (serogroups A, C, W, and Y; MMWR Recomm Rep 2013;62:1).

Meningococcal serogroup B (MenB vaccine) should be administered only to patients with asplenia, complement deficiencies, or eculizumab use, or to those who are microbiologists who work with *N. meningitidis*.

Vaccine response: Seroresponse to meningococcal vaccination has been studied only in HIV-infected children, adolescents, and young adults. In this population, vaccine efficacy varied by serogroup and was lower among those with CD4% <15% (Pediatr Infect Dis J 2010;29:391).

Streptococcus pneumonia

RISK: All patients with HIV infection. Risk for invasive pneumococcal infection was 50- to 100-fold greater than in patients without HIV infection in the pre-HAART era (Ann Intern Med 2000;132:182; JID 1996;173:857; JAIDS 2001;27:35; Am J Respir Crit Care Med 2000;162:2063). The risk of invasive pneumococcal disease has decreased substantially in the United States following introduction of Prevnar-7 for children, apparently due to the herd immunity effect (AIDS 2010;24:2253).

PREVENTING EXPOSURE: There are no evident means to decrease risk of exposure to *S. pneumoniae* besides routine handwashing and vaccination.

ANTIMICROBIAL PRIMARY PROPHYLAXIS: There is no recommended chemoprophylaxis for *S. pneumoniae*.

POST-EXPOSURE PROPHYLAXIS: Not described.

VACCINATION: HIV-infected individuals who have never received pneumococcal vaccination should receive the 13-valent PCV-13 vaccine (Prevnar-13). Following initial vaccination, those with CD4 counts of ≥200 cells/mm^3 should then receive the 23-valent pneumococcal polysaccharide vaccine (Pneumovax, PPV-23) ≥8 wks later. For those with CD4 counts of <200 cells/mm^3 vaccination can still be considered, but response may be suboptimal. If an individual has already received a dose of PPV-23, PCV-13 may be administered ≥12 mos after PPV-23 vaccination. After ≥5 yrs from receipt of initial PPV-23, patients should receive a second PPV-23 vaccination. Finally, a third PPV-23 vaccination should be administered at age 65 if ≥5 yrs have elapsed since last vaccination (MMWR Morb Mortal Wkly Rep 2012;61:816).

VACCINE RESPONSE: Studies of efficacy of pneumococcal vaccine in HIV-infected persons have shown variable results. A CDC report indicated 49% efficacy (Arch Intern Med 2000;160:2633), but others found poor efficacy in immunosuppressed hosts (NEJM 1986;315:1318; JAMA 1993;270:1826). A controlled study in Uganda found increased rates of pneumonia in vaccine recipients (Lancet 2000;355:2106), but a subsequent report indicated that vaccine recipients had a reduction in all-cause mortality (AIDS 2004;18:1210). The most complete and recent analysis was a review of 16 studies and concluded there is "only moderate support" for vaccination (HIV Med 2010;10:1468). Patients with low CD4 counts have a poor antigenic response (JID 2004;190:707), but those who respond to ART have a good serologic response (Vaccine 2006;24:2563).The best evidence for benefit of pneumococcal vaccination are data showing that it reduces the high rates of pneumococcal bacteremia in patients with HIV infection (Vaccine 2004;22:2006; Arch Intern Med 2005;165:1533). One case-control study found that the major factors in reducing risk were ART (OR −0.23) and pneumococcal vaccination (OR 0.44) (CID 2007;45:e82), but much of the decrease in invasive pneumococcal infections in adults, including those with HIV infection, is attributed to the herd effect of Prevnar-7, which is licensed only for children (JAIDS 2010;55:128). A randomized trial of Prevnar given to HIV-infected adult patients with pneumococcal bacteremia was highly effective in preventing recurrent pneumococcal sepsis and death, with a 74% efficacy rate ($P = 0.002$) (NEJM 2010;362:812). However, subsequent studies have shown Prevnar-7 to be only slightly more immunogenic than Pneumovax in adults with HIV infection (JID 2010;202;1114). Data supporting a PCV-13 →PPV-23 prime-boost vaccination strategy was initially inferred from studies demonstrating a more robust immune response with PCV-7 followed by PPV-23 vaccination (Vaccine 2002;20:545). More recent data support similar findings among HIV-infected patients receiving a PCV-13 → PPV-23 schedule (Sci Rep 2016 Sep 1;6:32076).

Treponema pallidum (Syphilis)

RISK: Syphilis is a sexually acquired infection. Rates of syphilis have been increasing in recent years, driven largely by higher incidence among MSM, among whom patterns of risky sexual behaviors appear to be increasing in parallel (AIDS 2010;24:1907; Sex Transm Dis 2005;32:458).

PREVENTING EXPOSURE: Providers should regularly screen for behaviors leading to increased risk of syphilis and other STIs. There are many provider- and patient-focused risk assessment tools to use in counseling HIV-infected patients on sexual risk-reduction strategies (MMWR Recomm Rep 2015;64:1). Regular STI screening (at least annually and more frequently depending on individual level of risk) should be incorporated into routine HIV care practices.

ANTIMICROBIAL PRIMARY PROPHYLAXIS: There is no recommended primary chemoprophylaxis for *T. pallidum*.

POST-EXPOSURE PROPHYLAXIS: HIV-infected patients who have had a sexual exposure to an individual with any stage of syphilis within 90 days should receive syphilis treatment per recommendations for the general population (MMWR Recomm Rep 2015 Jun 5;64:1). Those exposed >90 days should also receive treatment if follow-up is uncertain and syphilis serologies are not available.

VACCINATION: Not available.

Infections Due to Viruses

Cytomegalovirus

RISK: Overall CMV seroprevalence in the United States is approximately 50% (CID 2010;50:1439) but is higher among subpopulations, including MSM, injection drug users, and those with exposure to young children (specifically those in day care). Transmission can occur via sexual, respiratory, perinatal, and/or blood/tissue exposure.

PREVENTING EXPOSURE: CMV-seronegative, HIV-infected patients should (1) engage in safe sexual practices with latex condoms (2) minimize prolonged exposure to day care settings, (3) practice optimal handwashing practices, and (4) receive only CMV-antibody negative or leukocyte-reduced blood products unless needed in an emergency setting when other products are not available.

ANTIMICROBIAL PRIMARY PROPHYLAXIS: In the pre-ART era, the use of oral ganciclovir prophylaxis was employed. This practice is no longer recommended, and oral ganciclovir is no longer available in the United States. Valganciclovir primary prophylaxis is also not recommended as a randomized clinical trial failed to show efficacy in CMV disease prevention (HIV Clin Trials 2009;10:143). In the pre-ART era, routine ophthalmologic screenings every 3–4 mos were recommended for those with CD4 counts of <50 cells/mm^3. There is no CMV vaccine currently available.

POST-EXPOSURE PROPHYLAXIS: Not indicated.

VACCINATION: Not available.

Hepatitis A Virus

RISK: HAV risk is highest in MSM; injection and noninjection drug users; persons with chronic liver disease, including chronic HBV and HCV; and travelers to countries with endemic HAV (MMWR 2002;51[RR-6]:61). Susceptibility is defined by negative total HAV antibody, which is present in 30% of American adults. Some authorities recommend HAV vaccination for all nonimmune patients, as defined by negative total anti-HAV antibody.

PREVENTING EXPOSURE: HAV-antibody negative, HIV-infected patients should (1) wash and peel fruits and vegetables, especially in endemic regions; 2) avoid drinking tap water when traveling to developing countries; and (3) avoid sex practices that involve oral contact with feces, and consider use of dental dams if such exposure is anticipated.

ANTIMICROBIAL PRIMARY PROPHYLAXIS: There is no recommended primary chemoprophylaxis for HAV.

POST-EXPOSURE PROPHYLAXIS: If exposed to HAV within 2 wks and not previously vaccinated, administer a single dose of single-antigen Hepatitis A vaccine or IVIG (0.02 mL/kg).

VACCINATION: HAV vaccine: Havrix 1440 or VAQTA 50. If Hepatitis B vaccination is also indicated, combination HAV/HBV vaccine (Twinrix) can be used. Anti-HAV seroresponse should be measured at 1 mo post-vaccination, and, if not seroprotective, HAV vaccine should be readministered when CD4 is >200 cells/mm^3.

INDICATION: (1) Chronic liver disease, travelers to countries where HAV is endemic or epidemic, injection and noninjection drug users, or MSM; plus (2) seronegative for HAV.

VACCINE SCHEDULE: 0.5 mL IM × 2 separated by 6–18 mos (depending on the vaccine).

Hepatitis B Virus

RISK: The prevalence of chronic HBV in HIV-infected persons is reported at 6–15% among MSM, 10% among IDUs, and 4–6% among heterosexuals (J Hepatol 2006;44 Suppl 6) and has slowly declined since the pre-ART era (Clin Infect Dis 2010;50:426). The prevalence of HBV antibody indicating prior infection is 24–76% (J Hepatol 2006;44 S6; MMWR 2008;57 RR-8:S1). In countries (such as the United States) with low HBV endemicity, transmission is primarily through sexual exposure or injection drug use.

PREVENTING EXPOSURE: Patients with HIV should be counseled to 1) use condoms during sexual intercourse; (2) use only clean needles if injecting drugs, and consider use of a clean needle exchange program; and (3) be aware of the potential risks of HBV transmission when receiving tattoos and/or body piercings.

ANTIMICROBIAL PRIMARY PROPHYLAXIS: There is no recommended primary chemoprophylaxis for HBV.

POST-EXPOSURE PROPHYLAXIS: Recommendations for the use of HBV vaccine and/or hepatitis B immune globulin for post-exposure prophylaxis are identical to that of the general population (MMWR 2006,56(RR-16), Appendix B)

VACCINE: HBV vaccine is available as single-antigen formulation (Recombivax HB and Engerix B) and in combination with HAV vaccine as Twinrix. The recommended dose for single antigen vaccine is 20 μg HBsAg for Engerix B and 10 μg for Recombivax (MMWR 2018 RR 67(1);1–31).

INDICATION: HIV-infected patients without anti-HBsAg and with anti-HBs of <10 IU/mL, including those with isolated anti-HBc Ab (JAIDS 2003;34:439). It is preferable to initiate series when CD4 is >350 cells/mm^3, but vaccination should not be deferred if CD4 is <350 cells/mm^3.

VACCINE SCHEDULE: 0, 1, and 6 mos. Alternative schedules include: 0, 1, 2, and 6 mos; 0, 1, 2, and 12 mos. The vaccine schedule for Twinrix (HAV/HBV) is 0, 1, and 6 mos, or 0, 1, 2, and 12 mos, or accelerated schedule 0, 7, 21–30 days, and 12 mos. Patients with isolated anti HBcAb should be vaccinated with only one dose of HBV vaccine, and anti-HBs titers should be evaluated 1 month later to assess for seroresponse. If anti-HBs titers are <100 IU/mL, a complete HBV vaccination series should be restarted.

EFFICACY: Vaccine seroresponse should be assessed 1 month after completion of series. The achievement of anti-HBs titers of >10 mIU/mL is considered an appropriate serological response. Unfortunately, seroresponse to the standard CDC recommended vaccine regimen have been low (18–72%) compared to those without HIV (>90%) and appear to correlate with lower CD4 counts and detectable HIV RNA (Vaccine 2000;18:1161; AIDS 1994;8:558, Ann Intern Med 1988;109:101; AIDS 1992;6:509; AIDS Resp Ther 2006;3:9; AIDS Rev 2009;11:157; Vaccine 2005;23:2902; CID 2005;41:1045; CID 2004;38:1478). If patients do not respond to initial series, a three-dose revaccination series should be reinitiated. Of note, a study reported a response rate of 51% in patients given the double dose after failure to respond to the standard dose series (JID 2008;197:292).

ALTERNATIVE DOSING STRATEGIES: Higher response rates are noted with increased doses, frequency, and with intradermal vaccination. A trial comparing standard vaccine with four IM doses of 40 µg (instead of 20 µg) at weeks 0, 4, 8, and 24 was 82%, and four intradermal injections of low doses (4 ng) at weeks 0, 4, 8, and 24 showed responses of 77% (JAMA 2011;305:1432). A similar study, conducted in Thailand among those with CD4 of >200 cells/mm^3, found higher antiHBs titers (but not overall response) among those receiving a double-dose HBV vaccination at 0, 1, 4, 6 mos, compared to the standard three-dose regimen (PLoS One 2013;8:e80409). Finally, a study evaluating a double-dose strategy at standard dosing intervals (0, 1, 6 mos) found higher response rates compared to standard dosing (64.3% × 39.3%), but this was only found in those with CD4 of ≥350 cells/mm^3 (Vaccine 2005;23:2902).

Hepatitis C Virus

RISK: HCV may be transmitted through percutaneous exposure to blood products, through sexual exposure, or through vertical transmission. The most common means of transmission in the United States remains injection drug use, though there has been a recent increase in incidence of sexually acquired HCV among MSM (AIDS 2010;24(12):1799).

PREVENTING EXPOSURE: HIV-infected patients should be counseled to (1) avoid using injection drugs and, if necessary, engage in care in a comprehensive substance abuse treatment program; (2) avoid sharing needles; (3) use only clean needles if injecting drugs, and consider use of a clean needle exchange program; and (4) use barrier protection (condoms) during sexual intercourse.

ANTIMICROBIAL PRIMARY PROPHYLAXIS: There is no recommended primary chemoprophylaxis for HCV.

POST-EXPOSURE PROPHYLAXIS: Not indicated.

VACCINATION: Not available.

Herpes Simplex Virus

RISK: Seropositivity for HSV-1 and HSV-2 are high in the HIV population, approximately 90% and 50–90%, respectively (Sex Transm Infect 2004;80:77; CID 2006;43:347). Acquisition occurs through shedding on mucosal surfaces and can occur from those with or without active lesions.

PREVENTING EXPOSURE: HSV-2 seronegative patients with HIV should be counseled to (1) use barrier protection (condoms) during sexual intercourse; (2) consider asking new sexual partners to be tested for HSV-2 serology; (3) avoid mucosal contact with individuals with active HSV lesions; and (4) consider prophylactic valacyclovir (500–1000 mg/d) for the HSV-2 infected partner, which has been shown to decrease transmission by 48% in the general population (NEJM 2004;350:11). Note that suppressive anti-HSV therapy has not been shown to decrease infectivity to HSV-seronegative partners who are not on ART and thus is not recommended (JID 2013;208:1366).

ANTIMICROBIAL PRIMARY PROPHYLAXIS: There is no recommended primary chemoprophylaxis for HSV-1 or HSV-2 for HIV-infected patients.

POST-EXPOSURE PROPHYLAXIS: Not described.

VACCINATION: Not available.

Human Herpes Virus 8

RISK: HHV-8 seroprevalence is low in the general population (1–5%) but is higher among those with HIV and highest in general among MSM (20–77%) (NEJM 2000;343:1369; Int J Cancer 2016;138:45). HHV-8 is shed in saliva and genital secretions and occurs during asymptomatic infections.

PREVENTING EXPOSURE: There are no recommended means to prevent HHV-8 exposure.

ANTIMICROBIAL PRIMARY PROPHYLAXIS: There is no recommended primary chemoprophylaxis for HHV-8.

POST-EXPOSURE PROPHYLAXIS: Not described.

VACCINATION: Not available.

Human Papilloma Virus

RISK: HPV is the most common STI in the United States (STD 2013;40:187). Prevalence of any genital HPV in 18- to 59-yr-olds was 42.5%, and, in high-risk HPV (types 16 and 18) it was 22.7% from 2013 to 2014 in US surveys (NCHS Data Brief 2017;280; MMWR 2010;59:630). HPV infection increases risk of HIV acquisition in women (HR 2.06) and probably in men (AIDS 2012;26(17).

PREVENTING EXPOSURE: Reduce number of sexual partners and use barrier protection (not fully protective, as HPV spread by any skin that is infected and not covered by barrier).

ANTIMICROBIAL PRIMARY PROPHYLAXIS: Not available or recommended.

POST-EXPOSURE PROPHYLAXIS: Not available or recommended.

VACCINATION: HPV vaccines licensed in the United States are the bivalent Cervarix vaccine (2vHPV), quadrivalent Gardasil vaccine (4vHPV), and 9-valent Gardasil-9 (9vHPV). Only 9vHPV is currently commercially available. All three vaccines protect against HPV types 16 and 18 that account for 70% of cervical cancers. The 4vHPV also protects against HPV types 6 and 11, which cause 90% of genital warts. 9vHPV also protects against types 31, 33, 45, 52, and 58. Pre-vaccination screening for HPV is not recommended. These are not live vaccines. Pregnancy is a contraindication.

INDICATIONS: See Advisory Committee on Immunization Practices (ACIP) recommendations for non-HIV infected persons. All immunocompromised patients, including PLHIV with any CD4 count, should be vaccinated between ages 9 and 26, with greatest benefit if given before sexual debut. The vaccines are available for eligible persons <19 yrs through Vaccines for Children program (800-232-4636).

VACCINE SCHEDULE: Each of the three available vaccines can be given in three 0.5 mL doses IM at 0, 1–2, and 6 mos, and 9vHPV is also approved for children aged 9–14 as a two-dose schedule at mos 0 and 6–12, and for children aged 15–26 as a three-dose schedule, at mos 0, 2, and 6.

EFFICACY: Vaccine efficacy of the quadrivalent vaccine for preventing genital warts is 60% (NEJM 2011;364:401). Vaccine efficacy in women for preventing genital infection or lesions involving HPV types in the vaccine approach 100% with a 3- to 4-yr follow-up (NEJM 2007;356:1928; BMJ 2010;341:c4455; Cancer Prev Res 2009;2:868). One report showed a 78% reduction in anal intraepithelial neoplasia (a precursor of anal cancer) in vaccine recipients (Jessen H. 2010 IAS, Vienna:Abstr. THLBB101), and some have strongly advocated routine use of the quadrivalent vaccine in MSM up to 26 yrs (Vaccine 2010;28:6858; Lancet 2010;10:815). A cost analysis of this strategy concluded it would be cost-effective for MSM aged 12–26 yrs (Lancet 2010;10:845).

Influenza A and B

RISK: PLHIV are at a four- to eightfold increased risk for acute lower respiratory tract infection with influenza and more likely to have severe influenza, pneumococcal co-infection, influenza type B infection, longer hospitalization, and mortality (CID 2017;doi 10.1093/cid/cix903: Emerg Infect Dis 2013;19:1766; CID 2014;58:1241).

PREVENTING EXPOSURE: PLHIV should follow same preventative actions as non HIV-infected persons to avoid exposure to respiratory viruses. They should be counseled to avoid close contact with sick people, practice frequent hand hygiene, and clean and disinfect objects and surfaces that may be contaminated with viruses. If ill with an influenza-like illness, it is recommended that steps be taken to avoid spreading infection: cover nose and mouth when coughing or sneezing, practice frequent hand hygiene, and stay away from work and crowded places while ill and for at least 24 hrs after fever resolves (without use of antipyretics).

ANTIMICROBIAL PRIMARY PROPHYLAXIS/POST-EXPOSURE PROPHYLAXIS: Primary and post-exposure prophylaxis are secondary in importance to vaccination for influenza prevention and should not be considered a substitute for vaccination (CID 2009;48:1003).

INDICATIONS:

Primary: Can be considered in all PLHIV when influenza virus is circulating in the community and patient has not had adequate time following vaccination to mount immune response (i.e., first 2 wks) or in whom vaccination is contraindicated, unavailable, or expected to have low effectiveness due either to patient immune response or mismatch of vaccine to circulating strain. Greatest benefit expected for those at highest risk due to severe immunocompromise.

Post-exposure/expected exposure: Recommended for all residents of nursing homes and long-term care facilities (irrespective of HIV or vaccination status) that are experiencing influenza outbreaks. Can be considered in PLHIV when influenza virus is circulating in the community and patient has not had adequate time following vaccination to mount immune response (i.e., first 2 wks) or in whom vaccination is contraindicated, unavailable, or expected to have low effectiveness. PLHIV who are household contacts of suspected or confirmed influenza cases should receive chemoprophylaxis.

Primary regimen: Local antiviral susceptibility patterns should be reviewed annually to determine most favorable regimen. See www.cdc.gov/flu in United States.

Duration: If indicated, chemoprophylaxis should be initiated at the onset of sustained community influenza activity, as determined by local public health authorities. For persons given chemoprophylaxis while awaiting adequate immune response, course is 2 wks beyond vaccination (2 wks in adults, 6 wks in children requiring two-part vaccination). If no protection from vaccination is expected, chemoprophylaxis should be continued for the duration that influenza is circulating in the community. For household contacts requiring chemoprophylaxis, duration is 10 days.

VACCINATION: Inactivated, recombinant, and live influenza vaccines may be available depending on year and circulating strains, and each covers chosen strains of influenza A +/- influenza B.

INDICATIONS: Inactivated or recombinant influenza vaccine is recommended for all PLHIV; PLHIV are considered by the CDC to be a priority population for vaccination. Live vaccine formulations are contraindicated.

VACCINE SCHEDULE: Annually.

EFFICACY: Antigenic response is weaker in PLHIV (Vaccine 2011;29:1359; CID 2011;52:138) but improved with "high-dose" vaccine (Ann Int Med 2013;158:19) and with higher CD4 count.

JC Polyomavirus

RISK: JCV seroprevalence in the general population approaches 50–70% by adulthood (APMIS 2013;121:685; J Infect Dis 2009;199:837). Transmission is thought to be primarily respiratory and is usually asymptomatic. Risk for progressive multifocal leukoencephalopathy (PML) is higher at lower CD4 counts (<200 cells/mm^3) and is expected to be higher among HIV-infected patients undergoing solid organ transplant, chemotherapy treatment, and/or certain humanized monoclonal antibodies, including rituximab (J Clin Oncol 2006;24:4123).

PREVENTING EXPOSURE: There are no recommendations regarding proven methods of exposure prevention as JCV is usually acquired asymptomatically in childhood.

ANTIMICROBIAL PRIMARY PROPHYLAXIS: There is no recommended primary chemoprophylaxis for JCV.

POST-EXPOSURE PROPHYLAXIS: Not described.

VACCINATION: Not available.

Varicella zoster virus

RISK: VZV seroprevalence in the United States population surpasses 95% and is even higher among those born before 1980 (JID 2008;197 Suppl 2:S147). Serologic tests for varicella correlate well with a history of varicella but not with vaccination for varicella (Infect Control Hosp Epidemiol 2007;28:564). Lifetime risk of VZV reactivation (herpes zoster) in the general population is 15–20% but is >15 times higher in the HIV population (J Infect Dis 1992;166:1153; J Acquir Immune Defic Syndr 2005;40:169). Herpes zoster incidence is highest among HIV-infected patients with CD4 <200 cells/mm^3 but can occur at any CD4 count (J Acquir Immune Defic Syndr 2005;40:169). Primary VZV infection is spread through airborne viral droplet transmission, whereas individuals with active herpes zoster can transmit VZV through direct contact with non-crusted zoster lesions.

PREVENTING EXPOSURE: VZV-seronegative, unvaccinated, HIV-infected individuals should avoid exposure to individuals with primary varicella and/or herpes zoster. VZV-seronegative, unvaccinated, HIV-uninfected household contacts should be vaccinated.

ANTIMICROBIAL PRIMARY PROPHYLAXIS: Chronic antiviral chemoprophylaxis is not recommended.

POST-EXPOSURE PROPHYLAXIS:

- Varicella vaccine is recommended within 3–5 days of exposure among seronegative, unvaccinated individuals, without contraindications to immunization (see below).
- VariZIG: Dose: 125 IU/10 kg (to 625 IU) IM. In the United States, VariZIG is only available through a treatment investigational new drugs application (FFF Enterprises, Temecula, CA, 800-843-7477). Use for HIV-infected patients if close exposure occurs to an individual with active varicella (risk is highest) or herpes zoster (risk is lowest) and (1) previously unvaccinated, (2) no history of chickenpox or herpes zoster, (3) seronegative to VZV, (4) born after 1980, and (5) within 10 days of exposure. Note that serologic evidence of immunity is recommended

for persons born before 1980 who are immunocompromised (MMWR 2007;56:RR-4:1). There are no published data regarding VariZIG efficacy in patients with HIV infection.

- Antiviral post-exposure prophylaxis: Can consider use of acyclovir or valacyclovir prophylaxis beginning 7–10 days after exposure but there are no data to support this strategy in HIV-infected patients (Pediatrics 1993;92:219).

VACCINATION: Live attenuated varicella vaccine:

FORMULATIONS: For adults there is only one licensed formulation available in the United States: single antigen live varicella vaccine (Varivax). Schedule: 2 doses (0.5 mL) separated by 4–8 wks. Recommended for HIV-infected children with CD4% >15%, and may be considered in HIV-infected, VZV-seronegative adults with CD4 >200 cells/mm^3.

Other absolute contraindications include CD4 count of <200 cells/mm3, patients on immunosuppressive chemotherapy or high-dose steroids, other congenital or acquired immune deficiencies, and active tuberculosis.

HERPES ZOSTER VACCINE: For prevention of herpes zoster (shingles) in patients with a history of primary varicella.

FORMULATIONS: There are two licensed formulations available in the United States: (1) live attenuated zoster vaccine (Zostavax) and (2) recombinant zoster vaccine (Shingrix).

1. Live attenuated zoster vaccine (Zostavax): Dose: 0.65 mL as a single dose. Recommended for persons >60 yrs of age, but contraindicated in patients with HIV infection with CD4 counts of <200 cells/mm^3 (MMWR 2008;57:RR-5:1). A large study of immunocompetent adults older than 60 yrs showed vaccine efficacy in preventing zoster of 55% (JAMA 2010;305:160). Patients with HIV infection who are >60 yrs and have a CD4 count of >200 cells/mm^3 are now included in the CDC recommendations. A review of this vaccine given

to HIV-infected patients with a CD4 count >400 cells/mm^3 showed safety, but only a modest immune response (Human Vaccine 2010;6:318). If the vaccine causes infection, the patient should receive acyclovir.

2. Recombinant zoster vaccine (Shingrix): Dose: 0.5 mL, two doses recommended at 0 and 2–6 mos. Given the only very recent approval of the recombinant zoster vaccine, there are no specific recommendations regarding its use in the HIV population, but because it is not contraindicated in immunocompromised patients, this has led to expectations for future widespread use in the HIV population. The vaccine was evaluated in two randomized clinical trials (≥50 yrs and ≥70 yrs old) with efficacy of risk reduction of zoster of 97% and 90%, respectively (NEJM 2015;372:2087; NEJM 2016;375:1019).

Cryptosporidiosis

SOURCE DOCUMENT: Cryptosporidiosis NIH DHHS Guidance-last updated June 14, 2013; last reviewed June 2017 (http://aidsinfo. nih.gov/guidelines)

EPIDEMIOLOGY: Cryptosporidiosis was a common cause of chronic diarrhea in patients with advanced HIV infection in the pre-HAART era and continues to be an important opportunistic pathogen in AIDS patients in developing countries and in patients with advanced HIV infection due to delayed diagnosis or inadequate ART. The most common species is *C. parvum;* less common are *C. hominis* and *C meleagridis*. Diarrhea is usually caused by one species although it may be caused mixed species. Cryptosporidiosis has become an infrequent enteric pathogen in patients with early-stage disease or those receiving ART with immune response. The major risk is advanced HIV infection with a CD4 count of <100/mm^3. The usual source is ingestion of food or fluids contaminated with stool or water sources including pools, lakes, and water supplies, despite chlorination. Person-to-person transmission is infrequent and is most common in sexually active MSM.

CLINICAL EXPRESSION: Most common is acute watery diarrhea that is often accompanied by cramps, nausea, and vomiting. About one-third have fever. Involvement of the biliary tract is common, leading to sclerosing cholangitis and pancreatitis. Disease patterns described in patients with AIDS include asymptomatic carriage (5%), self-limited diarrhea of <2 mos duration (29%), chronic diarrhea lasting >2 mos (60%), and fulminant, severe cholera-like diarrhea with >10 L/d. Pulmonary disease has been reported but is not often diagnosed.

DIAGNOSIS: The standard test is microscopic examination of stool or tissue using acid-fast stain. Immunofluorescence staining appears to be 10× more sensitive compared to acid-fast stain and is now the gold standard test. Additional staining tests include EIA and immunochromatographic tests which detect stool antigens. Polymerase chain reaction (PCR) testing is the most sensitive and can detect as few as 5 oocytes. A single specimen is usually adequate for a patient with severe diarrhea, but repeat testing is advised for those with less severe symptoms. Microscopic exam of small bowel pathology sections is useful in patients with enteritis.

PREVENTION: Patients at risk should be counseled to avoid potentially contaminated food and water; to practice careful hygiene with handwashing after handling pets, soil contact, or diapering babies; to avoid eating raw oysters, drinking water during travel to developing countries, and oral–anal contact; and to use condoms with penile–anal contact. This risk is magnified by CD4 counts of <100 cells/mm^3 and notably reduced with immune response to ART. Rifabutin and possibly clarithromycin/azithromycin when taken for M. avium prophylaxis might confer some protection against cryptosporidiosis.

TREATMENT: Most important is ART with immune reconstitution to a CD4 count of >100 cells/mm^3. Symptomatic disease may be severe and require aggressive oral and intravenous rehydration plus electrolyte replacement. Total parenteral nutrition may be used in patients with severe diarrhea with nutritional deficiencies. Treatment of severe diarrhea should include tincture of opium (more effective) or loperamide. Antimicrobials recommended include nitazoxanide (500–1,000 mg po bid × 14 days with food) or paromomycin 500 mg po qid × 14–21 days. However, there is limited efficacy of these drugs in immunocompromised patients, and immune reconstitution remains paramount.

SPECIAL CONSIDERATIONS: In pregnant women, initiation of ART is important both in restoring immunity and in preventing maternal to child transmission. Loperamide use may be associated with birth defects and should be avoided during the first trimester unless benefits outweigh potential risk. Paromomycin and nitazoxanide can be considered after the first trimester in severe symptoms.

Mycobacterium avium Complex Infection

SOURCE DOCUMENTS: Guidelines for the Prevention and Treatment of Opportunistic Infections in HIV-infected Adults and Adolescents: Disseminated *Mycobacterium avium* Complex disease; last reviewed June 14, 2017 at http://aidsinfo.nih.gov/guidelines)

EPIDEMIOLOGY: M. avium complex (MAC) is ubiquitous and is thought to be acquired via inhalation or ingestion. Person-to-person transmission is less likely. No specific environmental exposure or activity has been defined as a risk. The incidence of disseminated MAC in patients with a CD4 cell count of <100 cells/mL in the absence of ART and MAC prophylaxis is 20–40%. The incidence of disseminated MAC in the HAART era has decreased by more than 10-fold to 2.5 cases per 1,000 person years. Risk factors include CD4 <50 cells/mL, HIV VL >100,000 copies/mL, and previous opportunistic and MAC infection (AIDS 2010;24:1549).

PRESENTATION: The usual symptoms of MAC infection include fever, night sweats, weight loss, fatigue, diarrhea, and abdominal pain. Lab tests at presentation frequently include anemia and an elevated alkaline phosphatase. Physical exam often shows hepatosplenomegaly and/or diffuse generalized lymphadenopathy. Localized infections such as pneumonitis, osteomyelitis, pericarditis, lymphadenitis, soft tissue abscesses, genital ulcers, or central nervous system (CNS) involvement are seen commonly in patients who have received ART with improved immune function or as a manifestation of immune reconstitution inflammatory syndrome (IRIS).

DIAGNOSIS: Isolation of MAC from blood cultures, lymph nodes, bone marrow, or other sterile body sites helps in diagnosis. In addition to microscopic exam and staining for acid-fast bacilli, clinical specimens are inoculated in solid media like Middlebrook 7H11 and in liquid media such as BACTEC 12B broth. Growth of MAC can take 2–4 wks in solid media and 7–14 days using BACTEC system. Identification of species is done by DNA probes or high performance liquid chromatography (HPLC). Blood cultures have >90% sensitivity in disseminated disease. Respiratory and stool specimens have poor sensitivities, 22% and 20%, respectively, but good positive predictive value (60%) for bacteremia (JID 1994;169:289).

PROPHYLAXIS: US Department of Health and Human Services (DHHS) guidelines recommend starting prophylaxis to prevent MAC disease if CD4 is <50 cells/mL. No specific measures are recommended to prevent environmental exposure.

PREFERRED: Azithromycin 1,200 mg weekly or clarithromycin 500 mg bid.

Prior to starting prophylaxis, disseminated MAC should be ruled out by clinical assessment, and AFB blood cultures should be ordered if necessary. Routine screening with respiratory and stool cultures is not recommended to rule out MAC infection.

ALTERNATIVE: Rifabutin 300 mg/d for those who cannot tolerate macrolides, but TB should be excluded before using rifabutin.

DISCONTINUATION: When CD4 count is >100 cells/mL for >3 mos. Two randomized placebo controlled studies have shown that risk of acquiring MAC after discontinuing prophylaxis is minimal. This helps reduce pill burden and potential drug–drug interactions.

The 2016 IAS-USA panel (JAMA 2016;316:191) recommends against primary prophylaxis for MAC if effective ART is initiated immediately and viral suppression is achieved since studies have shown no significant mortality difference once MAC disease develops irrespective of whether patients have received MAC prophylaxis or not (JID 2015;212:1366).

TREATMENT: Initial treatment should be with two or more drugs to prevent and delay the development of drug resistance. Susceptibility testing for macrolides is recommended.

PREFERRED:

1. Clarithromycin 500 mg po bid plus ethambutol 15 mg/kg/d po is the preferred regimen.
2. Azithromycin 500–600 mg/d plus ethambutol 15 mg/kg/d po may be substituted due to intolerance or drug interactions with clarithromycin.

ADDITIONAL THIRD AGENT: The addition of rifabutin 300 mg/d po is suggested when there is a high MAC load (>200 CFU/mL), advanced immunosuppression (CD4 <50 cells/mL), or absence of effective ART.

Randomized clinical trials have shown that addition of rifabutin improved survival and delayed emergence of resistance (CID 1999;28:1080).

Alternative additional agents include (1) amikacin 10–15 mg/kg/d IV; (2) streptomycin 1 g/d IV or IM; (3) moxifloxacin 400 mg/d po; (4) levofloxacin 500 mg/d po. However, no controlled trials have tested their efficacy.

STARTING ART: ART should be started as soon as possible after 2 wks of MAC treatment to reduce pill burden, drug interactions, and risk of IRIS initially.

ACTG 5164 was a randomized trial that showed early ART (within 14 days) in patients with acute OIs had less progression to death and no increase in adverse events as compared to deferred ART (within 45 days) (PLoS ONE 4:e5575).

RESPONSE TO THERAPY: Clinical improvement with decline in fever and symptoms should be noted within 2–4 wks. Blood cultures should be obtained at 4–8 wks in patients who fail to show clinical response. Therapeutic response may be expected to be delayed in patients who have more extensive disease and/or very advanced immunosuppression at baseline.

Drug Side Effects and Interactions

Clarithromycin/azithromycin: Can cause nausea, vomiting, abdominal pain, and transaminitis. A clarithromycin dose of >1g has been associated with increased mortality and is not recommended.

Protease inhibitors (PIs) can increase clarithromycin levels and efavirenz can decrease its levels. Azithromycin does not have significant interactions with them.

A comparative trial for treatment of MAC bacteremia showed clarithromycin superior in time to clearance of cultures, but another trial indicated these drugs were comparable when used with ethambutol (CID1998;27:1278).

Rifabutin: Can cause uveitis, arthralgias. It also a substrate and inducer of cytochrome P450 3A4 and can cause complex drug interactions with cobicistat, non-nucleoside reverse transcriptase inhibitors (NNRTIs) and PIs, thus requiring dose adjustments.

DISCONTINUATION OF SECONDARY PROPHYLAXIS: Criteria include at least 12 mos of complete treatment along with improvement in clinical symptoms and CD4 count of >100 cells/ mL for ≥6 mos.

Secondary prophylaxis should be reinstituted if CD4 count is <100 cells/mL. Primary prophylaxis should be reinstituted if the CD4 count decreases to <50 cells/mL.

TREATMENT FAILURE: This is defined by lack of clinical response and persistence of positive blood cultures after 4–8 wks of recommended treatment. Repeat drug susceptibility testing must be done in patients with relapsed disease. Based on sensitivity testing, new regimen that would include at least two new, previously unused agents should be started (e.g., a fluoroquinolone, amikacin, rifabutin, or ethambutol). The benefit of using macrolides despite development of resistance is unknown. Clofazimine is not recommended as trials have shown no efficacy and increased mortality with its use. Also important is use of appropriate ART regimen.

Treatment in Pregnancy

Clarithromycin has been associated with increased birth defects in certain animal studies; its use in first-trimester in humans showed increased risk of spontaneous abortion in one study so its use is not recommended in pregnant women. Azithromycin is recommended for primary prophylaxis and ethambutol plus azithromycin for secondary prophylaxis.

IRIS: IRIS is a relatively common feature of MAC treatment and occurs most commonly in the first 8 mos post-treatment, especially in mos 1–3 after initiating ART. Most common signs are fever and a focal inflammatory reaction such as lymphadenitis, pneumonitis, pericarditis, osteomyelitis, thoracic spine abscess, keratitis, peritonitis, skin abscesses, or the like. The incidence of MAC IRIS is reported at 3%, with three main clinical presentations: peripheral lymphadenitis, thoracic disease, and intraabdominal disease. Blood cultures are usually negative, but it is important to rule out therapeutic failure. Management of MAC IRIS includes continuation of ART and MAC therapy. Mild symptoms can be treated with nonsteroidal antiinflammatory drugs (NSAIDs); for severe disease, prednisone (20–60 mg/d) with slow taper can be used.

Pneumocystis jirovecii (Formerly P. carinii) Pneumonia

CLASSIFICATION AND NOMENCLATURE: Prior to 2002, the ubiquitous fungus *Pneumocystis jirovecii* was classified as a protozoan with the official name of *P. carinii*. Further investigation led to the discovery of two distinct species: *P. carinii* now refers strictly to a species which is specific to rats, while *P. jirovecii* is the opportunistic human pathogen. However, the abbreviation PCP continues to be used to refer to pneumocystis pneumonia.

EPIDEMIOLOGY: The majority of children develop serologic evidence of exposure by the age of 4 yrs. Disease can represent reactivation of latent disease or reinfection, as suggested by occasional outbreaks.

   PCP was the leading OI in patients with AIDS in the pre-HAART era, but rates of this infection since the beginning of the HAART era in 1996 have decreased substantially with the combination of ART and PCP prophylaxis. Most cases now occur in patients with undiagnosed HIV infection and in those with known HIV infection who are not receiving adequate ART and PCP prophylaxis. The major risk is a CD4 count of <200 cells/mL, previous PCP, or other factors that correlate with advanced HIV such as thrush, weight loss, and high HIV VLs.

CLINICAL FEATURES: PCP should be suspected in any patient with known or suspected HIV infection, a CD4 count of <200/mL, and typical clinical findings. The usual presentation is subacute onset and gradual progression of exertional dyspnea, nonproductive cough, fever, and chest pain. These symptoms evolve over several days or weeks. Physical exam is often negative except for fever, tachypnea, and tachycardia, with or without diffuse bilateral fine rales. Rarely, extrapulmonary disease is seen and is associated with use of pentamidine for prophylaxis. Many patients show other signs of advanced HIV infection including thrush and wasting. Patients with suspected PCP should have blood gases and HIV serology if HIV infection has not been confirmed.

RADIOGRAPHIC FINDINGS: Chest imaging usually shows diffuse bilateral, symmetrical interstitial infiltrates but can be normal during early stages. Less common findings include unilateral or apical infiltrates, cysts, pneumatoceles, adenopathy, effusion, or pneumothorax. Up to 18% of patients with PCP have a second process, including bacterial pneumonia or TB. A computed tomography (CT) scan is helpful if chest radiography is equivocal or normal.

LABORATORY FINDINGS: Hypoxemia is the cardinal finding of PCP. Blood gas testing typically shows reduced arterial O_2 and an increased alveolar-arterial (A-a) gradient that may be mild (A-a gradient <35 mm Hg), moderate (A-a gradient 35–45 mm Hg), or severe (A-a gradient >45 mm Hg). Post-exercise oxygen desaturation may facilitate the diagnosis in mild cases. Elevations of lactate dehydrogenase (>500 mg/dL), and 1,3 β-d-glucan are both sensitive but nonspecific.

Definitive diagnosis is usually established by demonstrating typical organisms in broncho-alveolar lavage (BAL) fluid or less sensitive induced sputum specimens. Biopsies are also highly sensitive (whether bronchoscopic, transbronchial, or via open biopsy), while spontaneously expectorated sputum is not recommended due to very low yield. Several stains are useful for detecting the characteristic cystic and trophic forms or cell walls of *P. jirovecii*. Sensitivity depends on the organism load, specimen quality, specimen source, and microbiology skill. Organisms remain detectable for several days after initiation of therapy; therefore, treatment should not be delayed in order to make the diagnosis.

PCR is highly sensitive and is increasingly utilized for diagnosis, although specificity can be as low as 85%. Although usually performed on BAL specimens, it has the advantage of being able to detect organisms in upper respiratory samples, including induced sputum and oral washes. A newer quantitative PCR may be a better at distinguishing between colonization versus infection.

PREVENTION: Indications for primary PCP prophylaxis: (1) CD4 count <200 cells/mL or CD4% <14%, (2) history of thrush, or (3) history of an AIDS-defining infection.

PROPHYLAXIS REGIMENS: TMP/SMX is the preferred agent due to efficacy and additional protection against toxoplasmosis and several bacterial infections when given at the recommended dose of 1 DS tab po daily. Lower dose of one SS tab daily or 1 DS tablet 3 times/week is also effective and may be better tolerated.

ALTERNATIVE PCP PROPHYLAXIS REGIMENS: (1) Dapsone100 mg/d; (2) dapsone 50 mg/d + pyrimethamine 50 mg/week + leucovorin 25 mg/week; (3) atovaquone 1,500 mg/d po with meals; (4) aerosolized pentamidine 300 mg by nebulization with a Respigard II nebulizer given monthly (the efficacy of other devices is unproven; also does not protect against toxoplasmosis).

STOPPING PCP PROPHYLAXIS: This is indicated when the CD4 count has been >200 cells/mL for >3 mos. Patients with suppressed VL and CD4 100–200 cells/mL remain at low risk for PCP.

TREATMENT: All courses are for 21 days. TMP/SMX remains the first-line agent and must be adjusted for renal function. Deterioration or lack of improvement within the first several days is common, and regimen should not be changed due to failure for at least 4–8 days.

MILD TO MODERATE DISEASE: Preferred: TMP/SMX 2 tabs tid (or total 5 mg/kg/dose tid based on TMP component). *Alternatives*: (1) Dapsone 100 mg po daily + TMP 15 mg/kg/d divided q8h; (2) primaquine 30 mg/d base po + clindamycin 450 mg po q6h; (3) atovaquone 750 mg po bid with food (less effective compared to TMP/SMX).

MODERATE TO SEVERE DISEASE: Preferred: TMP-SMX 5 mg/kg/dose (TMP component) IV q8h × 21 days. *Alternatives*: (1) Primaquine 30 mg/d base po + clindamycin 600 mg IV q6h; (2) pentamidine 4 mg/kg/d IV (reduce to 3 mg/kg/d for side effects)

Treatment with corticosteroids is associated with decreased mortality in severe disease. Patients with PaO_2 of <70 on room air or A-a gradient of ≥35 mm HG should receive prednisone 40 mg po bid × 5 days, then 40 mg/d × 5 days, then 20 mg/d for 11 days (or methylprednisolone at 75% of prednisone dose).

Secondary prophylaxis should begin as soon as the 21-day regimen is completed and is identical to primary prophylaxis in dosing and discontinuation.

Comments on Management

RELATIVE EFFICACY OF TREATMENTS: ACTG 108 showed TMP/SMX, TMP/dapsone, and clindamycin to be equally effective for mild to moderate PCP. A review of 1,122 HIV-infected patients in Denmark showed comparable 3-mo survival rates for HIV-associated PCP with TMP/SMX (85%), primaquine/clindamycin (81%), and IV pentamidine (76%). Aerosolized pentamidine should not be used for PCP therapy.

Resistance of *P jirovecii* to sulfonamides is suggested by mutations on the dihydropteroate synthase gene, but there does not appear to be an association with therapeutic failure. Patients who develop PCP despite TMP/SMX prophylaxis do not require alternate therapy.

ADVERSE DRUG REACTIONS: Adverse reactions to TMP/SMX for PCP have been reported in up to 80% of patients primarily rash (30–50%), leukopenia (30–40%), azotemia ((1–5%), hepatitis (20%), and thrombocytopenia (15%). Most can be treated through using antihistamines for rashes, antipyretics for fever, and antiemetics for nausea. The side effects of dapsone and primaquine include methemoglobinemia and hemolysis; pentamidine when administered systemically can cause hypoglycemia, hypotension, cardiac dysrhythmia, azotemia, and electrolyte abnormalities.

PREGNANCY: Therapy is identical to standard dosing, although primaquine should be avoided due to risk of maternal hemolysis. Folic acid 0.4 mg/d can be given to reduce risk of neural tube defect from TMP/SMX. However, addition of folinic acid has led to increased treatment failure and mortality; therefore folate supplementation should only be given within the first trimester.

4

Antiretroviral Therapy

Goals of Antiretroviral Therapy

The following goals of antiretroviral therapy (ART) follow the 2018 Department of Health and Human Services (DHHS) Guidelines.

CLINICAL GOALS: Reduce HIV-associated morbidity and mortality. Prolong life and improve quality of life.

VIROLOGIC GOALS: Maximal and durable suppression of plasma HIV RNA.

IMMUNOLOGIC GOALS: Restore and preserve immunologic function.

EPIDEMIOLOGIC GOALS: Prevent HIV transmission

Recommendations for Antiretroviral Therapy

Recommendations follow the 2018 DHHS Guidelines, the 2018 International Antiviral Society (IAS) USA, the 2015 British HIV Association (BHIVA) Guidelines (2016 Interim Update), the 2018 European AIDS Clinical Society (EACS), and the 2018 Update to the 2016 World Health Organization (WHO) Guidelines.

When to Start Antiretroviral Therapy

Patient readiness is the main determinant for initiating ART in most cases. Lower CD4 count and the presence of certain comorbid

TABLE 4.1 Antiretroviral drugs approved by the US Food and Drug Administration (FDA) for the treatment of HIV infection

Generic Name (Abbreviation)	Brand Name	Manufacturer	FDA Approval Date
Zidovudine (AZT, ZDV)	Retrovir	GlaxoSmithKline (ViiV)	March 1987
Didanosine (ddI)	Videx	Bristol-Myers Squibb	October 1991
Zalcitabine (ddC)[a]	Hivid	Hoffmann-La Roche	June 1992
Stavudine (d4T)	Zerit	Bristol-Myers Squibb	June 1994
Lamivudine (3TC)	Epivir	GlaxoSmithKline (ViiV)	November 1995
Saquinavir (SQV hgc)	Invirase	Hoffmann-La Roche	December 1995
Ritonavir (RTV)	Norvir	Abbvie	March 1996
Indinavir (IDV)	Crixivan	Merck	March 1996
Nevirapine (NVP)	Viramune	Boehringer Ingelheim	June 1996
Nelfinavir (NFV)	Viracept	Pfizer (ViiV)	March 1997
Delavirdine (DLV)[a]	Rescriptor	Pfizer (ViiV)	April 1997
Zidovudine/ Lamivudine (AZT/ 3TC)	Combivir	GlaxoSmithKline (ViiV)	September 1997
Saquinavir (SQV)[a]	Fortovase	Hoffmann-La Roche	November 1997
Efavirenz (EFV)	Sustiva	Bristol-Myers Squibb	September 1998
Abacavir (ABC)	Ziagen	GlaxoSmithKline (ViiV)	February 1999
Amprenavir (APV)[a]	Agenerase	GlaxoSmithKline (ViiV)	April 1999
Lopinavir/ritonavir (LPV/r)	Kaletra	Abbvie	September 2000
Zidovudine/ Lamuvudine/ Abacavir (AZT/ 3TC/ABC)	Trizivir	GlaxoSmithKline (ViiV)	November 2000

TABLE 4.1 Continued

Generic Name (Abbreviation)	Brand Name	Manufacturer	FDA Approval Date
Tenofovir DF (TDF)	Viread	Gilead Sciences	October 2001
Enfuvirtide (ENF)	Fuzeon	Hoffmann-La Roche	March 2003
Atazanavir (ATV)	Reyataz	Bristol-Myers Squibb	June 2003
Emtricitabine (FTC)	Emtriva	Gilead Sciences	July 2003
Fosamprenavir (FPV)	Lexiva	GlaxoSmithKline (ViiV)	November 2003
Abacavir/Lamivudine (ABC/3TC)	Epzicom	GlaxoSmithKline (ViiV)	August 2004
Tenofovir DF/ Emtricitabine (TDF/FTC)	Truvada	Gilead Sciences	August 2004
Tipranavir (TPV)	Aptivus	Boehringer Ingelheim	June 2005
Darunavir (DRV)	Prezista	Tibotec (Janssen)	June 2006
Tenofovir DF/ Emtricitabine/ Efavirenz (TDF/ FTC/EFV)	Atripla	Gilead Sciences/ Bristol-Myer Squibb	July 2006
Maraviroc (MVC)	Selzentry	Pfizer (ViiV)	August 2007
Raltegravir (RAL)	Isentress	Merck	October 2007
Etravirine (ETR)	Intelence	Tibotec (Janssen)	January 2008
Rilpivirine (RPV)	Edurant	Tibotec (Janssen)	May 2011
Tenofovir DF/ Emtricitabine/ Rilpivirine (TDF/ FTC/RPV)	Complera	Gilead Sciences/ Janssen	August 2011
Tenofovir DF/ Emtricitabine/ Elvitegravir/ cobicistat (TDF/ FTC/EVG/c)	Stribild	Gilead Sciences	August 2012

(continued)

TABLE 4.1 Continued

Generic Name (Abbreviation)	Brand Name	Manufacturer	FDA Approval Date
Dolutegravir (DTG)	Tivicay	ViiV Healthcare	August 2013
Abacavir/Lamivudine/ Dolutegravir (ABC/ 3TC/DTG)	Triumeq	ViiV Healthcare	August 2014
Atazanavir/cobicistat (ATV/c)	Evotaz	Bristol-Myers Squibb/Gilead Sciences	January 2015
Darunavir/cobicistat (DRV/c)	Prezcobix	Janssen Pharmaceuticals/ Gilead Sciences	January 2015
Tenofovir alafenamide/ Emtricitabine/ Elvitegravir/ cobicistat (TAF/ FTC/EVG/c)	Genvoya	Gilead Sciences	November 2015
Tenofovir alafenamide/ Emtricitabine/ Rilpivirine (TAF/ FTC/RPV)	Odefsey	Gilead Sciences/ Janssen	March 2016
Emtricitabine/ Tenorovir alafenamide (FTC/ TAF)	Descovy	Gilead Sciences	April 2016
Raltegravir, once daily (RAL)	Isentress HD	Merck	May 2017
Dolutegravir/ Rilpivirine (DTG/ RPV)	Juluca	ViiV Healthcare/ Janssen	November 2017
Bictegravir/ Emtricitabine/ Tenofovir alafenamide (BIC/ FTC/TAF)	Biktarvy	Gilead Sciences	February 2018

TABLE 4.1 Continued

Generic Name (Abbreviation)	Brand Name	Manufacturer	FDA Approval Date
Ibalizumab	Trogarzo	TaiMed Biologics	March 2018
Darunavir/ cobicistat/ Emtricitabine/ Tenofovir alafenamide (DRV/ c/FTC/TAF)	Symtuza	Janssen Pharmaceuticals/ Gilead Sciences	July 2018
Doravirine (DOR)	Pifeltro	Merck	August 2018
Doravirine/ Lamivudine/ Tenofovir DF (DOR/3TC/TDF)	Delstrigo	Merck	August 2018

aOut of market: No longer marketed or not available for general use.

TABLE 4.2 Classes of antiretroviral therapy (ART) drugs and examples of commonly used drugs in each class

Classes of ART Drugs and Examples of Commonly Used Drugs in Each Class	
Anti-CD4 monoclonal antibody Ibalizumab (IBA)	Binds to domain 2 of CD4 receptor causing a conformational change in the receptor preventing viral fusion and entry.
CCR5 co-receptor antagonist Maraviroc (MVC)	Binds to CCR5 and thereby, prevents HIV-1 from entering target cell.
Fusion inhibitor Enfurvitide (ENF)	Blocks gp41 transformation thereby preventing viral fusion and entry

(continued)

TABLE 4.2 Continued

Classes of ART Drugs and Examples of Commonly Used Drugs in Each Class

Nucleos(t)ide reverse transcriptase inhibitor (NRTI) Abacavir (ABC) Didanosine (ddI) Emtricitabine (FTC) Lamivudine (3TC) Stavudine (d4T) Tenofovir disoproxil fumarate (TDF)* Tenofovir alafenamide (TAF)* Zidovudine (AZT, ZDV)	Nucleotide/nucleoside analogs that act during viral DNA synthesis that leads to chain termination.
Non-nucleoside reserve transcriptase inhibitor (NNRTI) Doravirine (DOR) Efavirenz (EFV) Etravirine (ETR) Rilpivirine (RPV)	Binds to viral reverse transcriptase resulting in conformational changes and loss of enzymatic function.
Integrase strand transfer inhibitor (INSTI) Bictegravir (BIC) Dolutegravir (DTG) Elvitegravir (EVG) Raltegravir (RAL)	Binds to viral integrase causing conformational change and preventing insertion of viral DNA into host genome.
Protease inhibitor (PI) Darunavir (DRV) Atazanavir (ATV) Fosamprenavir (FPV) Lopinavir (LPV) Nelfinavir (NFV) Saquinavir (SQV) Tipranavir (TPV)	Bind and intact with viral protease inhibiting its ability to cleave polyprotein products of translation, preventing formation of mature virus.

*Tenofovir is a nucleotide analog, the rest are nucleoside analogs.

TABLE 4.3 Comparison of guideline recommendations for initiating antiretroviral therapy

Guidelines (Reference)	Recommendations (Strength of Recommendations)
2018 DHHS (March 27, 2018 revision)	*Treat All*, regardless of CD4 count (A1a)
2018 IAS-USA (JAMA 2018;320:379–396)	Chronic HIV infection: *Treat All*: As soon as possible after diagnosis.(A1a) AIDS or malignancy: Start within 2 wks of specific antimicrobial therapy for an AIDS-defining infection(A1a). Start immediately in setting of newly diagnosed malignancy(BIIa).
2015 British HIV Association (August 2016)	Chronic HIV infection: *Treat All* (1A) AIDS or a major infection: Start within 2 wks of specific antimicrobial therapy for an AIDS-defining infection, or with serious bacterial infection and a CD4 count <200 cells/µL (1B) Primary HIV infection: Immediate ART (1A)
2018 EACS (version 9.1, October 2018)	Chronic HIV infection: *Treat All*, irrespective of CD4 count, but the lower the CD4 count, the greater the urgency to start immediately Primary HIV infection: *Treat All*. Immediate treatment initiation advised on: 1. Acute infection 2. Severe or prolonged symptoms 3. Neurological disease 4. Age >50 yrs 5. CD4 count <350 cells/µL

(continued)

TABLE 4.3 Continued

Guidelines (Reference)	Recommendations (Strength of Recommendations)
2016 WHO (June 2016)	Age >19 yrs old: *Treat All*, at any CD4 count, regardless of WHO clinical stage(Strongly recommend, moderate quality evidence). Those with severe or advanced disease (WHO clinical stage 3 or 4) and CD4 count ≤ 350 cells/mm^3 are a priority (strongly recommend, moderate-quality evidence)
	Age 10–19 yrs old: *Treat all*, at any CD4 count, regardless of WHO clinical stage(Conditionally recommend, low quality evidence). Those with severe or advanced disease (WHO clinical stage 3 or 4) and CD4 count ≤ 350 cells/mm^3 are a priority (strong recommendation, moderate-quality evidence)
	Age 1 to <10 yrs old: *Treat all*, at any CD4 count, regardless of WHO clinical stage (conditionally recommend, low-quality evidence). Those aged ≤2 yrs or <5 yrs and with severe or advanced disease (WHO clinical stage 3 or 4) or CD4% <25% or CD4 count ≤750 cells/mm^3 are a priority, as are those 5 yrs old or older with severe or advanced disease (WHO clinical stage 3 or 4) or CD4% or CD4 count ≤350 (strong recommendation, moderate-quality evidence)
	Age <1 yr old: *Treat All*, at any CD4 count (strongly recommend, moderate-quality evidence)
	Pregnant and breastfeeding women: *Treat All*, at any CD4 count (strongly recommend, moderate-quality evidence)

conditions can increase the strength of recommendation, as well as the urgency to initiate ART. Several guidelines that deal with the treatment of HIV infection are nearly unified in endorsing that all HIV-infected persons should be treated irrespective of CD4 count, with a few caveats (Table 4.3).

Earlier recommendations relied on observational and cohort studies as the basis for the decision as to when to start ART. The *INSIGHT START* trial (N Engl J Med 2015;373:795) is one of the earliest randomized prospective trials that evaluated HIV-infected patients from 35 countries with CD4 counts of >500. This study enrolled 4,685 treatment-naïve participants who were randomized to either start receiving ART immediately or to wait until their CD4 count was <350. This trial demonstrated a 57% reduction in serious non-AIDS events or death in the early treatment arm. Most (59%) of the clinical events in the ART-deferred arm occurred while their CD4 counts were still high (>500 cells/mm^3). This study, in addition to the *TEMPRANO ANRS 12136* trial (N Engl J Med 2015;373:808), which showed similar benefits of early ART initiation in Cote d'Ivore, expanded the findings of *HPTN 052* (N Engl J Med 2011;365:493) and led to changes in treatment guidelines globally. Current guidelines from virtually all major global sources, including the WHO, recommend initiating treatment in patients defined as "ready" for what may be a lifelong treatment. The only difference in the various guidelines are the stratification of recommendations by strength of evidence or by prioritization of those with lower CD4 counts, AIDS-defining illnesses/advanced clinical HIV disease or comorbidities such as pregnancy, Hepatitis B (HBV), and HIV-associated nephropathy (Table 4.3). Guidelines from the US (2018 DHHS Guidelines and 2018 IAS-USA Guidelines) both recommend treatment of all HIV-infected individuals regardless of CD4 count. It is important to emphasize that the urgency for HIV treatment, the strength of the recommendations, and the quality of the evidence to support the recommendations correlate inversely with the CD4 count. Other conditions beyond "patient readiness" that contribute to the urgency of ART treatment include patient age, transmission risk, comorbidities, CD4 slope, HIV viral load (VL), and pregnancy.

The *INSIGHT START* and *TEMPRANO* trials led to the revision of most guidelines, including the 2018 DHHS and 2018 IAS-USA Guidelines, to recommend initiating ART for virtually all patients with HIV infection. Other studies that support the use of ART to prevent morbidity and mortality include the *NA-ACCORD* cohort study, which combined data for 22 cohorts in North America with >8,000 patients and 61,798 patient years of follow-up. This study showed a significant survival advantage with ART initiated at a CD4 count of 350–500 as opposed to waiting until below this threshold (odds ratio [OR] = 1.7; p <0.001) and with a CD4 count of >500 versus waiting until CD4 <500 (OR 1.94; p <0.001) (N Engl J Med 2009;360:1815). Other cohort studies also showed a survival benefit of ART initiated at higher CD4 counts including the *HIV-CASUAL Collaboration* study (AIDS 2010;24:123), which combined data from 12 cohorts with 62,760 HIV-infected patients included. This study showed an OR for survival that correlates inversely with CD4 count relative to no therapy: <100 cells/mm^3, 200–350 cells/mm^3, and >500 cells/mm^3 had ORs of 0.29, 0.55, and 0.77, respectively.

Early ART and Reducing HIV-related Immune Activation

The health consequences of immune activation have been implicated as a cause of morbidity and mortality associated with HIV infection. These include most of the non–AIDS-defining conditions that are now the dominant complications associated with HIV infection, such as cardiovascular disease, accelerated aging, liver, bone and metabolic disorders, non–AIDS-associated cancers, and neurocognitive dysfunction (N Engl J Med 2006;355:2283; Annu Rev Med 2011;62:141; BMJ 2009;338:3172). These complications are seen at all CD4 strata, and they correlate with elevations in biomarkers of immune dysfunction such as hsCRP, IL-6, and D-dimer (Curr Opin HIV AIDS 2010;5:498; PLoS Med 2008;5:e203). ART reduces the levels of these markers but not to normal levels (AIDS 2010;24:1657; PLoS Med 2008;5:e203; CID 2009;48:350; PLoS Med 2006;42:426).

Early ART in Preventing Sexual Transmission

There is a strong association between VL and probability of HIV transmission (N Engl J Med 2000;342:921). This was confirmed by *HPTN 052*, a large multinational trial comparing early versus deferred ART in HIV-infected patients with seronegative partners, which demonstrated 96% reduction in sexual transmission to the uninfected partner (N Engl J Med 2011;365:493). Two subsequent studies evaluating the risk of HIV transmission in discordant couples, the *PARTNER* Study and the *Opposites Attract Study*, both demonstrated a transmission risk estimate of zero when the HIV infected partner had a VL <200. After reviewing this data, the CDC released a letter on September 27, 2017, concluding, "When ART results in viral suppression, defined as less than 200 copies/mL or undetectable levels, it prevents sexual HIV transmission." It went on to explain, "This means that people who take ART daily, as prescribed, and achieve and maintain an undetectable VL have effectively no risk of sexually transmitting the virus to an HIV-negative partner." Finally, the letter noted that the limitation of this strategy was getting all HIV infected individuals, particularly gay and bisexual men living with HIV, access to care and treatment.

Early ART in Preventing Perinatal Transmission

It is well-established that ART in pregnancy prevents perinatal HIV transmission. When maternal HIV VL is suppressed (<50 c/mL) by the time of delivery, use of combination ART during pregnancy has dramatically reduced maternal-to-child transmission from approximately 20–30% down to 0.1–0.5% (Clin Infect Dis 2010;50:585; AIDS 2008;22:973).

Early ART in Lowering ART Resistance Risk

Reservations about early therapy in the past were often based on concerns about potential long-term complications of ART drugs and the prediction of increasing HIV resistance over time. However, the

30-plus years of experience with more than 30 ART drugs has taught us that current regimens are generally well tolerated, and long-term toxicity has become less concerning, including reduced use of drugs with predictable long-term consequences such as d4T, ddI, ddC, and IDV. Concerns about increased rates of resistance have been quelled by sequential testing showing that the rates of transmitted resistance are lower, presumably as results of better and earlier ART treatment (JAIDS 2009;51:450).

Summary of Benefits of Antiretroviral Therapy

See JAMA 2016;316:191.

1. Reduces mortality, serious AIDS-related and non–AIDS-related complications
2. Prevents development of AIDS and improves overall survival
3. Prevents progression of HIV-associated nephropathy
4. May reduce cardiovascular risk
5. Reduces incidence of Kaposi sarcoma and lymphoma
6. Improves cognitive function of those with HIV-associated neurocognitive disorder (HIV dementia)
7. Prevents acceleration of HBV and hepatitis C (HCV) infections
8. Reduce the risk of development of TB
9. Prevents HIV transmission

Special Co-Factor Considerations

The 2018 DHHS Guidelines have identified the following conditions as increasing the urgency for initiating ART, regardless of CD4 count:

Pregnant women: The purpose is to prevent perinatal transmission as well as to treat the mother.

HIV-associated nephropathy (HIVAN): since this condition may be seen at relatively high CD4 counts, the preventive benefits of ART are well established.

HBV co-infection: provide suppressive therapy for both HIV and HBV with drugs that are active against both viruses. Treating either infection alone risks development of resistance in the other virus and often leads to suboptimal drug therapy.

Acute or early HIV infection: There is increasing evidence that initiating ART during acute HIV infection has long-term benefits, including (1) reduction in transmission at a time of great risk (Ann Intern Med 2007;46:591; AIDS 2011;25:941), (2) reduction in symptoms of acute infection, and (3) reduction in the virologic set point and/or the rate of progression (J Infect Dis 2007;195:1762; J Infect Dis 2010;202:S2:S278; PLoS One 2012;7:e33948).

What Antiretroviral Regimen to Start

The Initial Regimen

Regimens recommended by virtually all guidelines are based on combinations that are most extensively used, well-studied, and have the best tolerability, accompanied by the least toxicity profile. This generally consists of regimens that combine two nucleoside/nucleotide reverse transcriptase inhibitor (NRTI) with an integrase strand transfer inhibitor (INSTI), a non-nucleoside reverse transcriptase inhibitor (NNRTI), or a protease inhibitor (PI) with a pharmacokinetic (PK) enhancer (booster). Tables 4.4 to 4.7 summarize the recommendations of the 2018 DHHS Guidelines, the 2018 IAS-USA Guidelines, the 2018 EACS Guidelines, and the 2015 BHIVA Guidelines(2016 Interim Update). The WHO Guidelines are found in and discussed in further details in Chapter 5.

Selection of the Two NRTIs

For more than a decade, NRTIs have been part of any ART combination regimen due to their inherent efficacy and relatively better tolerability compared with other earlier HIV drugs. Several dual or

TABLE 4.4 Recommended initial antiretroviral therapy (ART) regimen, 2018 DHHS Guidelines (October 2018)

Recommended Initial Regimens for Most People with HIV
Regimens with established durable virologic efficacy, favorable
  tolerability and toxicity profiles, and ease of use.

INSTI + 2 NRTIs:
- BIC/TAF/FTC (AI)
- DTG/ABC/3TC[a], *if HLA-B*5701 negative (AI)*
- DTG + tenofovir[b]/FTC[a] (*AI for both TAF/FTC and TDF/FTC*)
- RAL[c] + tenofovir[b]/FTC[a] (*AI for TDF/FTC, AII for TAF/FTC*)

Recommended Initial Regimens in Certain Clinical Situations
Regimens are effective and tolerable but have some disadvantages
  when compared with the above regimens or have less supporting
  data from randomized clinical trials. However, in certain clinical
  situation, one of these regimens may be preferred.

*Boosted PI + 2 NRTIs: (in general, boosted DRV is preferred over
boosted ATV)*
- (DRV/c or DRV/r) + tenofovir[b]/FTC[a] (*AI for DRV/r and AII for DRV/c*)
- (ATV/c or ATV/r) + tenofovir[b]/FTC[a] (*BI*)
- (DRV/c or DRV/r) + ABC/3TC[a], *if HLA-B*5701 negative (BII)*
- (ATV/c or ATV/r) + ABC/3TC[a], *if HLA-B*5701 negative and HIV RNA
  <100,000 c/mL (CI for ATV/r and CIII for ATV/c)*

NNRTI + 2 NRTIs:
- DOR/TDF/FTC or DOR + TAF/FTC
  EFV + tenofovir[b]/FTC[a] (*BI for EFV/TDF/FTC and BII for EFV + TAF/
  FTC*)
- RPV/ tenofovir[b]/FTC[a] – *if HIV RNA <100,000 c/mL and CD4 >200
  cells/mm³ (BI)*

INSTI + 2 NRTIs:
- EVG/c/tenofovir[b]/FTC (*AI for both TAF/FTC and TDF/FTC*)
- RAL[c] + ABC/3TC[a], *if HLA-B*5701 negative and HIV RNA <100,000 c/
  mL (CII)*

Regimens to consider when ABC, TAF, and TDF cannot be used:
- DTG + 3TC
- DRV/r + RAL (bid), *if HIV RNA <100,000 c/mL and CD4 >200 cells/
  mm³ (CI)*
- DRV/r(once daily) + 3TC[a] (*CI*)

TABLE 4.4 Continued

[a] 3TC may be substituted for FTC, or vice versa, if a non-fixed dose NRTI combination is desired.

[b] TAF and TDF are two forms of tenofovir approved by FDA.

[c] RAL can be given as 400 mg bid or 1,200 mg (two 600 mg tablets) once daily.

Note: Recommendations for those who are pregnant or of childbearing potential (May 30, 2018). These recommendations were generated after a report of neural tube defects in four infants born to women taking DTG in Botswana:

- A negative pregnancy test is recommended prior to initiating DTG.
- The risks and benefits of DTG use should be discussed with all women who are pregnant, desire to become pregnant, or are of childbearing potential.
- ARV-naïve or considering switch to DTG:
  - Do not start a DTG-based regimen in those who are pregnant and <8 wks from last menstrual period (LMP).
  - If pregnant and >8 wks from LMP, use DTG or other ARV drug.
  - Do not start a DTG-based regimen in those who desire pregnancy or are not using effective contraception.
  - DTG can be used in those who do not desire pregnancy and are using effective contraception.
- Currently taking DTG:
  - Switch DTG to alternative if pregnant and <8 wks from LMP. Do not stop DTG without replacing it with an effective ART.
  - Can continue DTG in those who are pregnant and >8 wks from LMP.
  - Switch DTG to alternative in those who desire pregnancy or who are not using effective contraception.
  - Continue DTG in those who do not desire pregnancy and are using effective contraception.

triple ART co-formulations containing one or more NRTI were commercially available as early as 1997.

Current guidelines favor tenofovir/FTC (either TDF/FTC or TAF/FTC) as their recommended NRTI pair based on ease of administration, potency, experience, tolerability, and toxicity. ABC/3TC is considered an alternative NRTI pair except when paired with dolutegravir, where it becomes recommended. Both are co-formulated and given as one

TABLE 4.5 Recommended initial antiretoviral therapy (ART) regimens, 2018 IAS-USA

Generally recommended initial regimens

Regimen	Ratings
BIC/TAF/FTC	AIa
DTG/ABC/3TC	AIa
DTG + TAF/FTC[a]	AIa

Recommended initial regimens for individuals for whom generally recommended regimens are not available or not an option

DRV/c + TAF(or TDF)/FTC[a]	AIa
DRV/r + TAF(or TDF)/FTC[a]	AIa
EFV/TDF/FTC	AIa
EVG/c/TAF(or TDF)/FTC[a]	AIa
RAL + TAF(or TDF)/FTC[a]	AIa for TDF
RPV/TAF(or TDF)/FTC [a](if RNA <100,000 and CD4 >200)	AIa

TDF is not recommended for those with or at risk for kidney or bone disease.

[a]In setting when TAF/FTC is not available or there are large cost differences, TDF (with FTC or 3TC) remains an effective and generally well-tolerated option. Note that this is particularly the case if the patient does not have or is at high risk for kidney or bone disease.

pill daily. TDF/FTC has been the mainstay NRTI pair for quite some time due to its efficacy and tolerability when combined in an ART regimen. TAF/FTC has been more recently approved and is available in several single-tablet combination regimens including combination with boosted elvitegravir (Genvoya), rilpivirine (Odefsey), and bictegravir (Biktarvy). TAF/FTC is overtaking TDF/FTC due to co-formulation advantages, as well as reduced bone and renal toxicities, compared to TDF/FTC in 48 wk studies.

3TC and FTC: Virtually all regimens include either 3TC or FTC, which are similar except for their half-life; both have few side effects. Both are active against HBV (with the potential for a severe flare of HBV if withdrawn or HBV resistance develops). Both also select for the M184V mutation. Continued use of either 3TC or FTC in the

TABLE 4.6 Initial combination antiretroviral therapy (ART) Regimen, 2018 European AIDS Clinical Society (Guidelines Version 9.1)

Recommended Regimens	Alternative Regimens (To Be Used When None of the Preferred Regimen is Feasible or Available, Whatever the Reason)
2 NRTIs + INSTI • ABC/FTC/DTG[a] • (TAF/FTC or TDF/FTC) + DTG • (TAF/FTC or TDF/FTC) + RAL **2 NRTIs + NNRTI** • (TAF or TDF)/FTC/RPV **2 NRTIs + boosted PI** • (TAF/FTC or TDF/FTC) + (DRV/c or DRV/r)	**2 NRTIs + INSTI** • ABC/3TC[a] + RAL • (TAF or TDF)/FTC/EVG/c **2 NRTIs + NNRTI** • ABC/3TC[a] + EFV • TDF/FTC/EFV **2 NRTIs + boosted PI** • (TAF/FTC or TDF/FTC) + (ATV/c or ATV/r) • ABC/3TC[a] + (DRV/c or DRV/r) • ABC/3TC[a] + (ATV/c or ATV/r) **INSTI + boosted PI** • RAL + (DRV/c or DRV/r) **INSTI + 3TC** • DTG + 3TC

[a]ABC contraindicated if HLA-B[a]5701 positive.

presence of the M184V mutation provides residual but reduced activity against HIV and does not risk acquiring additional NRTI resistance mutations. In addition, the presence of M184V mutation reduces viral fitness (i.e., viral ability to replicate). Although the clinical significance of this is unknown.

TDF/FTC is co-formulated as Truvada. It is also co-formulated with EFV (Atripla), with RPV (Complera), and with EVG/cobicistat (Stribild) to allow one pill, once daily dosing. In a trial comparing TDF/FTC versus AZT/3TC each in combination with EFV, the TDF/FTC recipients had superior results at 144 wks in terms of

TABLE 4.7 Recommended choice of antiretroviral therapy (ART), 2015 British HIV Association Guidelines (Interim Update August 2016)

	Preferred	Alternative
NRTI backbone	Tenofovir and FTC	ABC and 3TC[a,b]
Third agent (alphabetical order)	ATV/r DRV/r DTG EVG/c[c] RAL RPV[d]	EFV

[a]ABC contraindicated if HLA-B*5701 positive.

[b]Use recommended only if baseline VL <100,000 c/mL, except when in combination with DTG.

[c]TDF/FTC/EVG/c fixed dose combination (FDC) should not be initiated in people with CrCl <70 mL/min.

[d]Use recommended only if baseline VL <100,000 c/mL.

viral suppression to <50 c/mL (80% vs. 70%), CD4 count improvement (mean 312 vs. 271 cells/mm³), discontinuation due to adverse reactions (4% vs. 9%), limb fat atrophy by dual-energy X-ray absorptiometry (DEXA) scan, and a number of M184V mutations (N Engl J Med 2006;354:251; JAIDS 2006; 43:535). A comparative trial (ACTG 5202) of TDF/FTC versus ABC/3TC, each with either ATV/r or EFV, showed an increased rate of virologic failure in the ABC/3TC recipients with a baseline VL of >100,000 c/mL (N Engl J Med 2009; 361:2230). There was no significant difference in virologic outcomes noted in patients with baseline VL of <100,000 c/mL, although there were differences in safety endpoints favoring TDF/FTC (Ann Intern Med 2011; 154:445). Other comparative trials noted no difference in outcomes between TDF/FTC vs. ABC/3TC (AIDS 2009;23:1547). The disadvantages of TDF include poor central nervous system (CNS) penetration (of uncertain significance), renal toxicity, and greater loss of bone mineral density compared to other agents. The potential for renal toxicity makes TDF an unsuitable option if there is preexisting renal disease, particularly with a creatinine clearance of <50 mL/min. Use of TDF requires regular monitoring of renal function in all patients. Guidance on methods to monitor bone mineral density in TDF recipients are unclear, but caution is advised in patients with osteoporosis or osteopenia. TDF and FTC are both active against HBV, making this a preferred dual NRTI backbone in combination with a third antiretroviral agent to treat HIV/HBV co-infections (N Engl J Med 2007;356:1445; Hepatology 2006;44:1110; Clin Infect Dis 2010;51:1201).

TAF/FTC is co-formulated as Descovy. It is also available as a once-daily fixed dose combination (FDC) pill with cobicistat-boosted EVG (Genvoya), with RPV (Odefsey), with BIC (Biktarvy), and with DRV/cobicistat (Symtuza). In two large phase 3, randomized, double-blind studies the combination of TAF/FTC with EVG/cobicistat demonstrated similar efficacy as TDF/FTC/EVG/cobicistat and had reduced bone and renal negative effects. The requirement of only 10 mg of TAF provides an advantage of easier co-formulation with other agents. TAF/FTC is currently recommended as a first-line drug option in the 2018 DHHS, 2018 IAS-USA, and 2018 European (EACS) guidelines.

ABC/3TC is co-formulated as Epzicom, for once-daily administration in combination with a third agent. It is also co-formulated with DTG (Triumeq) in one pill and dosed once daily. Initially, ABC use was complicated by potentially serious hypersensitivity reaction (HSR), but this risk has been essentially eliminated by pretreatment testing for HLA-B5701 (N Engl J Med 2008; 358:568). ABC has the advantage over TDF of having no renal toxicity, but the disadvantage of possible reduced potency in patients with a baseline VL of >100,000 c/mL (see ACTG 5202: Ann Intern Med 2011; 154:445) and a possible increased risk of cardiovascular events. Both disadvantages are inconsistent across studies, making conclusions difficult. The most recent guidelines note that there is no decrease in potency at VL of >100,000 c/mL when used in combination with DTG. Although some recommend use of ABC/3TC in combination with other agents only if baseline VL is <100,000 c/mL, the British guidelines list ABC/3TC as an alternative for these reasons except when used in combination with dolutegravir, where ABC/3TC is recommended at any VL. There is a cautionary note for ABC use in patients with multiple cardiovascular disease risk factor in all of the guidelines. The main evidence for the risk of myocardial infarction (MI) is derived from data gathered from the D:A:D retrospective analysis of 33,347 patients, which found an OR for MI with ABC use of 1.9 (p <0.003) compared to other ART agents (Lancet 2008;371:1417). Similar associations were also shown in the SMART, STEAL, and a number of other studies. But in other studies, including a meta-analysis by the US Food and Drug Administration (FDA), this association with MI has not been observed. The DHHS Guidelines state that no consensus has been reached on this association or a potential mechanism to explain this association. The ABC/3TC (Epzicom) package insert states that the data are inconclusive.

AZT/3TC is co-formulated as Combivir and has been extensively used since 1997. It is now generic. This combination is no longer recommended for initial therapy due to decreased virologic and CD4 response compared to a TDF/FTC backbone, the need for twice-daily dosing, and greater toxicities and side effects including GI intolerance, fatigue, bone marrow suppression, lipoatrophy, and lactic acidosis. It is listed in the WHO guidelines as an alternative regimen largely due to the fact that it is generic. The pivotal randomized controlled trial GS934 compared AZT/3TC with TDF/FTC, each combined with EFV, and showed TDF/FTC recipients had better outcome in terms of viral suppression (80% vs. 70% for VL <50 c/mL, $p = 0.02$) and increase in CD4 count (190 cells/mm^3 vs. 158 cells/mm^3, $p = 0.002$) after 48 wks of follow-up (NEJM 2006; 354:251).

ddI+3TC or ddI+FTC: ddI-containing regimens have fallen out of favor due to their extensive toxicities including pancreatitis, peripheral neuropathy, and lactic acidosis. There is also a possible association with non-cirrhotic portal hypertension. In addition, clinical experience with this combination is limited, and most trials of ddI with either 3TC or FTC have been either been noncomparative or have used nonstandard comparators. One trial using a combination of ddI, FTC, and EFV given once daily demonstrated good viral suppression (Antivir Ther 2003; 8 Suppl 1:594).

AZT, d4T, and ddI: Thymidine analogs and ddI are not recommended in the US and European guidelines primarily due to their mitochondrial toxicities. These agents are still used in combination with 3TC in resource-limited countries due to economic considerations and are considered generally safe, so long as there is adequate monitoring for toxicities.

NRTI pairings to avoid: 3TC+FTC (redundant antiviral activity), AZT+d4T (antagonistic), ddI+d4T (potentiation of toxicities), TDF+ddI (high rate of virologic failure, resistance, increased ddI toxicity, and blunted CD4 response).

AZT/3TC/ABC: This combination is no longer recommended by the guidelines due to its inferiority to AZT/3TC+EFV in treatment-naïve patients (N Engl J Med 2004; 350:1850). It should be noted that this "triple nucleoside regimen" was a preferred regimen for treatment-naïve patients until the release of the ACTG 5095 results in 2003.

Selection of the Initial Third ART Drug

Regimen selection is based on efficacy, safety, tolerability, genetic barrier to resistance, and ease of use. In addition, it is important to take into consideration each individual's co-morbidities and concomitant medications, as well as the potential for drug–drug interactions. More recently, INSTI-based regimens have been preferred by most guidelines due to their high efficacy, favorable safety profile, and, with regard to DTG and RAL, minimal to no significant CYP3A4-associated drug interactions.

Integrase Strand Transfer Inhibitor (INSTI): Raltegravir (RAL) was the first INSTI approved for commercial use in 2007. Thereafter, three other INSTIs have been discovered and approved for use: namely, elvitegravir (EVG), dolutegravir (DTG), and, more recently, bictegravir (BIC). INSTIs have a rapid and potent antiviral activity that subsequently reduces the time in which viral suppression occurs. All these agents are highly efficacious, well-tolerated, and have demonstrated at the least noninferiority to other regimens using other classes, including PI- and NNRTI-based ones. DTG demonstrated superiority to DRV/r (Lancet 2014; 383:2222) and ATV/r (Lancet HIV 2017; 4:e536) and is the first agent to demonstrate superiorly against EFV in clinical trials (N Engl J Med 2013; 369:1807).

Dolutegravir (DTG) was approved based on three Phase 3 trials: SPRING-2, SINGLE, and FLAMINGO. In the SPRING-2 study, DTG was found to be noninferior to RAL when in combination with investigator-chosen NRTIs (Lancet Infect Dis 2013; 13:927). In SINGLE, DTG, in combination with ABC/3TC, demonstrated superiority to EFV/TDF/FTC, which was largely attributed to a higher discontinuation rate due to adverse events (AEs) (mainly neuropsychiatric side effects) in the EFV arm (N Engl J Med 2013; 369:1807). Similarly in the FLAMINGO trial, DTG with NRTIs was superior to DRV/r with NRTIs due to a higher discontinuation rate in the DRV/r group (Lancet 2014;383:2222). It should be noted that in VL of >100,000 c/mL, DTG had a higher rate of response than DRV/r. DTG has also been found to be superior to ATV/r mostly due to the ATV/r-arm having higher discontinuation rates due AEs in the ARIA trial (Lancet HIV 2017;4:e546). As noted earlier, DTG was the first backbone drug to demonstrate superiority to an EFV-based regimen. DTG is well-tolerated, with the most frequent side effects being headaches and insomnia. The ability to take DTG with or without food, its relatively few drug interactions, its co-formulation with ABC/3TC in a single-tablet regimen, and its high efficacy and tolerability has led both US and European guidelines to list DTG as a preferred agent.

Bictegravir (BIC) is co-formulated with TAF/FTC in a single FDC pill. The two registrational studies that led to the approval of BIC both compared it to DTG. BIC/TAF/FTC, as a once-daily FDC, was compared to DTG/ABC/3TC in GS-US-380-1489 (Lancet 2017;390:2063), while it was compared to DTG plus TAF/FTC in GS-US-380-1490 (Lancet 2017;390:2073). In both trials, BIC was found to be non-inferior to DTG after 48 wks of follow-up. There was no treatment-emergent resistance that developed to any of the study drugs. AEs were similar between groups.

Elvitegravir (EVG) requires cobicistat, a cytochrome P450 inhibitor, to be administered once daily. It is currently only co-formulated in a single-tablet regimen with cobicistat and TDF/FTC or TAF/FTC. In Phase 3 randomized clinical trials, EVG/c/TDF/FTC has been shown to be non-inferior to EFV/TDF/FTC (Lancet 2012; 379:2439) and to ATV/r plus TDF/FTC (Lancet 2012; 379:2429). EVG/c/TAF/FTC has been demonstrated to be non-inferior to EVG/c/TDF/FTC, but with reduced bone and renal effects (Lancet 2015; 385:2606). Although long-term data are still pending, the reduced renal and bone effects with EVG/c in combination with TAF/FTC is encouraging. Based on these data and use of cobicistat, both combinations using EVG/c are recommended in certain clinical situations and as an alternative in the DHHS and European guidelines, respectively.

Raltegravir (RAL) is the first commercially available INSTI. RAL can now be administered as 400 mg twice daily or 1200 mg once daily. In the STARTMRK study, RAL was compared to EFV, with each arm combined with TDF/FTC, in 566 treatment-naïve patients (Lancet 2009; 374:796). At 48 wks, HIV viral suppression (VL <50 c/mL) was seen in 86% of RAL recipients versus 82% of EFV recipient and therefore was non-inferior to the EFV arm. Notable is that RAL recipients had a significantly shorter time to viral suppression (though of no clear clinical significance), significantly fewer side effects leading to drug discontinuation, higher CD4 count response, and less hyperlipidemia (J Infect Dis 2011; 203:1204). At years 4 and 5, RAL was superior to EFV driven largely by discontinuations due to adverse events. RAL is a potent integrase inhibitor with few drug interactions and an excellent tolerability profile. Its main disadvantage is its low barrier to resistance, with cross-resistance to EVG, but not to DTG, as well as the lack of available a FDC and thus requiring higher pill burden over its competitors.

NNRTIs: ACTG 5142 is an important study assessing the relative merits of NNRTI versus ritonavir-boosted PI (PI/r)-based ART regimens. At 96 wks, the combination of EFV plus two NRTIs was found to be virologically superior (89% vs. 77% for VL <50 c/mL,

p = 0.006) compared to a PI/r-based one. However, ritonavir-boosted lopinavir (LPV/r) recipients had a greater increase in median CD4 count (285 cells/mm^3 vs. 240 cells/mm^3, p = 0.01), and failure with LPV/r resulted in fewer major resistant mutations (0 vs. 16) (N Engl J Med 2008; 358:2095). This barrier to resistance seen with LPV/r applies to other PI/r-based ART regimens including DRV/r, ATV/r, FPV/r, and SQV/r. The protection generally applies to the accompanying NRTI, as well. By contrast, virologic failure on EFV- or NVP-based ART regimens commonly results in resistance to EFV and NVP, as well as against some of the co-administered NRTIs. Recently, a new non-nucleoside reverse transcriptase inhibitor, Doravirine, active against NNRTI mutations such as the K103N and a number of others, has been evaluated in treatment-naïve patients in combination with TDF/3TC and was non-inferior to TDF/FTC/EFV; Doravirine had a lower rate of resistance, less neuropsychiatric side effects, and a favorable lipid profile in comparison to efavirenz. It has also been demonstrated to be non-inferior to DRV/r in treatment-naïve patients. Doravirine was approved by the FDA in 2018.

Efavirenz (EFV) has the advantage of having been extensively used since its FDA approval in 1998. EFV is part of the first one pill, once daily triple combination therapy with TDF/FTC (Atripla) that was approved in 2006. At that time, Atripla was the only single pill 3-in-1 drug agent to treat HIV infection, and therefore earlier guidelines preferred it due to its convenience factor. Recent availability of several well-tolerated once-daily FDC ARTs supplanted EFV-based regimens, and it is now an alternative agent. The main toxicity of EFV noted in current guidelines is the higher incidence of suicidality compared to other regimens based on the analysis of four ACTG trials (Ann Intern Med 2014;161:1–10). This has not been corroborated in observational studies. In addition, the potential teratogenic effects of EFV have been a major concern in the past that precluded its use during the first trimester of pregnancy or in women of childbearing potential. More recent data found no evidence of increased risk of congenital abnormalities associated with first-trimester exposure to EFV (AIDS 2014; 28:S123). Other major concerns with EFV are its low genetic barrier to resistance and its common neuropsychiatric side effects. The frequency of baseline resistance to EFV is comparatively high, and there is a possibility of minor resistant variants that may predict failure but are missed with standard genotypic resistance testing at baseline (J Infect Dis 2010;201:662). The uncertainty about long-term psychiatric complications with EFV (JAIDS 2006; 29:865; J Int AIDS Soc 2014; 17–4 Suppl 3:19512) and its metabolic consequences including hyperlipidemia (AIDS 2009; 23:1109; JAIDS 2010; 55:39) remain concerns.

Rilpivirine (RPV) is co-formulated with TDF/FTC (Complera), TAF/FTC (Odefsey), and with DTG (Juluca). The phase 3 ECHO and THRIVE studies (AIDS 2016; 30:251) for RPV showed that this agent was non-inferior to EFV, with both arms combined with TDF/FTC, with virologic suppression to <50 c/mL of about 76–77% on both arms. But in those people with baseline HIV VL of >100,000 c/mL, there was a higher rate of virologic failures in the RPV arm (22% failures) compared to EFV arm's 12% at 96 wks follow-up. RPV was nevertheless better tolerated than EFV, with significantly fewer discontinuations due to AEs (3.0% vs. 11%, P <0.001). RPV in combination with TAF/FTC was based on a couple of switch studies showing that RPV/TAF/FTC was non-inferior to RPV/TDF/FTC (Lancet HIV 2017; 4:e195; Lancet HIV 2017; 4:e205). The SWORD-1 and SWORD-2 studies are two identical phase 3 switch trials that evaluated dual ART with RPV/DTG as a once-daily FDC pill regimen (Lancet 2018;doi:10.1016/S0140-6736(17)33095-7) and compared it to a current ART regimen. The open-label, multicenter studies showed that RPV/DTG was non-inferior to the current ART regimen with suppression maintained over 48 wks follow-up (94.7% vs. 94.9%) and, more recently, 100 weeks. RPV is a well-tolerated agent with a favorable safety profile, but concerns for higher failures with high baseline VL limit its use in certain situations.

Doravirine (DOR) is available alone (Pifeltro), and co-formulated with TDF/3TC (Delstrigo). The drug was recently approved by the FDA based on two phase 3 studies, DRIVE-FORWARD and DRIVE-AHEAD (Lancet HIV 2018 May;5(5):e211–e220; Clin Infect Dis

2018 Aug 31. [Epub ahead of print]). In DRIVE-FORWARD, DOR was compared to DRV/r in combination with investigator selected NRTIs. At 48 weeks, DOR was non-inferior to the DRV/r (84% vs. 80% HIV RNA <50 c/mL). Protocol-defined virologic failure was seen in 5% and 6% of patients treated with DOR and DRV/r but only 1 patient developed resistance to DOR. There was no resistance in the DRV/r arm. Adverse events were similar in both arms but there was a higher rate of diarrhea with DRV/r (13% vs. 5%). Lipids increased in the DRV/r arm and slightly decreased in the DOR arm; there were similar increases in HDL in both arms. DOR was demonstrated to be non-inferior to EFV in the DRIVE-AHEAD study (84.3% vs. 80.8%, respectively). NNRTI resistance development was similar in both arms. There were higher rates of drug-related AEs in the EFV arm compared to DOR (63% vs. 31%). Neuropsychiatric symptoms were significantly lower in the DOR arm, and DOR had more favorable lipid changes compared with EFV. In vitro, DOR has activity against the K103N mutation as well as other NNRTI mutations. Overall, DOR is a well-tolerated agent with similar efficacy to DRV/r and EFV, but with favorable safety and lipid profiles compared to those agents.

PIs: Multiple ritonavir-boosted PIs appear comparably potent based on randomized clinical trials in treatment naïve HIV patients demonstrating similar virologic outcomes (VL <50 c/mL by intention-to-treat analysis at 48 wks or more). The flagship trials comparing PI/r versus LPV/r are:

- *KLEAN*: FPV/r vs. LPV/r (Lancet 2006; 365:476)
- *GEMINI*: SQV/r vs. LPV/r (J AIDS 2009; 50:367)
- *CASTLE*: ATV/r vs. LPV/r (Lancet 2008; 372:646)
- *ARTEMIS*: DRV/r vs. LPV/r (AIDS 2008; 22:1389)

The two PI-based regimens that are currently favored in the guidelines for treatment naïve patients are boosted darunavir (either DRV/r or DRV/c) and boosted atazanavir (either ATV/r or ATV/c). Both DRV/r and ATV/r have proved non-inferiority or superiority to LPV/r in viral suppression, with better tolerability and fewer lipid effects in the ARTEMIS and CASTLE trials, respectively. A more recent ACTG 5257 trial comparing DRV/r, ATV/r, and RAL demonstrated similar efficacy among the three groups but higher discontinuation in the ATV/r group due to AEs (Ann Intern Med 2014; 161:461).

With regards to current guidelines, DRV/r and ATV/r remain in the preferred option category of the British HIV association guidelines, but are not recommended for most in the US guidelines. European guidelines have DRV/r as a preferred option, only if in combination with TAF/FTC or TDF/FTC; otherwise, DRV/r and ATV/r are now alternative regimens.

Darunavir (DRV) is recommended in the European guidelines and recommended in certain clinical situations in the US guidelines. In ACTG 5257, the ritonavir-boosted darunavir (DRV/r)-containing arm demonstrated similar efficacy to ATV/r and RAL, with a lower discontinuation rate as compared to ATV/r but similar to RAL (Ann Intern Med 2014; 161:461). Its potency and tolerability were apparent from the ARTEMIS trial, whereby 79% of 343 treatment naïve patients who were given once-daily DRV/r had VL of <50 c/mL at 96 wks (AIDS 2009; 23:1679). Viral suppression in those with baseline VL of >100,000 c/mL was 76% and in those with baseline CD4 counts of <200 cells/mm^3 was 79%. DRV/r was better tolerated from a GI standpoint than LPV/r and had less hyperlipidemia side effects than LPV/r. However, DRV/r was found to be inferior to DTG in the FLAMINGO study, largely due to higher discontinuation rates related to AEs (Lancet 2014; 383:2222). Another disadvantage of DRV/r is the potential for rashes, which can sometimes be treatment-limiting.

Cobicistat-boosted darunavir (DRV/c) in combination with TDF/FTC in a single-arm Phase 3 trial had similar efficacy, pK, and tolerability outcomes compared to historical data using DRV/r (800 mg/100 mg once-daily dosing) (J Int AIDS Soc 2014; 17(4 Suppl 3):19772). Based on these data, DRV/c was approved by the FDA and is listed as recommended in certain situations in the DHHS guidelines. DRV/c when given in combination with TDF/FTC is not recommended for use in patients with a creatinine clearance rate (CrCl) of <70 mL/min.

A single-tablet regimen of DRV co-formulated with cobicistat, TAF, and FTC has been approved for use in the United States and the European Union under the trade name Symtuza. This was based on the AMBER trial, which compared this single-tablet regimen with DRV/c + TAF/FTC in treatment naïve patients, and the EMERALD trial, which evaluated those switching from a boosted PI + TDF/FTC to the single-table regimen. Both studies demonstrated high virologic suppression rates with the single-table regimen.

Atazanavir (ATV): ATV/r was compared to EFV in ACTG 5202, which included 928 subjects who were randomized to take either TDF/FTC or ABC/3TC with either EFV or ATV/r. Virologic outcomes at 96 wks were similar between EFV and ATV/r, with hazard ratio for virologic failure of 1.01 for EFV recipients and 1.13 for ATV/r recipients although prespecified definitions for equivalence were not met (*p* = NS) (Ann Intern Med 2011; 154:445). However, there were marked differences in the frequency of resistance mutations: the frequency of EFV resistance mutations in patients failing EFV therapy was 68/126 (54%), while only 7/38 (5%) among those who failed ATV/r developed major PI-resistant mutations. The companion NRTIs were also protected from NRTI resistance mutations among ATV/r recipients during virologic failure—NRTI resistance emerged in 12% versus 37% (*p* = 0.0003). Nevertheless, ATV/r had a higher discontinuation rate due to side effects when compared with DRV/r and RAL in ACTG 5257 (Ann Intern Med 2014; 161:461). Of these, 48% were due to jaundice or elevated bilirubin levels. This led to ATV/r being moved to the recommended in certain clinical situations section of the current guidelines. Other disadvantages of ATV/r include potential jaundice or scleral icterus, the need to take a meal with each dosing, the need for gastric acidity for adequate bioavailability, the possibility of both nephrolithiasis (although rare) and nephrotoxicity, drug interactions with concurrent use of TDF or EFV, the need for dose adjustment with hepatic insufficiency, and poor CNS penetration (unclear significance). In the ARIA study, ATV/r was compared with DTG, with a virologic suppression rate of

71% (vs. 82% in DTG arm). The difference was driven by both lower virologic response and higher discontinuation rates related to AEs in the ATV/r arm (Lancet HIV 2017; 4:e536).

Cobicistat-boosted atazanavir (ATV/c) has been demonstrated to be non-inferior to ATV/r when combined with TDF/FTC (J Infect Dis 2013; 208:32). Both ATV/r and ATV/c had similar toxicities (including renal and bilirubin effects) and had similar discontinuation rates. Based on these data and the relative lack of experience with ARV/c, the DHHS guidelines have listed it as recommended in certain situations for patients with a CrCl of >70 mL/min.

CCR5 Co-receptor Antagonist: Generally not used as a first-line agent mainly due to the need to determine if the virus is an R5 variant prior to use. There is only one CCR5 antagonist available in commercial use, and it is Maraviroc (MVC).

Maraviroc: The MERIT trial in both guidelines compared MVC against EFV, both in combination with AZT/3TC patients with R5 virus as screening (J Infect Dis 2010; 201:803). The once-daily MVC was stopped early due to excessive rates of virologic failure. At 48 wks (n = 721), MVC was inferior to EFV for suppression to <50 c/mL, but overall results were not significantly different when adjusted for erroneous baseline tropism screening using the more sensitive tropism assay, which is in current use. The main difference in outcome after the tropism adjustment was the reason for failure. More MVC discontinuations were for viral failure (12% vs. 4%), and more EFV discontinuation were for adverse reactions (4% in MVC arm vs. 14% in EFV arm). The 96-wk results of this trial showed similar rates of suppression with <50 c/mL in 59% of MVC recipients versus 63% of EFV recipients (HIV Clin Trials 2010; 11:125). Other analyses of the MERIT data found that MVC recipients had greater CD4 cell increases at 96 wks (medial 212 vs. 171 cells/mm^3 increase) (HIV Clin Trials 2010; 11:125), better lipid profiles (HIV Clin Trials 2011; 12:24), and slightly better impact on markers of immune activation (PLoS One 2010; 5:e13188). It is not listed as an initial drug option in the DHHS guidelines for ARV-naïve patients due to the need for CCR5 tropism testing, twice-daily dosing, and the perceived lack of benefit over other regimens.

Individualized Selection of the Initial Regimen

Previous discussions dealt primarily with relative potency of available agents. Selection of an appropriate regimen also requires consideration of patient-specific issues. These include the following:

- Prior resistance test results
- Co-morbidities, including cardiovascular, renal, hepatic, or metabolic disease, as well as mental health disorders
- Concurrent drugs
- Pregnancy or pregnancy potential
- Patient preference, including issues of pill burden, number of doses, and food requirements
- Baseline test results, including VL (whether >100,000 c/mL or not) and HLA-B*5701 test results if ABC is being considered.
- HBV co-infection
- Acute HIV infection: If treatment is to be given before resistance test results are available, a DTG- or PI/r-containing regimen is commonly recommended

Initiating ART with HIV-Associated Complications

Many patients with advanced disease present with HIV-associated complications, and nearly all require ART as well as management of the complications. This raises the question of timing of the initiation of ART. There are several complicating interrelated variables that need to be considered, including (1) the risk of immune reconstitution syndrome (IRIS); (2) the urgency of starting ART based largely on the CD4 count; and (3) the complications incurred by treating two or more conditions simultaneously in terms of drug interactions, drug toxicity, and pill burden. The impression given in the early analyses was dominated by the philosophy that ART is rarely a therapeutic emergency and that IRIS is a confusing and potentially serious complication. These considerations justified a delay in starting ART. However, several studies have addressed this issue and the emerging consensus is as follows:

- *ART should be started immediately* for conditions that represent important complications of advanced HIV infection and have no good therapeutic intervention other than ART. These includes progressive multifocal leukoencephalopathy (PML), microsporidiosis, cryptosporidiosis, HIV-associated nephropathy, and HIV-associated dementia.
- *ART is usually started within 2 wks* for conditions where there is effective therapy but risk of IRIS is present, such as in mycobacterium avium complex (MAC), pneumocystis pneumonia (PCP), cryptococcal meningitis, and toxoplasmosis. This recommendation is largely based on results of ACTG 5164 (PLoS One 2009; 4:e5575), a randomized trial of 283 treatment naïve HIV infected patients with a median CD4 count of 29 cells/mm^3 and a new AIDS-defining non-tuberculosis opportunistic infection (OI). Participants were randomized to early ART (within 14 days) or delayed ART (after OI treatment is completed). Results showed a significant benefit with early ART based on the study endpoint of AIDS progression or death (OR 0.51; 95% confidence interval [CI] 0.27–0.94). The median time to initiate ART in this trial was 12 days in the early ART group and 45 days in the delayed ART group. A subsequent report on this study suggested that the early ART did not increase the risk of IRIS with non-tuberculosis OIs (PLoS One 2010; 5:e11416). Initiation of ART in patients with cryptococcal meningitis is debated based on a study from Zimbabwe that showed a mortality rate of 88% with ART given within 72 hrs compared to 54% in those with ART delayed to 10 wks (Clin Infect Dis 2010; 50:1532). This study had very high mortality rate, making it difficult to interpret and generalize its findings, but many would avoid early initiation of ART in patients with cryptococcal meningitis, especially in those with elevated intracranial pressure.

Treatment of HIV-2 Infection

See HIV Med 2010;11:611; CID 2011;52:1780.

Background

Viral Load: There are two commercially available HIV-2 quantitative VL assays in the US (HIV-2 RNA PCR quantitative, University of Washington Laboratory Medicine, CPT code 87539, 800-713-5198; and the New York State Department of Health, 518-473-6007).

Choice of ARTs: There are several ongoing controlled trials of ART for HIV-2 infection or HIV-1/2 co-infection, but no results are available yet. Recommendations are largely based on anecdotal observations from clinical and in vitro reports.

- *NRTI*: HIV-2 is generally sensitive to NRTIs but is relatively resistant to AZT. It also has a low barrier to resistance to NRTIs and has high rates of K65R mutations (Leukemia 1997;11 Suppl 3:120; HIV Med 2010; 11:611).
- *NNRTI*: HIV-2 is inherently resistant to this class due to Y188L polymorphisms (Antiviral Ther 2004;9:3) causing an altered binding pocket resulting in high rates of failures reported with HIV-2 and HIV-1/2 co-infection (AIDS 2010; 24:1043).
- *PI*: PI-based ART is preferred, but it is critical to select agents well and follow closely since options after failure are limited: NNRTIs are inactive and NRTIs have low barrier to resistance. Most active PIs are LPV, DRV, and SQV (AAC 2008; 52:1545); less effective PIs due to their weaker binding are ATV, NFV, and TPV (AAC 2008; 52:1545; JAC 2006; 57:709). Clinical experience with PI-based ART is somewhat worse with HIV-2 or HIV-1/2 compared to HIV-1 (AIDS 2010; 24:1043; Trop R Soc Med Hyg 2010; 104:151). The best and most extensive experience is with LPV/r (AIDS 2009; 23:1171; AIDS 2006; 20:17). However, a single proV47A mutation confers LPV resistance but hypersensitivity to SQV that may be useful for sequencing (AAC 2008; 52:1545; JAC 2006; 57:709).

- *INSTI*: Integrase inhibitors including RAL, EVG, and DTG are generally active against HIV-2 (JAC 2008; 62:914; AIDS 2010; 24:2753; PLoS One 2012; 7:e45372; Retrovirology 2015; 12(10)). Resistance develops to INSTIs on therapy generally in the same pathway as in HIV-1. Published clinical experience has generally been favorable but is variable and has been unable to identify a preferred regimen (Eur J Med Res 2009;14 Suppl 3:47; Antivir Res 2010;86:224; Antiviral Ther 2012;17:1097; J Clin Virol 2009;46:176; AIDS 2008;22:665; AIDS 2008;22:109; JAC 2008;62:941; AIDS 2014;28:2329; BMC Infect Dis 2014;14:461).
- *MVC*: HIV-2 appears capable of using other co-receptors and therefore MCV should not be used (J Virol 2005; 79:1686; J Virol 1998; 72:5425).
- *ENF*: HIV-2 is resistant to ENF in vitro (Antiviral Ther 2004; 9:57).

Treatment Recommendations for HIV-2 Infection

See 2018 DHHS Guidelines; Clin Infect Dis 2011;52:780.

- *Patients with untreated HIV-2 or HIV-1/2 infection* who require ART should be treated with two NRTIs and either a boosted PI or an INSTI based on limited experience, including one series showing a good response in 17 of 29 (59%) HIV-2 monoinfected adults (AIDS 2009;23:1171; HIV Med 2010;11:611; Clin Infect Dis 2011;52:1257; J Clin Virol 2015;64:12). The largest published series includes 126 treated with LPV/r combined with 3TC, and either AZT or TDF (Clin Infect Dis 2011;52:1257). The mean CD4 count increase in this group was 12 cells/mm^3/mo, and the mean VL in detectable patients at 1 yr was 2.2 log$_{10}$ c/mL.
- *Monitoring for response to therapy*: Standard methods can be used to monitor response if VL assay access is available (see earlier discussion). However, some patients may have

an undetectable baseline VL. If unable to monitor VL response, then HIV-2's unique resistance mutations make therapy challenging (J Infect Dis 2009;199:1323; HIV Med 2010;11:611). The recommendation is to follow CD4 count and clinical response with the understanding that it is a poor indicator of virologic response or failure (AIDS 2008;22:457).

Factors That Influence Probability of Prolonged Viral Suppression

Regimen Potency and Tolerability

The current three-drug regimens recommended by the 2018 DHHS guidelines and the 2018 IAS-USA guidelines have all demonstrated virologic efficacy in clinical trials. All of these recommended regimens utilize a backbone consisting of two NRTIs in combination with a third agent. With the exception of the co-formulated ABC/3TC/DTG regimen, the DHHS guidelines recommend tenofovir (either TAF or TDF)/FTC as the primary dual NRTI backbone. ABC/3TC is recommended with DTG, given the data discussed later. However, ABC/3TC is an alternative when used in other combinations due to lower efficacy in the setting of higher VLs noted in ACTG 5202, as well as due to concern for increased cardiovascular risk and hypersensitivity in patients positive for the HLA B*5701 allele. With more clinical real-life experience data arriving, TAF may supplant TDF due to its more favorable kidney and bone profile.

The recent changes in the recommended regimens in the DHHS guidelines were driven by both the toxicities and tolerability with certain combinations, as well as differential efficacy levels between regimens. Integrase Inhibitors have become first-line agents due to their superior efficacy and tolerability. DTG was demonstrated to be superior to EFV, DRV/r, and ATV/r in head-to-head randomized clinical trials (N Engl J Med 2013;369:1807; Lancet Infect Dis 2013;13:927; Lancet 2017;4:e546). In ACTG 5257, RAL was superior to DRV/r and ATV/r due to a combination of factors including virologic efficacy and better tolerability (Ann Intern Med 2014;161:461). ATV/r had more people discontinue the drug due to intolerance, leading it to be downgraded to an alternative agent in most guidelines.

Prior to the trials demonstrating DTG superiority over EFV-based regimens, EFV had been demonstrated to be superior to LPV/r in ACTG 5142 and non-inferior to ATV/r in ACTG 5202, as described next.

ACTG 5142 and ACTG 5202: These are the major trials comparing EFV with PI/r-based ART regimens. ACTG 5142 demonstrated that EFV was superior to LPV/r in virologic suppression, but failure with EFV was associated with higher rates of NNRTI resistance (48%), while there were no major PI mutations with LPV/r failure. Subsequently, ATV/r proved virologically superior to LPV/r in the CASTLE study, setting the stage for ACTG 5202 Table 4.8, which compared EFV versus ATV/r in 928 treatment naïve patients (Ann Intern Med 2011;154:445). Virologic suppression was comparable between EFV and ATV/r, and, as with other studies of ritonavir-boosted PIs, PI resistance mutations were infrequent despite treatment failure with PIs.

TABLE 4.8 ACTG 5202 results at 96 wks – EFV + 2 NRTI vs. ATV/r + 2 NRTI (Ann Intern Med 2011;154:445)

	ABC/3TC +		TDF/FTC +	
	ATV/r *(n = 465)*	*EFV* *(n = 463)*	*ATV/r* *(n = 464)*	*EFV* *(n = 465)*
Virologic failure				
Total	16.6%	14.7%	11.0%	10.2%
Baseline VL >100,000	23.1%	17.5%	12.8%	9.5%
Major resistance mutation				
NNRTI	<1%	65%*	0	56%*
PI	<1%	0	0	0
NRTI	14%	40%	9%	23%

*p value <0.05.

Regimen Tolerability

Treatment Adherence

In a study by Paterson and colleagues (Ann Inten Med 2000;133:21), an adherence rate of >95% was required to achieve an 80% probability of virologic suppression to <400 c/mL at 24 wks. With 90–95% adherence, the probability of suppression dropped to 50%. However, while multiple studies have confirmed the importance of adherence (AIDS 2001;15:2109; Clin Infect Dis 2001;33:386; Clin Infect Dis 2002;34:115; AIDS 2004;35:S35), this early report is less relevant today, with the use of more potent agents such as boosted PIs, integrase inhibitors, and NNRTIs with long half-lives. More recent work has shown that adherence requirements vary depending on the regimen, which reflects regimen potency, pharmacokinetic properties, class or agent susceptibility, and within-class cross-resistance mutational patterns. Substantial experience shows that adherence to recommended regimens will achieve durable virologic suppression unless there is *transmitted resistance*. Some nuances of these conclusions include:

- *Resistant Strains are Less Fit than Wild-Type*: Transmitted resistance may be apparent with baseline testing, but resistant strains often have a competitive disadvantage over wild-type virus. The resistant strains in the latent pool emerge only with antiviral pressure. Thus, relevant historical data include prior resistance tests, antiretroviral history, and infecting source data.
- *Resistance Mutations are restricted* in the minority pool to latently infected reservoirs and may contribute to virologic failure despite good treatment adherence.
- *The role of resistance mutations* in reducing replication competence is poorly understood.
- *PI/r-based regimens have a higher genetic barrier to resistance* due to a combination of pharmacokinetics and other factors such as multiple PI mutations required for high level resistance.

Unlike NNRTI-based regimens, antiviral activity can often be achieved following virologic failure to PI/r-based regimens by simply improving adherence. This accounts for the relative safety of using DRV/r, ATV/r, or LPV/r monotherapy (AIDS 2008;22:385; JAC 2010;65:2436; AIDS Rev 2010;12:127; Antivir Ther 2011;16:59; AIDS 2010;24:2365; AIDS 2009;23:279).

- *Resistance testing is commercially available* for five of the six classes of antiviral drugs for HIV-1. The exception is CCR5 antagonists.
- *Persistence of Resistant Strains*: It is assumed that resistant strains persist for the lifetime of the patient, although this has been debated in the context of single-dose NVP to prevent perinatal transmission (N Engl J Med 2010;363:1499).
- *EFV has a pharmacologic barrier to resistance*: the long half-life prevents resistance with missed doses, as demonstrated in the FOTO trial with Five (days) On and Two (days) Off (HIV Clin Trials 2007;8:19). More recently, a study evaluated 100 virologically suppressed patients taking ART (PI/r in 29, NNRTI in 71) for 4 days and then stopping for 3 days (J Antimicrob Chemother 2017 Nov 25. Epub ahead of print). At 48 wks, 96% were still virologically suppressed; three virologic failures all resuppressed with daily therapy. Nevertheless, the dataset is small and current guidelines do not recommend this strategy at this time.
- *Genetic barrier*: EFV, NVP, ETR, 3TC, FTC, RAL, and some unboosted PIs and ENF have a lower barrier to resistance compared to MVC, DTG, and boosted PIs that have a higher barrier to resistance.
- *Cross-resistance is agent-within-class specific*: The K103N causes resistance to EFV and NVP, but not to ETR, RPV, and DOR; the 138K RT mutation, selected by RPV, causes cross-resistance to ETR. These patterns affect in-class sequencing decisions.
- *M184V Mutations*: This mutation is somewhat unique since it reduces activity of 3TC and FTC, but continued use

does not risk additional resistance mutations (J Infect Dis 2007;19:1537).

- *Importance of Adherence to Initial Regimen*: The greatest challenge to patients for virologic control and preventing development of mutant resistance strains is adherence to the initial regimen, since the level of HIV viremia is at its highest prior to initial therapy. Thus, baseline VL often correlates with risk of virologic failure and resistance.

- *Adherence and Resistance*: Though poor adherence predicts virologic failure, it does not necessarily predict resistance. The highest risk of resistance to an unboosted PI-based regimen is virologic failure in the face of good adherence (JAIDS 2002;30:278; AIDS 2000;14:357; AIDS 2001;15:1701). In one study, 23% of patients with virologic failure attributed to resistance had 92–100% adherence based on unannounced pill counts (AIDS 2003;17:1925). In another study, 88% of patients with resistance mutation had taken >70% of prescribed doses (Clin Infect Dis 2003;37:1112). Both reports found virologic failure but virtually no resistance mutations with consumption of <60% of prescribed doses with unboosted or boosted PI-based ART. The assumption is that the drug level was inadequate to select resistant strains. Later findings suggest this association between adherence and resistance is related to drug class and to specific agents (AIDS 2006;20:223). As noted, virologic failure and resistance are less likely to occur with boosted PIs compared to unboosted PIs due presumably to the pharmacologic barrier (JAIDS 2008;47:397; Clin Infect Dis 2006;43:939).

Guidance to Improve Adherence

1. *Common strategies and observations*:
   - Establish patient readiness before initiating treatment (but recognize relative urgency).
   - Use a standardized approach to assess adherence, but note that self-reported nonadherence is reliable.

- Use the entire healthcare team to reinforce adherence messaging to patient.
- Realize that healthcare professionals are poor predictors of who will adhere.
- Adherence may decrease with time, becoming significantly worse at 6–12 mo than it is initially (Topics HIV Med 2003;11:185).
- Address obvious issues of convenience: pill burden, frequency of daily administration, food or fasting requirements, tolerance, and pill size (See Table 4.9).

2. *Factors that predict reduced adherence* include side effects, mental illness, active substance abuse, complex regimens, stigma, low level of literacy, comorbidities such as TB, asymptomatic status of patient when treatment begins, poverty issues (homelessness, transportation problems), poor understanding of regimen, and inadequate pharmacy service (Topics HIV Med 2003;11:185).

3. *Adherence review and recommendations of the British HIV Association:*
   - *Treatment simplification*: A review of 53 clinical trials with 14,264 participants failed to show significant correlation between pill count and viral suppression (AIDS 2006;20:2051). A review of the HIV literature on the benefit of fewer daily doses found only one study demonstrating a better outcome with once-daily ART (JAMA 2002;288:2868). However, once-daily regimens are generally preferred by patients.
   - *Education on ARTs*: Two reports found a benefit with educational sessions (JAIDS 2003;34:191; Patient Educ Couns 2003;50:187). Other reports found no benefit with individual counseling by a trained counselor or group support (JAIDS 2003;34:174; J Assoc Nurse AIDS Care 2003;14:52).
   - *Use of dose time alarm*: One large randomized study found that there were significantly more virologic failures in

TABLE 4.9 Convenience factor

Class	Once Daily	Pill Burden	No Food Effect
NRTI [a]	ABC TDF TAF FTC 3TC ddI	1/day: ABC/3TC TDF/FTC TAF/FTC 2/day: AZT/3TC	ABC TDF TAF FTC 3TC d4T AZT
INSTI	BIC DTG EVG/c RAL (1,200 mg)	1/day: BIC DTG EVG/c RAL (1,200 mg) 2/day: RAL (400 mg)	BIC DTG RAL
PI/r [a] or PI/c	DRV/r or DRV/c ATV/r or ATV/c LPV/r FPV/r	1/day: DRV/c, ATV/c 2/day: ATV/r, DRV/r 3/day: FPV/r 4/day: LPV/r 6/day: SQV/r 8/day: TPV/r	LPV/r FPV/r
NNRTI	EFV NVP RPV ETR[b] DOR	1/day: EFV, RPV, DOR 1 or 2/day: NVP 2/day: ETR	NVP DOR
CCR5 antagonist		2/day: MVC	MVC

[a] Data provided for NRTI are limited to combination formulations. The PI data are limited to boosted PIs, and pill burden includes the ritonavir dose except in LPV/r.

[b] ETR is usually dosed bid but its half-life supports once-daily dosing.

patients using dose time alarms compared to controls (XV Int'l AIDS Conf 2004, Abstr. LbOrB15). The presumed reason was that patients depended on the alarm, which sometimes failed.

- *Practice with placebo*: One controlled trial with a 5-wk training period found a modest and transient benefit (AIDS 2006;20:1295).
- *Directly observed therapy (DOT)*: Several studies found improved virologic outcome using DOT with methadone maintenance (Clin Infect Dis 2004;38[suppl 5]:S409; Clin Infect Dis 2004;38[suppl 5]:S414; Clin Infect Dis 2006;42:1628; Clin Infect Dis 2007;45:770; Public Health Rep 2007;122:472). However, a meta-analysis of 12 studies that satisfied methodological criteria and were published before July 2001 showed no benefit (Lancet 2009;374:2064).

Measuring Adherence

Physician estimate is notoriously unreliable (Ann Intern Med 2000;133:21). Patient self-report is most reliable when there is acknowledgment of poor adherence; when queries are nonjudgmental of poor adherence, with simple standardized surveys for doses taken in past 3 days or 1 wk taken at each clinic visit; and when the queries are impersonal, as with a form or computer program (JAIDS 2006;46 Suppl 1:S149). Pharmacy records can be very useful (AIDS Behav 2008;12:86) and have been shown to correlate with virologic outcome (PLoS Med 2008;5:e109).

Adherence Recommendations

1. Data do not support frequent, intensive, or prolonged contact with an adherence specialist. Use of the entire HIV medicine team of healthcare providers appears more effective than an adherence specialist.
2. Regimens should not be simplified if simplification reduces potency.
3. Medication alarms may reduce adherence because people may overly depend on them, and they often fail.

4. Critical factors to adherence are patient understanding of the regimen, a good provider–patient relationship, and a drug regimen that addresses the patient's needs as much as possible.

5. Pharmacy records and pill counts are especially effective for documenting good or bad adherence.

Rapidity of VIROLOGIC Response

The trajectory of the VL response predicts the nadir plasma VL and, subsequently, the durability of HIV response. There are exceptions: Data indicate that the dose response slope is class dependent and possibly dictated by the stage in viral lifecycle at which the agent is active (Nat Med 2008;14:762). The VL response to Integrase Inhibitor-based ART is substantially more rapid compared to EFV in the first 6 wks of treatment, although results at 24 and 48 wks were similar. The median time to HIV RNA of <50 was 28 days with DTG and 84 days with EFV (NEJM 2013;369:1807). In fact, newer regimens using dual NRTI + INSTI (either DTG or BIC) result in viral suppression rates that easily exceed 75% by the first month of treatment (Lancet 2017;390:2063; Lancet 2017;390:2073). At the other end, an older large review found that the median time to a VL of <50 c/mL in treatment-naïve patients was 13.5 wks (Int J Sex Transm Dis AIDS 2006;17:522), reflecting the lesser potency of older ART regimens. To achieve an optimal and durable virologic response, treatment-naïve patients treated with ART are expected to respond as follows:

- VL decline by at least 0.7–1.0 $\log_{10}$ c/mL at 1 wk (Lancet 2001;358:1760; JAIDS 2002;30:167).
- VL decline by at least 1.5–2.0 $\log_{10}$ c/mL to <5,000 c/mL at 4 wks (AIDS 1999;13:1873; JAIDS 2000;25:36). One review of 656 treatment naïve patients given ART found that a VL reduction to <1,000 c/mL by wk 4 predicted an 82–95% probability of VL suppression of <50 c/mL at wk 24 (JAIDS 2004;37:1155).

- VL decline to <500 c/mL at 8–16 wks and <50 c/mL at 16–24 wks (Ann Intern Med 2001;135:954; JAIDS 2000;24:433).

Failure to achieve these goals suggests lack of antiviral potency, nonadherence, resistance, or inadequacy of drug levels due to drug interactions, poor absorptions, and the like.

Monitoring Response to Therapy

One of the main goals of ART is to achieve maximal and durable suppression of HIV RNA. In this regard, monitoring response to therapy is pertinent to achieving this goal (see Table 4.10).

TABLE 4.10 Monitoring response to therapy

Assays

HIV RNA	• Baseline • 2–4 wks (but not later than 8 wks) after ART initiation • 4–8 wks interval until VL <200 c/mL • Every 3–6 months once suppressed	• More frequently with treatment failure • Expected VL decline by: • 0.7–1.0 $\log_{10}$ c/mL at 1–2 wks • 1.5–2.0 $\log_{10}$ c/mL at 4 wks • <200 c/mL by 24–48 wks

CD4	• Baseline
	• Every 3–12 months thereafter
		• Expected CD4 increase:
		  • 30–70 cells/mm^3 by month 4
		  • 100–150 cells/mm^3 by first year
		• No clearly established methods to increase CD4 response beyond HIV suppression. Interferon and steroids decrease CD4 cell count substantially.

Virologic Response Definitions

See 2018 DHHS Guidelines.

Virologic suppression: A confirmed HIV RNA level below the LLOQ of available assays. Sustained virologic suppression occurs when a VL of <50 c/mL is sustained and confirmed with VL measurements at 3- to 6-mo interval. The more recent guidelines note that the frequency of this 3- to 4-mo interval can be decreased in patients with an established pattern of good adherence and consistent HIV suppression for at least 2–3 yrs. Sequence analysis of HIV clones from patients with sustained VL <50 c/mL show no sequence evolution with emergence of resistance mutation (JAMA 2005;293:817; J Infect Dis 2004;189:1444; J Infect Dis 2004;189:1452; J Virol 2006;80:6441; PLoS Path 2007;3:3122).

Virologic failure: The inability to achieve or maintain a suppression of viral replication to an HIV RNA level of <200 c/mL. The frequency of virologic failure has evolved over time. In a 2004 analysis of 12 reports with 1,197 patients in the United States, 62% failed to achieve the goal of VL <50 c/mL by 24 wks (Clin Infect Dis 2004;38:614). A review of 14,264 treatment-naïve patients in clinical trials between 1994 and 2004 found that 45% failed to achieve a VL of <50 c/mL at 48 wks, but this improved to 36% failure by 2003–2004 (AIDS 2006;20:2051). More recent studies show virologic failure rates that substantially declined to 5–10% in both clinical trials and cohorts (AIDS 2015;29:373; Clin Infect Dis 2016;63:268).

- *Virologic failure and resistance*: The VL predicts the probability of resistance developing since mutation rates are a function of replication rates, and continued drug exposure drives strain selection with additional resistance mutation at rates that are dependent on the VL (replication rate). This means that the rate of new resistance mutations will be in the order of magnitude greater with a VL of 100,000 c/mL as opposed to a VL of 1,000 c/mL, even though both represent virologic failure (JAIDS 2002;30:154; JAIDS 2001;27:44; AIDS 1999;19:1035; AIDS 1999;13:341).

Incomplete virologic response: Two consecutive plasma HIV RNA levels of >200 c/mL after 24 wks on an ART regimen in a patient who has not yet had documented virologic suppression on this regimen. A patient's baseline HIV RNA level may affect the time course of response, and some regimens may take longer than others to suppress HIV RNA levels.

Virologic rebound: Confirmed HIV RNA of ≥200 c/mL after virologic suppression.

Virologic blip: After virologic suppression, an isolated detectable HIV RNA level, usually <200 c/mL, that is followed by a return to virologic suppression. One study of patients with sustained VL <50 c/mL measured VL every 2–3 days for 3–4 months. Blips were found to be very common (9/10 patients), low-level (median of 79 c/mL), transient (isolated events), unrelated to clinical events (illness, vaccination, etc.), inconsistent (noted in only one of duplicate samples), and appeared to represent a statistical variation around the mean VL of <50 c/mL (JAMA 2005;293:817). This suggests that most blips are unconfirmed with repeat testing and are sampling errors. The frequency of blips caused both the ACTG and the DHHS to change their definition of virologic failure to a "confirmed VL>200 c/mL." Blips are not usually associated with subsequent virologic failure (2018 DHHS guidelines), but repeated blips can be associated with virologic failure.

Low-level viremia: Confirmed detectable HIV RNA <200 c/mL. Though with unclear clinical implication, in one analysis persistent low-level viremia has been weakly associated in virological failure with an adjusted hazard ratio (aHR) of 1.38 (AIDS 2015;29:373). In this same study, a VL of 200–499 c/mL was strongly associated with virologic failure with an aHR of 3.97 (95% CI between 3.05–5.17).

Immunologic Failure

There is no consensus definition. The expected increase is about 100 cells/mm^3 at 1 yr with baseline levels <350 cells/mm^3, and increases on an average of about 50 cells/mm^3/yr in the second and third years. Median CD4 increase expected is 250–300 cells/mm^3 over 5 yrs (Lancet 2007;370:470; Clin Infect Dis 2007;44:441). Initiation of treatment with CD4 counts of <200 cells/mm^3 is associated with a reduced immunologic response (Clin Infect Dis 2007;44:441; JAIDS 2004;36:702), with some studies showing a plateau of 350–500 cells/mm^3 at 4–6 yrs, indicating a limited immunologic reserve with late treatment start (JAIDS 2007;45:515). Other larger cohort studies show continuing increases in the mean CD4 counts to a level of >600 cells/mm^3 even with late starts (Lancet 2007;370:407). Persistently low CD4 counts are infrequently complicated by AIDS-defining complications if there is complete viral suppression. In most cases, intensification or changes in the ART regimen in the face of viral suppression has not been proved effective in restoring the CD4 count.

CD4 count increases despite virologic failure: Multiple studies have shown that suboptimal virologic response to ART is commonly associated with increases in CD4 counts. This has consistently been shown in several large "salvage" studies (RESIST, POWER, BENCHMRK, TORO), in which most of the patients in the control group were given an optimized background regimen (i.e., without the investigational agent) and had increases in median CD4 count despite incomplete viral suppression. However, the CD4 count increase was significantly less than in those who achieved good virologic suppression (N Engl J Med 2003;348:2175; Lancet 2006;368:406; JAIDS 2007;46:24; JAIDS 2007;46:125). Several large studies also showed that OIs are uncommon with a VL of <5,000 c/mL regardless of the CD4 count (see Table 4.11).

HIV RNA levels and CD4 slope: The CD4 response correlates inversely with viral suppression. The CD4 increase has a biphasic pattern—initial increase by mean values between 50 and 120 cells/mm^3 during the first 3 months, thereafter increasing by 2–7 cells/mo (J Infect Dis 2006;94:29; JAMA 2002;288:222; J Infect Dis 2002;185:471; JAMA 2004;292:1911). Early studies suggested that the HIV RNA level was the strongest predictor of the rate of CD4 decline in untreated patients (Ann Intern Med 1997;126:946), but subsequent studies suggest that this association may have

TABLE 4.11 Flagship salvage trials: 48-wk results

Agents	Citation	Trial	N	VL <50 OBR (%)	Mean CD4 Count in OBR[a]
ENF	J AIDS 2005	TORO	661	8	+90
TPV/r	Lancet 2006	RESIST	1,486	10	+18
DRV	Lancet 2007	POWER	255	10	+19
RAL	N Engl J Med 2008	BENCHMRK	703	33	+54
MVC	N Engl J Med 2008	MOTIVATE	1,049	17	+45
ETR	Lancet 2007	DUET	1,203	40	+73
DTG	J Infect Dis 2014	VIKING-3	183	63	+110

OBR, optimal background regimen

[a]Mean CD4 count increase (cells/mm^3) in the OBR group with virologic failure rates of 60–92%.

been overstated (JAMA 2006;296:1498). These studies suggest that CD4 slope is primarily regulated by immune activation attributed to HIV viral replication, but possibly also influenced by co-morbidities (such as TB, HSV, CMV, etc.) and translocation of gut microbes and microbial products (Nat Med 2006;12:1365; Nat Rev Immunol 2004;4:485). Nevertheless, it should be noted that the only therapeutic intervention with major and sustained impact on outcome and CD4 increase is ART. This conclusion is supported by repeated studies showing that viral suppression is associated with a prompt increase in CD4 counts (without any apparent effect on co-pathogens, or intestinal gut-associated lymphoid tissue, GALT), studies showing that there are no alternative interventions to increase CD4 response in patients with VL/CD4 discordance, and treatment interruption trials in which discontinuation of ART caused a prompt increase in VL and rapid CD4 count decline averaging 30–80 cells/mo during the first 2 months. There is no consensus, since some authorities have argued that the original data are correct, and reanalysis of the MACS data found that baseline VL strongly predicted long-term prognosis (JAMA 2007;297:2346).

Discordant CD4 count and HIV RNA levels: Virologic suppression is associated with immune recovery, and the magnitude of the CD4 count increase correlates with viral suppression. However, there are substantial individual variations, and discordant changes in both directions are relatively common (J Infect Dis 2001;183:1328; Clin Infect Dis 2002;35:1005). Most discordant results are enigmatic. An exception is treatment with a combination of TDF and full-dose ddI, which is associated with a blunted CD4 response and should not be used (AIDS 2004;18:2442). Some studies have shown superior CD4 count increases with DTG, RAL, MVC, or PI-based ART compared to NNRTI-based regimens (N Engl J Med 2013;368:1807; JAIDS 2010;55:39; PLoS One 2010;5:e13188 J Infect Dis 2010;201:803; Antivir Ther 2009;14:771). Medications that most often cause reduced CD4 count are interferon and corticosteroids.

The approach to CD4/VL discordance: Decisions regarding antiviral therapy are governed by HIV RNA levels: (1) viral suppression appears to reduce the frequency of OIs independent of the CD4 count, and (2) there are no interventions with ART known to confer additional benefit (other than avoiding use of ddI + TDF, and possibly AZT). It is possible that RAL, MVC, or a PI-based ART would be superior for CD4 response compared to NNRTI-based therapy, but there are no clinical data supporting therapeutic switches. Interleukin (IL)-2 increases CD4 count but without apparent clinical benefit (AIDS 2005;19:279; AIDS 2006;20:405; JAIDS 2006;42:140).

Clinical Failure

Clinical failure is defined as the occurrence or reoccurrence of an AIDS-defining opportunistic complication after 3 months or more of ART. IRIS should not be considered as evidence of clinical treatment failure.

When to Modify Therapy

Guidelines for Modifying Antiretroviral Regimens

There are multiple reasons for which initial ART regimens are changed including drug toxicity, virologic failure, or due to miscellaneous issues such as cost, access, or convenience.

Changes due to toxicity: Single-agent substitution can be made assuming there has been adequate virologic response and the substitution is rational on the basis potency and prior resistance resting (see Table 4.12).

Changes due to convenience: ART may be changed to improve convenience based on pill burden or dosing frequency (Table 4.9), drug interactions (such as the need for methadone or rifampin), or due to side effects (such as substitution of RAL for ENF).

Changes due to virologic failure: 2018 DHHS guidelines have simplified and defined virologic failure as the inability to achieve or maintain suppression of viral replication to HIV RNA level <200 c/mL. This was based on findings from a few retrospective studies which showed that, as a threshold for virologic failure, VL <200 c/mL and VL <50 c/mL had the same predictive value for subsequent viral rebound of >200 c/mL (AIDS 2015;29:373; Antivir Ther 2015;20:165), although some studies suggest that detectable viremia can be predictive of future viral rebound (Lancet Infect Dis 2013;13:587; Clin Infect Dis 2013;57:1489). Thus, the therapeutic goal remains at VL <50 c/mL since this appears to be indicative of absence of viral replication based on studies showing lack of sequence evolution (J Virol 2006;80:6441; J Virol 209;83:8470) and data suggesting that blips are not caused by replicating virus and therefore are clinically inconsequential (JAMA 2005;293:817; J Virol 2004;78:968).

Risk Factors for Virologic Failure

1. *Suboptimal adherence*: this is the most important factor in large studies (AIDS 2001;15:185).

TABLE 4.12 Monitoring for adverse drug reactions (ADRs) (Clin Infect Dis 2014;58:1 and 2018 DHHS Guidelines)

Test	Frequency	Comments
CBC w/ differential	• Entry to care • On ART start or change • Every 6 months	• If on AZT, repeat at 2–8 wks, then every 3–6 months
Chemistry	• Entry to care • On ART start or change, then 2–8 wks on ART • Every 3–6 months	• Includes electrolytes, BUN, creatinine, eGFR, liver function tests • Some experts monitor serum phosphate with TDF use
Fasting lipids	• Entry to care • On ART start or change • Every 6 months if abnormal • Every 12 months if normal	• Includes total cholesterol, LDL-C, HDL-C, and triglycerides • Interpret in context of Framingham risks and ART agent-specific risks
Glucose (fasting), or hemoglobin A1c	• Entry to care • On ART start or change • Every 12 months if normal	• Test every 3–6 months, if last test was abnormal
Urinalysis	• Entry to care • On ART start or change • Every 6 months, if on TDF or TAF • Otherwise, every 12 months	

2. *Date of initiation of ART*: patients treated in the pre-HAART era often took suboptimal regimens associated with high failure rates and higher rates of resistance (J Infect Dis 2008;197 Suppl 3:261).

3. *Agent-specific risks*: NNRTIs, RAL, 3TC, and FTC are more prone to resistance mutations than are RTV-boosted PIs, DTG, or MVC (See Table 4.13).

4. *High baseline VL* (>100,000 c/mL): This is an issue, although most of the currently recommended regimens appear to be almost equally effective in patients with high or low baseline VL.

5. *Advanced HIV disease* as indicated by low CD4 count or an AIDS-defining illness.

6. *Failure of the drug to reach the site of viral infection* due to problems with adherence, drug interactions, and drug toxicities. Factors that affect drug pharmacology include renal disease, hepatic disease, and genetics of drug metabolisms especially related to the cytochrome P450 metabolic pathways.

7. *Co-morbidities* that substantially affect adherence such as depression, substance abuse, poverty, and co-morbid medical conditions.

8. *Lack of access to continuous therapy* due to interruptions in pharmacy supply, drug payment issues, and idiosyncrasies of the healthcare system.

9. *Transmitted drug resistance* that is in the latent pool and not detected with baseline testing (JAMA 2011;305:1327).

Evaluation of Virologic Failure

An evaluation of virologic failure should include:

- *Comprehensive review of adherence-related issues* including detailed review of the regimen using pills or pill charts, timing of doses, assessment of food or drug interactions, review of drug access, and review of toxicities. Pharmacy records are valuable when available (AIDS Care 2010;10:1189).

TABLE 4.13 Frequency of resistance mutation associated with virologic failure

Class	Agent	Trial	Virologic Failure (%)	Resistance[a]
PI/r[b]	LPV/r	ACTG 5142 (N Engl J Med 2008;358:2095)	94/253 (37)	0/76
		ARTEMIS (AIDS 2008;22:1389)	49/346 (14)	0/18
		CASTLE (Lancet 2009;374:376)	26/443 (6)	0/8
	ATV/r	ACTG 5202 (Ann Intern Med 2011;154:445)	140/465 (30)	1/140
		CASTLE (Lancet 2009;374:376)	25/440 (6)	2/10
	DRV/r	ARTEMIS (AIDS 2008;22:1389)	34/343 (10)	0/10
	FPV/r	SOLO (AIDS 2004;18:1529)	22/322 (7)	0/22
INSTI	RAL	STARTMRK (Lancet 2009;374:796)	27/281 (10)	4/8 (50%)
		BENCHMRK (N Engl J Med 2008;359:355)	105/462 (23)	64/94 (68%)
	EVG	GS-US-236-0103 (Lancet 2012;379:2429)	36/353 (10)	4/12 (33%)
		GS-US=236-0102 (Lancet 2012;379:2439)	39/348 (11)	7/14 (50%)
	DTG	SINGLE (N Engl J Med 2013;369:1807)	18/414 (4)	0/18
		SPRING-2 (Lancet 2013;381:735)	20/411 (5)	0/8
		FLAMINGO (Lancet 2014;383:2222)	2/242 (<1)	0/2
		SAILING (Lancet 2013;382:700)	21/354 (6)	0/4
		GS-US-380-1489 (Lancet 2017;390:2063)	8/293 (3)	0/4
		GS-US-380-1490 (Lancet 2017;390:2073)	4/325 (1)	0/4
	BIC	GS-US-380-1489 (Lancet 2017;390:2063)	3/314 (1)	0/1
		GS-US-380-1490 (Lancet 2017;390:2073)	14/320 (4)	0/7

Class	Agent	Trial	Virologic Failure (%)	Resistance[a]
NNRTI	EFV	ACTG 5142 (N Engl J Med 2008;358:2095)	60/250 (24)	11/46 (24%)
		ACTG 5202 (Ann Intern Med 2011;154:445)	129/465 (28)	49/126 (39%)
		SINGLE (N Engl J Med 2013;369:1807)	17/419 (4)	4/17 (24%)
		GS-US-236-0102 (Lancet 2012;379:2439)	51/352 (14)	8/17 (47%)
		MERIT (J Infect Dis 2010;201:803)	13/361 (4)	9/13 (69%)
	DOR	DRIVE-AHEAD (Clin Infect Dis 2018 August 31[Epub ahead of preint])	22/364 (6.0%)	7/22
		DRIVE-FORWARD (Lancet HIV 2018 May;5(5):e211-e220)	19/383 (5%)	1/19
CCR5 antagonist	MVC	MERIT (J Infect Dis 2010;201:803)	29/360 (8)	13/29[c] (45%)

[a] Resistance = Number of major resistance mutations to the agent noted/number of sensitivity tests done in virologic failures.

[b] Total for PI/r = 1/323 (0.3%).

[c] X4 virus 9/29 (31%); R5 resistance 4/29 (14%).

Note: Data based on virologic failure as per protocol of individual studies.

- *Medical history review*, including sequential CD4 counts, VLs, concurrent medications, and comorbidities. It is essential to review the patient's history of prior and current antiretroviral (ARV) use, as well as the reasons for any ARV change or discontinuation.
- *Current and prior resistance tests*: Most important in this assessment are the results of all current and prior resistance tests and prior antiretroviral exposure, as well as responses, including failures and toxicities, if present. It must be emphasized that resistance mutations, once selected, are archived in the latent pool and will reemerge under selective pressure (J Infect Dis 2003;188:1433; JAMA 2011;305:1327). Therefore, any resistance mutations that have been documented at any time are assumed to persist, and a history of virologic failure while on therapy with drugs that have low genetic barriers to resistance (3TC, FTC, EFV, NVP, and RAL) should raise the possibility of resistance, which is still best documented with resistance testing performed during therapy.

Important Principles to Consider During Drug Selection for Virologic Failure

- *Address issues that prevent an adequate response to the prior or current regimens*: The major concern is adherence. Other issues include potency of the regimen, drug interactions, and pharmacologic issues.
- *Use at least two and preferably three agents* from at least two classes that are active based on a review of current and prior test results and treatment history.
- *The change in therapy should be rapid.* This is to avoid accumulation of additional resistance mutation which will further restrict future options (AIDS 2007;21:721). Exceptions are with 3TC and FTC.
- *Do not stop therapy except for toxicity.*
- *Do not add a single drug to a failing regimen.*

Resistance Tests

These tests are most accurate for evaluating resistance to drug classes being taken at the time the test is performed or within 4 wks of discontinuation of therapy. Transmitted mutations persist longer than acquired mutations. The duration of persistence depends on the effect of the mutation on replication capacity. For example, thymidine analog mutations (TAMs) and NNRTI mutations generally persist, whereas the strains with PI mutations or the M184V mutation are more quickly replaced by wild-type virus. Resistance assays do not reliably detect minority species (i.e., <20% of the viral population) (JAMA 2011;305:1327) and therefore are better at indicating what drug not to use and best for drugs that are currently being taken. Always consider prior resistance test results and treatment history, including duration of therapy in the presence of virologic failure and agent-specific genetic barriers to resistance (high barrier with most boosted PIs and thymidine analogs; low barrier with 3TC, FTC, RAL, and NNRTIs). For suppressed patients who have a history of treatment experience but no accessible genotypes, use of technology evaluating resistance mutations in proviral DNA, the so-called *archive genotype*, may be helpful, but may not reveal all mutations the patient has had in previous genotypes (HIV Clin Trials 2006;17:29; HIV Med 2012;13:517).

The sensitivity of resistance testing after ART is discontinued depends on the time off treatment and the drug being evaluated. Wild-type virus tends to reemerge as early as 4 wks after discontinuation, especially with respect to PI mutations. Therefore, 4 wks after drug discontinuation is the anticipated maximal duration of resistance test validity, at least for PI-based regimens. Some mutations, such as NNRTI mutations or TAMs, may persist for 9–12 months or longer (J Clin Lab Anal 2002;16:76), possibly because they do not alter replication capacity (J Med Virol 2003;69:1). The M184V mutation exerts a stronger influence on replication capacity (AAC 2003;47:3377) and may become undetectable within 5–20 wks after discontinuation (AAC 2002;46:2255; AAC 2004;48:644). With newer drugs used in highly treatment-experienced patients, the response rates are often dependent on the number of active drugs in the regimen, as well as on the number of resistance mutations affecting response to the newer agent(s).

Strategies for Virologic Failure

In the first decade of highly active ART (HAART), the probability of success was greatest with the initial regimen and decreased with each successive regimen. This has since changed, with more recent drug developments and the discovery of more potent agents in various drug classes. In salvage trials, a larger proportion of patients attain full virologic suppression despite extensive drug resistance. The goal of treatment remains full virologic suppression to <50 c/mL to prevent resistance, stop disease progression, and preserve future treatment options. This goal is very much achievable with most patients (AIDS 2010;24:2469; N Engl J Med 2009;360:1815).

First Regimen Failure: In most cases, the usual regimen change after virologic failure of the initial regimen is to switch to an alternative regimen based on resistance tests, preferably performed on treatment or within 4 wks of changing or stopping ART. The lack of resistance despite failure typically suggests nonadherence. Resuppression for PI/r-based ART can usually be achieved by improved adherence.

FTC and 3TC Resistance: With virologic failure, an early NRTI resistance mutation that can appear with most regimens containing either 3TC or FTC is the M184V mutation, which reduces activity of 3TC and FTC. Some residual antiviral activity is nevertheless retained, possibly due to decreased replication capacity associated with M184V mutation. The mutation also results in an increase in activity of AZT, d4T, and TDF without risk of further NRTI resistance mutation. For this reason, it is sometimes recommended that 3TC or FTC be continued despite resistance, but in such cases these drugs should not be counted as active components of an antiviral regimen.

Virologic Failure without Resistance Mutations: If the test was performed on therapy, the usual cause of failure is failure of the drug to reach the target due to inadequate adherence, or, less often, due to drug interactions, noncompliance with food requirements, and the like. This is most commonly seen with boosted PI-based ART and usually means the regimen will be successful if properly taken.

PI-based Regimen with Virologic Failure: Patients failing PI-based regimens frequently have no PI resistance mutations, in which case the cause of failure is usually nonadherence. Options are (1) correct problems in adherence, drug interactions, or other pharmacologic issues that might account for suboptimal response; (2) add RTV boosting (applies only to unboosted FPV or ATV); (3) intensify with an additional agent; or (4) change to a new regimen. The response should be monitored with VL testing at 2–4 wks after a new regimen. Multiple studies show that virologic failure on PI/r-based ART in patients without preexisting PI mutations is not associated with primary PI resistance mutation. The NRTIs given concurrently are also somewhat protected, although NRTI resistance can still occur, especially to 3TC or FTC as seen in ACTG 5142 (N Engl J Med 2008;358:2095).

NNRTI-based Regimen with Virologic Failure: Virologic failure with EFV usually results in a K103N mutation with cross-resistance to NVP but retained susceptibility to ETR and RPV. Switch options usually include ETR as well as PI/r, INSTI, and MVC. DOR, a recently approved NNRTI with retained activity in the presence of K103N and other nutations, could also be considered, however, there is no clinical data evaluating its use in virologic failure. The favored mutation with NVP resistance is 181C, which substantially reduces activity of EFV and ETR. The favored mutation with RPV is 138K, which reduces ETR activity (AAC 2011;55:600). The switch to ETR for virologic failure or toxicity is generally straightforward (AIDS 2011;25:143). The switch from EFV to RPV is more complicated due to the long half-life of EFV and drug interactions of RPV. However, in clinical trials, patients have been shown to maintain suppression with this EFV-to-RPV switch (HIV Med 2012;13:517). It should be emphasized that there is no benefit and perhaps some potential harm to continue EFV or NVP in the face of virologic failure with resistance. There is no benefit because, once resistance has occurred, there is no residual antiviral effect and no negative effect on viral fitness (J Med Virol 2003;69:1; J Infect Dis 2005;192:1537). The potential harm is the accumulation of an NNRTI resistance mutation that will impair effectiveness of second-generation NNRTIs, such as ETR and RPV.

NRTI Resistance Virologic Failure: A dual NRTI combination is a standard component of the initial regimen in virtually every guideline. Historically, NRTI-containing regimens were usually superior to most available "NRTI-sparing" combinations (Tables 4.14 and 4.15). FTC or 3TC have been often continued even in the presence of the M184V mutation due to good tolerability, documented antiviral effects attributable to the reduction in replication capacity and/or partial antiviral effects, and increased activity of AZT, d4T, and TDF. However, the OPTIONS trial demonstrated that optimized regimens without NRTI were non-inferior to regimens containing NRTIs in treatment-experienced patients failing their current regimen if they had several fully or partially active drugs available for their new optimized regimen, and the continuous phenotypic susceptibility score (cPSS) was >2 (Ann Intern Med 2015;163:908). The selection of the backbone is still based on resistance testing, consideration of co-morbid conditions (e.g., renal impairment, cardiovascular risk factors, HBV coinfection), and avoidance of incompatible or toxic combinations (e.g., AZT+d4T, ddI+d4T, and ddI+TDF).

Integrase Resistance with Virologic Failure: Although initially only used in treatment-experienced patients, integrase inhibitors (INSTI) have rapidly become the favored agents in initial therapy due to their efficacy and wide tolerability. Despite this widespread use of INSTI, virologic failure has been relatively rare with this class. Resistance has occurred in relatively few antiretroviral-naïve patients failing treatment with INSTI. When used in combination therapy (not monotherapy), no resistance has been documented with failure on DTG in naïve patients. Additionally, DTG has been demonstrated to be effective at twice the daily dose in patients with INSTI resistance (J Infect Dis 2013;207:740; J Infect Dis 2014;210:354). Continued RAL or EVG therapy with resistance mutation confers no therapeutic benefit and may lead to acquisition

TABLE 4.14 Nucleoside/nucleotide reverse transcriptase inhibitor (NRTI)-sparing regimens in treatment-naïve patients

Trial	Regimen (Dose in mg)	Duration (Wks)	N^a	Comments
CTN 177 JAIDS 2009;50:335	LPV/r 533/133 bid + NVP 200 bid vs. LPV/r + AZT/3TC vs. NVP + AZT/3TC	96	26	High rate ADRs—only 6/26 (23%) reached 96 wks; No benefit vs. controls
ACTG 5142 N Engl J Med 2008;358:2095	LPV/r 533/133 bid + EFV 600 qd vs. (EFV or LPV/r) + 2 NRTIs	96	250	Virologic failure 26% (similar in all 3 groups); More resistance mutation in NRTI-free arm
A4001078 JAIDS 2013;62:164	MVC 150 ad + ATV 300/100 qd vs. ATV/r + TDF/FTC	48	60	VL<50 at 48 wks: MVC 75% vs. TDF 84%; Grade 4 hyperbilirubinemia: MVC 15% vs. TDF 5%
ACTG 5262 AIDS 2009;23:1605	DRV/r 800/100 qd + RAL 100 bid	48	112	No comparator group; 21/28 failures had baseline VL>100,000 c/mL; 5/21 had integrase resistance

(continued)

TABLE 4.14 Continued

Trial	Regimen (Dose in mg)	Duration (Wks)	N^a	Comments
ANRS 121 AIDS 2011;25:2113	(EFV or NVP) + (LPV/r or IDV/r) vs. NRTI containing regimen	24	117	Virologic failure higher with NRTI sparing (28% vs. 12%), and more EFV resistance mutations; Not Recommended
ACTG 5110 JAC 2009;25:2113	LPV/r 533/133 bid + NVP 200 bid vs. LPV/r + (AZT or d4T) Vs. LPV/r + ABC	48	101	VL>200 c/mL in 3-6% (all 3 groups). Significant increase in toxicity with LPV/r + NVP ($p = 0.007$)
MIDAS JAIDS 2013;64:167	MVC 150 qd + DRV/r 800/100 qd	96	24	Virologic failure 8.3% at wk 48, and 10% at week 96. Majority of failures had baseline VL>100,000 No resistance seen
RADAR PLoS One 2014;9:e106221	DRV/r 800/100 qd + RAL 300 bid vs. DRV/r 800/100 bid + TDF/FTC	48	42	VL<48: RAL 62% vs. TDF 83.7% at 48 wks Most discontinuations due to lost to follow-up; No resistance seen

Study	Regimen	Weeks	N[a]	Results
SPARTAN HIV Clin Trials 2012;13:119	ATV 400 bid + RAL 300 bid vs. ATV/r + TDF/FTC	24	63	VL<50: 84% RAL vs. 76% TDF RAL resistance mutations in 4 Grade 4 hyperbilirubinemia: RAL arm 21% vs. TDF arm 0%
PROGRESS AIDS Res Hum Retroviruses 2013;29:256	LPV/r 400/100 + RAL 400 qd vs. LPV/r + TDF/FTC	96	101	VL<50: 66% RAL vs. 68.3% TDF Similar ADRs Most participants had low baseline VL. Decrease GFR & BMD in TDF arm
NEAT 001/ANRS 143 Lancet 2014;384:1942	DRV/r 800/100 qd + RAL 400 bid vs. DRV/r + TDF/FTC	96	401	Treatment failure rates: RAL 19% vs. TDF 15%, noninferior; Similar AEs; No resistance in TDF arm 15/55 had INSTI resistance in RAL arm—associated with baseline VL

[a] N = total in NRTI-sparing arm

TABLE 4.15 Nucleoside/nucleotide reverse transcriptase inhibitor (NRTI)-sparing regimens as antiretroviral therapy (ART) switch and/or for treatment-experienced patients

Trial	Regimen (Dose in mg)	Duration (Wks)	N[a]	Comments
ACTG 5116 AIDS 2007;21:325	LPV/r 533/133 bid + EFV 600 qd vs. EFV + 2 NRTIs	96	226	NRTI-sparing regimen showed higher rates of virologic failure (12% vs. 6%), and toxicity (17% vs. 4%).
No Nuke ANRS 108 HIV Med 2008;9:625	(IDV/r or LPV/r) + NVP vs. NRTI-containing regimen	48	100	Study goal was reversal of d4T or AZT lipodystrophy; NRTI-sparing arm retained viral suppression and increased subcutaneous fat.
ACTG 5110 JAC 2009;63:998	LPV/r 533/133 bid + NVP 200 bid vs. LPV/r + NVP + ABC	48	101	NRTI-sparing group: maintained viral control and reduced lipodystrophy but had earlier ADRs (p<0.007)
MULTINEKA Clin Infect Dis 2009;49:892	LPV/r 400/100 bid + NVP 200 bid vs. LPV/r + 2 NRTIs	48	34	VL<50 c/mL maintained with slight improvement in lipodystrophy.
Monotherapy regimens	DRV/r, LPV/r	—	—	See Table 4.18

TRIO Clin Infect Dis 2009;49:1441	RAL + ETR + DRV/r	48	103	Extensive baseline resistance; Not a switch study; VL<50 at 48 wks: 86%
KITE AIDS Res Hum Retroviruses 2012;28:1196	LPV/r 400/100 bid + RAL 400 bid vs. LPV/r + 2 NRTIs	48	40	VL<50: 92% RAL vs. 88% NNRTI; AEs similar but higher triglycerides in RAL arm
LATTE Lancet ID 2015;15:1145	CBG[b] + RPV IM vs. EFV + 2 NRTI, after 24 wks CBG[b] or EFV + 2 NRTIs	96	181	VL<50 results: 24 wk. induction—87% CBG po vs. 74% EFV po; 48 wk: 82% CBG IM vs. 71% EFV; 96 wk: 76% CBG IM vs. 63% EFV
ETR + RAL JAC 2014;69:742	ETR 200 mg + RAL 400 mg bid (Switch study)	48	25	Baseline 84% with prior virologic failure; VL<50: 84% at 48 wks
ETR + RAL Antiviral Res 2015;113:103	ETR 200 mg + RAL 400 mg bid (Switch study)	48	25	Prospective open-label; All remained suppressed at median 722 days follow-up
RAL + DRV/r HIV Clin Trials 2016;17:38	RAL 400 bid + DRV/r 800/100 qd (Observational switch study)	48	82	VL<50: 92.7%; Reduction in lipid levels & tubular proteinuria

(*continued*)

TABLE 4.15 Continued

Trial	Regimen (Dose in mg)	Duration (Wks)	N^a	Comments
PROBE JAIDS 2016;72:46	DRV/r 800/100 qd + RPV 25 qd vs. DRV/r + 2 NRTI	48	30	VL<50: RPV 96.7% vs. NNRTI 93.4%; NRTI arm had greater reduction in bone stiffness
DOMONO Lancet HIV 2017;4:e547	DTG 50 mg qd monotherapy (Immediate vs. delayed switch design)	48	95	DTG mono: noninferior at 24 wk, but virologic failure continued to occur leading to DTG resistance (8% with VF;3 of 8 VF developed INSTI resistance)
SWORD 1 & 2 Lancet 2018	DTG 50 mg + RPV 25 mg qd vs. current ART regimen (CAR) (Early vs. late switch design)	48	513	VL<50: DTG 94.7% vs. CAR 94.9%; DTG/RPV: more AEs resulting in withdrawal (3% vs. <1%)

^{a} N = total in NRTI-sparing arm.

^{b} Cabotegravir (CBG) is a long-acting experimental INSTI currently not approved by the US Food and Drug Administration for commercial use; comes in IM or PO (oral form is given in 3 doses over 24 wks).

of additional integrase inhibitor mutations which may limit the activity of other integrases, including DTG (JAC 2009;64:1087).

Using MVC for Salvage: This CCR5 antagonist offers an option for patients with extensive treatment experience and resistance, but, due to the need for a R5 tropic virus (ascertained through a tropism assay) to be useful, it may be better utilized in a treatment naïve or less treatment-experienced patient setting. Unfortunately, approximately 50–60% of patients with extensive treatment experience have dual/mixed (DM) or X4 tropic virus and therefore are not candidates for MVC therapy (Clin Infect Dis 2007;44:591). MVC also has many drug interactions, so dose adjustments of MVC are commonly needed.

Using INSTI for Salvage: The integrase inhibitors offer an option with several advantages, including high potency, excellent tolerability, and minimal drug interactions. Drug susceptibility to INSTI is virtually assured in patients who have not been previously treated with integrase inhibitors. Both RAL and EVG are highly efficacious but susceptible to virologic failure due to the development of resistant mutations (Retrovirology 2017;14:36). In the SAILING trial (Lancet 2013;382:700), DTG demonstrated superiority over RAL (VL<50 c/mL at week 48, DTG 71% vs. RAL 64%, p = 0.03) in treatment-experienced, INSTI-naïve patients with baseline resistance to two or more ART classes. DTG used twice daily with an optimized background regimen in treatment-experienced patients with raltegravir or elvitegravir resistance in the open label VIKING-3 trial achieved VLs of <50 in 69% of patients at 24 wks. More recently, in resource-limited settings, patients failing an NNRTI regimen with at least 1 active NRTI, DTG + 2 NRTIs was compared to LPV/r + 2NRTIs. The study was stopped by the Independent Data Monitoring Committee after review of 24 wks' data and subsets of 36 wks' data which revealed differences in virologic nonresponse and protocol-defined virologic failure favoring the DTG arm (HIV RNA <50: 82% DTG; 69% LPV/r). No resistance was seen in the DTG arm compared with three patients in the LPV/r arm.

Using Ibalizumab for Salvage: This anti-CD4 receptor monoclonal antibody is first in its class and was fast-track approved by the

FDA for the treatment of multidrug-resistant HIV infection. It is administered as an IV infusion every 2 wks. In a Phase 3 study of treatment-experienced patients with multidrug-resistant HIV and limited treatment options, 40 patients were treated with ibalizumab in combination with an optimized background: 43% of patients achieved a VL of <50 at 24 wks. At 48 wks, 16/27 patients who continued on the study after week 24 retained an HIV RNA <50. Based on these data, the drug was approved as an option to use in combination for the treatment of HIV infected patients with MDR HIV. It should be noted that in the registrational trial for Iblaizumab, patients could co-enroll in a Phase 3 trial evaluating an attachment inhibitor, fostemsavir, in heavily treatment-experienced patients with limited treatment options. At 24 wks, 54% of patients receiving fostemsavir achieved virologic success with an HIV RNA of <50. Fostemsavir is currently in late-stage clinical development and could represent another potential agent for treatment-experienced patients once approved.

Extensive Drug Resistance: There are now more than 30 ART drugs from seven different classes (Table 4.1 and Table 4.2), allowing nearly all patients multiple HIV treatment options, as seen in the TRIO trials (Clin Infect Dis 2009;49:1441; Drugs 2010;70:1629). This report showed that 90% of patients with "triple class resistance" had a VL of <200 c/mL at 24 wks on a regimen containing RAL, ETR, and DRV/r. Nevertheless, there will always be patient situations in which no good options are available. In such patients, the strategy would be to have them participate in clinical trials that target multiclass failure patients, possibly with access to a new drug class or an alternative novel strategy. If virologic suppression is not attainable, the goal of therapy should be viral suppression to the greatest extent possible, with the goal of increasing or at least maintaining the CD4 count, since this ultimately determines the risk for most of the HIV-associated complications. It is of note that multiple studies have found that CD4 count tends to be stable or increase modestly on ARTs despite a VL indicating virologic failure (AIDS 1999;13:1035). In fact, a review of six seminal salvage trials (POWER, RESIST, TORO, DUET, MOTIVATE, BENCHMRK) in which patients in the control groups, who took only an optimized background regimen (OBR), experienced substantial increases in mean CD4 count despite virologic failure rates of 60–80% Table 4.11. A review of RESIST, POWER, DUET, and BENCHMRK trials demonstrated high failure rates in the OBR group (mean 54%), but the mean CD4 count at 1 yr increased by 38 cells/mm^3 (though in the group getting the test drug it was 103 cells/mm^3). It should still be emphasized that the goal of therapy is still a VL of <50 c/mL.

Continuing ART in the face of virologic failure has the benefit of reducing risk of clinical failure but at the cost of increasing resistance and decreasing future options. Prior studies show that continuing the same regimen with a VL of >1,000 c/mL results in an average loss of about one drug option per year (Scand J Infect Dis 2005;37:890; Clin Infect Dis 2006;43:1329). Decisions to continue ART in cases of virologic failure were based on CD4 count and limited available options at the time the study was conducted. A concern with stopping ART is the possibility of rapid virologic rebound and CD4 decline, as shown in the SMART trial (see Table 4.16).

Summary of Recommendations for Extensive Resistance

1. The regimen should include at least two, preferably three active agents.
2. FTC or 3TC are often continued despite resistance (but they do not count as active drugs). Use of other NRTIs to which the virus is resistant is arbitrary, but some studies show efficacy when options are limited (JAIDS 2011;57:4).
3. First-generation NNRTIs (NVP or EFV) should be permanently stopped once resistance is observed. Second-generation NNRTIs (RPV or ETR) may be options depending on resistance test results and the ability to deal with RPV and EFV interactions.
4. Make optimal use of current and historic resistance test results.
5. With extensive resistance and limited options, consider infrequently used agents such as ENF or the TRIO combination

(RAL+ETR+DRV/r) (Drugs 2010;70:1629). Other options include MVC or newer INSTIs such as DTG, or possibly Ibalizumab (a newly approved anti-CD4 monoclonal antibody). Recycling drugs with prior resistance has no established merit.

6. When necessary, seek access to investigational drugs through clinical trials or expanded access programs.

7. If at least two active agents are not available, the goal of treatment is to (a) reduce VL as much as possible and for as long as possible, (b) maintain or increase the CD4 count, (c) reduce drug toxicity, and (d) limit use of drugs likely to lead to resistance mutations that may limit future treatment options. Note that patients with a VL <10,000 c/mL usually can maintain a stable or even increasing CD4 count on ART (AIDS 1999;13:1035).

8. The urgency of decisions in patients with limited options is usually driven by the risk of progression, which is largely reflected by the CD4 count.

9. Mega-HAART, recycling, dual PIs, and treatment interruptions are all historic strategies for managing patients with extensive drug resistance, are antiquated, and are not recommended.

Treatment Strategies in Selected Situations

Stopping Haart

Effects of a Failing Regimen: Most patients with virologic failure that cannot be corrected with salvage regimens should not discontinue ART since this would result in a prompt increase in VL averaging $0.8\text{--}1.0 \log_{10}$ c/mL to pretreatment baseline levels with a concurrent rapid decrease in CD4 count averaging 85–100 cells/mm^3 in 3 months (N Engl J Med 2003;349:837; J Infect Dis 2000;181:946). Thus, despite virologic failure, defined by the 200 c/mL threshold, the failing regimen often has significant activity. The attempt to determine the ART agents that are responsible for this residual activity suggest a debated role for 3TC (and FTC by inference) and possibly other NRTIs and PIs, but apparently not with EFV or NVP (J Infect Dis 2005;192:1537). Nevertheless, continuation of antiviral agents in the face of ongoing viral replication has obvious risk related to cost, toxicity, and resistance. With regard to resistance, the EuroSIDA study showed that continued use of a failing regimen resulted in an average of 2 new resistance mutations and a loss of 1.25 active antiviral agents per 6 months (AIDS 2007;21:721), which could have an important impact on future options (J Infect Dis 2003;188:1001). A similar study in 106 heavily pretreated patients continuing a failing regimen demonstrated that 23% and 18% developed at least one new NRTI and one new PI mutation, respectively, at 1 yr (Clin Infect Dis 2006;43:1329–36). The usual recommendation is not to discontinue ART, but to tailor the regimen to the individual patient based on critical need (CD4 count), the potential for selection of further resistance mutations that could affect future options, and the ability to achieve partial virologic control. Prior studies suggest clinical and immunological benefit when the VL is maintained at <10,000 c/mL (Curr Opin Infect Dis 2001;14:23; N Engl J Med 2001;344:472). With regard to agent selection, 3TC or FTC is usually retained due to M184V's effect on viral fitness. PI/r therapies are often favored with selection based on the combination of genotype and phenotype sensitivity tests interpreted by an expert. RAL and EFV are usually avoided unless there is likelihood of a fully suppressive regimen. The concern is resistance to these and the fear of resistance developing to next-generation INSTIs, such as DTG and BIC. There is no evidence that EFV or NVP contribute to residual activity in the face of resistance. Continuation of either EFV or NVP in virologic failure risks acquisition of new NNRTI mutations that could potentially reduce susceptibility to ETR and RPV. Recommendations for the use of specific agents in nonsuppressive regimens cannot be made based on available data.

Stopping NVP and EFV-based ART: These drugs have long half-lives. As a result, discontinuation of EFV- or NVP-containing regimens result in the equivalence of a prolonged monotherapy with drugs that have low barriers to resistance (J Infect Dis 2006;42:401). Methods to avoid resistance include staggering discontinuation with continuation of NRTIs for a period of time following discontinuation of the NNRTI or substituting the NNRTI with a PI/r for 2–4 wks prior to discontinuation of the entire regimen.

NVP: This drug autoinduces hepatic CYP3A4 metabolism over 2–4 wks to reduce its half-life from 45 to 25 hrs (J Infect Dis 1995;171:537). With a single dose of NVP used to prevent perinatal transmission, resistance mutations have been reported in 15–75% of treated women due to prolonged exposure to subtherapeutic levels of NVP (J Infect Dis 2005;192:24). Resistance was significantly reduced with the use of 3–7 days of AZT/3TC continued after administration of single-dose NVP (J Infect Dis 2006;193:482), although 5/39 (13%) do still develop primary resistance mutations despite use of AZT/3TC. On the basis of this observation, as early as 2008, pregnant HIV-positive women are recommended to take a single dose of NVP with a 7-day "tail" of AZT/3TC, while acknowledging that this does not totally eliminate the risk of NVP resistance since the right duration of the NRTI tail is unknown. The risk of developing NNRTI resistance after discontinuation of a suppressive NVP-based regimen may be lower than that seen with single-dose NVP, assuming that VL is suppressed at time of discontinuation. Nevertheless, the concerns discussed later (in the EFV section) also apply to NVP. Some have suggested that the "tail" should be up to 2 wks for NVP, particularly in the first 1–2 wks prior to autoinduction of metabolic pathways (AIDS 2007;21:1673). Another issue relating to this is the reintroduction of NVP after discontinuation. The recommendation is to repeat the low dose (200 mg/day) lead-in for 2 wks if the time off NVP exceeds 2 wks.

EFV: The half-life of EFV ranges from 36 to 100 hrs, significantly longer than that of NVP. The major metabolic pathway is CYP2B6, and there are significant variations in the half-life that are governed largely by polymorphisms at codon 516 of the CYP2B6 gene (Clin Infect Dis 2006;42:401; Clin Infect Dis 2007;45:1230; J Infect Dis 2011;203:246). The result is that therapeutic levels can be detected for more than 21 days after the drug is discontinued in some patients (AIDS 2005;19:716; Clin Infect Dis 2006;42:401). The risk of EFV resistance with discontinuation of all agents in EFV-based ART was 16% in SMART and anecdotally reported by others (Lancet 2006;368:459; AIDS 2007;21:1673; Clin Infect Dis 2008;46:1601). Recommendations to prevent resistance in this situation are to continue the two NRTIs for 1–2 wks ("NRTI tail" method) or to substitute a PI-based regimen for 3–4 wks (AIDS 2007;21:1673). Despite this recommendation, it should be noted that the half-life of EFV is highly variable based on genetic variation in EFV metabolism, and the appropriate duration of this is not known, making the "NRTI tail" method unpredictable and the PI substitution method more attractive.

Treatment Strategies in the Setting of Immunologic Failure

Immunologic failure refers to unexplained failure to achieve and maintain an adequate CD4 count despite virologic suppression. There is no consensus definition: some define it as failure to achieve an increase to selected thresholds that represent risk for HIV-related complications such as 50, 100, or 200 cells/mm^3; some use a suboptimal CD4 cell response, such as an increase of <50 cells/mm^3/yr; and some use thresholds of 350 or 500 cells/mm^3 at 4–7 yrs. In a review of 53 therapeutic trials with 14,264 treatment-naïve patients, the median CD4 count increase at 1 yr with good viral suppression was 180–200 cells/mm^3 (AIDS 2006;20:205). Immune recovery was significantly greater with boosted PIs than with NNRTI-based ART (+200 cells/mm^3 vs. 179 cells/mm^3).

Factors contributing to poor CD4 response include interferon or prednisone therapy; advanced age; co-infection with HTLV-1, HTLV-2, HCV, or HIV-2; and serious co-morbidities.

Antiretroviral drugs: The CD4 response is somewhat lower with EFV-based ART compared to alternative regimens including PI/r, MVC, and INSTIs. The difference is often statistically significant in large trials of treatment naïve patients, but there appears to be no medical consequence. AZT-based regimens may have reduced response based on studies showing CD4 increase after switching to ABC or TDF (N Engl J Med 2006;354:251). The combination of TDF and ddI has been associated with a blunted CD4 response (Clin Infect Dis 2005;19:569).

Risk for OIs: The risk of an OI in patients with virologic suppression is substantially reduced despite a blunted CD4 response (J Infect Dis 2005;192:1407; AIDS 2006;20:371). The best documentation comes from the ClinSurv Study (J Infect Dis 2011;203:364), which analyzed data from 1,318 patients with VLs of <50 c/mL and CD4 counts of <200 cells/mm^3. There were only 42 new OI events with 5,038 patient-years follow-up. Although PCP prophylaxis is still recommended in this group, the risk of PCP is very low. One study found zero cases of PCP per 1,000 patient-years follow-up in patients with a CD4 count of 100–200 cells/mm^3 (Clin Infect Dis 2010;51:611).

Interventions: Options to improve the CD4 response include changing the ART regimen. As previously noted, the CD4 response with EFV-based ART is somewhat less robust than that with INSTI-, DRV/r-, LPV/r-, or MVC-based ART regimens among those with viral suppression to <50 c/mL. Nevertheless, this difference is of unclear clinical significance, and there has been no convincing benefit with drug switches. The usual approach is to ignore the issue based on the ClinSurv data. Another option is treatment intensification with additional antivirals despite effective viral suppression, but this approach has not succeeded in increasing the CD4 count (PLoS One 2011;6:e14764). There have also been attempts to supplement the regimen with an agent known to stimulate CD4 production. IL-2 increases the CD4 count (Arch Intern Med 2007;167:597), but this was not associated with any clinical benefit in two large clinical trials (ESPRIT and SILCAAT) with 5,706 patients randomized (N Engl J Med 2009;361:1548). Some studies suggest a genetic basis for the blunted CD4 response in some patients (J Infect Dis 2006;194:1098; JAIDS 2006;41:1). There are no management recommendations, and the highest priority remains virologic suppression with adequate attention to concurrent medications (steroids, etc.) and co-morbidities that may be contributing.

Other Strategies: Treatment Interruption, Monotherapy, and NRTI-Sparing Regimens

Intermittent Treatment Interruptions

The rationale for intermittent treatment interruption had been to reduce drug cost, toxicity, and inconvenience while maintaining viral suppression. However, the SMART trial demonstrated that CD4-based treatment interruption using a CD4 threshold of 350 cells/mm^3 for interruption and 250 cells/mm^3 for reinitiation was associated with a significantly higher risk of OIs and death compared to continuous ART (J Infect Dis 2008;97:1145) (See Table 4.16).

Scheduled Interruptions

The STACCATO trial attempted the alternative-weeks strategy (also called WOWO for "week-on, week-off") with various regimens;

TABLE 4.16 Results of the SMART Trial (N Engl J Med 2006; 355:2283)

	Interrupted ART N = 2,720		Continuous ART N = 2,752	
	N	Event Rate (Per 100 Person-Year)	N	Event Rate (Per 100 Person-Year)
Primary end point	120	3.3	47	1.3*
Death any causes	55	1.5	30	0.8*
Serious OI	13	0.4	2	0.1*
Major cardiovascular, hepatic, renal	65	1.8	39	1.1*
Cardiovascular	46	1.3	31	0.8*
Hepatic	9	0.2	2	0.1*
Renal	10	0.3	7	0.2*
Grade 4 Event	173	5.0	148	4.2*

*$P \leq 0.05$.

virologic failure occurred in 53% in the experimental treatment group compared to 5% of controls treated with continuous ART (Lancet 2006;368:459). This study also showed a high rate of new resistance mutations in the WOWO group (Clin Infect Dis 2005;40:728). A subsequent trial with an 8 wks on and 8 wks off strategy was used in the DART study, but this was stopped early due to excessive HIV-related complications in the intermittent treatment arm (Lancet 2010;395:123). Another intermittent study is called FOTO, "five [days] on, two off." With its long half-life, EFV presumably maintains its antiviral activity over the weekend. The initial experience with 20 participants in the FOTO trial has shown continued viral suppression in 19 of 20 taking NNRTI-based ART at 1 yr (HIV Clin Trials 2007;8:256). This strategy should be reserved for patients in clinical trials until more data can be accumulated about its safety and efficacy. Treatment interruption is NEVER recommended, especially if it results in virologic rebound.

Monotherapy

The basic standard of at least two active drugs (preferably three) was established in 1996 with the inception of the HAART era, shown in the Merck 035 trial (N Engl J Med 1997;337:734). The combination of AZT/3TC+IDV achieved viral suppression (<50 c/mL) in 80% of patients compared to 43% given IDV, and zero given AZT/3TC. Attempts to find exceptions have included several trials of monotherapy using agents with high efficacy and high resistance mutation thresholds. The goals are to reduce pill burden, cost, and side effects.

Boosted Protease Inhibitor (PI/r) Monotherapy: Results of 11 trials investigating this approach are summarized in Table 4.17, which includes six studies on LPV/r bid, two with DRV/r, and three small trials with ATV/r. The format for 9 of the 11 studies was to achieve virologic suppression (VL <50 c/mL) on a standard three-drug regimen and then to discontinue NRTIs, leaving patients on boosted PI monotherapy, usually with continuation of the standard

TABLE 4.17 Monotherapy trials with boosted protease inhibitors

Trial	Design[a]	Duration (Wks)	Regimen	N	VL<50 c/mL (%)
LPV/r					
MONARK AIDS 2008;22:385	Treatment-naïve	48	LPV/r bid	83	67
OK-04 J AIDS 2009;51:147	Induction-maintenance	96	LPV/r bid LPV/r + 2N	100 98	77 78
KalMo HIV Clin Trials 2009;10:368	Induction-maintenance	96	LPV/r bid Current therapy	30 30	80 87
SHCS AIDS 2010;24:2347	Induction-maintenance	[b]	LPV/r bid Current therapy	42 18	75 100
STAR 2011 CROI Abstract 584	NRTI failure	48	LPV/r bid LPV/r + TDF + 3TC	100 100	64 82
M03-613 J Infect Dis 2008;198:234	Induction-maintenance	96	LPV/r bid EFV + AZT/3TC	104 51	48 61
DRV/r					
MONOI-ANRS 136 J Antimicrob Chemother 2012;67:691	Induction-maintenance	96	DRV/r qd DRV/r + 2 NRTIs	113 112	88 84

(continued)

TABLE 4.17 Continued

Trial	Design[a]	Duration (Wks)	Regimen	N	VL<50 c/mL (%)
MONET HIV Med 2012;13:398	Induction-maintenance	144	DRV/r qd DRV/r + 2 NRTIs	127 129	75 69
ATV/r					
ATARITMO AIDS 2007;21:1309	Induction-maintenance	24	ATV/r qd	27	93
Karolinski J Acquir Immune Defic Syndr 2007;44:417	Induction-maintenance	72	ATV/r qd	15	83
ACTG 5201 J Infect Dis 2009;199:866	Induction-maintenance	48	ATV/r qd	34	88

[a] Induction-maintenance design consisted of randomization after patients attain VL <50 c/mL.

[b] Study discontinued due to excessive failure rates in the monotherapy arm (6 vs. 0) including five with high HIV levels in cerebrospinal fluid.

three-drug regimen as the comparator (control group). In the past, monotherapy has been attempted mainly with PI/r-based therapy on the assumption that resistance would be unlikely, and, if necessary, virologic control could be achieved by restarting NRTIs. Conclusions regarding these data are based on the results in Table 4.17 and a review by Perez-Valero and Arribas (Curr Opin Infect Dis 2011;24:7):

- *Relative Merits*: (1) the best results have been with DRV/r given once daily in the MONET Trial, (2) trials with ATV/r have been too small to allow for conclusion, and (3) the most extensive data are with LPV/r given twice daily.
- *Benefit*: a large proportion of patients can maintain suppression with DRV/r or LPV/r using an induction-maintenance approach.
- *Risks*: LPV/r monotherapy is associated with higher rates of low-level viremia (VL 50–500 c/mL) and higher rates of virologic failures than standard therapy, but most virologic failures can be "rescued" with reintroduction of two NRTIs, and resistance mutations are relatively rare. The SHCS Trial (AIDS 2010;24:2347) suggests that LPV/r monotherapy fails to protect the CNS. This concern may also apply to DRV/r, but it has not been studied.
- *HIV Guideline Recommendations*: Guidelines generally do NOT recommend PI/r monotherapy except for the European AIDS Clinical Society Guidelines, which state that it can be tried in adherent, suppressed patients who have NRTI toxicity or other contraindications to standard ART.

Dolutegravir Monotherapy: Because DTG has a high resistance mutation threshold, and resistance has not been documented in clinical trials with ART-naïve patients, some have proposed using DTG as monotherapy. Resistance mutations that arise to DTG in vitro result in significant decreases in enzymatic activity and viral replication leading to the question of whether clinical resistance will develop to DTG (Retrovirology 2013;10:22). Similar to boosted PI monotherapy, this strategy is based on the concept of reducing cost. DTG monotherapy has been evaluated in several small induction maintenance studies and one small case series of monotherapy for treatment initiation (JAC 2016;71:1632; JAC 2016;71:1046; JAC 2016;71:1975; JAIDS 2016;72:e12). Other reports have demonstrated the development of DTG resistance in the context of baseline INSTI resistance (JAC 2016;71:1948; Antivir Ther 2016;21:481). The DOMONO Trial (Lancet HIV 2017;4:e547) is a randomized non-inferiority study conducted in Netherlands evaluating DTG monotherapy as maintenance therapy after at least 6 months suppression with combination therapy. This switch study showed DTG monotherapy was non-inferior to combination ART at 24 wks, but virologic failure continued to occur thereafter, leading to DTG resistance (8%, or 8 of 95 subjects developed virologic failure, with 3 of 8 failures associated with resistance mutations). Therefore, current DHHS Guidelines do not recommend use of DTG monotherapy.

Nucleoside-Sparing Regimens

Standard treatment of all treatment-naïve patients and most treatment-experienced patients consists of using a dual NRTI backbone. However, there are multiple clinical settings in which use of these drugs is considered ill-advised, primary due to safety concerns and sometimes due to resistance. Multiple NRTI-sparing regimens have been studied (Tables 4.14 and 4.15). Most of the older studies show limited benefit compared to standard therapy. However, more recent studies have shown more promising results. It is apparent that population characteristics and the specific regimens chosen for that population can have a significant impact on the success of the strategy. As more data become available, this may become a reasonable strategy for specific patient populations. It should be noted that 3TC and FTC are rarely contraindicated since they have excellent tolerability, no well-characterized long-term metabolic complications, and continued albeit reduced activity in the presence of the M184V mutation. Continued use of 3TC or FTC does not lead to additional resistance nor eliminate antiviral activity (JAIDS

2010;54:51; AIDS 2006;20:795; J Virol 2008;80:201; J Infect Dis 2005;192:1537).

Regimen Switch and Simplification

The DHHS Guidelines define "switch and simplification" as a regimen change to achieve reduction in pill burden or frequency of administration, improve tolerability, improve potency, or to respond to new data or treatment recommendations. The ultimate goal is to use a regimen that provides long-term viral suppression and to maintain a good quality of life with as minimal risk as possible. Data to support this approach come from studies demonstrating that long-term adherence to ART correlates with reduced adherence demands, reduced pill burden, and better patient satisfaction (N Engl J Med 2006;354:251; AIDS Res Hum Retroviruses 2007;23:1505; JAIDS 2004;36:808). The best candidates for this type of regimen change are those without a history of treatment failure or with known susceptibility to the agents in the new regimen.

- *Within-class substitutions*: Examples include the desire to eliminate thymidine analogs (AZT, d4T) and ddI in favor of less toxic agents or more convenient pill combinations. Another example is the switch from LPV/r to an alternative boosted PI to simplify the regimen, reduce LPV/r-associated intolerance side effects, or improve potency (as with switch to ATV/r or DRV/r).
- *Out-of-Class substitution*: Examples include switches to lower pill burden combinations. This includes switching to newer single-tablet regimens as they becomes available.
- *Toxicity*: an example is ENF switches, which were common and usually successful in maintaining viral suppression when newer agents such as RAL, MCV, and ETR became available (JAC 2009;64:1341).
- *Cost*: This has not been a primary issue in the past due to limited options but has become more important as more ART options become available, and some agents are now available in generic form.

There is growing evidence that an ART switch to a two-drug regimen can maintain virologic suppression. Strategies with clinical trials data supporting the use of two-drug regimens include utilizing a boosted PI (either ATV/r or DRV/r) in combination with 3TC, and an integrase inhibitor (DTG or CBG) in combination with RPV. Another combination under evaluation is dolutegravir in combination with 3TC. The PADDLE study evaluated this combination in 20 ART-naïve patients with a 90% success rate at 48 wks. This was followed by ACTG 5353 where 120 ART-naïve patients were treated with DTG and 3TC. At 24 wks, 90% of patients had an HIV RNA of <50. There were three protocol-defined virologic failures, all of whom had undetectable levels of DTG at time points during the trial indicating nonadherence. Only one subject developed resistance. DTG+3TC has also been evaluated as a switch strategy in virologically suppressed patients. The LAMIDOL study found that 103/104 patients remained suppressed after 24 wks, and the ASPIRE study demonstrated non-inferiority of DTG/3TC to continuing a baseline ART regimen in 89 patients. The GEMINI studies, two large Phase 3 trials comparing DTG/3TC to DTG+TDF/3TC in 1441 treatment naïve patients, recently reported noninferiority of the two arms with no development of resistance in either arm. This data led the DHHS guidelines to list DTG/3TC as a regimen to consider if regimens with current NRTIs are not optimal.

Dose Adjustments of Antiretroviral Drugs

Dose Adjustment for Hepatic Insufficiency

See 2018 DHHS Guidelines.

NRTIs: Minimal effect because these drugs have limited first-pass metabolism and low protein binding. They are primarily eliminated by renal excretion. No dose adjustment with liver disease except for ABC. Generally ABC is avoided, or use of 200 mg bid dosing should be considered.

NNRTIs (EFV, NVP, ETR, RPV, DOR): Liver dysfunction has a minimal effect on trough levels of EFV, NVP, ETR, RPV and DOR. Avoid NVP with Child-Pugh Class B or C due to risk of hepatotoxicity. RPV and DOR have not been evaluated in patients with Child-Pugh Class C disease.

Integrase Inhibitors (RAL, EVG, DTG, BIC): No dose adjustment for Child-Pugh Class A and B; Recommendation is to avoid in Class C due to the lack of data.

Protease Inhibitors: These are extensively metabolized by the Cytochrome p450 enzymes. Recommendations are as follows:

- *NFV or LPV/r*: Standard dose, but use with caution.
- *IDV*: Recommended dose is 600 mg every 8 hrs. Limited data.
- *FPV*: Treatment-naïve: Child-Pugh Class A or B, Use 700 mg bid (unboosted); Class C, Use 350 mg bid; treatment-experienced: Class A, Use 700/100 mg bid; Class B, 450/100 mg/day; and Class C, 300 mg bid + RTV 100 mg/day.
- *ATV*: Child-Pugh Class B, Use 300 mg/day dosing without RTV or COBI boosting; Child-Pugh Class C, avoid.
- *DRV/r*: Use with caution; not recommended with severe liver disease.
- *TPV/r*: Use with caution with Child-Pugh A. Contraindicated with Child-Pugh Class B or C.

CCR5 Antagonist (MVC): No recommendations; MVC levels are likely to increase in liver disease.

Dose Adjustment for Renal Insufficiency

See 2018 DHHS Guidelines.

NRTIs: All require dose adjustment except ABC (See Table 4.18).

NNRTIs (EFV, NVP, ETR, RPV, DOR): No dose adjustment for mild renal disease; use with caution with moderate to severe renal disease. DOR requires no adjustment in severe renal disease but has not been studied in end stage renal disease and dialysis.

TABLE 4.18 Nucleoside/nucleotide reverse transcriptase inhibitor (NRTI) dosing in renal insufficiency

Drug	Usual Daily Dose	Dosing in Renal Insufficiency (CrCl in mL/min)		
		30–49	15–29	<15 or on HD
ABC	300 mg po bid	No dose adjustment necessary		
3TC[a]	300 mg po qd, or 150 mg po bid	150 mg q24h	150 mg × 1 dose, then 100 mg q24h	150 mg × 1 dose, then 50 mg q24h (use 25 mg q24h if <5 or on HD)
FTC	200 mg po qd (capsule), or 240 mg (24 mL) qd (solution)	200 mg cap q48h 120 mg sol'nq24h	200 mg cap q72h 80 mg sol'n q24h	200 mg cap q96h; 60 mg sol'n q24h
TDF	300 mg po qd	300 mg q48h[b]	300 mg 2×/wk	Not recommended
TDF/FTC	1 tablet po qd	1 tablet q48h[b]	Not recommended	
TAF/FTC	1 tablet po qd	No adjustment	Not recommended	
AZT	300 mg po bid	No dose adjustment necessary		100 mg tid, or 300 mg qd

qd, once daily; bid, twice daily; tid, three times daily; cap, capsule; sol'n, solution (liquid).

[a] Many providers do not dose-adjust 3TC below 100–150 mg q24 hrs since this requires the use of liquid 3TC and may impact adherence. At higher than recommended doses, 3TC is generally well tolerated.

[b] Consider switch to TAF formulation.

Integrase Inhibitors (RAL, EVG, DTG, BIC): No dose adjustment with RAL or DTG. As EVG is co-formulated with TDF or TAF, and BIC is co-formulated, TDF/FTC/EVG/c is not recommended for use in patient with a CrCl of <70 mL/min, while TAF/FTC/EVG/c and BIC/TAF/FTC/BIC is not recommended for use in those with a CrCl of <30 mL/min.

Protease Inhibitors

- *DRV/r, LPV/r, FPV, or IDV:* Use standard dose.
- *ATV:* With hemodialysis, use ATV/r 300 mg/100 mg daily for treatment-naïve patients; avoid ATV and ATV/r in treatment-experienced patients with HD due to reduced concentrations.

CCR5 Antagonist (MVC): Use 300 mg bid without potent CYP3A inducers or inhibitors. Not recommended if postural hypotension is present or with potent CYP3A inhibitors.

THERAPEUTIC DRUG MONITORING (TDM) is a potential method for determining appropriate drug dosing for HIV-infected patients with issues that are problematic, including adherence, drug interactions, pregnancy, concentration-dependent toxicities, interpatient variability, and/or altered physiology due to hepatic, renal, or GI complications. TDM cannot be readily performed with NRTIs because the in vivo correlates are with intracellular concentrations rather than plasma concentrations, although plasma concentrations can be meaningful. There may also be interest in drug concentrations in other compartments such as the CNS, genital tract, and the like. Nevertheless, TDM for clinical care is not recommended by the DHHS Guidelines for several reasons:

- Lack of large prospective studies showing improved outcomes
- Lack of consistent data indicating clinically significant levels that correlate with therapeutic response or toxicity
- General unavailability of reliable laboratory resources to do this work

TABLE 4.19 Suggested minimum concentrations for drug-susceptible HIV-1 (Adopted from 2014 DHHS Guidelines)

Drug	Concentration (ng/mL)	Drug	Concentration (ng/mL)
APV	400	LPV	1,000
ATV	150	MVC	>50
DRV	3,300	NFV	800
EFV	1,000[a]	NVP	3,000
ETR	275	RAL	72
FPV	400	SQV	100–250
IDV	100[b]	TPV	20,500

[a] Cmin >4,000 ng/mL associated with central nervous system toxicity.

[b] Cmax >10,000 ng/mL associated with toxicity.

- Requirement of fastidious technique for collecting and processing specimens
- Substantial intrapatient variation

Clinical trial data show that even with highly qualified labs and careful techniques, results may vary enormously. In one study with an average of 40 samples per drug per patient, the coefficient of variation for drug levels was 44% for PIs and 25% for NNRTIs (Clin Infect Dis 2006;42:1189). Nevertheless, there are exceptions and some high-quality labs have shown the clinical utility of TDM, including dose adjustment of EFV to prevent CNS toxicity (Antivir Ther 2011;16:189) or to monitor PI-based ART (JAC 2009;64:109).

Summary of Pivotal Antiretroviral Trials

Trials that Demonstrated Benefits of Early ART

HPTN 052 (N Engl J Med 2011;365:493), *N* = 1763: This study enrolled HIV-1 discordant couples where they were randomized 1:1 to start ART either immediately (Early treatment arm) or after CD4 count declined to 250 cells/mm³ (Delayed treatment arm). This study proved that early initiation of ART reduced rates of sexual HIV-1 transmission (Hazard ratio of 0.04 in early treatment group) and clinical events.

INSIGHT START (N Engl J Med 2015;373:795), N = 4,685: This study formed the primary basis for a shift in ART treatment guidelines to the current recommendation of treating all HIV-1 infected patients regardless of CD4 count. This study had a mean follow-up of 3 yrs and demonstrated that immediate ART initiation had superior outcomes compared to the deferred-initiation group (waiting until CD4 drops below 500 cells/mm^3) in terms of serious AIDS-related (lower 0.20 vs. 0.72 per 100 person-year; p <0.001) and serious non–AIDS-related events (lower 0.42 vs. 0.67 per 100 person-year; p = 0.04).

TEMPRANO ANRS 12136 (N Engl J Med 2015;373:808), N = 2056: Conducted between 2008 and 2015 in Ivory Coast, this trial demonstrated that early immediate ART lowered rates of severe illness compared to deferred ART (treatment initiated based on the WHO criteria for starting ART). This study supported the findings in the START trial.

Treatment Strategy Trials

See also the section on "Intermittent Treatment Interruptions."
SMART (N Engl J Med 2006;355:2283), N = 5,472: This large multinational trial demonstrated that episodic ART therapy guided by CD4 counts significantly increased risk of OIs and death from any cause, compared to continuous ART.

Landmark Trial that Brought About the Era of HAART

Merck 035 (N Engl J Med 1997;337:734), N = 97: This trial was the first randomized controlled trial to demonstrate the superiority of combination ART with three active agents. The combination of AZT/3TC+IDV achieved virologic suppression (VL<50 c/mL) in 80% of patients compared to only 43% given IDV monotherapy and none in the AZT/3TC group. This also started the strategy of having a dual NRTI backbone as part of ART regimens.

Comparative Trials that Form the Basis of Current ART Guidelines

The trials are listed in chronological order.

ACTG 5142 (N Engl J Med 2008;358:2095), *N* = 757: First study to demonstrate NNRTI superiority over a PI/r regimen. EFV + 2 NRTI was virologically superior to LPV/r-based regimens (VL<50 at 96 wks; 89% vs. 77%; *p* = 0.006).

ACTG 5202 (Ann Intern Med 2011;154:445), *N* = 1857; EFV and ATV/r had similar efficacy when used with either ABC/3TC or TDF/FTC. The ABC/3TC arms had higher failures compared to the TDF/FTC arms when baseline VL was >100,000 c/mL (18.8% vs. 10.5%, *p* <0.05).

STARTMRK (Lancet 2009;374:796), *N* = 566: First of the integrase inhibitor class to demonstrate efficacy, RAL was found to be non-inferior to EFV in treatment naïve HIV-1 patients (VL <50 at 48 wks: 86.1% vs. 81.9%). RAL had fewer AEs than EFV (44% vs. 77%, *p* <0.0001).

GS-US-236-0102 (Lancet 2012;379:2439), *N* = 700: EVG/c demonstrated non-inferiority to EFV (VL <50 at 48 wks: EVG/c arm 87.6% vs. EFV arm 84.1%). Both treatment arms were combined with TDF/FTC.

GS-US-236-0103 (Lancet 2012;379:2429), *N* = 1017: EVG/c demonstrated non-inferiority to ATV/r (VL <50 at 48 wks: EVG/c arm 89.5% vs. ATV/r 86.8%). Both treatment arms were combined with TDF/FTC.

SPRING-2 (Lancet Infect Dis 2013;13:927), *N* = 827: DTG demonstrated non-inferiority to RAL-based regimens (VL <50 at 96 wks; DTG 81% vs. RAL 76%). DTG and RAL were combined with investigator-selected backbone NRTI (either ABC/3TC or TDF/FTC).

SINGLE (N Engl J Med 2013;369:1807), *N* = 844: This is the first trial that demonstrated the superiority of any ART regimen when compared to EFV. DTG was found to be superior to EFV (VL <50 at 48 wks; DTG/ABC/3TC 88% vs. EFV/TDF/FTC 81%; p = 0.003).

FLAMINGO (Lancet 2014;383:2222), *N* = 484: DTG demonstrated superiority to DRV/r (VL <50 at 48 wks; DTG 90% vs. DRV/r 83%; p = 0.025). This is the first INSTI in a randomized clinical trial to show superiority to DRV/r-based regimens.

ACTG 5257 (Ann Intern Med 2014;161:461), *N* = 1809: DRV/r, ATV/r, and RAL demonstrated similar efficacy but higher discontinuation in the ATV/r group due to AEs.

ARIA (Lancet HIV 2017;4:e546), *N* = 499: DTG demonstrated superiority to ATV/r (VL <50 at 48 wks; DTG 82% vs. ATV/r 71%; p = 0.005). The difference was driven by higher virologic response and lesser discontinuation due to AEs in the DTG arm.

GS-US-380-1489 (Lancet 2017;390:2063), *N* = 631: BIC co-formulated with TAF/FTC demonstrated non-inferiority to DTG co-formulated with ABC/3TC (VL <50 at 48 wks; BIC 92.4% vs. DTG 93.0%; p = 0.78). No treatment-emergent resistance developed in either treatment arm.

GS-US-380-1490 study (Lancet 2017;390:2073), *N* = 742: BIC demonstrated noninferiority to DTG (VL <50 at 48 wks; BIC 89% vs. DTG 93%; p = 0.12). Both arms were co-formulated with TAF/FTC. There was no treatment-emergent resistance in either arm.

Trials on Treatment-Experienced HIV-1 Patients

See also Table 4-11.

BENCHMRK (N Engl J Med 2008;359:355), *N* = 699: RAL was found superior to placebo when combined with an OBR for resistant HIV-1 infection.

ANRS 139 TRIO (Clin Infect Dis 2009;49:1441), *N* = 103: Combination therapy with DRV/r + ETR + RAL demonstrated efficacy in treatment-experienced patients with 90% achieving a VL of <50 c/mL at wk 24 and 86% at week 48.

SAILING (Lancet 2013;382:700), N = 715: In treatment-experienced but INSTI-naïve patients, DTG demonstrated superiority over RAL (VL <50 at 48 wks; DTG 71% vs. RAL 64%; p = 0.03) when combined with investigator-selected background therapy. There was significantly less treatment-emergent INSTI resistance in the DTG arm in those who fail therapy (4 vs. 17 patients, p = 0.003).

VIKING-3 (J Infect Dis 2014;210:354), N = 183: A single-arm, open-label study on ART-experienced adults with INSTI resistance that demonstrated the efficacy of DTG (50 mg bid) + OBR with a 63% suppression rate (VL <50 c/mL) at week 48. Mean CD4 change from baseline was +110 (40–190) cell/mm^3 at week 48.

VIKING-4 (Antivir Ther 2015;20:343), N = 30: In HAART-experienced patients with extensive baseline resistance to all approved anti-retroviral classes, DTG (50 mg bid) was found superior to placebo when combined with an OBR. At 48 wks, 40% of DTG + OBR had a VL of <50 c/mL.

5

HIV in Resource-Limited Settings

Current Status of the HIV Pandemic

In 1997, global HIV incidence peaked at 3.3 million new infections per year (Lancet HIV 2016;3:e361--e87). Highly active antiretroviral therapy (HAART) had just been announced at the International AIDS Society meeting in Vancouver, and this successful treatment approach was subsequently rapidly deployed throughout the United States and Europe; HIV was for the first time no longer a death sentence. However, in sub-Saharan Africa, the pandemic continued to flourish, with 1.8 million deaths from HIV by 2005 (Lancet HIV 2016;3:e361–e87).

ART was far out of reach for most people in resource-limited settings, with a year of first-line ART costing about $10,000 in 2000 (JAMA 2016;316:1139–1140).

In 2003, U.S. President George W. Bush announced the President's Emergency Plan for AIDS Relief (PEPFAR), a $15 billion, 5-year plan to combat HIV/AIDS globally. This bilateral funding initiative, together with other funding initiatives such as UNAIDS; The Global Fund to Fight AIDS, Tuberculosis, and Malaria; and the privately funded Bill and Melinda Gates Foundation, drastically changed the funding landscape for HIV/AIDS initiatives, particularly in sub-Saharan Africa and Asia.

PEPFAR 1.0 from 2003 to 2008 was focused on decreasing the high mortality rate due to HIV in resource-limited settings by providing ART to the sickest persons to avert AIDS. PEPFAR 2.0 then focused on transition of health programs to local ownership for sustainability. PEPFAR 3.0 has focused on achievement of HIV epidemic control.

From 2003 to 2017, PEPFAR spent more than US$72 billion to combat HIV/AIDS, tuberculosis (TB), and other opportunistic infections (OIs) (PEPFAR Funding. U.S. President's Emergency Plan for AIDS Relief, 2017; accessed February 26, 2018, at https://www.pepfar.gov/documents/organization/252516.pdf). In 2000, only 50,000 people were receiving ART in sub-Saharan Africa; as of 2017, PEPFAR funds ART for 13.3 million people (2017 Latest PEPFAR Results. U.S. President's Emergency Plan for AIDS Relief, 2017; accessed February 26, 2018, at https://www.pepfar.gov/documents/organization/276321.pdf).

HIV treatment has drastically changed since 2003. At that time, ART was costly, had multiple side effects, and was only indicated for the sickest persons to avert death or onset of AIDS. Over the following decade, drug prices fell, side-effect profiles improved, and several important trials demonstrated the benefit of expanding treatment access. First-line ART has dropped from $10,000 per year to less than $100 in 2016 (JAMA 2016;316:1139–1140). Despite expanded treatment access and decreases in AIDS-related mortality, global HIV prevalence has continued to increase, with an estimated 38.8 million persons living with HIV in 2015 (Lancet HIV 2016;3:e361–e87).

In 2014, UNAIDS announced the ambitious goals of 90-90-90 to achieve epidemic control: 90% of HIV-infected persons should know their status, 90% of those are on ART, and 90% of those are virally suppressed (UNAIDS. 90-90-90 An ambitious treatment target to help end the AIDS epidemic. Geneva: Joint United Nations Programme on HIV/AIDS; 2014). Although this ultimately means only 73% of HIV-infected persons are on ART and virally suppressed, modeling exercises predict that, combined with treatment as prophylaxis (TasP) and halting of vertical mother-to-child transmission (MTCT), this is sufficient to halt viral spread. Trials such as HPTN052 (NEJM 2011;365:493–505) demonstrated the efficacy of TasP, while START (NEJM 2015;373:795–807) and

TEMPERANO (NEJM 2015;373:808–822) highlighted the benefits of early ART compared to deferred ART. Based on these trials and other evidence, in 2015, the World Health Organization (WHO) expanded treatment eligibility to all HIV-infected persons (Guideline on When to Start Antiretroviral Therapy and on Pre-Exposure Prophylaxis for HIV. World Health Organization, 2015; accessed February 26, 2018, at http://apps.who.int/iris/bitstream/10665/186275/1/9789241509565_eng.pdf?ua=1), and many countries have since followed suit.

Current global priorities focused on strategies to achieve the three 90s include, to meet the first 90 goal, targeted testing, index client testing, universal routine testing to increase testing yield; to meet the second 90 goal, health systems strengthening, community health initiatives, differentiated service delivery, and task-shifting to improve linkage to treatment and care; and, to meet the third 90 goal, point-of-care (POC) diagnostics, more durable antiretroviral (ARV) regimens, and novel adherence support strategies to achieve long-lasting viral suppression.

Diagnosis of HIV

Who to Test

In the era of epidemic control, 90-90-90, and Treat All, a renewed emphasis has been placed on finding all HIV-infected individuals and linking them to care (Consolidated guidelines on HIV testing services. World Health Organization, 2015; accessed February 26, 2018, at http://apps.who.int/iris/bitstream/10665/179870/1/9789241508926_eng.pdf?ua=1&ua=1).

Most resource-limited countries employ a combination of universal routine testing and targeted testing strategies. Universal routine testing stipulates that all patients presenting to healthcare facilities, regardless of reason, should be offered HIV testing. Targeted testing is a strategy whereby populations at significant risk of HIV acquisition are offered testing in the community so as to maximize positivity yield and case finding and thus make maximal progress toward 90-90-90. This may include *key populations* and *priority populations*. Key populations are groups experiencing particularly high HIV incidence, including sex workers, men who have sex with men (MSM), people in prisons, people who inject drugs, and transgendered people (Consolidated guidelines on HIV testing services. World Health Organization, 2015; accessed February 26, 2018, at http://apps.who.int/iris/bitstream/10665/179870/1/9789241508926_eng.pdf?ua=1&ua=1).

Priority populations are those that have unique vulnerability or particularly high risk of HIV acquisition and may include infants and children, adolescents and youth, pregnant women, couples or partners, men, and other vulnerable populations (Consolidated guidelines on HIV testing services. World Health Organization, 2015; accessed February 26, 2018, at http://apps.who.int/iris/bitstream/10665/179870/1/9789241508926_eng.pdf?ua=1&ua=1).

HIV Testing

HIV testing may occur in a variety of settings, including

- Voluntary counseling and testing centers
- Targeted testing in high-prevalence areas
- Provider-initiated counseling and testing
- Mobile outreach testing
- HIV testing at the workplace or in the community
- HIV testing campaigns

Novel strategies currently being rolled out include index client testing, whereby persons newly identified as HIV-positive are asked about their sexual or drug-injecting partners. Those individuals are then sought out and also offered HIV testing. HIV self-testing has recently been adopted as a novel strategy to reach persons who may not want to test at routine testing service points.

HIV Diagnostic Tests

In resource-limited settings, POC rapid diagnostic tests (RDTs) (sensitivity 99–100%, specificity 99–100%) are often used for initial testing and screening, with more robust laboratory tests such as enzyme immunoassays (EIA) (sensitivity 100%, specificity 99–100%) for confirmatory tests. Western blot or other advanced assays may be used in the case of discordant results between RDTs and EIAs. Both RDTs and EIAs are able to detect HIV-1, HIV-2, and co-infection. RDTs detect the presence of antibodies from 21 days after infection, whereas current fourth-generation EIAs detect p24 antigen from 14 days after infection (HIV Assays: Laboratory Performance and Other Operational Characteristics. Report 18. World Health Organization, 2015; accessed February 26, 2018, at http://www.who.int/diagnostics_laboratory/evaluations/hiv/150819_hiv_assay_report18_final_version.pdf?ua=1).

Dried blood spot (DBS) polymerase chain reaction (PCR) is used for early infant diagnosis (EID) and is also being explored for viral load (VL) assessment and drug resistance screening for people on therapy as DBS does not require cold chain storage. Nucleic acid testing (NAT) is also now being used for EID and can detect the presence of HIV nucleic acid as early as 10 days after infection (HIV Assays: Laboratory Performance and Other Operational Characteristics. Report 18. World Health Organization, 2015; accessed February 26, 2018, at http://www.who.int/diagnostics_laboratory/evaluations/hiv/150819_hiv_assay_report18_final_version.pdf?ua=1).

WHO Guidelines and Treatment Recommendations

When to Start Antiretroviral Therapy

In 2013, the WHO released consolidated guidelines on the use of antiretroviral drugs for treating and preventing HIV infection (Consolidated guidelines on the use of antiretroviral drugs for treating and preventing HIV infection: recommendations for a public health approach. World Health Organization, 2013; accessed February 26, 2018, at http://www.who.int/hiv/pub/guidelines/arv2013/en/). These guidelines were updated in 2016 with the inclusion of new recommendations. The new recommendations were lifelong ART for all children, adolescents, and adults, including pregnant and breastfeeding women, regardless of the CD4 cell count. Additional recommendations in the 2016 guidelines included the use of an integrase inhibitor as first-line ART, reduced dose of efavirenz, differentiated approaches to HIV care, and use of pre-exposure prophylaxis (Consolidated guidelines on the use of antiretroviral drugs for treating and preventing HIV infection: recommendations for a public health approach—second edition. World Health Organization, 2016; accessed February 26, 2018, at http://www.who.int/hiv/pub/arv/arv-2016/en/). In 2017, the WHO issued further guidelines for managing advanced HIV disease and rapid initiation of ART (Guidelines for managing advanced HIV disease and rapid initiation of antiretroviral therapy. World Health Organization, 2017; accessed February 26, 2018, at http://www.who.int/hiv/pub/guidelines/advanced-HIV-disease/en/).

The "Treat All" recommendation was a change from the 2013 consolidated guidelines where the treatment threshold had been a CD4 count of <500 cells/mm^3. Evidence for starting ART earlier is presented in the summary of the Global Trials section. For adolescents and adults aged 19 yrs and older, ART is strongly recommended regardless of the CD4 cell count, with a priority for adults with severe or advanced HIV disease and adults with CD4 count of ≤ 350 cells/mm^3. Lifelong ART for all pregnant and breastfeeding women living with HIV at any CD4 count was another new recommendation in the 2016 consolidated guidelines (Consolidated guidelines on the use of antiretroviral drugs for treating and preventing HIV infection: recommendations for a public health approach—second edition. World Health Organization, 2016; accessed February 26, 2018, at http://www.who.int/hiv/pub/arv/arv-2016/en/). Furthermore, the WHO recommended that ART should be initiated for all children living with HIV regardless of the WHO clinical stage and at any

CD4 count, with a priority for all children aged 2 yrs and younger or children younger than 5 yrs with WHO stage 3 or 4 or a CD4 count of ≤ 750 cells/mm^3.

Who to Treat

Once a person is identified as HIV-positive, the WHO now recommends immediate staging with a CD4 count and clinical assessment. All HIV-infected individuals should be offered immediate antiretroviral treatment.

In the era of 90-90-90 and Treat All, as of 2016, 36.7 million people were estimated to be living with HIV and 19.5 million (53%) had access to antiretroviral treatment. Current progress toward 90-90-90 is estimated at 70% of people living with HIV (PLHIV) knowing their status, 77% of PLHIV aware of their status are on treatment, and 82% of PLHIV on treatment are virally suppressed. Meanwhile, annual AIDS-related mortality has fallen from its peak of 1.9 million in 2005 to 1 million in 2016 (UNAIDS. Global AIDS Update 2017: Ending AIDS. Geneva: Joint United Nations Programme on HIV/AIDS; 2017).

This represents the first time in the history of the HIV pandemic that more than half of the PLHIV in the world have access to ART, which is largely responsible for the large decline in AIDS-related mortality (see Table 5.1).

What to Start: First-Line ART

Dolutegravir (DTG) and efavirenz 400 mg/d are new drugs in the WHO 2016 consolidated guidelines. A number of countries in sub-Saharan Africa have already introduced DTG as part of their first-line ART, and others are already moving in that direction (Transitioning to new antiretroviral drugs in HIV programmes: clinical and programmatic considerations: Technical update. World Health Organization, 2017; accessed February 26, 2018, at http://www.who.int/hiv/pub/toolkits/transition-to-new-arv-technical-update/en/).

TABLE 5.1 First-line regimens for treating adults, pregnant or breastfeeding women, adolescents, and children

First-line ART	Preferred First-line Regimens	Alternate First-line Regimens[a]
Adults	TDF + 3TC (or FTC) + DTG* TDF + 3TC (or FTC) + EFV	AZT +3TC + EFV (or NVP) TDF + 3TC (or FTC) + DTG[b] TDF + 3TC (or FTC) + EFV$_{400}$[b,c] TDF + 3TC (or FTC) + NVP
Pregnant or breastfeeding women	TDF + 3TC (or FTC) + DTG* TDF + 3TC (or FTC) + EFV	AZT +3TC + EFV (or NVP) TDF + 3TC (or FTC) + NVP
Adolescents	TDF + 3TC (or FTC) + DTG* TDF + 3TC (or FTC) + EFV	AZT +3TC +EFV (or NVP) TDF + 3TC (or FTC) +DTG[b] TDF + 3TC (or FTC) + EFV$_{400}$[b,c] TDF + 3TC (or FTC) + NVP
Children 3 yrs to 10 yrs	2 NRTIs + DTG[d] 2 NRTIs + LPV/r ABC + 3TC + EFV	ABC + 3TC + NVP AZT + 3TC +EFV (or NVP) TDF + 3TC (or FTC) + EFV (or NVP)
Children <3 yrs	ABC (or AZT) + 3TC + LPV/r	ABC (or AZT) + 3TC +NVP

*Women and adolescent girls of childbearing potential with consistent and reliable contraception and who are fully informed of the benefits and risks can use DTG. WHO recommends a "woman-centered approach" that involves discussing the risks and benefits of ART with the woman and allowing her to participate in the choice of her ART.

[a] ABC or boosted protease inhibitors (ATV/r, DRV/r, LPV/r) can be used in special circumstances.

[b] Safety and efficacy data on the use of DTG and EFV400 in pregnant women, people with HIV/TB co-infection, and adolescents <12 yrs are not yet available.

[c] EFV at lower dose (400 mg/d).

[d] DTG is recommended for children 6 yrs of age and older and weighing >15 kg. Data for younger children are expected in 2019. RAL is approved for infants starting at birth.

3TC, lamivudine; ABC, abacavir; AZT, zidovudine; DRV, darunavir; DTG, dolutegravir; EFV, efavirenz; FTC, emtricitabine; LPV, lopinavir; NVP, nevirapine; r, ritonavir; TDF, tenofovir.

Adapted from the WHO 2016 Consolidated guidelines on the use of antiretroviral drugs for treating and preventing HIV infection (World Health Organization, 2016; accessed February 26, 2018, at http://www.who.int/hiv/pub/arv/arv-2016/en/) and Updated recommendations on first-line and second-line antiretroviral regimens and post-exposure prophylaxis and recommendations on early infant diagnosis of HIV: interim guidance, World Health Organization, 2018; accessed July 31, 2018, at http://www.who.int/hiv/pub/guidelines/ARV2018update/en/).

DTG has a lower potential for drug interactions and a higher genetic barrier to resistance. Two formulations of single-dose DTG are part of the WHO prequalified list (Essential medicines and health products: prequalification of medicines. Prequalified lists of medicines/finished pharmaceutical products. World Health Organization, 2017; accessed February 26, 2018, at https://extranet.who.int/prequal/content/prequalified-lists/medicines). These recommendations were updated in July 2018, following the report of four cases of neural tube defects in women who conceived while on DTG-based regimens. In the updated recommendations, men and women who are not of childbearing potential, do not desire to get pregnant, and have access to reliable and effective contraception should be treated with tenofovir, lamivudine, and DTG. For women of childbearing potential who wish to get pregnant or do not have access to effective contraception, tenofovir, lamivudine, and efavirenz are recommended (Updated recommendations on first-line and second-line antiretroviral regimens and post-exposure prophylaxis and recommendations on early infant diagnosis of HIV: interim guidance, World Health Organization, 2018; Accessed July 31, 2018, at http://www.who.int/hiv/pub/guidelines/ARV2018update/en/).

When to Switch Therapies

If a patient is suspected to have treatment failure, VL testing should be performed, based on the new criteria for treatment failure (What's new in treatment monitoring: VL and CD4 testing. World Health Organization, 2017; accessed February 26, 2018, at http://www.who.int/hiv/pub/arv/treatment-monitoring-info-2017/en/).

VIROLOGIC FAILURE: Virologic failure is defined as having a VL of >1,000 copies/mL based on two consecutive VL measurements in a 3-mo interval, with adherence support following the first VL test after at least 6 mos of starting a new ART regimen

IMMUNOLOGICAL FAILURE: For adults and adolescents, immunological failure is defined as a CD4 count of ≤ 250 cells/mm^3 following clinical failure or persistent CD4 levels <100 cells/mm^3

For children younger than 5 yrs, immunological failure is defined as persistent CD4 levels <200 cells/mm^3. For children older than 5 yrs, it is persistent CD4 levels <100 cells/mm^3.

CLINICAL FAILURE: For adults and adolescents, clinical failure is defined as a new or recurrent clinical event indicating severe immunodeficiency after 6 mos of effective treatment.

For children, clinical failure is defined as a new or recurrent clinical event indicating advanced or severe immunodeficiency after 6 mos of effective treatment.

Third-Line ART

WHO encourages countries to develop their own guidelines for third-line ART, which should include drugs with minimal risk of cross-resistance. These include integrase strand transfer inhibitors (INSTIs), second-generation non-nucleoside reverse transcriptase inhibitors (NNRTIs), and protease inhibitors (PIs) (Consolidated guidelines on the use of antiretroviral drugs for treating and preventing HIV infection: recommendations for a public health approach—second edition. World Health Organization, 2016; accessed February 26, 2018, at http://www.who.int/hiv/pub/arv/arv-2016/en/).

Monitoring ART Efficacy and Toxicity

Laboratory monitoring of clients living with HIV is essential to ensure quality care, monitor virological response to treatment, and prevent treatment failure. Symptom-directed laboratory tests can also help detect ART toxicities. In the current era of Test and Treat, CD4 count is not essential for starting ART; however, CD4 count can help determine the clinical status of an HIV-infected individual and determine what prophylaxis is required. VL is the recommended monitoring approach for diagnosing treatment failure. CD4 count and immunological criteria lack sensitivity to detect treatment failure, and reliance on these measures could result in undetected virologic failure,

TABLE 5.2 Recommended second-line regimens

Population		Failing First-line Regimen	Preferred Second-line Regimen	Alternative Second-line Regimen
Adults and adolescents (including women and adolescent girls who are of childbearing potential or pregnant)		2 NRTIs + EFV (or NVP)	2 NRTIs + DTG[a]	2 NRTIs + DRV/r
		2 NRTIs + DTG	2 NRTIs + ATV/r or LPV/r	
Children	Less than 3 yrs	2 NRTIs + LPV/r	2 NRTIs + RAL	Maintain the failing LPV/r-based regimen and switch to 2 NRTIs + EFV at 3 yrs of age
		2 NRTIs + NVP	2 NRTIs + LPV/r	2 NRTIs + RAL
	3 yrs to less than 10 yrs	2 NRTIs + LPV/r	2 NRTIs + DTG[b]	2 NRTIs + RAL
		2 NRTIs + EFV (or NVP)	2 NRTIs + DTG[c]	2 NRTIs + ATV/r
		2 NRTIs + DTG	2 NRTIs + ATV/r or LPV/r	

[a] Women and adolescent girls of childbearing potential with effective contraception who are fully informed of the benefits and risks can use DTG.

[b] In children for whom approved DTG dosing is available. RAL should remain the preferred second-line regimen for the children for whom approved DTG dosing is not available.

[c] ATV/r or LPV/r should remain the preferred second-line treatment for the children for whom approved DTG dosing is not available. This applies to children for whom approved DTG dosing is available.

Adapted from the WHO 2016 Consolidated guidelines on the use of antiretroviral drugs for treating and preventing HIV infection (World Health Organization, 2016; accessed February 26, 2018, at http://www.who.int/hiv/pub/arv/arv-2016/en/) and Updated recommendations on first-line and second-line antiretroviral regimens and post-exposure prophylaxis and recommendations on early infant diagnosis of HIV: interim guidance, World Health Organization, 2018; accessed July 31, 2018, at http://www.who.int/hiv/pub/guidelines/ARV2018update/en/).

with subsequent accumulation of resistance mutations. If VL testing is not routinely available, CD4 count and clinical monitoring can be used with targeted VL testing to confirm treatment failure. Where VL testing is available, the WHO recommends stopping routine CD4 count monitoring, a policy that would result in cost savings. While drug resistance testing is routinely used prior to starting ART and in patients with suspected treatment failure, the WHO at the moment does not recommend routine use of resistance testing because of the cost. Instead, the WHO recommends routine surveillance for HIV drug resistance (HIV-DR) in populations initiating ART and in populations on ART for 12 mos and 48 mos (Consolidated guidelines on the use of antiretroviral drugs for treating and preventing HIV infection: recommendations for a public health approach—second edition. World Health Organization, 2016; accessed February 26, 2018, at http://www.who.int/hiv/pub/arv/arv-2016/en/). Table 5.3 describes the routine laboratory tests that the WHO recommends for managing HIV-infected patients.

Treatment and Prophylaxis of Opportunistic Infections and Other Comorbid Conditions

Tuberculosis

DIAGNOSIS OF TUBERCULOSIS: The traditional test of choice in resource-limited settings for diagnosis of pulmonary tuberculosis has been sputum smear staining for acid-fast bacilli (AFB). Sputum AFB smears are relatively cheap, require minimal training to perform, have a quick turnaround time, and are also used for monitoring of individuals during treatment. A major drawback of sputum smears is its low sensitivity of diagnosis—as low as 30%—in PLHIV. Additional disadvantages include: Mycobacterium tuberculosis cannot be differentiated from nontuberculous mycobacteria, drug-susceptibility testing cannot be performed, and smear positivity may reflect dead, rather than viable, bacilli. Mycobacterial culture, the gold standard for diagnosis of active tuberculosis, is not

TABLE 5.3 Laboratory Tests for HIV screening and monitoring and approaches to screening for co-infections and noncommunicable diseases

Phase of HIV Management	Recommended	Desirable
HIV diagnosis	HIV testing (serology for adults and children 18 mos or older); DNA PCR for children younger than 18 mos; CD4 cell count; TB symptom screening	HBV (HBsAg) serology; HCV serology; Cryptococcus antigen if CD4 cell count ≤ 100 cells/mm^3; STI Screening; Pregnancy test to allow for PMTCT; Assessment of major non-communicable chronic diseases and comorbidities
ART initiation		Hemoglobin testing for starting AZT; Pregnancy test; Blood pressure measurement; Serum creatinine and estimated glomerular filtration rate (eGFR) for starting TDF; Alanine aminotransferase for NVP; Baseline CD4 count
Receiving ART	HIV VL (at 6 mos and 12 mo after initiating ART and every 12 mos thereafter); CD4 cell count every 6 mos until patients are stable on ART	Serum creatinine and eGFR for TDF; Pregnancy test, especially for women of childbearing age not receiving family planning and on treatment with DTG or low-dose EFV

(*continued*)

TABLE 5.3 Continued

Phase of HIV Management	Recommended	Desirable
Suspected treatment failure	Serum creatinine and eGFR for TDF; Pregnancy test, especially for women of childbearing age not receiving family planning and on treatment with DTG or low-dose EFV	HBV (HBsAg) serology (before switching ART regimen if this test was not done or if the result was negative at baseline and the patient was not vaccinated thereafter)

Adapted from the WHO 2016 Consolidated guidelines on the use of antiretroviral drugs for treating and preventing HIV infection (World Health Organization, 2016; accessed February 26, 2018, at http://www.who.int/hiv/pub/arv/arv-2016/en/).

available for routine use in most resource-limited settings. Although *M. tuberculosis* can be definitively identified and drug-susceptibility testing performed with mycobacterial culture, the assay is limited by its expense, requirement for laboratory infrastructure, and long turnaround time. It may take up to 6 wks for *M. tuberculosis* to grow on culture and an additional 4–6 wks for drug susceptibility results to be finalized.

Rapid molecular tests for diagnosis of active tuberculosis are increasingly used as the test of choice in resource-limited settings. Xpert MTB/RIF (or "GeneXpert") utilizes PCR for identification of *M. tuberculosis* and simultaneous detection of rifampin resistance. The test may provide results in as little as 2 hrs and is relatively easy to perform. In sputum smear-positive individuals, the sensitivity of diagnosis is >98%. Sensitivity is lower in those who are sputum-smear negative (as low as 70%) but may increase to >90% if up to three specimens in total are tested. An additional benefit is that extrapulmonary specimens, such as cerebrospinal fluid, lymph node aspirates, and pleural biopsy samples (but not pleural fluid), may undergo testing by Xpert MTB/RIF. In addition, studies are under way for validating testing in stool samples of children with presumptive tuberculosis, given the difficulties in diagnosis in this population. Although major limitations in widespread use of Xpert MTB/RIF include the expenses for procurement and maintenance as well as the requirement for an adequate power supply, significant price reductions have been negotiated for resource-limited settings. An important caveat is that, since the assay is a molecular test, it will detect dead *M. tuberculosis* bacilli and consequently should not be used for routine monitoring while individuals are on treatment.

Another POC molecular test for diagnosis of active tuberculosis involves detection of urinary lipoarabinomannan (LAM), a lipopolysaccharide found in the cell wall of *M. tuberculosis* and secreted into the systemic circulation in pulmonary and extrapulmonary TB. Although relatively inexpensive, urine LAM testing has only been shown to have adequate sensitivity (approximately 66%) for diagnosis of tuberculosis in severely ill HIV-infected individuals with CD4 counts of <50 cells/μL. The assay has decreased sensitivity in those with higher CD4 counts and in HIV-uninfected individuals. The microscopic observation drug-susceptibility (MODS) assay, another inexpensive test developed for use in resource-limited settings, is able to speciate *M. tuberculosis* (MTB) in sputum specimens and simultaneously provide drug susceptibility results in 7–10 days after incubation. The major disadvantages of MODS are the need for laboratory infrastructure as well as technical training of personnel. Line probe assay (LPA) is a molecular test involving amplification of nucleic acid for detection of tuberculosis. Not only can LPA differentiate MTB from nontuberculous mycobacteria, but it can also be used for first- and second-line drug susceptibility testing. Additional advantages include the rapid turnaround time, as quickly as 2 hrs, and the ability for it to be performed directly on sputum specimens or indirectly on culture isolates. Drawbacks include its expense and the need for trained laboratory personnel. In resource-limited settings, LPA is most appropriately used in national mycobacterial reference laboratories for rapid detection of drug-resistant tuberculosis.

TREATMENT OF TUBERCULOSIS: The recently updated 2017 WHO guidelines for treatment of drug-susceptible tuberculosis continue to recommend that individuals with pulmonary tuberculosis be treated with a 6-mo regimen, consisting of a 2-mo intensive phase with isoniazid, rifampin, ethambutol, and pyrazinamide, and a 4-mo continuation phase of isoniazid and rifampin. Daily therapy should be provided in both the intensive and continuation phases: intermittent regimens (e.g., twice- or thrice-weekly) are not recommended due to the associated risks of treatment failure, relapse, and acquired drug resistance. Ethambutol is added to isoniazid and rifampin in the continuation phase in settings in which there is a high level of isoniazid monoresistance (Guidelines for treatment of drug-susceptible tuberculosis and patient care. World Health Organization, 2017; accessed February 26, 2018, at http://apps.who.int/iris/bitstream/10665/255052/1/9789241550000-eng.pdf?ua=1).

Evidence for the timing of initiation of ART in ART-naïve, HIV-infected individuals with pulmonary TB comes from three high-quality trials: SAPiT (NEJM 2011;365:1492–1501), CAMELIA (NEJM 2011;365:1471–1481), and ACTG 5221 STRIDE (NEJM 2011;365:1482–1491). These trials conclusively demonstrated a mortality benefit in early initiation of ART in HIV-infected individuals with low CD4 counts. For individuals with higher CD4 counts, the risks of immune reconstitution inflammatory syndrome (IRIS) and drug toxicities were not outweighed by any mortality benefit. Thus, all ART-naïve HIV-infected individuals with CD4 counts <50–100 cells/μL should begin ART within 2 wks after beginning antituberculosis therapy. For those with higher CD4 counts, ART should be initiated by 8 wks—that is, before the continuation phase of treatment for TB commences. Although there is some data suggesting that HIV-infected individuals who are treated for at least 8 mos with a rifampin-containing regimen have improved outcomes as compared to those treated for 6 mos or less, recommendations at the time of this writing are that PLHIV be treated for tuberculosis for the same duration of 6 mos, as in the case of HIV-uninfected individuals.

In our era of Treat All, it is imperative that individuals with newly diagnosed HIV be screened appropriately for OIs prior to initiation of ART. Unmasking TB-associated IRIS causes a great deal of morbidity and is likely the major cause of early mortality after initiating ART. TB-associated IRIS may present in any organ system but is most severe in the central nervous system (CNS). ART should generally be continued in most cases of TB-IRIS; consultation with a specialist is necessary in severe cases. Corticosteroids are usually reserved for life-threatening IRIS, such as CNS involvement or impending respiratory failure due to a rapidly enlarging pleural effusion or massive mediastinal lymphadenopathy.

Extrapulmonary tuberculosis is treated with the same regimen as that for pulmonary TB; the duration is increased to 9–12 mos for TB of the CNS. Due to its mortality benefit, a 6- to 8-wk course of corticosteroids is indicated during the intensive phase of treatment for tuberculous meningitis. Of note, early initiation of ART in HIV/TB co-infected individuals with TB meningitis is not warranted and is associated with high morbidity. In these individuals, ART should be initiated after the continuation phase has commenced. Evidence supporting the use of corticosteroids for tuberculous pericarditis is weaker than that for TB meningitis; the WHO recommendation for their use in this case is more guarded.

An important update in the 2017 WHO guidelines is that the category II regimen (5HRZES/1HRZE/2HRE) is no longer recommended. This regimen is associated with acquired drug resistance, poor treatment success rates, and development of irreversible toxicities to streptomycin. Rather than retreating individuals who have failed first-line treatment with the category II regimen, drug-susceptibility testing should be performed to determine whether appropriate treatment for drug-resistant TB is warranted. In the case of multidrug-resistant TB (MDR-TB)—tuberculosis that is resistant to at least isoniazid and rifampin—a new short-course regimen of 9–11 mos has been recommended by the WHO for eligible individuals, including children and PLHIV who are unlikely to harbor resistance to fluoroquinolones or second-line injectable drugs. Unfortunately, pregnant women and those with extrapulmonary TB are not eligible for the short-course regimen at this time. Specialist consultation should be obtained for treatment of drug-resistant TB.

ISONIAZID PREVENTIVE THERAPY: Adults and adolescents living with HIV who do not report any of the symptoms of current cough, fever, weight loss, or night sweats are unlikely to have active TB disease and should be offered isoniazid preventive therapy (IPT). WHO recommends at least 6 mos of IPT in individuals who are unlikely to have active TB, and at least 36 mos of IPT in individuals living in settings of high TB transmission rate in whom active TB has been safely ruled out. Children who are >12 mos of age should receive 6 mos of IPT if they have no contact with a TB case and are unlikely to have active TB based on symptom screening, while children who are <12 mos of age should only receive IPT if they have contact with a TB case and evaluation shows no TB disease. In addition, children who complete TB treatment should receive IPT for an additional 6 mos (Consolidated guidelines on the use of antiretroviral drugs for treating and preventing HIV infection: recommendations for a public health approach—second edition. World Health Organization, 2016; accessed February 26, 2018, at http://www.who.int/hiv/pub/arv/arv-2016/en/).

INFECTION CONTROL: Each healthcare facility should have a TB infection control plan that includes administrative, environmental, and personal protection measures for health workers and caregivers to reduce TB transmission within the facility. The WHO has published details of the infection control measures (WHO policy on TB infection control in health-care facilities, congregate settings and households. World Health Organization, 2009; accessed February 26, 2018, at http://www.who.int/tb/publications/2009/infection_control/en/).

Cryptococcal Meningitis

The WHO published a rapid advice on diagnosis, prevention, and management of cryptococcal disease in resource-limited settings in 2011 (Rapid advice: Diagnosis, prevention and management of cryptococcal disease in HIV-infected adults, adolescents and children. World Health Organization, 2011; accessed February 26, 2018, at http://www.who.int/hiv/pub/cryptococcal_disease2011/en/). The guidance emphasizes early diagnosis of cryptococcal disease to improve mortality, early ART initiation, and use of optimal antifungal treatment regimens to improve survival, clinical, and neurological outcomes.

DIAGNOSIS OF CRYPTOCOCCAL MENINGITIS: The recommended approach to diagnosis cryptococcal meningitis in HIV-infected adults, adolescents, and children is with a prompt lumbar puncture (LP) with measurement of cerebrospinal fluid (CSF) opening pressure and rapid CSF cryptococcal antigen (CrAg) test or a rapid serum cryptococcal antigen test. The CrAg assay may be performed either with a latex agglutination test or lateral flow assay. CSF India ink examination is another method of diagnosing cryptococcal meningitis (Consolidated guidelines on the use of antiretroviral drugs for treating and preventing HIV infection: recommendations for a public health approach—second edition. World Health Organization, 2016; accessed February 26, 2018, at http://www.who.int/hiv/pub/arv/arv-2016/en/); Rapid advice: Diagnosis, prevention and management of cryptococcal disease in HIV-infected adults, adolescents and children. World Health Organization, 2011; accessed February 26, 2018, at http://www.who.int/hiv/pub/cryptococcal_disease2011/en/).

PREVENTION OF CRYPTOCOCCAL DISEASE: The WHO does not recommend routine use of antifungal primary prophylaxis for cryptococcal disease in HIV-infected adults, adolescents, and children with a CD4 count of <100 cells/mm^3 and who are CrAg-negative or where CrAg status is unknown. Pre-emptive antifungal therapy may be used if serum CrAg is positive in patients with a

CD4 count of <100 cells/mm^3 and where this population has a high prevalence (>3%) of cryptococcal antigenemia (Consolidated guidelines on the use of antiretroviral drugs for treating and preventing HIV infection: recommendations for a public health approach—second edition. World Health Organization, 2016; accessed February 26, 2018, at http://www.who.int/hiv/pub/arv/arv-2016/en/).

INDUCTION, CONSOLIDATION, AND MAINTENANCE TREATMENT REGIMENS: The rapid advice on cryptococcal disease recommends at least 2-wk induction therapy with amphotericin B combined with either flucytosine or fluconazole. In situations where amphotericin B is not available, a combination of high-dose (800 mg/d) fluconazole with flucytosine or high-dose (1,200 mg/d) fluconazole monotherapy are suggested as alternate therapeutic options. Once CSF cultures cleared, an 8-wk consolidation treatment phase with fluconazole 400–800 mg/d is recommended, followed by the maintenance with oral fluconazole 200 mg/d for >12 mos. In addition, the WHO recommends a minimum package of toxicity prevention, monitoring, and management to minimize the side effects of hypokalemia and nephrotoxicity with amphotericin B. This includes pre-emptive hydration and electrolyte replacement and toxicity monitoring (Rapid advice: Diagnosis, prevention and management of cryptococcal disease in HIV-infected adults, adolescents and children. World Health Organization, 2011; accessed February 26, 2018, at http://www.who.int/hiv/pub/cryptococcal_disease2011/en/). Patients with raised intracranial pressure need serial LPs to reduce the intracranial pressure. Antifungal maintenance therapy may be discontinued when patients are stable and adherent to ART with evidence of immune reconstitution (>100/mm^3) for 3 mos and have been on fluconazole maintenance therapy for at least 1 yr.

UPDATED GUIDELINES: The WHO guidelines for treatment of cryptococcal meningitis[1] changed in March 2018 based on the results of the ACTA (Advancing Cryptococcal Meningitis Treatment for Africa)

Trial[2] presented in 2017[3] and published March 2018. ACTA was an RCT demonstrating that one-week induction therapy for cryptococcal meningitis with Amphotericin B plus flucytosine was non-inferior to two-week induction therapy and resulted in improved outcomes. WHO guidelines now recommend the following regimens for treatment of cryptococcal meningitis:

INDUCTION THERAPY:

- Preferred: Amphotericin B plus flucytosine for 1 week
- Alternative: High-dose fluconazole plus flucytosine for 2 weeks
- Alternative: Amphotericin B fluconazole plus fluconazole for 2 weeks

CONSOLIDATION THERAPY:

- Fluconazole for 8 weeks.

References

1. Guidelines for the diagnosis, prevention and management of cryptococcal disease in HIV-infected adults, adolescents and children. World Health Organisation, 2018. (Accessed 26 February 2018, at http://apps.who.int/iris/bitstream/10665/260399/1/9789241550277-eng.pdf?ua=1.)

2. Molloy SF, Kanyama C, Heyderman RS, et al. Antifungal Combinations for Treatment of Cryptococcal Meningitis in Africa. The New England journal of medicine 2018;378:1004–17.

3. Molloy S, Kanyama C, Heyderman R, Loyse A, Kouanfack C, Chanda D, Mfinanga S, et al. A randomized controlled trial for the treatment of HIV-associated cryptococcal meningitis in Africa: oral fluconazole plus flucytosine or one week amphotericin-based

therapy vs two weeks amphotericin-based therapy. The ACTA Trial. 9th IAS Conference on HIV Science. Paris 23–26 July, 2017. Abstract 5573.

Opportunistic Infection Prophylaxis

CO-TRIMOXAZOLE PROPHYLAXIS: Co-trimoxazole (CTX) is recommended for adults with severe or advanced HIV clinical disease (WHO stage 3 or 4, including pregnant women, and/or with a CD4 count ≤350 cells/mL). CTX may be discontinued when CD4 count is >350 cells/mL and patients are virally suppressed. In settings where malaria and severe bacterial infections are highly prevalent, the WHO recommends CTX regardless of the WHO stage or CD4 count. Furthermore, CTX is recommended for infants, children, and adults with HIV, irrespective of clinical and immune conditions. In settings with low prevalence of both malaria and severe bacterial infections, CTX may be discontinued in children older than 5 yrs who are clinically stable with evidence of immune recovery and/or viral suppression on ART (Consolidated guidelines on the use of antiretroviral drugs for treating and preventing HIV infection: recommendations for a public health approach—second edition. World Health Organization, 2016; accessed February 26, 2018, at http://www.who.int/hiv/pub/arv/arv-2016/en/).

Hepatitis B

The WHO recommends that adults, adolescents, and children with chronic hepatitis B and clinical evidence of cirrhosis (or cirrhosis based on the noninvasive AST to platelet ratio index (APRI) (APRI>2 in adults) should be treated regardless of alanine amino transferase (ALT) levels, hepatitis B e antigen (HBeAg) status, or HBV DNA levels. Additional information is available in the WHO guidelines (Guidelines for the prevention, care and treatment of persons with chronic hepatitis B infection. World Health Organisation, 2015;

accessed February 26, 2018, at http://www.who.int/hiv/pub/hepatitis/hepatitis-b-guidelines/en/).

Noncommunicable Diseases in HIV Infection

As PLHIV are now living longer even in resource-limited settings, we must turn our attention to noncommunicable diseases in HIV-infected individuals. Additional details are available from the WHO (Package of Essential Noncommunicable Disease Interventions for Primary Health Care in Low-Resource Settings. World Health Organization, 2010; accessed February 26, 2018, at http://www.who.int/nmh/publications/essential_ncd_interventions_lr_settings.pdf).

HIV Prevention

In the past decade, the field of HIV prevention has seen multiple new developments. In addition to standard interventions such as safe sex counseling and condom use, new evidence for male circumcision, treatment as prevention (TasP), and oral pre-exposure prophylaxis has emerged. Furthermore, the field of vaccines continues to evolve, with hope for both preventative and therapeutic vaccines.

Behavioral Interventions

Counseling and education about measures to prevent HIV acquisition remain the cornerstone of HIV prevention. Such measures have been demonstrated to increase condom use and decrease partner concurrency in heterosexual couples (Sex Trans Infect 2013;89:620–627) as well as reduce self-reported unprotected anal sex among MSM. (Cochrane Database of Systematic Reviews 2008:Cd001230). However, many studies have shown only modest or minimal effectiveness of such behavioral interventions in resource-limited settings (Int J Adolesc Med Health 2004;16:303–323).

Condoms

Male condoms remain one of the standards of HIV prevention, yet they are not always used consistently or correctly. Meta-analyses have estimated that consistent male condom use reduces HIV incidence by 70–80% (Cochrane Database of Systematic Reviews 2002:Cd003255; Exp Rev Pharmacoeconom Outcomes Re 2016;16:489–499).

Topical Interventions

Vaginal and rectal microbicides are attractive preventative measures as they could be applied immediately prior to sex. The CAPRISA 004 trial in 2010 demonstrated that a tenofovir-containing vaginal gel reduced HIV incidence by 39%. (Science 2010;329:1168–1174). However, the subsequent VOICE trial (NEJM 2015;372:509–518) and FACTS 001 trial (FACTS 001 Phase III trial of pericoital tenofovir 1% gel for HIV prevention in women; abstract 26LB. Program and abstracts of the 2015 Conference on Retroviruses and Opportunistic Infections (CROI) Seattle) demonstrated no reduction in HIV incidence with use of precoital vaginal tenofovir gel, though efficacy appeared to be linked to adherence. (NEJM 2015;372:509–518). In addition to tenofovir, dapivirine, an NNRTI, has been investigated as a long-acting vaginal ring in the MTN-020—ASPIRE Study (NEJM 2016;375:2121–2132) and the Ring Study (NEJM 2016;375:2133–2143), which demonstrated a 27% and 31% reduction in HIV incidence, respectively. Efficacy again increased with adherence in both trials.

Rectal microbicides are also under investigation to prevent HIV acquired during penetrative anal sex. Phase I [MTN-007 (PloS One 2013;8:e60147), CHARM-01 (PloS One 2015;10:e0125363), and CHARM-02 (AIDS Res Hum Retroviruses 2015;31:1098–1108)] and Phase II [MTN-017 (CID 2017;64:614–620)] trials of anal tenofovir gel have demonstrated it to be safe and acceptable. Dapivirine (MTN-026) and maraviroc (CHARM-03) are also currently being evaluated as rectal microbicides.

Treatment as Prevention and U=U

In 2011, HPTN 052 demonstrated that between HIV sero-discordant heterosexual partners, HIV sexual transmission does not occur if the HIV-infected person is virally suppressed (NEJM 2011;365:493–505). This gave rise the concept of *Treatment as Prevention* (TasP), the idea that if all HIV-infected persons are successfully treated (i.e., achieve viral suppression), this will prevent spread of HIV.

In 2016, the PARTNER trial demonstrated HIV transmission does not occur between heterosexual and MSM couples having condomless sex if the HIV-infected person is suppressed to VL of <200 copies/mL (*JAMA*. 2016;316(2):171-181). In 2018, the follow-up trial, PARTNERS 2, conclusively affirmed this finding (Rodgers A, et al. Risk of HIV transmission through condomless sex in MSM couples with suppressive ART: The PARTNER2 Study extended results in gay men. Abstract presented at AIDS 2018, Amsterdam, Netherlands. Available at: https://programme.aids2018.org/Abstract/Abstract/13470).

Taken together, HPTN 052 and PARTNER 1 & 2 gave rise to the concept of *Undetectable = Untransmittable*, known as U=U. The U=U public health message is being broadly disseminated and has broad implications for patient adherence, serodiscordant couples, HIV prevention, and de-criminalization of HIV-infected persons.

Pre-exposure Prophylaxis

Oral pre-exposure prophylaxis (PrEP) offers multiple advantages for HIV prevention; it can be taken discreetly, offers high rates of protection, and does not require negotiation with partners, unlike barrier methods and microbicide gels. The first key trial was the 2010 iPrex trial, which demonstrated a 44% reduction among MSM and transgender women taking daily tenofovir/emtricitabine (TDF/FTC) (NEJM 2010;363:2587–2599). The 2012 Partners PrEP trial among sero-discordant couples in Kenya and Uganda demonstrated decreased HIV acquisition risk by 67% with TDF alone and 75%

with TDF/FTC (NEJM 2012;367:399–410). However, the subsequent FEM-PrEP trial among high-risk African women showed no difference between placebo and those taking TDF/FTC; subsequent analysis showed that <40% of women in the intervention arm had evidence of recent pill use (NEJM 2012;367:411–422). The 2012 TDF2 trial demonstrated 62% efficacy of TDF/FTC in preventing HIV acquisition among sero-discordant couples in Botswana (NEJM 2012;367:423–434). Further meta-analyses have demonstrated that the effectiveness of PrEP is tightly correlated with adherence and that the highest PrEP effectiveness is achieved when adherence is >70%. PrEP is also associated with few safety risks, and there is no evidence of behavioral risk compensation (AIDS (London, England) 2016;30:1973–1983).

PrEP is currently being rolled out in various resource-limited settings, including South Africa and Kenya. It has potential for limiting HIV acquisition among high-risk key populations who require discreet methods of HIV prevention.

HIV Vaccines

Successful production of an effective HIV vaccine will be a critical tool to help end the pandemic, yet this goal continues to elude researchers for multiple reasons: the HIV virus demonstrates extreme mutability and an ability to evade the immune system, and standard approaches of neutralizing antibodies have not proved effective (J Immunol Res 2015;2015:560347). Current vaccine research focuses on three main approaches: induction of broadly neutralizing antibodies, induction of CD8 T-cell mediated immunity, and combination approaches. The 2009 RV144 study has demonstrated the greatest efficacy to date: 16,402 participants received a recombinant canary pox vector vaccine (ALVAC-HIV [vCP1521]) plus two booster injections of a recombinant glycoprotein 120 subunit vaccine (AIDSVAX B/E) and demonstrated a vaccine efficacy of 31.2% (NEJM 2009;361:2209–2220).

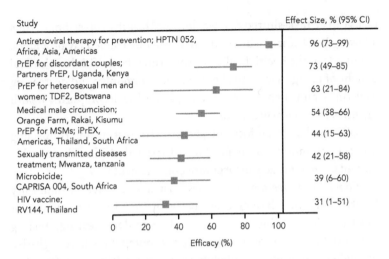

Study	Effect Size, % (95% CI)
Antiretroviral therapy for prevention; HPTN 052, Africa, Asia, Americas	96 (73–99)
PrEP for discordant couples; Partners PrEP, Uganda, Kenya	73 (49–85)
PrEP for heterosexual men and women; TDF2, Botswana	63 (21–84)
Medical male circumcision; Orange Farm, Rakai, Kisumu	54 (38–66)
PrEP for MSMs; iPrEX, Americas, Thailand, South Africa	44 (15–63)
Sexually transmitted diseases treatment; Mwanza, tanzania	42 (21–58)
Microbicide; CAPRISA 004, South Africa	39 (6–60)
HIV vaccine; RV144, Thailand	31 (1–51)

Efficacy (%)

FIGURE 5.1 Efficacy of HIV biomedical prevention strategies from randomized clinical trials.

Abdool Karim S, Abdool Karim Q. Antiretroviral prophylaxis: a defining moment in HIV control. Lancet. 2011;378:e23–e25

Current research focuses on both the search for a preventative vaccine, which would protect individuals against HIV infection, as well as a therapeutic vaccine, which could assist HIV-infected individuals in controlling their infection and thus lessen the need for ART (Figure 5.1).

Differentiated Service Delivery Models of HIV Care

As resource-limited countries strive to adopt the WHO Treat All and UNAIDS 90-90-90 goals, it is clear that existing healthcare systems are likely to become overwhelmed by the demand created by these initiatives. In many countries, healthcare systems lack the physical infrastructure, the human resource capacity, and the commodities needed to absorb the extra demand for health services. Hence, in recent years, the global health community has explored *differentiated service delivery* (DSD) models of care, whereby routine health-related tasks can be task-shifted to lower levels of health professionals, thus allowing healthcare to be conducted either by trained lay providers, or outside of the health facility, or sometimes both. This has the dual benefit of bringing care to clients in the community and decreasing wait times and client inconvenience, as well as decongesting health facilities to serve acute needs.

DSD models often focus on shifting HIV testing and counseling into the community or on novel ways to provide ART refills to stable patients; some models incorporate both elements.

Community testing initiatives usually involve community health workers (CHWs) offering tests in locations outside of health facilities; this can involve door-to-door testing, testing at health fairs or in the workplace, or at "hotspots" where high-risk individuals congregate. Individuals testing positive are referred or escorted to the health facility for evaluation and ART initiation, whereas clients testing negative may be referred for preventative measures.

For patients stable on ART treatment (usually defined as adults on the same ART regimen for >12 mos with a suppressed VL and no active OIs or comorbidities), a variety of DSD models exist to provide routine clinical checkups and to dispense antiretroviral refills. The International AIDS Society (IAS) classifies DSD models into four categories (Differentiated Care. International AIDS Society, 2018; Accessed 23 February 2018, at http://www.differentiatedcare.org/):

Health care worker (HCW) managed groups are groups of 25–30 clients who meet every 2–3 mos to discuss their health, encourage adherence, and receive ART refills. They are seen by a HCW for a clinic visit at least once yearly and more frequently as needed. These groups are usually appropriate for urban and peri-urban areas. To date, more than 30,000 clients in South Africa participate in HCW-managed adherence groups (Trop Med Intl Health 2016;21:743–749), and group participants have demonstrated improved viral suppression and retention in care compared to standard facility-based care (JIAS 2017;20:21649).

Facility-based individual models of care allow for fast tracking of patients who present for ART refills without waiting to see a clinician. In this model, a nurse or pharmacist performs a quick health check, and medications are dispensed; the client still comes for a complete check-up once or twice a year. Studies from Uganda have demonstrated that these models of care are cost-effective (PloS one 2011;6:e18193), decrease client-waiting time (AIDS Behav 2013;17:274–283), and improve client ART adherence (Global Health Action 2014;7:24198).

Client-managed groups consist of stable ART clients who form small groups of 4–10 clients. They meet on a monthly basis outside of the facility and provide updates on adherence and symptoms. One client then presents to the facility with information on the entire group and undergoes a routine clinical exam; that client also provides updates on all the other members to the facility. The presenting client then picks up refills for all group members and distributes them at the next group meeting. Thus, each client rotates through the clinic on a routine basis while providing updates on other group members and efficiently distributing refills to the group. This model has been implemented for the past decade as Community ART Groups (CAGs) by Medecins Sans Frontieres in Mozambique, where they demonstrated that CAG clients had excellent retention outcomes (92% at 4 yrs) (Trop Med Intl Health 2014;19:514–521) and 35% less loss-to-follow up (JAIDS 2016;73:e11–22).

Out-of-facility individual DSD models provide a method to distribute ART refills to stable ART clients outside of health facilities. ART may be delivered to a client at his or her home by a CHW or picked up by the client at a fixed distribution point in the community. Two research clinical trials in Uganda (Lancet 2009;374:2080–2089), and Kenya (JAIDS 2010;55:483–490) showed that home-based ART delivery was equivalent but not superior to standard facility care in terms of virological failure or mortality, but home-based delivery resulted in less health service utilization and patient costs.

Some models seek to combine various services; for example, the University of Maryland Community HIV Epidemic Control (CHEC) model uses CHWs to offer HIV testing in the community, link persons to care and treatment, and deliver ART refills to stable clients in their home. A pilot study of this model in Zambia showed 3–5-fold improvement in pregnant women initiated and retained on ART (JAIDS 2017;74:96).

Important Global Trials

HPTN 052: Prevention of HIV-1 infection with early antiretroviral therapy (NEJM 2011;365:493–505).

Summary: HPTN 052 was a large multicountry randomized controlled trial (RCT) designed to determine whether viral suppression decreased sexual transmission of HIV. A total of 1,763 sero-discordant couples in nine countries were assigned to either early ART (CD4 350–500) or delayed ART (CD4 <250 cells/mL or decline of AIDS-related symptoms). The HIV-negative partners were followed for linked HIV transmission, and the HIV-positive partners were followed for a clinical composite outcome of TB, bacterial infection, AIDS, or death. Thirty-nine HIV transmissions occurred (IR: 1.2 per 100 person-years), of which 28 were virologically linked to the infected partner. Only one linked transmission occurred in the early ART group (HR: 0.04, 95% CI, 0.01–0.27, p <0.001).

Sero-discordant couples initiated on early ART had a 96% relative reduction in the number of linked HIV-1 transmissions as compared to delayed therapy, likely due to sustained suppression of HIV-1 in genital secretions. Early ART was also associated with a relative reduction of 41% in HIV-related clinical events.

Take-away: Sero-discordant couples in which the HIV-infected partner is on ART have very low rates of transmission. This trial forms the cornerstone of evidence for the strategy of TasP: viral suppression in HIV-infected individuals prevents transmission to others in the community.

HPTN 052: Antiretroviral Therapy for the Prevention of HIV-1 Transmission (NEJM 2016;375:830–839).

Summary: Following the preceding results, ART was offered to all study participants. HIV-infected participants were followed for a total of 10,031 person-years and their partners for 8,509 person-years. Seventy-eight total infections occurred among HIV-negative partners; viral linkage was performed for 72 (92%) of these, and 46 (64%) were genetically linked: 3 in the early ART group and 43 in the delayed ART group. Early ART demonstrated a 93% relative reduction of HIV transmission compared to delayed ART (HR: 0.07; 95% CI, 0.02–0.22). No genetically linked infections occurred when the index HIV-infected partners were stably virally suppressed.

Take-away: HIV-1 is not sexually transmitted when the infected partner is stably virally suppressed. Appropriate treatment of the infected partner results in prevention of HIV transmission (i.e., TasP).

START: Initiation of Antiretroviral Therapy in Early Asymptomatic HIV Infection (NEJM 2015;373:795–807).

Summary: The Strategic Timing of Anti-Retroviral Therapy (START) trial was a large multicountry RCT to assess the benefit of early ART initiation versus delayed ART.

A total of 4,685 patients in 215 clinics in 35 countries were randomized to either an immediate-initiation group (CD4>500 cells/mL, immediate ART) or a deferred-initiation group (CD4<350 cells/mL or development of AIDS or other indication for ART). The composite endpoint included any serious AIDS-related or non–AIDS-related event and all-cause mortality.

Patients were followed for 3 yrs; in 2015, the study was halted by the Data Safety and Monitoring Board (DSMB) because the interim results clearly favored early initiation. The immediate initiation group had a 57% relative reduction in the primary endpoint (1.8% vs. 4.1%; HR: 0.43, 95% CI: 0.30–0.62, p <0.001). Patients in the early initiation group had a 72% relative reduction in serious AIDS-related events, primarily due to decreased rates of TB, Kaposi's sarcoma (KS), and malignant lymphomas. Early initiators also had a 39% relative reduction in serious non–AIDS-related events, primarily due to reduction in non–AIDS-defining cancers.

Immediate ART benefited patients even with CD4 counts of >500 cells/mL, indicating that early ART accrues benefits other than halting CD4 decline; when the results were stratified to those with higher CD4 counts, the benefit of ART in preventing TB and other OIs was just as strong.

Take-away: START demonstrated that early ART increases long-term survival and decreases occurrence of AIDS-related (primarily OIs) and non–AIDS-related (primarily malignancies) events. Taken in the context of prior evidence, the START and TEMPERANO trials together provide the final conclusive evidence for the strategy of Test and Treat (i.e., that all HIV-infected individuals should be commenced on ART immediately after diagnosis, regardless of CD4 count or WHO stage).

TEMPERANO: A Trial of Early Antiretrovirals and Isoniazid Preventive Therapy in Africa (NEJM 2015;373:808–822).

Summary: The TEMPERANO trial was a 2-by-2 factorial design conducted in Ivory Coast to simultaneously assess the benefits of early versus delayed ART and IPT versus no IPT. A total of 2,056 HIV-infected patients were randomized to deferred ART, deferred ART + IPT, early ART, or early ART + IPT. The composite endpoint was a combination of AIDS, AIDS-defining illness, non–AIDS-defining bacterial disease, and all-cause mortality at 30 mos. Patients receiving early ART had a 44% lower risk of death or severe HIV-related illness (HR: 0.56; 95% CI, 0.41–0.76) compared to deferred ART. Patients on IPT had a 35% lower risk of death or severe HIV-related illness (HR: 0.65; 95% CI 0.48–0.88) compared to those not on IPT. The efficacy of the interventions was primarily attributed to prevention of TB, while early ART also prevented invasive bacterial disease.

Take-away: TEMPERANO confirmed the findings of START that early ART is beneficial while also demonstrating the efficacy of IPT in TB-endemic areas.

iPrex: Preexposure Chemoprophylaxis for HIV Prevention in Men Who Have Sex with Men (NEJM 2010;363:2587–2599).

Summary: The iPrex trial was a multinational RCT designed to assess the efficacy of PrEP in MSM. A total of 2,499 MSM and transgender women were randomly assigned to receive either placebo or TDF/FTC once daily, along with risk-reduction counseling and condoms, and they were followed for 3,324 person-years. Thirty-six people in the TDF/FTC group compared to 64 people in the placebo group acquired HIV, for a 44% reduction in incidence of HIV (95% CI, 15–63; p = 0.005).

Thirty-six in the TDF/FTC group and 64 in the placebo group acquired HIV, indicating a 44% reduction in the incidence of HIV (95% CI, 15–63; P = 0.005). However, adherence was intermittent among participants on TDF/FTC. A subanalysis demonstrated that study participants with detectable blood levels of TDF/FTC compared to those with no detectable drug levels had a relative reduction in HIV risk of 92% (95% CI, 40–99; P <0.001).

A trend toward rising creatinine was seen among patients on TDF/FTC, but this was not significant and resolved after discontinuation. No statistically significant differences in grade 3 or 4 adverse events were observed between the two study groups.

Take-away: iPrex was the first trial to demonstrate the efficacy of oral PrEP, particularly for MSM. This strategy has been borne out in subsequent studies, including FEM-PREP, PARTNERS, and IPERGAY; however, all trials have demonstrated the critical role of adherence in efficacy. PrEP has since been rolled out as a key prevention measure in the developed world and Asia and is currently being deployed in sub-Saharan Africa.

COAT: Timing of Antiretroviral Therapy after Diagnosis of Cryptococcal Meningitis (NEJM 2014;370:2487–2498).

Summary: The COAT trial was an RCT conducted in Uganda and South Africa to determine the optimal timing of ART initiation in HIV-positive patients with cryptococcal meningitis. A total of 177 patients were enrolled and assigned to either early ART (1–2 wks) or deferred ART (5 wks after diagnosis). All patients were treated with amphotericin and fluconazole for 2 wks, followed by fluconazole consolidation therapy. Earlier ART was associated with significantly higher 26-wk mortality compared to deferred ART (HR: 1.73; 95% CI, 1.06–2.82, p = 0.03). Mortality benefit was particularly pronounced among patients with lack of CSF pleocytosis (CSF WBC <5 cells/mL) (HR: 3.87; 95% CI, 1.41–10.58). The trial was stopped early due to the significant observable difference between the two groups.

Take-away: Early ART is not indicated for ARV-naïve individuals with cryptococcal meningitis. Delay ART 4–6 wks after the start of antifungal therapy.

Timing of Initiation of Antiretroviral Therapy in Human Immunodeficiency Virus (HIV)—Associated Tuberculous Meningitis (Clin Infect Dis 2011;52:1374–1383).

Summary: This was a double-blind placebo RCT conducted in Vietnam to assess optimal timing of ART initiation in HIV-infected patients with TB meningitis. A total of 253 patients presenting with TBM received either early ART (within 7 days of diagnosis) or deferred ART (within 2 mos). Overall 9-mo mortality was high at 58%, but did not differ significantly between the two groups (HR: 1.12; 95% CI, 0.81–1.55). However, there were significantly more grade 4 adverse events in the early ART group compared to the deferred ART group (102 vs. 87, respectively; $P = 0.04$), supporting delayed ART for patients with TBM.

Take-away: ART should generally be started within 2 wks of a diagnosis of an AIDS-defining OI, particularly in patients with very low CD4 cells of <50 cells/mL. The exception to this rule is CNS infections, as CNS IRIS is far more likely to be fatal. In cryptococcal meningitis, COAT supports delaying ART to after 5 wks. In TB meningitis, OXTREC supports delaying ART to 8 wks.

Recommended General Reading

Abdool Karim SS, Naidoo K, Grobler A, et al. Integration of antiretroviral therapy with tuberculosis treatment. *NEJM* 2011;365:1492–1501. [SAPiT Trial assessing the timing of antiretroviral initiation in HIV-infected individuals with TB in South Africa.]

Blanc F-X, Sok T, Laureillard D, et al. Earlier versus later start of antiretroviral therapy in HIV-infected adults with tuberculosis. *NEJM* 2011; 365:1471–1481. [CAMELIA Trial assessing the timing of antiretroviral initiation in HIV-infected individuals with TB in Cambodia.]

Boehme CC, Nabeta P, Hillemann D, et al. Rapid molecular detection of tuberculosis and rifampin resistance. *NEJM* 2010; 363:1005–1015. [A major article on utilization of Xpert MTB/RIF in resource-limited settings in HIV-infected and uninfected individuals.]

Havlir DV, Kendall MA, Ive P, et al. Timing of antiretroviral therapy for HIV-1 infection and tuberculosis. *NEJM* 2011; 365:1482–1491. [ACTG 5211 STRIDE Trial at multiple sites assessing the timing of antiretroviral initiation in HIV-infected individuals.]

Lawn SD, Kerkhoff AD, Vogt M, et al. Diagnostic accuracy of a low-cost, urine antigen, point-of-care screening assay for HIV-associated pulmonary tuberculosis before antiretroviral therapy: a descriptive study. *Lancet Infect Dis* 2012; 3:201–209. [A major article on urine LAM testing in HIV-infected individuals in South Africa.]

Török ME, Yen NT, Chau TT, et al. Timing of initiation of antiretroviral therapy in human immunodeficiency virus (HIV)-associated tuberculous meningitis. *Clin Infect Dis* 2011; 52:1374–1383. [Vietnamese study demonstrating harms associated with early initiation of ART in TB meningitis.]

Van Deun A, Maug AK, Salim MA, et al. Short, highly effective, and inexpensive standardized treatment of multidrug-resistant tuberculosis. *Am J Respir Crit Care Med* 2010;182:684–692. [A trial in Bangladesh demonstrating superiority of short-course regimen for treatment of MDR-TB.]

World Health Organization Treatment of Tuberculosis. Guidelines for treatment of drug-susceptible tuberculosis and patient care. 2017 Update. Accessed at: http://apps.who.int/iris/bitstream/10665/255052/1/9789241550000-eng.pdf?ua=1 [Most recent WHO guidelines for treatment of drug-susceptible tuberculosis.]

6

Drug Information

DRUG PROFILES are listed alphabetically by generic drug names.

TRADE NAME and pharmaceutical company source are provided unless there are multiple manufacturers. Trade names are for United States brands.

COST is based on average wholesale price (AWP) according to Lexicomp and Mckesson (2018). Prices are generally given for generic products when generics are available.

Pharmacology, Side Effects, and Drug Interactions

Data are from Approved FDA labeling, American Hospital Formulary Service, Bethesda, MD; PDR 2018; published conference abstracts (CROI, IAC, ICAAC, IAS, HIV Pharm Workshop).

Creatinine Clearance (Cockcroft-Gault Equation)

Males: Weight (kg) × (140 – age)/72 × serum creatinine (mg/dL).

Females: Determination for males × 0.85.

Obese patients: Use lean body weight.

Formula assumes stable renal function: Assume creatinine clearance (CrCl) of 5–8 mL/min for patients with anuria or oliguria.

TABLE 6.1 Child-Pugh calculation

Points	1	2	3
Bilirubin (mg/dL)	<2	2–3	>3
Albumin (g/dL)	>3.5	2.8–3.5	<2.8
PT (seconds)	<4	4–6	>6
Ascites	Absent	Mild-mod	Severe
Encephalopathy*	Absent	Mild (1–2)	Severe (3–4)
INR	<1.7	1.7–2.3	>2.3

Child-Pugh A = 5–6 points, B = 7–9 points, C = 10–15 points

1 Personality change, decreased attention span, mild asterixis; uncoordinated; EEG slowing.

2 Lethargic; asterixis; EEG, slowing, triphasic.

3 Asleep; asterixis; EEG, slowing, triphasic.

4 Comatose, decerebrate, EEG, severe slowing.

Pregnancy and volume expansion: Glomerular filtration rate (GFR) may be increased in third trimester of pregnancy and with massive parenteral fluids.

Note: MDRD equation: 186 × serum creatinine (mg/dL) 1.154 × Age – 0.203 × (1.212 if Black) × (0.742 if female). This has not been validated in HIV-infected persons.

PATIENT ASSISTANCE PROGRAMS: Most pharmaceutical companies that provide this service require all of the following:

- Income eligibility criteria such as an annual income <$12,000 for an individual or <$15,000 for a family.
- Nonavailability of prescription drug payment from public or private third-party sources.
- A prescription and a letter of verification.

Note that most will provide a 3-mo supply subject to re-review after that time (see www.needymeds.org).

CLASSIFICATION FOR DRUG USE IN PREGNANCY BASED ON FDA CATEGORIES: Ratings range from "A" for drugs that

TABLE 6.2 US Food and Drug Administration (FDA) pregnancy classification

Category	Interpretation
A	*Controlled studies show no risk*: Adequate, well-controlled studies in pregnant women have failed to demonstrate risk to the fetus.
B	*No evidence of risk in humans*: Either animal findings show risk, but human findings do not, or, if no adequate human studies have been performed, animal findings are negative.
C	*Risk cannot be ruled out*: Human studies are lacking, and animal studies are either positive for fetal risk, or lacking as well. However, potential benefits may justify the potential risk.
D	*Positive evidence of risk*: Investigational or post-marketing data show risk to the fetus. Nevertheless, potential benefits may outweigh the potential risk.
X	*Contraindicated in pregnancy*: Studies in animals or humans, or investigational or post-marketing reports, have shown fetal risk that clearly outweighs any possible benefit to the patient.

have been tested for teratogenicity under controlled conditions, without showing evidence of damage to the fetus to "D" and "X" for drugs that are definitely teratogenic. The "D" rating is generally reserved for drugs with no safer alternatives. The "X" rating means there is absolutely no reason to risk using the drug in pregnancy.

PREGNANCY REGISTRY FOR ANTIRETROVIRAL DRUGS: This is a joint project sponsored by pharmaceutical companies and an advisory panel with representatives from the Centers for Disease Control (CDC), National Institutes of Health (NIH), obstetrical practitioners, and pediatricians. The registry allows anonymity of patients, and birth outcome follow-up is obtained by registry staff. Healthcare professionals should report prenatal exposures to

TABLE 6.3 Classification of controlled substances

Category	Interpretation
I	*High potential for abuse and no current accepted medical use*: Examples are heroin and LSD.
II	*High potential for abuse*: Use may lead to severe physical or psychological dependence. Examples are some opioids (e.g., oxycodone, hydrocodone, fentanyl), amphetamines, and short-acting barbiturates. Prescriptions must be written in ink or typewritten, and signed by the practitioner. Verbal prescriptions must be confirmed in writing within 72 hrs, and may be given only in a genuine emergency. No renewals are permitted.
III	*Some potential for abuse*: Use may lead to low-to-moderate physical dependence, or high psychological dependence. Examples are barbiturates and preparations containing small quantities of codeine. Prescriptions may be oral or written. Up to five renewals are permitted within 6 mos.
IV	*Lower potential for abuse*: Examples include chloral hydrate, phenobarbital, and benzodiazepines. Use may lead to limited physical or psychological dependence. Prescriptions may be oral or written. Up to five renewals are permitted within 6 mos.
V	*Subject to state and local regulation*: Abuse potential is low; a prescription may not be required. Examples are antitussive and antidiarrheal medications containing limited quantities of opioids.

antiretroviral agents to Antiretroviral Pregnancy Registry, Research Park, 1011 Ashes Drive, Wilmington, NC 28405; 800-258-4263; fax 800-800-1052; (www.apregistry.com). For interpretation of rates, it should be noted that the rate quoted for infants without exposure to antiretroviral agents is 2.7/100 live births and 2.09/100 live births for the first 7 days. Data are provided for antiretroviral agents with >200 first-trimester exposed live births.

TABLE 6.4 Hepatitis C drugs

Formulation/Manufacturer	Dose and Duration	Genotype	Side Effects*
Ledipasvir 90 mg/sofosbuvir 400mg tab (Harvoni)/Gilead	1 tab PO QD × 12wks (no cirrhosis or compensated cirrhosis)	1a, 1b, 4, 5, 6	Fatigue, headache, asthenia, diarrhea, and insomnia. <1% requiring discontinuation.
1) Dasabuvir 200 mg/ombitasvir 8.33 mg/paritaprevir 50 mg/ritonavir 33.33 mg XR tablet (Viekira XR) 2) Ombitasvir 12.5 mg/paritaprevir 75mg/ritonavir 50 mg tablet PLUS Dasabuvir 250 mg tablet (Viekira Pak)/Abbvie Note: This is an alternative regimen Genotype 4 (alternative): Paritaprevir/RTV	3 XR tablets PO QD PLUS RBV with food ×12 wks (Gen 1a; no cirrhosis). No RBV needed for Gen 1b.	1a, 1b, 4	Nausea, pruritus insomnia, and asthenia. 2% of patients discontinued treatment due to side effects.
Elbasvir 50 mg/grazoprevir 100 mg tablet (Zepatier)/Merck	1 tab PO QD ×12wks (no cirrhosis or compensated cirrhosis). If Gen1a & NS5A polymorphisms, add RBV, treat 16 wks)	1a, 1b, 4	Fatigue, headache, nausea, insomnia, and diarrhea. 1% of patients discontinued treatment due to side effects (comparable to placebo).

(*continued*)

TABLE 6.4 Continued

Formulation/Manufacturer	Dose and Duration	Genotype	Side Effects*
Sofosbuvir 400 mg/velpatasvir 100 mg tablet (Epclusa)/Gilead	1 tab PO QD ×12 wks (no cirrhosis or compensated cirrhosis)	1–6	Headache, fatigue, nausea, asthenia, and insomnia. 0.2% of patients discontinued treatment due to side effects.
Sofosbuvir 400 mg/velpatasvir 100 mg/voxilaprevir 100 mg tablet (Vosevi)/Gilead	1 tab PO QD x12wks (Alternative in patients with compensated cirrhosis with Y93H mutation).	3	Headache, fatigue, diarrhea, nausea, asthenia, insomnia. 0.2% of patients discontinued treatment due to side effects.
Glecaprevir 100 mg/pibrentasvir 40 mg tablet (Mavyret)/Abbvie	3 tabs QD × 8 wks (no cirrhosis). Treat for 12 wks, if compensated cirrhosis.	1–6	Headache, fatigue, and nausea. <1% discontinued treatment due to side effects.

Regimen	Dosing	Genotype	Side effects
Daclatasvir 30 mg, 60 mg, 90 mg tablet (Daklinza) (note: dose based on co-administered ARV)/Bristol-Meyer Squibb Sofosbuvir 400 mg tablet (Solvaldi)/Gilead Note: Alternative for G1b in patients w/o cirrhosis. For G3: add RBV if Y93H present.	Daklinza 1 tab (note: dose based on co-administered ARV) PLUS Solvaldi 1 tab PO QD × 12 wks (no cirrhosis) Treat for 24 wks as an alternative regimen in Gen 1a, 2, 3 compensated cirrhosis with or without RBV)	1a, 1b, 2, 3	Headache and fatigue. No discontinuation due to side effects if RBV not co-administered.
Simeprevir 150 mg capsule (Olysio)/Janssen Sofosbuvir 400 mg tablet (Solvaldi)/Gilead Note: Alternative for G1b w/o cirrhosis.	Olysio 1 capsule PO QD PLUS Solvaldi 1 tab PO QD ×12 wks (no cirrhosis) Treat for 24 wks as an alternative for compensated cirrhosis with or without RBV)	1a, 1b (avoid if Q80K mutation)	Nausea, headache, and fatigue. No discontinuation due to side effects.

TABLE 6.5 Antiretroviral–hepatitis C drug–drug interactions

	PI/r	NNRTIs	InSTI	NRTIs	MVC
Sofosbuvir	DRV/r: SD TPV/r: may decrease SOF; avoid.	EFV: SD RPV: SD	RAL: SD BIC: SD	TDF[a]/FTC: SD	No data; SD likely
Ledipasvir (/SOF)	ATV/r, DRV/r, LPV/ r: SD	EFV: Ledipasvir decreased 34% Use SD RPV: SD ETR, NVP: Ledipasvir may be decreased.	BIC: SD EVG/c: avoid when combined with TDF	TDF: SD, but avoid with CrCl; <60ml/min. Monitor for nephrotoxicity when combined with PI/r, PI/c TAF: use SD	No data: usual dose likely.
Simepravir (/SOF)	DRV: avoid; increased SIM PI/r and Cobi: avoid	EFV: avoid ETR, NVP: no data; avoid RPV: SD	RAL: SD DTG: SD EVG/c: avoid	TDF[a], ABC, FTC, 3TC, T-20: SD	No interaction: SD
Dasabuvir, ombitasvir, paritaprevir, ritonavir	Avoid: DRV/r, LPV/r, TPV/r, COBI ATV: 300 mg/d (without RTV)	EFV: Contraindicated; Avoid: RPV, NVP, ETR.	BIC, RAL:SD,DTG: SD EVG/c: avoid	TDF[a], FTC, 3TC, T-20: SD	MVC no data; avoid or consider 150 mg bid.

	PI/r	NNRTIs	InSTI	NRTIs	MVC
Daclatasvir (+SOF)	Decrease daclatasvir to 30 mg/d with ATV/r, ATV/c, IDV, NFV, SQV Daclatasvir 60 mg/d with ATV. FPV, FPV/r, DRV/r, DRV/c, LPV/r TPV/r: avoid.	EFV, ETR and (possibly NVP): increase daclatasvir dose to 90 mg/d RPV: daclatasvir 60 mg/d	BIC, DTG, RAL: daclatasvir 60 mg/d EVG/c or EVG/r: decrease daclatasvir dose to 30 mg/d	Daclatasvir 60 mg/d	Daclatasvir 60 mg/d; MVC standard dose.
Glecaprevir/ Pibrentasvir	Avoid PI/r and ATV.	Avoid EFV and ETR RPV: SD	EVG/c: SD Check LFTs RAL, BIC, RAL: SD	TAF & TDF: SD FTC & 3TC: SD	No data: standard dose likely.
Grazoprevir/ Elbasvir	ATV, DRV, LPV/r, SQV, TPV/r: increase grazoprevir/albasvir concentrations 2 to 8-fold and may increase risk of LFTs elevation. Avoid PI/r and COBI boosted regimens.	RPV: SD EFV: significant decrease in grazoprevir and elbasvir concentrations Avoid EFV, ETR, NVP.	RAL: SD DTG: SD EVG/c: Avoid	ABC, FTC, 3TC, TDF, TAF, T-20: SD	No data: standard dose likely.

(continued)

TABLE 6.5 Continued

	PI/r	NNRTIs	InSTI	NRTIs	MVC
Velpatasvir/ Sofosbuvir[b]	TPV/r: avoid ATV/r, DRV/r: SD COBI: SD	EFV, ETR, NVP: avoid RPV: SD	DTG: SD RAL: SD EVG/c: SD BIC: SD	TDF: use with renal function monitoring TAF may be considered.	No data: standard dose likely

SD standard dose.

[a]TAF may be considered, but no data.

[b]With voxilaprevir co-formulation, avoid ATV/r, ATV/c, LPV/r, Consider monitoring LFTs with EVG/c co-administration.

If ribavirin added to regimen, ddI and d4T contraindicated. Avoid AZT (additive anemia).

TABLE 6.6 HCV antiviral drug interactions

	Sofosbuvir	Ledipasvir	Simepravir	Dasabuvir/ Ombitasvir/ Paritaprevir/RTV	Daclatasvir	Velpatasvir/ Sofobuvir[a]	Glecaprevir/ Pibrentasvir[a]
Acid reducing agents	SD	May decrease ledipasvir. Separate antacid by 4 h; Famotidine 40 mg bid or omeprazole 20 mg/d (max dose)	SD	SD	SD	May decrease velpatasvir. Give velpatasvir 4h before antacid Famotidine 40 mg bid or omeprazole 20 mg/d (max dose)	SD

(continued)

TABLE 6.6 Continued

	Sofosbuvir	Ledipasvir	Simepravir	Dasabuvir/ Ombitasvir/ Paritaprevir/RTV	Daclatasvir	Velpatasvir/ Sofobuvir[a]	Glecaprevir/ Pibrentasvir[e]
CYP3A substrate w/narrow therapeutic index	SD	SD	May increase intestinal CYP3A4 substrates (oral midazolam)	Same contraindication with drugs listed for RTV.	SD	Atorvastatin and rosuvastatin may be increased. Rosuvastatin 10 mg/d (max dose) or use pravastatin	All Statins may be increased Use lowest dose with close monitoring. Do not exceed cyclosporine 100 mg/d.
CYP3A4 inhibitors (azole antifungal, macrolides)	SD	SD	May significantly increase simepravir levels. Avoid.	Paritaprevir dasabuvir may be increased. Dose not established	Decrease daclatasvir to 30 mg/d	SD	SD
Pgp and CYP34 inducers[c]	Avoid	Avoid	Avoid	Avoid	Avoid	Avoid	Avoid

Anti-convulsant[b]	Avoid	Avoid	Avoid	Avoid	Avoid	Avoid	Avoid carbamazepine
Ethinyl estradiol	SD	No interaction SD	No interaction SD	Contraindicated. Potential increased risk of ALT elevation.	SD	SD	Avoid. Potential increased risk of ALT elevation.
Amiodarone	Avoid	Avoid	Avoid	May increase amiodarone levels. Use with close monitoring.	Avoid	Avoid	No data

SD standard dose;

[a] bradycardia reported when sofosbuvir (in combination with ledipasvir, simepravir, velpatasvir, or daclastavir) was given with amiodarone.

[b] Carbamazepine, phenytoin, phenobarbital, oxcarbazepine.

[c] Rifampin, St. John's wort.

[d] Digoxin and topotecan levels may be increased. Monitor Digoxin levels. Avoid topotecan.

[e] Digoxin AUC increased, 48%; dabigatran AUC increased 138%. Use with monitoring & dose adjustment.

Abacavir (ABC)

TRADE NAME: Ziagen (GlaxoSmithKline and generic manufacturers).

CLASS: Nucleoside analog.

FORMULATIONS, REGIMEN, AND COST: Ziagen.

> *Forms:* 300 mg tab (generic available); 20 mg/mL oral solution.
> Regimen: 300 mg bid or 600 mg/d.
> AWP: $502/mo.
> *Trizivir:* AZT/ABC/3TC (300/300/150 mg tab).
> Regimen: 1 tab bid.
> AWP: $1,738/mo.
> *Epzicom (or Kivexa):* ABC/3TC (600/300 mg tab).
> Regimen: 1 tab qd.
> AWP: $1,395/mo.
> *Triumeq:* DTG/ABC/3TC (50/600/300 mg tab).
> Regimen: 1 tab qd.
> AWP: $3,118.62/mo

PATIENT ASSISTANCE: 866-728-4368.

FOOD: Take without regard for meals.

RENAL FAILURE: ABC—no dose adjustment; Trizivir, Epzicom, and Triumeq—not recommended with CrCl <50 mL/min; use separate components with dose adjustment.

HEPATIC FAILURE: Based on limited clinical data, 200 mg bid may be used for Child-Pugh class A (CP score 5–6). Some use standard dose. Contraindicated for classes B and C (CP score 7–12). No data in moderate to severe hepatic impairment.

ADVANTAGES: Co-formulated with dolutegravir, well tolerated, once-daily therapy, no food effect and excellent CNS penetration.

DISADVANTAGES: Hypersensitivity reaction in 5–8% of patients. Screening for HLA-B*5701 nearly eliminates the risk of this reaction, and should be performed prior to administration.

Reports from D:A:D and SMART studies suggest that ABC may be associated with an increased risk of cardiovascular disease (this is debated), and ACTG 5202 suggests that ABC/3TC may be inferior to TDF/FTC in treatment of patients with a baseline VL >100,000 c/mL when combined with EFV or ATV/r but not with DTG (see below).

POTENCY: With monotherapy, ABC reduced viral load 1.5–2.0 logs, significantly more than AZT, ddI, 3TC, and d4T. Most trials have shown good potency when combined with an INSTI, NNRTI. or PI/r. ACTG 5202 is a randomized trial comparing ABC/3TC to TDF/FTC combined with EFV or ATV/r. After enrollment of >1,800 participants, the study was stopped by the data and safety monitoring board (DSMB) due to excessive rates of virologic failure in ABC/3TC recipients with a baseline VL >100,000 c/mL (NEJM 2009;361:2230). The difference was highly significant ($p = 0.003$) and was independent of the third drug (EFV or ATV/r). However, virologic response with DTG plus ABC/3TC treatment of patients with baseline VL >100,000 c/mL were not inferior to EFV/TDF/FTC treated patients (Walmsley S et al., JAIDS 2015). Results of ACTG 5202 for patients with a baseline VL <100,000 c/mL showed no difference between these two NRTI pairs, which was surprising, although meta-analysis of 12 trials with 5,168 patients found TDF/FTC was superior in virologic outcome with baseline VL >100,000 c/mL ($p < 0.002$) and <100,000 c/mL ($p = 0.02$) (HIV Med 2009;10:527).

CLINICAL TRIALS:

Comparison of Non-nucleoside Reverse Transcriptase Inhibitors (NNRTIs) and NRTI Combinations (CNA 30024) compared AZT/3TC and ABC/3TC, each with EFV, in 699 treatment-naïve patients. At 48 wks VL was <50 c/mL in 69% and 70%, respectively, by ITT analysis (CID 2004;39:1038). ABC/3TC was associated with less anemia, nausea, and vomiting, but more hypersensitivity reactions. This paved the way to co-formulation (Epzicom).

Comparison of ABC/3TC once- vs. twice-daily: ESS 3008 compared twice-daily vs. once-daily ABC/3TC combined with a PI or NNRTI. Viral suppression was sustained at 48 wks in 81% in the once-daily group vs. 82% in the twice-daily group. Adherence was better in the once-daily group. (JAIDS 2005;40:422). (Note: The intracellular half-life is 12–21 hr, justifying once-daily dosing.).

BICOMBO: Comparison of ABC/3TC vs. TDF/FTC: 333 patients with virologic control while receiving a 3TC-containing regimen were randomized to TDF/FTC vs. ABC/3TC as the NRTI backbone (JAIDS 2009;51:290). Results at 48 wks showed virologic failure in 4 (2%) in the ABC/3TC group vs. none in the TDF/FTC group.

HEAT: Comparison of ABC/3TC + LPV/r vs. TDF/FTC + LPV/r in 688 treatment-naïve patients (AIDS 2009;23:1547). Virologic suppression at 48 wks was comparable, and rates of treatment limiting side effects, and changes in lipid profile were similar. CD4 count recovery among ABC/3TC recipients. (median increase 250/mm^3 vs. 247/mm^3) by week 96.

ACTG 5202: This was a 4 arm trial of 1,858 treatment-naïve patients randomized to receive blinded ABC/3TC vs. TDF/FTC, and open label EFV vs. ATV/r. The DSMB recommended early unblinding in the subset with a baseline VL >100,000 c/mL due to excessive virologic failures in the ABC/3TC vs. TDF/FTC recipients (15% vs. 7%; p <0.003) (NEJM 2009;361:2230). A more recent analysis showed a significantly lower virologic response rate in patients given ABC/3TC (Ann Intern Med 2011;154:445).

ASSERT: Open-label trial in 385 treatment-naïve, HLA-B*5701 negative patients randomized to ABC/3TC + EFV vs. TDF/FTC/EFV. At 96 wks ABC/3TC recipients had lower rates of viral suppression (VL <50 c/mL in 59% vs. 71%; p <0.05), a nonsignificant trend toward better renal function (change in GFR of + 1.48 vs. −1.15 mL/min/1.73 M^2 (p = NS) and less decrease in bone mineral density at hip and lumbar spine (hip: −2.17% vs. −3.55%) (JAIDS 2010;55:49; CID 2010;51:973).

ACTG 372A: ABC Intensification: The addition of ABC to patients who had stable HIV suppression failed to confer clinical or virologic benefit (HIV Clin Trials 2010;11:312).

TABLE 6.7 Major clinical trials of ABC in initial therapy

Study	Regimen	N	Dur (wks)	VL <50 (%)	VL <400 (%)
CNA 3014	AZT/3TC/ABC	164	48	60	66[a]
Curr Med Res Opin 2004;20:1103	AZT/3TC + IDV	165		50	50
CNA 3005	AZT/3TC/ABC	262	48	31	51
JAMA 2001;285:1155	AZT/3TC + IDV	265		45[a]	51
ACTG 5095	AZT/3TC/ABC	382	48	61	74[b]
NEJM 2004;350:1850	AZT/3TC + EFV±ABC	765		83[a]	89[b]
CNA 30024	ABC/3TC + EFV	324	48	70	
CID 2004;39:1038	AZT/3TC + EFV	325		69	
CNA 30021 (ZODIAC)	ABC (qd) + 3TC + EFV	384	48	66	—
JAIDS 2005;38:417	ABC (bid) + 3TC + EFV	386		68	—
ESS 30009	ABC/3TC + TDF	102	12[c]		51[c]
JID 2005;192:1921	ABC/3TC + EFV	169	48	71	75[a]
ESS 30008	ABC/3TC (qd) + 3rd agent	130	48	82	
JAIDS 2005;40:422	ABC/3TC (bid) + 3rd agent	130		81	
HEAT (Smith KY, et al., 17th Intern AIDS Conf. 2008:Abstr. LBPE1138)	ABC/3TC + LPV/r	343	96	60	
	TDF/FTC + LPV/r	345		58	
ALTAIR	EFV/TDF/FTC	114	48		95[a]
CID 2010;51:855	ATV/r + TDF/FTC	105			96[a]
	AZT + ABC + TDF/FTC	103			82

(continued)

TABLE 6.7 Continued

Study	Regimen	N	Dur (wks)	VL <50 (%)	VL <400 (%)
ACTG 5202 Ann Intern Med 2011;154:445	ABC/3TC + EFV or ATV/r	719	96		82
	TDF/FTC + EFV or ATV/r	767			89[a]
SINGLE JAIDS 2015;70:2015	ABC/3TC + DTG	414	96	80	
	TDF/FTC/EFV	419		72	

[a] Superior to comparitor (P <0.05).

[b] VL <200 c/mL.

[c] Study terminated due to high failure rate; VL <50 c/mL at 12 wks was 17% (TDF) vs. 50% (EFV). The triple NRTI arm had high rates of K65R and 184V resistance mutations.

TABLE 6.8 Results of HEAT (ABC/3TC + LPV/r vs. TDF/FTC + LPV/r) at 48 wks

	ABC/3TC + LPV/r n = 343	TDF/FTC + LPV/r n = 345
VL <50 c/mL	68%	67%
Response w/baseline VL >100K c/mL	63%	65%
CD4 count (cells/mm³)	+201	+173
Virologic failure (VL >50 c/mL)	12%	11%
GFR decreased	5%	5%
Suspected ABC HSR*	4%	1%

From AIDS 2009;361:2230.

HSR, hypersensitivity reactions.

Note that the patients were not prescreened for HLA-B*5701.

RESISTANCE: ABC selects primarily for L74V and, to a lesser extent, K65R. The M184V mutation by itself does not reduce in vitro or clinical activity, but when combined with 2 or 3 TAMs there is reduced activity, and with ≥4 TAMs there is no activity (Topics HIV Med 2006;14:125; Antiviral Ther 2004;9:37). Mutations at RT codons K65R and L74V lead to cross-resistance to ddI, and K65R leads to loss of susceptibility to TDF, especially when not accompanied by M184V. Each of these mutations results in a 2- to 4-fold decrease in susceptibility to ABC. Significant resistance requires multiple mutations, usually in addition to the M184V mutation (JAC 2010;65:307). In combination with TDF there is selection for 65R (AAC 2004;48:1413). The initial use of d4T or AZT drives TAMs, which reduce activity of all NRTIs. In contrast K65R protects against TAMs and enhances activity of AZT and d4T (AIDS 2007;21:405; JID 2004;189:837; JAIDS 2010;61:346). This is an additional reason for starting with ABC/3TC or TDF/FTC. However, such sequencing considerations have become less important in developed countries because of the declining use of d4T and AZT. They remain relevant in resource-limited settings.

RISK OF CARDIOVASCULAR DISEASE: *This is a controversial association with no consensus.* A retrospective review of the D:A:D observational cohort for cardiovascular disease risks associated with NRTI use included 33,347 patients and 157,912 patient-years of follow-up. There were 517 myocardial infarctions (MIs), including 192 in patients receiving ABC-containing regimens. The relative risk for recent ABC use was 1.9 (95% CI, 1.5–2.5) (Lancet 2008;371:1417). More recent analysis of the D:A:D database continues to show this association (JID 2010;201:318). Analysis of SMART data for 1019 patients who received continuous ABC and 2882 patients treated with alternative NRTIs found that the relative risk for acute myocardial infarction with ABC use was 4.3 (JID 2008;197:1133). Switching from ABC to TDF has also been noted to decrease augmentation index, a measure of arterial stiffness, and Framingham risk score by 2% (AIDS 2010;24:2403). The risk was observed only with use in the prior 6 mos, indicating that the risk resolves when ABC is stopped.

Arguing against this association are the following: (1) No likely pathophysiological mechanism is apparent; (2) markers of inflammation and coagulation do not correlate with ABC use (AIDS Res Ther 2010;7:9; AIDS 2010;24:f1; AIDS 2010;24:1657); (3) other studies including a pooled analysis of 14,683 treated patients (9,639 ABC recipients) have not shown this risk (Lancet 2008;371:1413); (4) an FDA review of 26 controlled clinical trials with 9,832 patients found no association between ABC use with AMIs (OR = 1.06) (Ding X. 2011 CROI, Abstr. 808; (5) ACTG 5001/ ALLRT, a retrospective analysis of 6 ACTG trials in 3,205 treatment-naïve patients followed; a total of 17,404 patient years with 36 MI events failed to show an ABC risk (CID 2011;52:429); and (6) it has also been argued that the association, if real, may reflect preferential use of ABC in patients with the metabolic syndrome or renal failure that are associated with increased cardiovascular events (JID 2010;201:315).

PHARMACOLOGY:

Bioavailability: 83%; alcohol increases ABC levels by 41% (clinical significance unknown). Good central nervous system (CNS) penetration.

$T^{1/2}$: 1.5 hr (serum); intracellular $T^{1/2}$: 12–21 hr. The active metabolite, carbovir triphosphate, has an intracellular half-life of >20 hrs (AIDS 2002;16:1196). CSF levels: Ranks class 3 in the four-class CNS penetration classification (Neurology 2011;76:693).

Elimination: 81% metabolized by alcohol dehydrogenase and glucuronyl transferase with renal excretion of metabolites; 16% recovered in stool, and 1% unchanged in urine. Metabolism does not involve the cytochrome P450 pathway. Plasma clearance correlates with body weight, suggesting the possibility of suboptimal levels in patients with greater body weight (Br J Clin Pharmacol 2005;59:183).

Dose modification in renal failure: None (Nephron 2000;87:186). Triumeq, Trizivir, and Epzicom should not be used when

CrCl <50 mL/min because of the need to reduce dosages of the 3TC components.

SIDE EFFECTS:

Hypersensitivity reaction (black box FDA warning): In an analysis of 30,595 participants in clinical trials and expanded access programs prior to screening for HLA-B*5701, 1,302 (4.2%) had definite or probable hypersensitivity reactions (HSR), and 19 were fatal, for a mortality rate of 0.03% (3/10,000) (Clin Ther 2001;23:1603). Of the 19 deaths, 6 occurred with re-challenge. The median time of onset was 9 days, and 90% occurred in the first 6 wks. Clinical features include fever (usually 39–40°C), skin rash (maculopapular or urticarial), fatigue, malaise, GI symptoms (nausea, vomiting, diarrhea, abdominal pain), arthralgias, cough, and/or dyspnea). The rash occurs in 70% who have HSR (CID 2002;34:1137). Laboratory changes may include increased CPK, elevated liver function tests, and lymphopenia. Nearly all true HSRs have symptoms involving ≥2 organs (Drug Saf 2006;29:811).

Susceptibility to this reaction has been associated with the MHC class I allele HLA-B*5701 haplotype (Lancet 2002;359:727; Lancet 2002;359:1121). The flagship study of HLA-B*5701 screening was the PREDICT trial in which 1956 patients were tested prior to use of ABC, with results communicated to physicians based on randomization. Patients who had suspected HSR had confirmatory patch tests for verification of this mechanism.

All patch test-confirmed cases had the HLA-B*5701 allele, giving a negative predictive value of 100% (NEJM 2008;358:568). Specificity was 30–55%. This suggests that a negative test provides near absolute assurance that the ABC HSR will not occur. There are no well confirmed published cases of ABC HSR in patients with negative tests for HLA-B*5701 (S. Mallal, personal communication, February 2011). The current recommendation for resource-rich countries are: (1) All patients who are to receive ABC should have this screening test, (2) Those with positive tests should never receive ABC, and (3) Those with negative tests who are given ABC should still be warned about ABC HSR, even though the risk is extremely low.

There are substantial geographic and ethnic differences in rates of HLA-B*5701, as shown below (J HIV Ther 2003;8:36; CID 2006;43:103):

US: White 8%, Asian 1%, African American 2.5%, Hispanic 2%.
South America: 5–7%.
Western Europe: 5–7%.
UK: 8%.
Middle East 1–2%.
India: 5–20%.
China: 0.
Japan: 0.
Thailand: 4–10%.
Australia: 8%.
Africa: <1%.
A review of tests of 9,720 patients in 272 European centers found a rate of.
5%: 6.5% in whites and 0.4% in blacks (Pharmacogenet Geonomics 2010;5:307).

Testing for HLA-B*5701 is offered by commercial labs at a cost of about $90–130, or it can be done in some local facilities, especially those with transplant programs. The test results usually require

TABLE 6.9 Results of PREDICT

	HLA-B*5701 Results	
	Known	Not Known
Clinically suspected HSR	3.4%	7.8%
Patch test confirmed	0	2.7%

From NEJM 2008;358:9.

3–10 days for reporting, the results are definitive (yes/no), and it never needs to be repeated (since it is a genetic test). Patients who have poorly confirmed HSR and a negative test can usually be rechallenged safely (Antivir Ther 2008;13:1019). Rechallenge with ABC in a patient with true hypersensitivity virtually always results in a reaction within hours, and may resemble anaphylaxis in 20% with hypotension, bronchoconstriction, and/or renal failure (AIDS 1999:13:999). Treatment of rechallenge reactions is supportive with IV fluids, ventilator support, dialysis, as required. Steroids and antihistamines are not effective. Rechallenge has been associated with death, but this is rare. HSR should be reported to the Abacavir Hypersensitivity Registry.

Patients prescribed ABC, including those with negative screening tests, should be warned to consult their provider immediately if they note two or more of the hallmark symptoms, including fever, skin rash, typical GI symptoms, cough, dyspnea, and/or constitutional symptoms, especially during the first month of therapy. A warning sheet is usually provided to the patient by the pharmacist. A possible solution in unclear cases with negative screening for HLA-B*5701 is administration under observation, because patients experiencing true ABC HSR will predictably experience worsening symptoms with continued dosing. The patch test used in the PREDICT study is not commercially available.

> *Other side effects*: Include nausea, vomiting, malaise, headache, diarrhea, or anorexia.
>
> *Lactic acidosis*: Patients taking ABC can presumably develop lactic acidosis, although this is rare because ABC, like 3TC, FTC, and TDF, has low affinity for mitochondrial DNA (J Biol Chem 2001;276:40847).

BLACK BOX WARNINGS: (1) ABC HSR; (2) lactic acidosis.

DRUG INTERACTIONS: Minimal drug–drug interactions. Alcohol increases ABC levels by 41%; ABC has no effect on alcohol levels (AAC 2000;283:1811). ABC AUC ↓40% with TPV/r co-administration; clinical significance unknown. Ribavirin has potential antagonism; lower rate of early virologic response in the treatment of HCV (avoid or use with caution). Methadone clearance increased is 22%; not clinically significant. Use standard dose.

PREGNANCY: Category C. The 2018 DHHS Guidelines for Antiretroviral Drugs in Pregnant HIV-Infected Women recommend. The Pregnancy Registry shows an adverse birth in 30/1088 (2.76%). No evidence of human teratogenicity. (www.apregistry.com; accessed April 6, 2018). Rodent teratogen test showed skeletal malformations and anasarca at 35 times the comparable human dose. Placental passage positive in rats. Studies in pregnant women show the ABC AUC is not altered, so the standard dose is appropriate (AIDS 2006;28:553).

Acyclovir (also includes famciclovir and valacyclovir)

TRADE NAMES: Zovirax (GlaxoSmithKline, acyclovir), Famvir (Novartis, famciclovir), Valtrex (GlaxoSmithKline, valacyclovir). All three are also available as generics.

CLASS: Synthetic nucleoside analogs derived from guanine.

FORMULATIONS, REGIMEN, AND COST:.

Acyclovir (Zovirax): Caps: 200 mg at $.98. Tabs: 400 mg at $2.17, 800 mg at $4.22. Suspension: 200 mg/5 cc at $445/473 mL. IV vials: 500 mg and 1 g at $5.40 and $10.98, respectively. 5% ointment: 15 g at $797.00 (utility limited); 5% cream: (5 g) $804 (utility limited).

Famciclovir (Famvir): Tabs: 125, 250, 500 mg; $5.81, $6.32, $12.69, respectively.

Valacyclovir (Valtrex): Tabs: 500 mg at $7.22, 1,000 mg at $12.64.

PATIENT ASSISTANCE PROGRAM: 866-728-4368 (acyclovir and valacyclovir).

INDICATIONS AND DOSES: For oral therapy, acyclovir, famciclovir, or valacyclovir are advocated by the CDC for treatment and prevention of HSV (MMWR 2010;59:RR-12). They are generally considered equivalent, although some authorities prefer valacyclovir and famciclovir for the immuno-suppressed host (Lancet 2001;353:1513). Acyclovir is the only available IV formulation in this class. Recommendations are based on 2018 NIH/CDC/IDSA OI guidelines, 2015 CDC STD guidelines, and 2010 CDC guidelines for treating HSV in patients with HIV co-infection (MMWR 2010;59 [RR12]:30–35) and the CDC-IDSA recommendations for treating VZV with HIV co-infection (MMWR 2004;53 [RR-15]:42–44). In vitro activity of various antivirals against herpes viruses are summarized below.

HERPES SIMPLEX: (MMWR 2010;59 [RR12]:30–35).
Initial Infection: All patients should be treated, even if the infection is mild.
  Acyclovir 400 mg po tid5–10 d.
  Famciclovir 500 mg po bid × 5–10 d.
  Valacyclovir 1 g po bid × 5–10 d.
Suppressive Therapy (with HIV co-infection):
  Acyclovir 400 mg po bid.
  Famciclovir 500 mg po bid.
  Valacyclovir 500– mg po bid.
Episodic HSV Infection (with HIV co-infection):
  Acyclovir 400 mg po tid × 5–10 d.
  Famciclovir 500 mg po bid × 5–10 d.
  Valacyclovir 1 g bid × 5–10 d.

Severe or Resistant Infection: Acyclovir 5–10 mg/kg IV q8h might be necessary. If lesions persist, test HSV for resistance (Arch Intern Med 2003;163:76). HSV strains resistant to acyclovir are usually sensitive to foscarnet, which can be given at 40 mg/kg IV q8h until lesions resolve. An infrequently used alternative is cidofovir 5 mg/kg/wk. Topical alternatives include imiquimod, or 1% cidofovir gel (must be compounded by pharmacy). Topical treatment should be given once-daily × 5d.

Genital HSV in Pregnancy: Most neonatal HSV infections are acquired from women without a history of genital HSV (NEJM 1997;337:509). The greatest recognized risk is HSV acquired near delivery (30–50%); the risk is low in women who have a history of recurrent HSV or who acquire HSV in the first half of pregnancy (JAMA 2003;289:203).

Pregnant women should be asked if they have a history of genital HSV, and some authorities routinely test pregnant women for type-specific HSV. The safety of acyclovir, famciclovir, and valacyclovir in pregnancy is not definitely established, but available data suggest that acyclovir is safe during the first trimester (Birth Defects Res A Clin Mol Teratol 2004;270:201). Recommendations based on these observations are:

Acyclovir po can be given to pregnant women with initial genital HSV or severe recurrent infection; IV acyclovir should be given for severe HSV.

Acyclovir po can be given to women who have a history of recurrent HSV to prevent recurrence in late pregnancy (Obstet Gynecol 2002;10:71; Am J Obstet Gynecol 2003;188:836; Obstet Gynecol 2003;102:1396).

Women without signs or symptoms of genital HSV or prodromal symptoms can deliver vaginally. C-section should be performed if there is evidence of genital HSV at onset of labor.

HERPES ZOSTER: Recommendations of the 2018 Guidelines from NIH, CDC, and IDSA for VZV in patients with HIV infection:

Dermatomal zoster: Valacyclovir 1 g po tid, or famciclovir 500 mg po tid, or acyclovir 800 mg po 5/d × 7–10 d; may require longer duration. Extensive cutaneous lesions or visceral VZV: Acyclovir 10–15 mg/kg IV q8h; change to po therapy when lesions start to regress using valacyclovir (1,000 mg

TABLE 6.10 Activity of antivirals against herpes viruses

	HSV	VZV	EBV	CMV	HHV 6–8
Acyclovir	+ +	+	+	—	—
Famciclovir	+ +	+	+	—	—
Valacyclovir	+ +	+	+	—	—
Ganciclovir	+ +	+	+ +	+ +[a]	+
Foscarnet	+	+	+ +	+ +[a]	+
Cidofovir	+	+	+ +	+ +[a]	+ +

[a] Performed well in clinical studies.

tid), famciclovir (500 mg tid), or acyclovir (800 mg 5 ×/d) to complete 10- to 14-day course.

Progressive outer retinal necrosis (PORN): Ganciclovir 5 mg/kg IV q12h + foscarnet 90 mg/kg IV q12h + ganciclovir 2 mg/0.05 mL given by intravitreal injection 2 ×/wk, and/or foscarnet 1.2 mg/0.05 mL intravitreal injection 2 ×/wk (plus ART).

Acute retinal necrosis (ARN): Acyclovir 10 mg/kg IV q8h × 10–14 d, then valacyclovir 1,000 mg po tid × 6 wk + ganciclovir 2 mg/0.05 mL given by intravitreal injection 2 ×/wk × 1–2 doses (plus ART).

VZV resistant to acyclovir: Foscarnet 90 mg/kg IV q12h.

Oral hairy leukoplakia (EBV): Indications to treat are unclear, but treatment is requested by some patients, usually for cosmetic reasons. One study of 18 patients given valacyclovir 1 g q8h × 28 days showed clinical and virologic response in 16 (89%), and virologic response in 16 (89%). Recurrence after 1 mo off treatment occurred in 2 of 12 patients (17%) (JID 2003;188:883). An alternative is topical 1% penciclovir cream (Oral Surg Oral Med, Oral Pathol, Oral Radid Endod 2010;110:611).

HIV: Acyclovir is reported to have a modest impact on the viral load with a decrease of about $0.5 \log_{10}$ c/mL in some reports (Lancet Infect Dis 2010;10:455; JAIDS 2008;59:77).

PHARMACOLOGY:

Bioavailability: Acyclovir, 15–20% with oral administration.

$T^{1/2}$: Acyclovir, 2.5–3.3 hr, CSF levels: 50% serum levels.

Elimination: Renal. Consult fda labeling for acyclovir dose adjustment in renal failure.

Famciclovir (VZV): CrCl 40–59 mL/min = 500 mg q12h; 20–39 = 500 mg q24h; <20 = 250 mg q24h (after HD on HD days).

Valacyclovir (VZV): CrCl 30–49 = 1 g q12h; 10–29 = 1 g q24h; <10 = 500 mg q24h (post-HD on HD days).

SIDE EFFECTS: Acyclovir, famciclovir, and valacyclovir are generally well tolerated.

IV Acyclovir: Irritation and phlebitis at infusion site, rash, nausea.

Albendazole

CLINICAL TRIALS: Albendazole (400 mg bid until CD4 >200/mm^3 × 6 mos) after initiation of ART is effective with microsporidiosis involving *Encephalitozoon* (Septata) intestinalis (Parasitol Res 2003;90 Suppl 1:S14; Gastroenterol Clin Biol 2010;34:450) but is not effective against E. bieneusi, which account for about 80% of cases of microsporidiosis in AIDS patients. These species can be distinguished by special stain (Uvitex-2B) EM or polymerase chain reaction (PCR) that is also used for species identification in disseminated microsporidiosis and intraocular infection with *E. cuniculi* (Int J Med Microbiol 2005;294:529; Ethiop Med J 2005;43:97). Some reports suggest fumagillin may be useful with *E. bieneusi* infection (Transpl Infect Dis 2009;11:83), but is not commercially available in the United States.

PHARMACOLOGY:

Bioavailability: Low (<5%), but absorption is increased 5-fold if taken with a fatty meal vs. in a fasting state. Should be taken with fatty meal.

$T^{1/2}$: 8 hrs.

Elimination: Metabolized in liver to albendazole sulfoxide, then excreted by enterohepatic circulation.

Dose modification in renal failure: None.

SIDE EFFECTS: Adverse reactions are infrequent and include reversible hepatotoxicity, GI intolerance (abdominal pain, diarrhea, nausea, vomiting), reversible hair loss, hypersensitivity reactions (rash, pruritus, fever), reversible neutropenia, and central nervous system (CNS) toxicity (dizziness, headache). Some recommend monitoring liver function tests every 2 wks. Rare fatal pancytopenia has been reported (Am J Trop Med Hyg 2005;72:291).

PREGNANCY: Category C. Albendazole is teratogenic and embryotoxic in rodents at doses of 30 mg/kg. Not recommended for use in pregnancy; ART is preferred for microsporidiosis.

Amphotericin B

TRADE NAME: Parenteral form, generic; oral form is no longer available from commercial sources but can be prepared by a pharmacy.

CLASS: Amphoteric polyene macrolide with activity against nearly all pathogenic and opportunistic fungi.

FORMULATIONS, REGIMEN, AND COST: Fungizone at $45.60/d/50 mg vial; Abelcet $240/d/100 mg; Amphotec no longer available; AmBisome $208/100 mg.

INDICATIONS AND DOSES: Sharply reduced general usage of conventional amphotericin in recent years due to concerns about nephrotoxicity and availability of alternatives, such as posaconazole, voriconazole, caspofungin, and lipid amphotericin formulations (CID 2006;42:1289). Due to higher rates of nephrotoxicity and infusion-related reaction; conventional amphotericin is can be considered for cryptococcal meningitis if cost is an issue with liposomal amphotericin.

ADMINISTRATION—ORAL: Oral suspension for thrush is no longer available commercially, but it can be prepared by a pharmacist to a strength of 5–10 mg/mL of amphotericin B. *Dose*: 1–5 mL qid; swish as long as possible, then swallow.

ADMINISTRATION—IV: Usual dose of conventional amphotericin B is 0.3–1.5 mg/kg/d given by slow IV infusion over ≥2–4 hrs (BMJ 2000;332:579). Some authorities advocate a test dose (1 mg in 50 mL DSW given over 30 minutes with cardiovascular monitoring for 4 hrs) as a test for hypersensitivity. The usual dose for cryptococcal meningitis is 0.7 mg/kg/d combined with flucytosine. Higher doses (1 mg/kg/d) of amphotericin appear to be more rapidly fungicidal (CID 2008;47:131). For infusion-related side effects, pre-medicate with nonsteroidal antiinflammatory drug (NSAID) + /– diphenhydramine or hydrocortisone 50–100 mg. Give meperidine for rigors.

LIPID PREPARATIONS OF AMPHOTERICIN B INCLUDE:

Abelcet (ABLC) (Sigma-Tau Pharmaceutical): Amphotericin B complexed with two phospholipids—DMPC and DMPG.

Amphotec (ABCD) (AlkoPharma): Amphotericin B colloidal dispersion with cholesterol sulfate is no longer available in the United States.

AmBisome (LAmB) (Gilead/Astellas Pharma US, Inc.): Liposomal amphotericin B is a true liposomal delivery system.

ADVANTAGES: Compared with amphotericin B, these formulations cause less nephrotoxicity and infusion-related reactions (NEJM 1999;340:764). Comparative trials vs.

TABLE 6.11 Acyclovir dose modification in renal failure

Usual Dose	Creatinine Clearance	Adjusted Dose
200 mg 5×/d	>10 mL/min	200 mg 5×/d
	≤10 mL/min	200 mg q12h
800 mg 5×/d	10–50 mL/min	800 mg q8h
	<10 mL/min	800 mg q12h
5–10 mg/kg IV q8h	25–50 mL/min	5–10 mg/kg q 12 hr
	10–24 mL/min	5–10 mg/kg q 24 hr
	<10 mL/min/HD	5 mg/kg q24h

amphotericin B consistently show that the lipid preparations are therapeutically equivalent and sometimes superior, especially AmBisome. The daily drug cost of liposomal amphotericin is significantly higher compared to conventional amphotericin B; however, with many infections the lipid formulations may be more cost-effective due to reduced rates of renal failure and dialysis (CID 2001;32:686; CID 2003;37:415; CID 2009;49:1721; Medicine 2010;89:236).

PHARMACOLOGY:

Bioavailability: Peak serum concentrations with standard IV doses are 0.5–2 µg/mL. There is no significant absorption with oral administration; CSF levels are 3% of serum concentrations.

$T^{1/2}$: 24 hr with IV administration, detected in blood and urine up to 4 wks after discontinuation.

Elimination: Serum concentrations in urine; metabolic pathways are unknown.

Dose adjustment in renal failure: None, but with chronic renal insufficiency consider lipid amphotericin unless ESRD on HD.

TABLE 6.12 Amphotericin for fungal infections associated with HIV infection

Fungus	Preferred	Amphotericin B Regimens
Aspergillosis	Voriconazole	Ampho B 1 mg/kg/d IV or Liposomal ampho B 5 mg/kg/d IV
Candidiasis • Thrush • Esophagitis	Azoles	Ampho B 0.3 mg/kg/d IV or Ampho B suspension 100 mg/mL with 1 mL gargled 4×/dAmpho B 0.3–0.7 mg/kg/d IV Lipid ampho B 3–5 mg/d IV
Coccidioidomycosis • Mild/moderate • Severe (non-meningeal) • Meningitis	Azole Ampho B Fluconazole	Ampho B 0.7–1.0 mg/kg/d IV Lipid ampho B 4–6 mg/kg/d IV until improved – then azole Ampho B intrathecal if high dose azoles fail
Cryptococcosis • Meningitis	Liposoma Ampho B + 5FC	Ampho B 0.7 mg/kg/d IV Liposomal ampho B 4–6 mg/kg/d IV Induction phase: a minimum of 2 wks
Histoplasmosis • Mild/moderate • Moderate/severe (non-meningeal) • Meningitis	Itraconazole Liposomal Ampho B Liposomal Ampho B	Liposomal ampho B 3 mg/kg/d IV Alternate: ampho B lipid complex 3 mg/kg/d IV Duration: 2 wks or when clinically improved Liposomal ampho B 5 mg/kg/d IV × 4–6 wks
Penicilliosis • Mild • Acute	Itraconazole Ampho B	Ampho B 0.6 mg/kg/d IV × 2 wks

From 2017 IDSA/NIH/CDC Guidelines for Prevention and Treatment of Opportunistic Infections in HIV-infected Adults and Adolescents.

SIDE EFFECTS:

Oral form: Rash, GI intolerance, and allergic reactions. Infusion-related toxicity with IV form is formulation, dose-related, and less severe with slow administration.

Fever and chills, usually 1–3 hrs post infusion and lasting for up to 4 hrs post infusion. Reduce with hydrocortisone (10–50 mg added to infusion, but only if necessary due to immunosuppression); alternatives that are now often preferred are meperidine, ibuprofen, or naproxen, prior to infusion.

Hypotension, nausea, vomiting, usually 1–3 hrs post infusion; may be reduced with Compazine.

Nephrotoxicity in up to 80% ± nephrocalcinosis, potassium wasting, renal tubular acidosis. Reduce with gradual increase in dose, adequate hydration, avoidance of concurrent nephrotoxic drugs, and possibly sodium loading. Discontinue or reduce dose with blood urea nitrogen (BUN) >40 mg/dL and creatinine >3 mg/dL. Lipid amphotericin preparations are less nephrotoxic, are preferred, and could be substituted.

Hypokalemia, hypomagnesemia, and hypocalcemia corrected with supplemental potassium, magnesium, and calcium.

Normocytic normochromic anemia with average decrease of 9% in hematocrit.

Phlebitis and pain at infusion sites: add 1,200–1,600 units of heparin to infusate.

DRUG INTERACTIONS: Increased nephrotoxicity with concurrent use of nephrotoxic drugs: aminoglycosides, cisplatin, cyclosporine, possibly tenofovir, foscarnet, cidofovir, methoxyflurane, vancomycin; increased hypokalemia with corticosteroids and diuretics. Potential for digoxin toxicity secondary to hypokalemia.

PREGNANCY: Category B. Not teratogenic in animals or humans. Preferred over azoles in first trimester, if equally effective.

TABLE 6.13 Relative merits of Amphotericin B formulations

Preparation	Amphotericin. B[c]	Amphotec ABCD[c]	Abelcet (ABLC)[c]	AmBisome (LAmB)[c]
Dose	0.5–1.2 mg/ kg/d	3–4 mg/ kg/d	2.5–5 mg/ kg/d	3–6 mg/ kg/d
C_{max} (ug/mL)	0.5–2	3.1	1.7	83
Usual cost (AWP) [b]	$45/d	N/A	$840/d	$728/d
Adverse reactions[a]			18%	
Chills	30%	53%	15–20%	18%
Fever >38⁵°C	16%	27%	10–20%	7%
Creatinine >2× base	30–50%	10–25%	15–20%	19%

From CID 2003;37:415; NEJM 1999;340:764; CID 2002;35:359.

[a] Comparison of ADR is based on AmBisome vs. Ampho, Amphotec vs. Ampho.

[b] AWP based on 0.7 mg/kg for Amphotericin; 5 mg/kg for lipid amphotericin.

[c] AmBisome is recommended for cryptococcal meningitis.

Alternative preparations: (CID 2009;49:1721; CID 2003;37:415; Medicine 2010;89:236; CID 2001;32:686; CID 2005;41:1448; CID 2010;50:291).

Amprenavir (APV)—see Fosamprenavir

Amprenavir is no longer available.

Ancobon—see Flucytosine

Androgel—see Testosterone

Atazanavir (ATV)

TRADE NAME: Reyataz (Bristol-Myers Squibb); Evotaz (ATV co-formulation with COBI).

CLASS: Azapeptide protease inhibitor (CID 2004;38:1599).

FORMULATIONS, REGIMEN, AND COST:

Forms: ATV caps, 100, 150, 200, and 300 mg; ATV 300 mg coformulation with cobicistat 150 mg (Evotaz).

Regimen: ATV 400 mg/d (PI-naïve only); ATV/r 300/100 mg/ d (preferred). Must use ATV/r 300/100 mg (boosted) with TDF. ATV/r 400/100 mg with EFV. ATV/r 400/100 mg with TDF + H2 blockers.

ATV/COBI 300/150 mg/d.

AWP cost per month: ATV/r 300/100 mg: $1,739.50/mo (plus RTV cost); ATV 400 mg/d: $1,755.91/mo.

ATV/COBI (Evotaz): 300/150 mg tab: $1,926.56/mo.

Food: Take with a meal.

Interactions: Requires gastric acidity; avoid proton-pump inhibitors (omeprazole, etc). Dosing separation required with antacids, H2 blockers, etc.; see warnings.

Renal failure: Standard doses except in patients on hemodialysis, who should receive only boosted ATV since levels are significantly lower (Agarwala S. 8th Internat Clin Pharm HIV Ther 2007; Abstr. 2). Avoid boosted-ATV in treatment-experienced patients with PI-resistant mutations undergoing HD.

Hepatic failure: With Child–Pugh score 7-9, dose is 300 mg/d (limited clinical data); avoid with Child-Pugh score >9.

Storage: Room temperature, 15–30°C.

PATIENT ASSISTANCE: 800-861-0048 (8 AM–5 PM CST, Mon.–Fri.).

WARNINGS: Avoid unboosted ATV with TDF, EFV, ETR, and NVP (JAC 2005;56:380); avoid buffered ddI (use ddI-EC). Caution with drugs that prolong QTC; with clarithromycin use half-dose clarithromycin, or alternative such as azithromycin.

Proton pump inhibitors (PPIs): Avoid if co-administration is needed. Give PPI (maximum dose omeprazole is 20 mg) 12 hr before ATV/r (PI treatment-naïve patients), or avoid PPI (treatment experienced patients) with ATV/r, and/or give ATV/r >10 hr after H2 blocker (HIV Med 2007;8:335).

H2 blockers: Take H2 blocker 2 hr after ATV/r.

Antacids: Give ATV/r 2 hr before, or ≥1 hr after.

Food requirement: Increases ATV AUC 70%.

Hepatitic disease: See dose modification below (Pharmacology).

ADVANTAGES: (1) Potency, especially with RTV or COBI boosting; (2) low pill burden among PIs and once-daily regimen; (3) negligible effect on insulin resistance and lipids, even with RTV boosting; (4) unique major resistance mutation (I50L) that does not cause PI cross-resistance, effects; (5) co-formulation with COBI.

DISADVANTAGES: (1) Higher rates of discontinuation due to jaundice and GI intolerance compared to DRV/r- and RAL-based regimen; (2) Indirect hyperbilirubinemia, medically inconsequential but may cause jaundice or scleral icterus (<5-7%); (3) drug interactions, see warnings; (4) requirement for a meal and gastric acid; and (5) need for RTV boosting when combined with TDF (or an NNRTI).

CLINICAL TRIALS:

TREATMENT-NAÏVE PATIENTS: *Switch studies: ATAZIP* trial consisted of 248 patients with viral suppression on LPV/r-based ART who were randomized to continue the same regimen or switched to ATV/r-based ART. Results at 48 wks showed higher rates of treatment failure with LPV/r (20% vs. 17%) (*P* = 0.002) and significant reductions in triglyceride and total cholesterol levels with ATV/r (JAIDS 2009;51:29).

Induction-maintenance: ACTG 5201 was a single-arm open label pilot study to determine efficacy of ATV/r monotherapy (300/100 mg/d) in patients who had achieved viral suppression to <50 c/mL for ≥48 wks on a regimen of PI-based ART (JAMA 2006;296:806). At 24 wks, 31/34 (91%) had a sustained virologic response. Resistance testing in the 3 patients with virologic failure showed no PI resistance mutations.

The *ARIES* trial randomized patients who had VL <50 c/mL on ATV/r + ABC/3TC to continued ATV/r (300/100 mg/d) or unboosted ATV (400 mg/d). At 84 wks (48 wks post randomization) the rates of continued viral suppression (VL <50 c/mL) were 181/220 (86%) in the unboosted ATV group and 169/209 (81%) in the ATV/r group. The overall rate of virologic failure was 2%, and there were no PI resistance mutations in those 8 patients. CD4 count increases and adverse reactions were similar in the two groups, but lipid profiles were better in the unboosted ATV group (AIDS 2010;24:2019).

ATV vs. ATV/r: BMS 089 compared ATV (400 mg) vs. ATV/r (300/ 100 mg/d in treatment-naïve patients. There was a clear pharmacologic advantage to boosting, though lipid levels were also higher. The study was underpowered to detect potential differences in virologic outcome (JAIDS 2008;47:161). The conclusion was that boosted ATV is preferred over unboosted ATV, and they are equivalent in terms of viral suppression and CD4 count recovery, but it also produced higher lipid changes and more jaundice. These changes were correlated with the sustained trough level achieved with RTV boosting.

CASTLE: ATV/r vs. LPV/r in treatment-naïve patients: This trial compared ATV/r (300/100 mg once-daily) vs. LPV/r (400/ 100 mg twice-daily) in 883 treatment-naïve patients (Lancet 2008;372:646). All patients also received TDF/FTC. Virologic suppression was comparable at 48 wks (78% vs. 76%), and ATV/ r performed better with respect to lipid changes, diarrhea, and quality of life (Lancet 2008;373:646). Efficacy was similar across baseline CD4 strata, but LPV/r performed numerically worse (63% vs. 78% w/baseline CD4 <50 cells/mm^3) (JAIDS 2010;53:323). Another analysis of CASTLE data concluded that ATV/r-based ART was more cost-effective than LPV/r-based ART (Scand J Infect Dis 2011;43:304).

ATV/r vs. EFV: ACTG 5202 was an open-label trial in which 1,400 participants were randomized to receive ATV/r vs. EFV, each combined with separately randomized TDF/FTC or ABC/3TC. Randomization was stratified by baseline VL less or greater than 100,000 c/mL. Participants with baseline VL >100,000 c/mL were unblinded after it was found that virologic suppression was greater in the TDF/FTC arm compared to the ABC/3TC arm (see Abacavir). Overall results at 96 wks showed similar rates of viral suppression to <200 c/mL between ATV/r and EFV arms: 83% vs. 85% respectively, and there was no significant difference when combining ATV/r with TDF/FTC (89%) vs. ABC/3TC (83%) (Ann Intern Med 2011;154:445). ATV/r was associated with less increase in LDL cholesterol and fewer major resistance mutations in failures: EFV 41/71 (65%) vs. ATV/r 12/83 (16%); the 12 resistance mutations included

11 184V mutations occurring in ATV/r-treated participants and one PI mutation (88N/S).

ACTG A5257: ATV/r vs. DRV/r or RAL: Randomized open-label trial, compared ATV/r (*n* = 605), DRV/r (*n* = 601), or RAL (*n* = 603), each given in combination with TDF/FTC. The groups were well matched at baseline with a median CD4 of 308 cells/mm^3 and VL 4.62 log/mL. At week 96, ATV/r, RAL, and DRV/r groups had similar virologic failure with 12.6%, 9%, and 14.9%, respectively. However, a significantly higher proportion of patients in the ATV/r arm discontinued treatment because of adverse events (jaundice, GI toxicities), with a 12.7% and 9.2% higher incidence of discontinuation compared to RAL and DRV/r, respectively.

NUC-SPARING REGIMEN: *ATV + RAL:* In the SPARTAN trial, patients receiving ART with virologic failure or intolerance were randomized to ATV 300 mg bid (unboosted) + RAL 400 bid (*N* = 63) vs. standard therapy with TDF/FTC + ATV/r (*n* = 31). Participants included were RAL-naïve and had no PI mutations and no proton pump inhibitor requirement. The study was stopped prematurely because of high rates of resistance among those failing therapy and high rates of jaundice. Results in 22 patients showed good pharmacologic data for both antivirals, but substantial individual variation in tolerance (Drug Monit 2010;32:782).

ATV + RAL + 3TC: A pharmacokinetic study of ATV + RAL + 3TC in 17 patients showed therapeutic levels of RAL, and virologic control was achieved with a regimen of ATV (600 mg) + RAL (800 mg) and 3TC or FTC (Jansen A. 2011 CROI;Abstr. 634).

Multiple HAART failures: BMS 045: Patients with ≥2 HAART failures with ≥1 PI, NRTI, or NNRTI were randomized to TDF/NRTI plus either LPV/r 400/100 mg bid, SQV/ATV 1200/400 mg/d, or ATV/r 300/100 mg/d with two NRTIs in each group. Results at 24 wks showed the SQV/ATV group did poorly, and these patients were given the option to change (AIDS 2006;20:711). Efficacy at 96 wks for the remaining two groups was similar, and patients taking ATV/r had less hyperlipidemia and grade 2–4 diarrhea than those on LPV/r (3% vs. 13%) with ATV/r.

TABLE 6.14 ATV clinical trials with treatment-naïve and in patients after virologic failure

Trial	Regimen	No	Dur (wks)	VL <50	VL <200–400
BMS 034:	ATV 400 mg/d + AZT/3TC	286	48	32%*	70%
Treatment-naïve	EFV + AZT/3TC	280		37%	64%
(JAIDS 2004;36:1011)					
BMS AI 424-008: Treatment-	ATV + AZT/3TC	181	48	33%	67%
naïve (Package label)	NFV + AZT/3TC	91		38%	59%
BMS AI 424-007: Treatment-	ATV + ddI + d4T	103	48	36%	64%
naïve (JAIDS 2003;32:18)	NFV + ddI + d4T	103		39%	56%
CASTLE:	ATV/r (300/100 mg/d) + TDF/FTC	440	96	74%‡	—
Treatment-naïve	LPV/r (400/100 mg bid)	443		68%	—
(Lancet 2008;372:646;	+ TDF/FTC				
JAIDS 2010;53:323)					
BMS 089: Treatment-naïve	ATV + d4T + 3TC	105	96	55%	70%
(JAIDS 2008;47:161)	ATV/r + d4T + 3TC	95		65%	75%
ALERT:	ATV/r + TDF/FTC	53	48	75%	79%
Treatment-naïve (AIDS Res Ther	FPV/r 1400/100 mg	53		83%	87%
2008;5:5)	+ TDF/FTC				

(continued)

TABLE 6.14 Continued

Trial	Regimen	No	Dur (wks)	VL <50	VL <200–400
BMS 043: Failed one PI regimen (CID 2004;38:1599)	ATV 400 mg/d + 2 NRTIs	144	24	59%	—
	LPV/r + 2 NRTIs	146		77%‡	—
BMS 045:† Failed ≥2 HAART regimens containing ≥1 PI (AIDS 2006;20:711)	ATV/r 300/100 mg/d + 2 NRTIs	120	96‡	56%	—
	LPV/r + 2 NRTIs	123		58%	—
	SQV/ATV 1200/400 mg/d + 2 NRTIs	115		38%‡	—
AI 424-009: Failed therapy (AIDS 2003;17:1339)	SQV/ATV 1200/400 mg/d + 2 NRTIs	34	48	—	41%
	SQV/ATV 600/1200 mg/d + 2 NRTIs	28		—	29%
	SQV/r 400/400 mg bid + 2 NRTIs	23		—	35%

	N	Wk		
ARIES: ATV vs. ATV/r after 36 wks on ATV/r (AIDS 2010;24:2019)				
ATV/r 300/100 qd + ABC/3TC	209	48	81%	86%
ATV 400 qd + ABC/3TC	210		86%	92%
ACTG 5202: (Ann Intern Med 2011;154:445)				
ATV/r + TDF/FTC or	702	96	—	90%
ATV/r + ABC/3TC				85%
EFV + TDF/FTC or	698		—	91%
EFV + ABC/3TC				91%
ACTG 5257: (Ann Intern Med 2014;161:461)				
ATV/r + TDF/FTC	605	96	87.4%	—
RAL + TDF/FTC	603		91%	—
DRV/r + TDF/FTC	601		85.1%	—

[a] Low frequency of VL <50 c/mL is attributed to use of inappropriate collection tube for VL testing (J Clin Virol 2006;35:420).

[b] Results for >1 $\log_{10}$ c/mL decrease or <400 c/mL.

[c] The SQV/ATV group did poorly and this arm was stopped.

TABLE 6.15 BMS 089-ATV vs. ATV/r

	ATV n = 94	ATV/r n = 103
Outcome at 48 wks		
VL <50/mL	70%	75%
CD4 count (median increase)	+ 189	+ 224
Pharmacokinetic substudy		
C trough (geometric mean ng/mL)	127	670
Inhibitory quotient	9	53
Lipid changes		
Total cholesterol (mg/dL)	+ 8%	+ 16%
Triglycerides (mg/dL)	+ 10%	+ 45%

From JAIDS 2008;47:161.

RESISTANCE: ATV/r selects for 13 mutations: *10F/I/V, 16E, 33F/I/V, 46I/L*, 54L/V/M/T, *I50L, 60E,* 62V, 71I/T/L, 82A/T, *84V, 85V,* 90M, and 93L. The mutations in italics are used in the ATV score. Virologic response with boosted ATV-based ART was noted in 100% of patients with 0 or 1 of these mutations, 80% of those with 2, 42% with 3, and none with ≥4 mutations (AIDS 2006;20:35). Another scoring system consists of 16E, 32I, 20I/M/R/T/V, 53L/Y, 64L/M/V, 71I/T/V, 85V, and 93L/M. One, two, or three mutations were associated with response rates of 67%, 6%, and 0%, respectively. The IAS-USA resistance profiles (2017) lists just three major ATV resistance mutations: 50L, 84V, and 88S with the notation that "often numerous mutations are necessary to substantially impact virologic response" (Top HIV Med 2015;23:132). The signature mutation is I50L in treatment-naïve patients treated with unboosted ATV, which does not cause cross-resistance with other PIs, including FPV, which has the signature mutation I50V. The I50L mutation reduces ATV activity by a median of 10-fold, reduces replication capacity to 0.3–42%, and increases susceptibility to other PIs (AAC 2005;49:3825), although the clinical significance of this is unknown. Among 78 virologic failures in clinical trials, 23 had both phenotypic resistance and the I50L mutation (JID 2004;189:1802). The

TABLE 6.16 CASTLE Trial: ATV/r vs. LPV/r in treatment-naïve patients 96-wk results

	ATV/r n = 440	LPV/r n = 443
VL <50 c/mL	74%	68%
Baseline CD4 <50/mm³	78%	58%[a]
Baseline VL >100,000 c/mL	74%	66%
CD4 count (median)[b]	+ 219	+ 219
Lipids (% increase)		
Cholesterol	+ 16%	+ 29%
LDL cholesterol	+ 32%	+ 40%
Triglyceride	+ 23%	+ 49%
Discontinued for adverse reaction	3%	5%
Resistance mutations with failure. Major PI	1/28	0/29
M184V	5	7

From JAIDS 2010;53:323.

[a] $P = <0.05$.

[b] 48-wk data.

I50L mutation is often associated with 71V, which increases susceptibility to other PIs in vitro (AAC 2005;49:3825).

PHARMACOLOGY:

Absorption: Requires food and gastric acid for optimal absorption, which is highly variable. Food increases AUC 70%. ATV trough levels >150 ng/mL correlate with virologic response (AIDS Patient Care STDS 2008;22:7). RTV boosting (300/100 mg) increases ATV AUC 3- to 4-fold and C_{min} by 10-fold (Clin Pharmacokin 2005;44:1035).

Distribution: Protein-binding 86%, CSF/plasma levels ratio is 0.002–0.02. Penetration into seminal fluid is poor, with a seminal/blood plasma ratio of 0.1 (AAC 2007;51:335). Ranks class 2 in the four-class scoring system for CNS penetration (Neurology 2011;76:693).

Serum half-life: 7 hrs.

Elimination: Inhibitor and substrate for cytochrome P450 3A4 and inhibitor of glucuronidation. Metabolized by the liver, and metabolites are excreted by the biliary tract; only 13% of unmetabolized drug is excreted in urine.

SIDE EFFECTS: Generally well-tolerated, but when compared to RAL and DRV/r resulted in a higher rate of tolerability discontinuation (12.7% and 9.2%, respectively).

Common: Reversible increase in indirect bilirubinemia due to UGT 1A1 inhibition in 22–47%; this is medically inconsequential but may cause jaundice (reported in 7%). The levels of unconjugated bilirubin correlate with ATV trough levels (HIV Clin Trials 2008;9:213). An increase in bilirubin of ≥0.3 serves as a surrogate marker for ATV adherence (AIDS 2005;19:1700). ATV/r appears safe in patients with advanced liver disease (AIDS 2011;25:1006). Nevertheless, there is a strong association between the genetic variants of ATV metabolism and ATV/r discontinuation (CID 2011;203:246). Analysis of CASTLE data at 96 wks found significantly more women than men discontinued ATV/r (22% vs. 15%) (JAC 2011;66:383).

Occasional: GI intolerance with nausea, vomiting, abdominal pain (one the reason for ATV/r discontinuation in ACTG A5257); rash (reported in 1–6%, and occasionally severe) (Can J Infect Dis Med Microbiol 2009;20:e10); increase in transaminase levels.

Prolongation of QTc and PR interval, including asymptomatic first-degree AV block. Studies with ATV/r 300/100 mg/d showed slight, but not significant increases in PR interval averaging 3 msec and no change at 1 mo (HIV Med 2006;7:317). PR interval monitoring should be performed in patients with conduction defects or with concurrent use with other drugs that alter cardiac conduction (e.g., verapamil, saquinavir, clarithromycin, diltiazem; use half dose of clarithromycin and diltiazem with slow titration or consider as alternative azithromycin).

Metabolic complications and lipodystrophy: ATV and, to a lesser extent ATV/r, appear to be "heart friendly" based on: (1) little or no effect on lipid levels (AIDS 2006;20:711; JAIDS 2005;39:174); (2) minimal or no effect on insulin resistance (AIDS 2006;20:1813);

(3) not associated with increased levels of biomarkers of CVD (AIDS 2010;24:2657); and (4) an observational study showing decrease in carotid intima-media thickness in patients on ATV/r (AIDS 2010;24:2797). ACTG 5224 compared rates of visceral fat accumulation in ACTG 5202 participants (McComsey C. 2011 CROI:Abstr. 77). ATV/r was associated with significantly more trunk fat than EFV.

ATV-associated renal disease—Urolithiasis: ATV occasionally causes urolithiasis that is presumably due to precipitation of the drug resulting in crystalluria in a fashion analogous to indinavir (NEJM 2006;355:2158; AIDS 2006;20:2131; AIDS 2007;12:1060; AIDS 2007;21:1215;CID 2007;45:e105). About 7% of ATV is excreted in the kidney, and ATV is poorly soluble. Spectrophotometry analysis of the stones shows crystals of ATV and no metabolites. The stones are yellow, friable, and radiolucent. The frequency in one report was 11/1134 patients or 1/100 patients; continued use of ATV in 6 patients with symptomatic stones was complicated by a recurrence in only one (CID 2007;45:e105). A EuroSIDA review of 6,843 HIV-infected patients for evidence of renal disease showed the risk of decrease in baseline CrCL >25% with ATV-based ART was an incidence risk ratio of 1.2/yrs (p <0.0003) (AIDS 2010;24:1667) after adjustment of factor associated with chronic kidney disease (CKD). This risk actually exceeded the rate of CKD associated with TDF use (incidence risk ratio 1.16/yr) (AIDS 2010;24:1667).

Interstitial nephritis with acute renal failure has been reported (Am J Kidney Dis 2004;44:e81; Virchows Arch 2007;450:665; Antivir Ther 2011;16:119). A review from EuroSIDA based on sequential data for 6,842 patients found 225 receiving ATV/r (3.3%) progressed to chronic renal disease for a relative risk of 1.21 (95% CI, 1.09–1.34; p = 0.0003) (AIDS 2010;24:1667).

BLACK BOX WARNINGS: None.

DRUG INTERACTIONS:

Avoid concurrent use with ATV/r: Astemizole, alfuzosin, bepridil, cisapride, ergotamine derivative, dexamethasone (at steady-state), dofetilide, eplerenone, flibanserin, fluticasone, indinavir, quinidine, irinotecan, ivabradine, lovastatin, midazolam, nevirapine, pimozide, proton pump inhibitors, propafenone, flecainide, amiodarone, rifampin, rifapentine, salmeterol, sildenafil (high dose for pulmonary hypertension), simvastatin, triazolam, ranolazine, terfenadine, silodosin, enzalutamide, mitotane, dospirenone (with ATV/c), and St. John's wort. Rivaroxaban, betrixaban, ticagrelor, vorapaxar (may increase oral anticoagulation, avoid.)

Dose adjustment needed with edoxaban, apixiban, and dabigatran based on renal function and indication. contraindicated with oral midazolam, but IV may be used with close monitoring.

Dose modification: ATV standard unless specified.

Rifabutin: 150 mg q24 or 300 mg 3×/wk. Consider rifabutin TDM.

Clarithromycin: ↑ clarithromycin AUC 94% and may cause QTc prolongation; use half dose clarithromycin or use azithromycin.

Oral contraceptive: Estradiol AUC ↑48% and norethindrone AUC ↑110%; consider alternative contraception with ATV (do not exceed 30 µg) or ATV/r (use at least 35 µg).

Statins: Rosuvastatin AUC ↑213%. Start with 5 mg. Pitavastatin, pravastatin or atorvastatin preferred. *Anticonvulsants*: carbamazepine, phenobarbital and phenytoin may ↓ levels of ATV substantially; avoid ATV/c and unboosted ATV; avoid or use ATV/r with caution. Consider valproic acid, or levetiracetam.

Sildenafil: Maximum of 25 mg q48h.

Vardenafil: No data; use ≤2.5 mg/24 hrs, and ≤2.5 mg/72 hrs with ATV/r.

Voriconazole has not been studied, but it is anticipated that co-administration with ATV/r may increase ATV levels and decrease voriconazole levels; avoid if possible (consider voriconazole TDM with co-administration).

Atovaquone/Proguanil: ATV/r ↓atovaquone AUC 46%; ↓proguanil 41%. Consider alternative malaria prophylaxis.

Diltiazem: ↑AUC 125%; use half dose, and monitor EKG.

Calcium channel blocker: Monitor EKG.

TABLE 6.17 Dose adjustments for ATV/r with other antiretrovirals

Drug	Effect on Co-administered Drug (AUC)	Effect on ATV (AUC)	Recommendation
ddI EC	↓ 34%	No change	ddI EC—must take on empty stomach and ATV with meal. Standard doses
TDF	↑ 37% (w/ ATV/r) ↑ 24% (w/ ATV)	↓ 25%	Use ATV/r 300/100 qd + TDF 300 mg/d
EFV	No change	↓ 74%	Use ATV/r 400/100 mg/d with food + EFV 600 mg/d. Avoid co-administration in PI-experienced patient
NVP	↑ C_{min} 46%	↓ C_{min} 41%	Avoid co-administration due to potential NVP toxicity
ETR	↑ 30–50%	↓ 14%	Avoid; clinical significance unclear
MVC	↑ 3.6×	-----	Use MVC 150 mg bid + ATV or ATV/r standard dose
DRV	No change	No change	ATV 300 qd + DRV/r standard dose
FPV	↑ 78%	↓ 33%	Insufficient data
LPV/r	No change	↑ 45%	LPV/r 400/100 bid + ATV 300 qd
SQV	↑ 449%	Not measured	Insufficient data; poor clinical response
IDV	---	---	Avoid; hyperbilirubinemia
RAL	↑ 41–72%	---	Use standard dose RAL + ATV/r 300/100 mg/d
TPV/r	↑ 11%	↓ 39%	Avoid
EVG	No change	--↓ 11%	EVG 85 mg/d + ATV/r 300/100 mg/d
DTG	↑62% (w ATV/r) ↑91% (w ATV)	No change	DTG 50 mg + ATV/r 300/100 mg/d or ATV 400 mg/d
BIC	↑310%	No data	BIC concentrations may be increased. Dose not established

H2 receptor antagonists (e.g., ranitidine, famotidine, cimetidine): Separate doses by as much time as possible, preferably; give ATV 2 hr before or 10 hr after H2 blockers.

Posaconazole: ATV AUC ↑ 2.5-fold. Posaconazole AUC ↑3.7-fold. Monitor for potential ↑adverse drug reaction.

Antacids and buffered medications: Give ATV 2 hr before or >1 hr after antacid. *Proton pump inhibitors* such as omeprazole should be avoided. Co-administration of 40 mg omeprazole with ATV/r 300/100 mg resulted in a 75% reduction in ATV AUC. This restriction applies to all PPIs. If PPI needed, *omeprazole* 20 mg (max dose) should be separated by 12 hrs, ATV (ATV/r 300/100) AUC decreased by 42%. Manufacturer states that it may be considered in PI-naïve patients, but it is best to avoid. This admonition does not apply to other PIs, except NFV.

Methadone: No interaction with unboosted ATV. With ATV/r, monitor for withdrawal.

Buprenorphine: AUC ↑93% and 66% with ATV and ATV/r, respectively. ATV may ↓ if unboosted. Use ATV/r with buprenorphine. Monitor for sedation.

Paclitaxel, Repaglinide: May be increased with ATV. Use with close monitoring.

Bosentan: Avoid with unboosted ATV. With ATV/r ↓ bosentan to 62.5 mg/d or qod after ATV/r has reach a steady state (>10 days).

PREGNANCY: Category B: The pharmacokinetics of ATV/r with standard dosing (300/100 mg/d) was reported in four studies: One showed the ATV AUC was not altered by pregnancy (AIDS 2007;21:2409), and three studies showed significant pregnancy-associated decreases of about 25% (Eley, 15th CROI, 2008; Mirochnick M. 16th CROI, 2009; Mirochnick M. JAIDS 2012; Epub Ahead: PMID21283017). Concurrent use of TDF is an important variable due to the effect of this agent on ATV levels. Perhaps the most relevant report is IMPAACT10426, designed to measure pharmacokinetics of ART agents in pregnancy. The authors of this report recommend a dose adjustment of ATV/r to 400/100 mg for pregnant women (Mirochnick M. JAIDS 2012;Epub Ahead: PMID 21283017). The dose adjustment becomes more critical in ART-experienced pregnant patients if ATV/r is combined with TDF. It is not known whether the increase in bilirubin levels noted with ATV will increase rates of hyperbilirubinemia in the neonate to clinically important levels. Transplacental passage is low (10–16%), and this has not been seen in clinical trials. The FDA approved ATV/r for use in pregnant women based on a trial of 41 HIV-infected pregnant women given ATV/r (300/100, or 400/100 mg/d in combination with AZT/3TC). The approval was supported by pharmacology data showing adequate levels in the second and third trimesters. The 2018 DHHS Guidelines for Antiretroviral Drugs in Pregnant Women recommend ATV/r as a preferred PI when combined with ABC/3TC orTDF/FTC. Use of unboosted ATV is not recommended in pregnancy. With TDF or H2 blocker co-administration, the recommended dose is ATV/r 400/100 mg/d in the second and third trimesters. Although PHACS analysis of atazanavir first trimester exposure (n = 222) found an association of skin and musculoskeletal birth defects (adjusted OR 1.93), the Antiretroviral Pregnancy Registry did not find an association with 1,235 births after first-trimester exposure (reports through July 31, 2017).

Atorvastatin

TRADE NAME: Lipitor (Pfizer and generic manufacturers).

CLASS: Statin (HMG-CoA reductase inhibitor).

FORMULATIONS, REGIMEN, AND COST: Tabs: 10 mg at $3.85, 20 mg at $5.50, 40 mg at $5.50, and 80 mg at $5.77.

> INDICATIONS AND DOSES: Elevated total and LDL cholesterol and/or triglycerides. Recommended statin for hyperlipidemia with PI-based ART by IAS-USA (JAIDS 2002;31:257) and HIVMA/ACTG (CID 2003;37:613). Atorvastatin use in a

double-blind study in HIV infected patients reduced markers of immune activation (JID 2011;203:756). A review of statin use and efficacy by HIV-infected patients also showed the favored agents in terms of use and efficacy in achieving NCEP goal were atorvastatin and rosuvastatin (CID 2011;52:387). With atorvastatin, the initial dose is 10 mg/d with increases at 2–4 wk intervals to maintenance doses of 10–80 mg/d (or 10–40 mg/d for patients on PIs due to drug interactions). Target dose should be based on recommended intensity of statin therapy (Stone NJ et al., Circulation 2014;129:S1–S45). Should be taken with or without food, preferably in the evening.

MONITORING: Blood lipids at ≤4-wk intervals until desired results are achieved, then periodically. Obtain transaminase levels at baseline, at 12 wks, and then at 6-mo intervals. Patients should be warned to report muscle pain, tenderness, or weakness promptly, especially if accompanied by fever or malaise. Obtain CPK for suspected myopathy.

PRECAUTIONS: Atorvastatin (and other statins) are contraindicated with pregnancy, breastfeeding, concurrent conditions that predispose to renal failure (e.g., sepsis, hypotension) and active hepatic disease. Alcoholism is a relative contraindication.

PHARMACOLOGY:

Bioavailability: 14%.

$T^{1/2}$: 14 hr.

Elimination: Fecal (biliary and unabsorbed), 98%; renal, <2%.

Renal failure: No dose adjustment.

Hepatic failure: Concentrations of atorvastatin are markedly elevated.

SIDE EFFECTS:

Musculoskeletal: Myopathy with elevated CPK plus muscle pain, weakness or tenderness, ± fever and malaise. Rhabdomyolysis with renal failure reported.

Hepatic: Use with caution. Elevated transaminases in 1–2%; discontinue if ALT and/or AST shows unexplained increase >3× upper limit of normal (ULN) × 2.

Miscellaneous: Diarrhea, constipation, nausea, heartburn, stomach pain, dizziness, headache, skin rash, impotence (rare), insomnia.

DRUG INTERACTIONS:

PI/r, PI/c, NNRTI: Potential for large increase in statin AUC with most PIs: Increase with NFV, 74%; LPV/r, 5.8×; SQV/r, 4.5×; TPV/r, 9×; FPV, 1.3×; DRV/r, 4×. Avoid with TPV/r; with other PI/r, PI/c, EVG/c start with 10 mg/d, and monitor clinically for myopathy or consider pitavastatin or pravastatin; avoid atorvastatin doses >40 mg/d with PIs. EFV decreases atorvastatin AUC 43%. ETR decreases atorvastatin AUC 37%. NVP: no data, but may decrease atorvastatin concentrations.

Others: Grapefruit juice increases atorvastatin levels up to 24%; avoid large amounts before or after administration.

Erythromycin: Atorvastatin levels increased by 40%.

Antacids: Atorvastatin levels decreased by 35%.

Other interactions with increased risk of myopathy: Azoles (ketoconazole, itraconazole), cyclosporine, fibric acid derivatives, niacin, macrolide antibiotics, nefazodone.

Niacin and gemfibrozil: Increased risk of myopathy; rhabdomyolysis reported only with lovastatin + niacin, but could occur with other statins.

PREGNANCY: Category X: contraindicated.

Atovaquone

TRADE NAME: Mepron (GlaxoSmithKline and generic manufacturer).

FORMULATIONS, REGIMEN, AND COST: 750 mg/5 mL: $1,378 per 210-mL bottle (21-days).

PATIENT ASSISTANCE PROGRAM: 866-728-4368.

INDICATIONS AND DOSE: PCP: Oral treatment of mild to moderate PCP (A-a O_2 gradient <45 mm Hg and P_AO_2 >60 mm Hg; less effective than TMP/SMX) and PCP prophylaxis in patients who are intolerant of TMP-SMX and dapsone; toxoplasmosis treatment (third-line) and prophylaxis (third-line). EFV, LPV/r, ATV/r decreases atovaquone by 75%, 74%, and 46%, respectively. Consider alternative ARVs.

PCP treatment: 750 mg (5 mL) twice-daily with fatty meals × 21 days.

PCP prophylaxis: 1,500 mg/d or 750 mg bid with fatty meals.

Toxoplasmosis treatment (alternative): 1,500 mg po bid with meals combined with either pyrimethamine 200 mg × 1, then 50 mg (<60 kg) or 75 mg (>60 kg) qd or sulfadiazine 1 g (<60 kg) or 1.5 g (>60 kg) qid. With atovaquone monotherapy, efficacy associated with serum concentration >18.5 µg/mL. Since measurement is not routinely available, the authors do not recommend monotherapy for CNS toxoplasmosis.

PHARMACOLOGY:

Bioavailability: Absorption of suspension averages 47% in fed state (with meals). Concurrent administration of fatty food increases absorption by 2-fold. There is significant individual variation in absorption. Administration with fatty food needs emphasis.

$T^{1/2}$: 2.2–2.9 days.

Elimination: Enterohepatic circulation with fecal elimination; <1% in urine.

CSF/plasma ratio: <1%.

Effect of hepatic or renal disease: No data.

SIDE EFFECTS: Rash (20%), GI intolerance (20%), diarrhea (20%). Possibly related headache, fever, insomnia. Life-threatening side effects: None. Percent requiring discontinuation due to side effects: 7–.9% (rash, 4%).

DRUG INTERACTIONS:

Rifampin: ↓ atovaquone by 54%, ↑ rifampin by 30%; avoid co- administration.

Tetracycline: ↓ atovaquone by 40%. Avoid or use with caution.

AZT: AUC increased 31% due to atovaquone inhibition of AZT gluconuridation (clinical significance unknown).

Atovaquone: AUC is reduced by 75% with concurrent EFV and LPV/r, and by 50% with ATV/r (AIDS 2010;24:1223). Levels of proguanil (relevant for the use of atovaquone/proguanil for malaria) were reduced by 38–43%. Consider as an alternative to EFV, LPV/r, and ATV/r. Interaction unlikely with BIC, DTG and RAL.

Warfarin: Possible increase in INR (Ann Pharmacother 2011;45:e3).

PREGNANCY: Category C. Not teratogenic in animals; limited experience in humans.

Atripla—see Efavirenz, Emtricitabine, and Tenofovir

Azithromycin

TRADE NAME: Zithromax (Pfizer and generic manufacturers).

CLASS: Macrolide antibiotic.

FORMULATIONS, REGIMEN, AND COST: Tabs: 250 mg tab at $7.78; 600 mg at $18.68; 1 g packet at $29.13. Z-Pak (generic) with 6 tabs (500 mg, then 250 mg/d × 4 days) at $46.70 (generic); Zmax (single-dose therapy), 2 g/60 mL at $160.21; Tri-Pak with 3 tabs (500 mg × 3 days) for exacerbations of bronchitis at $46.70; IV formulation as 500 mg vial at $7.20, suspension 200 mg/5 mL (22.5 mL) or 100 mg/5mL (15mL) at $34.88. 1% ophthalmic solution (2.5 mL) at $149.61.

ACTIVITY: *S. pneumoniae* (about 20–30% of *S. pneumoniae* strains are resistant to azithromycin and other macrolides in the United States), streptococci (not *Enterococcus*), erythromycin-sensitive *S. aureus, H. influenzae, Legionella, C. pneumoniae, M. pneumoniae, C. trachomatis, M. avium* complex (MAC), *N. gonorrhoeae* (2 g dose, but generally not recommended due to increased resistance); *T. pallidum* (resistance increasing), and *T. gondii* are generally sensitive. There is concern about increasing macrolide resistance by *S. pneumoniae* (AAC 2002;297:1016; JID 2000;182:1417; AAC 2002;46:265; AAC 2001;45:2147). However, multiple clinical trials show that in vivo activity with pneumococcal pneumonia is much better than in vitro results. For *MAC bacteremia*, one study found that azithromycin 600 mg/d was equivalent to clarithromycin 500 mg bid (CID 2000;31:1245) when used in combination with ethambutol. The VA trial found clarithromycin to be superior (CID 2000;31;1245). For *syphilis*, preliminary studies in patients without HIV infection showed that azithromycin (2 g po × (1) was equivalent to benzathine penicillin (2.4 mil units IM × (1) for treatment of early syphilis (NEJM 2005;353:1236). Studies have shown an explosive rise in *T. pallidum* resistance to azithromycin in San Francisco, from 0% to 56% in 2004 (CID 2006;42:337). *N. gonorrhoeae* has developed resistance to multiple antibiotics making cephalosporins the only recommended class in the US 2015 CDC Guidelines (www.cdc.gov/std/tg2015/). For pharyngeal GC the recommendation is ceftriaxone 250 mg IM plus azithromycin 1 g po × 1 (or alternatively doxycycline 100 mg bid × 7d). Test of cure recommended for pharyngeal GC.

PHARMACOLOGY:

Bioavailability: Absorption is ~30–40%. The 600 mg tabs and the 1 g powder packet may be taken without regard to food, but food improves tolerability.

$T^{1/2}$: 68 hrs; detectable levels in urine at 7–14 days; with the 1,200 mg weekly dose, the azithromycin levels in peripheral leukocytes remain above 32 µg/mL for 60 hrs.

Distribution: High tissue levels; low CSF levels (<0.01 µg/mL).

Excretion: Primarily biliary; 6% in urine.

Dose modification in renal or hepatic failure: Use with caution.

SIDE EFFECTS: GI intolerance (nausea, vomiting, pain); diarrhea: 14%. With 1,200 mg weekly dose, major side effects are diarrhea, abdominal pain, and/or nausea in 10–15%; reversible dose-dependent hearing loss is reported in 5% at mean day of

TABLE 6.18 Azithromycin regimens by condition

Indication	Dose[b]
M. avium complex (MAC) prophylaxis[a]	1,200 mg po per week or 600 mg po twice weekly (2018 IDSA/NIH/CDC Guidelines for Treatment and Prevention of Opportunistic Infections)
MAC treatment[a]	500–600 mg po qd + EMB ± rifabutin (2018 IDSA/NIH/CDC OI Guidelines; Alternative)
Pneumonia[a]	500 mg IV qd × ≥2 days (hospitalized patients), then 500 mg po qd × 7 to 10 days; outpatient: 1.5–2 g po over 1, 3 or 5 days
Sinusitis[a]	500 mg po × 1, then 250 mg po qd × 4 (Z-pak) or 500 mg po qd × 3 days (Tri-pak)
C. trachomatis[a] (nongonococcal urethritis or cervicitis)	1 g po × 1 or doxycycline 100 mg po bid × 7 days
Gonococcal urethritis or cervicitis	Ceftriaxone 250 mg IM ×1 + azithromycin 1 g po (2015 CDC Guidelines for STDs)
Toxoplasmosis	900–1200 mg po qd + pyrimethamine 200 mg po ×1, then 50–75 mg/d + leucovorin 10–20 mg/d × ≥ 6 wks then maintenance treatment with half dose of each

[a] FDA-approved indications.

[b] Caps must be taken ≥1 hr before or >2 hrs after a meal; food improves absorption and tolerance of tabs and powder.

onset at 96 days and mean exposure of 59,000 mg (package insert). Frequency of discontinuation in AIDS patients receiving high doses: 6%, primarily GI intolerance and reversible ototoxicity: 2%; rare: erythema multiforme, increased transaminases.

CONTRAINDICATIONS: Hypersensitivity to erythromycin.

DRUG INTERACTIONS: Preferred macrolide for PI, COBI, and NNRTI co- administration because it avoids the drug interactions of clarithromycin.

Azithromycin increases levels of *theophylline* and *Coumadin*. Concurrent use with antiretroviral agents, rifampin, and rifabutin is safe. Concurrent use with pimozide may cause fatal arrhythmias, and must be avoided.

PREGNANCY: Category B (safe in animal studies; no data in humans). Preferred macrolide for MAC prophylaxis and treatment in pregnancy.

Azoles

AZT—see Zidovudine

Bactrim—see Trimethoprim-Sulfamethoxazole

Bedaquiline

TRADE NAME: Sirturo (Janssen Therapeutics).

FORMULATIONS, REGIME, AND COST: 100 mg tablet/$ 191.49 per 100 mg tablet.

Indicated for the treatment of pulmonary MDR TB in combination with other active antimycobacterial agents. Bedaquiline should not be used for the treatment of latent TB, extra-pulmonary TB, or drug-sensitive TB.

Dosing Recommendations: 400 mg once-daily × 2 wks, then 200 mg 3×/wk for 22 wks. Take with food. Do not crush tablet. Avoid ETOH.

Hepatic impairment dosing: Mild to moderate haptic impairment: Usual dose. With Child-Pugh B, 20% decrease in bedaquiline and metabolite. Severe hepatic impairment: no data; use with close monitoring.

Renal impairment dosing: 10–50 mL/min: Usual dose likely <10 mL/min: No data. Use with caution; usual dose likely PD; HD; CVVHD: no data. Unlikely to be removed due to high protein binding.

PHARMACOLOGY: Bedaquiline is a diarylquinoline that inhibits mycobacterial ATP synthase.

Pharmacokinetic absorption: Bioavailability increased by 2-fold with standard meal (558 kcal; 22 g fat).

High protein binding: >99.9%.

Large volume of distribution: Vd = 164 L.

Metabolized via CYP3A4 into active metabolite (*N*-monodesmethyl metabolite is 4–6 times less active than bedaquiline). Excreted in feces with <0.001% excreted in urine.

Terminal $T^{1/2}$ of bedaquiline and metabolite is 5.5 mos.

SIDE EFFECTS: Common: nausea, arthralgia, and headache (>10%).

QTc Prolongation: Compared to placebo, Mean QTc prolongation 9.9 ms vs. 3.5 ms (placebo) at week 1 and 15.7 ms vs. 6.2 ms (placebo) at week 18. Discontinue bedaquiline if QTc >500 ms develops. Obtain EKG at baseline, 2, 12, and 24 wks after starting bedaquiline. Monitor closely in patients with risk factor for QTc prolongation (e.g., history of torsade de pointes, congenital long QT syndrome, hypothyroidism, bradyarrhythmias, uncompensated heart failure).

If potassium, calcium, or magnesium is low, it should be corrected before starting bedaquiline.

Hepatitis: More hepatic-related adverse drug reactions reported with bedaquiline-treated patients (8.9 vs. 1.2%). Monitor liver function tests (LFTs) at baseline, then monthly while on therapy. If LFTs >3× ULN, it should be repeated in 48 hrs. Discontinue bedaquiline if AST/ALT >8× ULN, AST/ALT elevation with >2× ULN total bilirubin elevation, or if AST/ALT elevation remains persistently elevated past 2 wks.

Occasional ADR: Compared to placebo, amylase elevation (2.5% vs. 1.2%); chest pain (11.4 vs. 7.4%%); anorexia (8.9 vs. 3.7%); rash (7.6% vs. 3.7%).

PREGNANCY: Pregnancy category B. No data human data. Not teratogenic in animal studies at 2-fold humans exposure. *Breast feeding*: No human data. In animal studies, bedaquiline concentrations were 6- to 12-fold higher in breast milk compared to plasma concentrations.

DRUG INTERACTIONS: Bedaquiline is metabolized by CYP3A4. In vitro bedaquiline does not inhibit or induce CYP 1A2, 2C9, 2C19, and 3A4. Bedaquiline does not inhibit CYP 2A6, 2D6, 2E1.

Ketoconazole: Bedaquiline AUC increased 22%. Co-administration for more than 14 days should be avoided unless the benefit outweighs the risk.

LPV/r: Bedaquiline AUC increased 22%. No significant effect on bedaquiline Cmax. Other HIV protease inhibitor and COBI may also increase bedaquiline concentrations. Monitor QTc with co-administration.

Rifampin: Bedaquiline AUC decreased by 52%. Avoid co-administration.

Rifapentine: No data. Significant reduction in bedaquiline likely. Avoid.

Rifabutin: No data. Bedaquiline concentrations may be decreased. Monitor closely with co-administration.

CYP3A4 inducer (e.g., carbamazepine, phenobarbital, phenytoin): May decrease bedaquiline concentrations. Avoid

Isoniazid: No change in INH and bedaquiline concentrations. Use standard dose.

Pyrazinamide: No change in pyrazinamide and bedaquiline concentrations. Use standard dose.

Ethambutol: No significant change in ethambutol concentrations. Use standard dose.

Kanamycin: No significant change in kanamycin concentrations. Use standard dose.

Ofloxacin: No significant change in ofloxacin concentrations. Use standard dose.

Cycloserine: No significant change in cycloserine concentrations. Use standard dose.

Nevirapine: No change in bedaquiline concentrations. Use standard dose.

Efavirenz: No data. PK modeling suggest a 52% reduction in bedaquiline concentrations. May require higher bedaquiline with co-administration.

NRTI, BIC, DTG, RAL, MVC: interaction unlikely. Use standard dose.

Agents that prolong QTc (e.g., TCA, macrolides, fluoroquinolones, clofazimine, certain antiarrhythmics): Additive QTc prolongation possible; use with caution.

RESISTANCE: One of the mechanism of bedaquiline resistance is modification of atpE target gene. MIC breakpoint has not been established. Patients who failed to convert their sputum or relapsed had post-baseline isolates with 4 to >8-fold increases in MIC (corresponding to 0.24 to >0.48 µg/mL measured by agar method; odds ratio [OR] 0.015–1.0 µg/mL measured by REMA method).

In a 2-yr follow-up study of a randomized placebo-controlled trial, acquisition of resistance to companion antimycobacterial agents developed in 1 patient treated with bedaquiline and 5 patients treated with placebo (4.8% vs. 21.7%; $p = 0.18$) (Diacon AH et al., AAC 2012;56:3271).

CLINICAL TRIALS:

In an ongoing placebo-controlled study, patients with MDR-TB were randomized to bedaquiline (n = 79) or placebo (n = 81) plus 5 other antimycobacterial drugs (e.g., ethionamide, kanamycin, pyrazinamide, ofloxacin, cycloserine/terizidone, or available alternative). Median time to sputum at week 24 was 83 days for bedaquiline-treated patients vs. 125 days for placebo-treated patients. At week 24, treatment success was 77.6% and 57.6% in bedaquiline- and placebo-treated patients, respectively (p = 0.014). At week 72, there was trend toward a higher treatment success in bedaquiline-treated patients (70.1% vs. 56.1%; p = 0.092). There was an unexplained increased in mortality observed in bedaquiline-treated patients (11.4% 9/79 vs. 2.5% 2/81). Mortality not associated with sputum conversion, HIV status, severity of disease, relapse rates, or sensitivity to other antimycobacterial drugs (Provisional CDC Guidelines for the Use and Safety Monitoring of Bedaquiline Fumarate (Sirturo) for the Treatment of Multidrug-Resistant Tuberculosis (MMWR 2013/62(RR09);1–12).

Benzodiazepines

Benzodiazepines are commonly used for anxiety and insomnia. They are also commonly misused and abused, with some studies showing that up to 25% of AIDS patients take these drugs. The decision to use these drugs requires careful consideration of side effects along with a discussion of the following issues with the patient:

EFV may cause false-positive urine tests for benzodiazepine. This is due to 8 hydroxy-EFV (CID 2009;48:1787).

Dependency: Larger than usual doses or prolonged daily use of therapeutic doses.

Abuse potential: Most common in those with abuse of alcohol and other psychiatric drugs.

Tolerance: Primarily to sedation and ataxia; minimal to antianxiety effects.

Withdrawal symptoms: Related to duration of use, dose, rate of tapering, and drug half-life. Features include (1) recurrence of pretreatment symptoms developing over days or wks, (2) rebound with symptoms that are similar to but more severe than pretreatment symptoms occurring within hours or days (self-limited), and (3) the "benzodiazepine withdrawal syndrome" with autonomic symptoms, disturbances in equilibrium, sensory disturbances, and more.

Daytime sedation, dizziness, incoordination, ataxia, and hangover: Use small doses initially and gradually increase. Patient must be warned that activities requiring mental alertness, judgment, and coordination require special caution; concomitant use with alcohol or other sedating drugs is hazardous. Patients often experience amnesia for events during the drug's time of action.

Drug interactions: Sedative effects are antagonized by caffeine and theophylline. Erythromycin, clarithromycin, fluoroquinolones, all PIs, cobicistat, cimetidine, nefazodone may reduce hepatic metabolism and prolong half-life. Midazolam and triazolam are thus contraindicated for coadministration. Lorazepam, temazepam, and oxazepam are safer alternatives. Rifampin and anticonvulsants (phenobarbital, phenytoin, carbamazepine) increase hepatic clearance and reduce half-life of midazolam and triazolam.

Miscellaneous side effects: Blurred vision, diplopia, confusion, memory disturbance, amnesia, fatigue, incontinence, constipation, hypotension, disinhibition, bizarre behavior.

Antiretroviral agents: Concurrent use of triazolam or midazolam with PIs or cobicistat is contraindicated. No interaction with NRTIs, BIC, DTG, RAL, and MVC expected.

SELECTION OF AGENT AND REGIMEN: Drug selection is based largely on indication and pharmacokinetic properties. Drugs with rapid onset are desired when temporary relief of anxiety is

TABLE 6.19 Azoles and antiretroviral agents: drug interactions

Antifungal	ART NNRTI	Effect AUC	Recommendation
Fluconazole	EFV	No effect	Standard doses
	ETR	ETR ↑86%	Caution
	NVP	NVP ↑110%	Risk hepatotoxicity— monitor[a]
	RPV	RPV may be ↑	Monitor QTc
Posaconazole	EFV	Posa ↓50%	Use alternative or monitor[a]
	ETR	ETR may ↑	Standard doses
	NVP	Posa may ↓; NVP may ↑	Use alternative or monitor
	RPV	RPV may be ↑	Monitor QTc
Itraconazole	EFV	Itra ↓35–44%	Monitor[a] May need ↑ itra dose
	ETR	Itra may, ETR may ↑	Monitor[a] May need ↑ itra dose
	NVP	Itra ↓61%, NVP may ↑	Monitor[a] May need ↑ itra dose
	RPV	RPV may ↑	Monitor QTc
Voriconazole	EFV	Vori ↓ 77%. EFV ↑ 44%	Vori 400 mg bid, EFV 300 mg/d
	ETR	ETR ↑ 36%	Standard doses and caution
	NVP	Vori may ↓↓, NVP may ↑	Avoid, Use alternative
	RPV	RPV may ↑	Monitor QTc
Isavuconazole	EFV, ETR, NVP	Isavuconazole may ↓	Monitor[a]
	RPV	RPV may ↑	Monitor QTc
	PI		
Fluconazole	ATV/r	No effect	Standard doses
	SQV	SQV ↑	Use Standard doses. No data for SQV/r
	TPV/r	TPV ↑50%	Flucon dose ≤200 mg/d

TABLE 6.19 Continued

Antifungal	ART NNRTI	Effect AUC	Recommendation
	Other PIs	—	Use standard dose
Posaconazole	ATV/r	ATV ↑146%	Monitor for ATV ADR
	ATV	ATV ↑268%	Monitor for ATV ADR
	FPV	Posa and APV ↓	Avoid
	RTV/. COBI	May ↑Posa	Monitor[a]
Itraconazole	LPV/r	Itra ↑	Itra dose >200/d requires monitor[a]
	SQV/r	Itra ↑, SQV ↑	Monitor[a]
	Other PIs and. COBI	Itra may ↑, PI may ↑	ATV/r, DRV/r, FPV/r, TPV/r. Dose itra ≤200 mg/d and/or monitor
Itraconazole/ Voriconazole	MVC	MVC ↑	MVC 150 mg bid
Isavuconazole	MVC	May increase MVC concentrations.	No data. With orthostatic hypotension, consider dose reduction MVC 150 mg bid
Azoles	RAL	No interactions	Standard doses
	EVG/c or EVG/r	Azoles and EVG may be increased	See dosing recommendations above
	DTG	Interaction unlikely	Usual dose
	BIC	BIC ↑61% with Vori	Usual dose likely

[a] Indicates monitoring azole blood levels.

TABLE 6.20 Comparison of benzodiazepines

Agent	Trade Name	Anxiety	Insomnia	T_{max} (hrs)	Mean Half-life (hrs)	Dose Forms	Regimens
Chlordiazepoxide	Librium	+	−	0.5–4.0	10	5, 10, 25 mg tabs	15–100 mg/d hs or. 3 to 4 doses
Clorazepate	Tranxene	+	−	1–2	73	3.75, 7.5, 15, 11.25, 22.5 mg tabs	15–60 mg/d hs or 2 to 4 doses
Diazepam	Valium	+	+	1.5–2.0	73	2, 4, 5, 10 mg tabs	15–60 mg/d hs or 2 to 4 doses
Flurazepam	Dalmane	−	+	0.5–2.0	74	15, 30 mg caps	15–30 mg/d, hs
Quazepam	Doral	−	+	2	74	7.5, 15 mg tabs	7.5–30 mg hs
Alprazolam	Xanax	+	−	1–2	11	0.25, 0.5, 1, 2 mg tabs. 0.5, 1, 2, 3 mg SR tabs	0.75–1.5 mg/d in 3 divided doses

Lorazepam	Ativan	+	+	2	14	0.5, 1, and 2 mg tabs	0.25–0.5 mg tid up to 4 mg/d
Oxazepam	Serax	+	+	1–4	7	10, 15, 30 mg caps	15–30 mg tid-qid
Temazepam	Restoril	–	+	1.0–1.5	13	15, 30 mg caps	15–30 mg qhs
Triazolam[a]	Halcion	–	+	1–2	3	0.125, 0.25 mg tabs	0.25 mg hs
Midazolam[a]	Versed	+	+	2 min	1–5	IV vial	0.03–0.06 mg/kg

[a] Concurrent use of oral midazolam or triazolam and cobicistat, all PIs are contraindicated. Single-dose IV midazolam may be considered with ATV, TPV/r, and LPV/r. Monitor closely.

needed. The smallest dose for the shortest time is recommended, and patients need frequent reevaluation for continued use. Long-term use should be avoided, especially in patients with a history of abuse of alcohol or other sedative-hypnotic drugs. Dose adjustments are usually required to achieve the desired effect with acceptable side effects. Long-term use (more than several weeks) may require an extended tapering schedule over 6–8 wks (20–30% dose reduction weekly) adjusted by symptoms and sometimes facilitated by antidepressants or hypnotics.

Biaxin—see Clarithromycin

Bictegravir (BIC)

TRADE NAME: Biktarvy (Fixed dose co-formulation: bictegravir/TAF/FTC).

CLASS: Integrase strand transfer inhibitor (InSTI).

FORMULATION, REGIMEN, AND COST: BIC/TAF/FTC 50 mg/25 mg/200 mg tablet.

> *Cost*: $3,534.78/mo.
> *Dose*: BIC/TAF/FTC 50 mg/25 mg/200 mg tablet with or without food. *Note*: must be taken with food with when co-administered with iron or calcium supplements.
> *Dose in renal impairment*: CrCL >30 mL/min: usual dose; CrCL <30 mL/min: BIC/TAF/FTC co-formulation not recommended.
> *Dosing with hepatic impairment*: Child-Pugh A or B: usual dose. Not recommended in severe liver impairment (Child-Pugh C) due to lack of data.

RESISTANCE: Emergence of resistance to bictegravir was not observed in clinical trials to date. High barrier to BIC resistance observed in vitro. In vitro, M50I, R263K, M50I + R263K, T66I,

S153F, and T66I + S153F resulted in a small reduction in susceptibility to BIC.

Clinical isolates with G140A/C/S, Q148 H/R/K, and complex INSTI resistance pattern with L74M, T97A, or E138 A/K had cross-resistance to BIC with more than 2.5-fold (above biological cutoff for BIC) reduction in susceptibility. G118R + T97A and M50I + R263K exhibited a 2.8-fold reduced susceptibility to BIC (AAC 2016;60:7086).

CLINICAL TRIALS: See Lancet 2017;390:2063; Lancet 2017;390:2073. BIC/TAF/FTC was approved based on two randomized, double-blind, multicenter, controlled studies that compared BIC/TAF/FTC to DTG/ABC/3TC (GS-US-380-1489) and DTG plus TAF/FTC (GS-US-380-1490).

In GS-US-380-1489, BIC/TAF/FTC was found to be noninferior to DTG/ABC/3TC after 48 wks with 92.4% of patients (n = 290 of 314) in the BIC/TAF/FTC group and 93.0% of patients (n = 293 of 315) in the DTG/ABC/3TC achieving HIV-1 RNA <50 copies/mL (difference –0.6%; p = 0.78). Similarly, in the GS-US-380-1490 study, HIV-1 RNA <50 copies per mL was achieved in 89% of patients (n = 286 of 320): in the BIC/TAF/FTC-treated patients and 93% (n = 302 of 325) in DTG + TAF/FTC-treated patients (difference –3.5%, 95% CI, –7.9 to 1.0, p = 0.12), There was no treatment-emergent resistance that developed to any of the study drugs.

PHARMACOLOGY:

Absorption/Distribution: High-fat meals increase BIC AUC by 24%. May be taken with or without food. Time to peak concentration 2–4 hrs; >99% protein binding.

Metabolism/Elimination: Metabolized via CYP3A4 and UGT1A1 then eliminated in urine (35%) and feces (60.3%).

SIDE EFFECTS:

In comparative clinical trials, adverse drug reactions (ADRs) associated with BIC/TAF/FTC were comparable to DTG + TAF/FTC- and

DTG/ABC/3TC-treated patients (except for nausea that occurred more frequently in the DTG/ABC/3TC-treated patients). The majority of side effects were grade 1 with only 1% discontinuation rate in patients treated with BIC/TAF/FTC.

Reported side effects: Diarrhea (3–6%), nausea (3–5%), headache (4–5%), fatigue (2–3%), abnormal dreams (<1–3%), dizziness (2%), insomnia (2%).

Reported laboratory abnormalities: Increase in amylase (>2.0 × ULN) in 2%, AST/ALT (>5.0 × ULN) in 1–2%, CK (≥10 × ULN) in 4%, neutropenia (<750 mm^3) in 2%, LDL elevation in 2% observed in clinical trials.

BIC inhibition of serum creatinine tubular secretion resulted in a median 0.10 mg/dL increase of Scr without affecting GFR.

DRUG INTERACTIONS:

BIC is a substrate of CYP3A4 and UGT1A1. In vitro BIC inhibits OCT2 and MATE1 drug transporter.

BIC concentrations may be significantly decreased with carbamazepine, oxcarbazepine, phenobarbital, phenytoin, rifabutin, rifampin (contraindicated), rifapentine, and St. John's Wort co-administration. Avoid co-administration.

Enzalutamide amd mitotane may decrease BIC concentrations. Avoid

Dofetilide concentrations may be significantly increased. Contraindicated.

Co-administered Drug	BIC concentrations (AUC)	Co-administered drug concentration	Recommendation
Ledipasvir/ sofosbuvir	↔	No clinically significant change	Use standard dose
Sofosbuvir/ velpatasvir/ voxilaprevir	↑7%	No clinically significant change	Use standard dose
Rifampin	↓75%	—	Contraindicated
Rifabutin	↓38%	—	Avoid

Co-administered Drug	BIC concentrations (AUC)	Co-administered drug concentration	Recommendation
Voriconazole	↑61%	—	Clinical significance unknown. Use standard dose.
Iron supplement. when given with food	↓16%	—	Use BIC usual dose with food
Calcium supplement when given with food	↔	—	Use BIC usual dose with food
Magnesium/ Aluminum/ Calcium cations-containing antacid, laxatives, buffered medications, and sucralfate	↓ 79% (simultaneous). ↓13%. (2 hrs after BIC)	—	Take BIC on empty stomach, and then give cations 2 hrs *after* BIC.
Metformin	—	↑39%	Use with close monitoring. Avoid with CrCL <45 mL/min.
Midazolam	—	↔	Use standard dose
Norelgetromin/ Norgestrel/ Ethinyl estradiol	—	No clinically significant change	Use standard dose

PREGNANCY: No human data. Not teratogenic in rat studies given 36× human exposure. Spontaneous abortion and decreased body weight observed in rabbits given 1.4× human exposure.

Bupropion

TRADE NAME: Wellbutrin, Wellbutrin SR, Wellbutrin XL, Zyban (GlaxoSmithKline) and generic.

CLASS: Atypical antidepressant.

FORMULATIONS, REGIMEN, AND COST: Tabs: 75 mg at $0.79, 100 mg at $1.06, 150 mg and 300 sustained-release at $5.21. Wellbutrin comes in 75 and 100 mg tabs; Wellbutrin SR-12h comes in 100, 150, and 200 mg tabs; and Wellbutrin XL-24h comes in 150, 300, and 450 mg tabs.

INDICATIONS AND DOSES: Depression: 150 mg/d × 4 days, then 300 mg/d (XL formulation) or 150 mg bid (SR formulation); antidepressant effect may require 4 wks.

Zyban for smoking cessation: Dose same as SR formulation × 7–12 wks.

PHARMACOLOGY:

Bioavailability: 5–20%.

$T^{1/2}$: 8–24 hrs.

Elimination: Extensive hepatic metabolism to ≥6 metabolites, two with antidepressant activity; metabolites excreted in urine.

Dose modification in renal or hepatic failure: Not known, but dose reduction may be required.

SIDE EFFECTS: Seizures, which are dose-dependent and minimized by gradual increase in dose; dose not to exceed 450 mg/d. Use with caution in seizure-prone patients and with concurrent use of alcohol and other antidepressants.

Other side effects: Agitation, insomnia, restlessness; GI: anorexia, nausea, vomiting; weight loss: noted in up to 25%; rare cases of psychosis, paranoia, depersonalization.

DRUG INTERACTIONS: LPV/r decreases bupropion AUC 57% (Hogeland et al., CPT 2007;81:69); no seizures reported with PI co-administration. Avoid bupropion with MAO inhibitors; pimozide, tamoxifen, thioridazine.

BuSpar—see Buspirone

Buspirone

TRADE NAME: BuSpar (Bristol-Myers Squibb) and generics.

CLASS: Nonbenzodiazepine-nonbarbiturate antianxiety agent; not a controlled substance.

FORMULATIONS, REGIMEN, AND COST: Tabs: 5 mg tab at $0.77, 7.5 mg tab at $1.09, 10 mg tab at $1.35, 15 mg tab at $1.99, 30 mg tab at $3.63.

INDICATIONS AND DOSES: Anxiety: 5 mg po tid; increase by 5 mg/d every 2–4 days. Usual effective dose is 15–30 mg/d in 2–3 divided doses. Onset of response requires 1 wk, and full effect requires 4 wks. Total daily dose should not exceed 60 mg/d.

PHARMACOLOGY:

Bioavailability: >90% absorbed when taken with food.
$T^{1/2}$: 2.5 hrs.
Elimination: Rapid hepatic metabolism to partially active metabolites; <0.1% of parent compound excreted in urine.
Dose adjustment in renal disease: Dose reduction of 25–50% in patients with anuria.

Hepatic disease: May decrease clearance and must use with caution.

SIDE EFFECTS: Sleep disturbance, nervousness, headache, nausea, diarrhea, paresthesias, depression, increased or decreased libido, dizziness, and excitement. Compared with benzodiazepines, there is no risk of dependency, it does not potentiate CNS depressants including alcohol, it is usually well-tolerated by elderly, and there is no hypnotic effect, no muscle relaxant effect, less fatigue, less confusion, and less decreased libido but nearly comparable efficacy for prevention of anxiety (not effective for acute anxiety attacks). Nevertheless, the CNS effects are somewhat unpredictable, and there is substantial individual variation; patients should be warned that buspirone may impair ability to perform activities requiring mental alertness and physical coordination, such as driving.

DRUG INTERACTIONS: Rifampin decreases buspirone AUC 90%, avoid; NNRTIs may also decrease buspirone (Lamberg TS et al., Br J Clin Pharmacol 1998;45:381; Drugs 2011;71:11).

PREGNANCY: Category B.

Caspofungin

TRADE NAME: Cancidas (Merck) and generic manufacturer.

CLASS: Polypeptide antifungal; echinocandin glucan synthesis inhibitor.

FORMULATIONS, REGIMEN, AND COST: 50 mg vial $269.40; 70 mg vial $122.22.

> ACTIVITY: Active against nearly all *Candida* spp, although somewhat higher concentrations are needed for *C. parapsilosis* and *C. guilliermondii*. Most fluconazole-resistant strains are sensitive (Am J Med 2006;119:993). Active against most *Aspergillus* spp; the combination of caspofungin

with voriconazole or amphotericin is synergistic or additive against *Aspergillus* spp. (CID 2003;36:1445; Cancer 2006;107:2888; Med Mycol 2006;44(Suppl):373). No activity against *C. neoformans*.

INDICATIONS:

Invasive aspergillosis, in patients intolerant of voriconazole or amphotericin B, caspofungin plus posaconazole has been used for invasive aspergillus refractory to standard treatment (Mycosis 2011;54 Suppl 1:1439).

Candidemia and other serious Candida infections, including *Candida* esophagitis refractory and resistant to azoles. FDA-approved for oropharyngeal, esophageal, and disseminated candidiasis and for invasive aspergillosis. Reliable activity against azole-resistant *candida sp.* including *C. albicans*, *C. glabrata*, *C. krusei* and, *C. tropicalis*; makes caspofungin and other echinocandins (micafungin and anidulafungin) the preferred first-line agent for candidemia (Pappas PG et al., 2016 IDSA Clinical Practice Guidelines for the Management for Candidiasis CID 2016; The 2018 IDSA/FDA/CDC Guidelines for Opportunistic Infections list caspofungin and other echinocandins) as alternative options in fluconazole-refractory oral or esophageal candidiasis. A major concern is expense.

Dose: 70 mg IV on day 1, then 50 mg/d.

Dose with renal failure: Standard.

Dose in obese patients: 70 mg/d.

Dose with hepatic failure: With Child-Pugh score of 7–9, give standard loading dose of 70 mg, then 35 mg/d. Use with caution with Child-Pugh score >9.

PHARMACOLOGY:

Absorption: N/A; IV only.

$T^{1/2}$: 9–11 hr.

Distribution: Poor CNS, ocular, and urinary penetration.

Elimination: Metabolized by hydrolysis and acetylating; <2% excreted unchanged in urine.

SIDE EFFECTS: Excellent safety profile; rare side effects are rash, facial swelling, nausea, vomiting, headache, fever, phlebitis, hypokalemia, increased alkaline phosphatase. Rare patients have histamine release symptoms with rash, fever, pruritus, and sensation of warmth that accompanies infusion.

DRUG INTERACTIONS: *Cyclosporin* increases caspofungin AUC 35%; co-administration is not recommended due to increase in liver enzymes. *Tacrolimus* levels reduced 20% with caspofungin; monitor tacrolimus levels. *Phenytoin, carbamazepine, phenobarbital, dexamethasone, ETR, EFV,* and *NVP* may decrease caspofungin; consider increasing dose to 70 mg/d with invasive disease. *Rifampin* decreases caspofungin by 30%; increase caspofungin dose to 70 mg/d or consider micafungin.

PREGNANCY: Class C: Embryotoxic with skeletal abnormalities in rats and rabbits; limited experience in humans. Amphotericin B is preferred.

Cidofovir

TRADE NAME: Vistide (Gilead Sciences).

FORMULATIONS, REGIMEN, AND COST: 1% gel (not commercially available but can be compounded by pharmacy); 375 mg in 5 mL vial at $888.

> PATIENT ASSISTANCE PROGRAM AND REIMBURSEMENT HOTLINE: 800-226-2056.
> ACTIVITY: Active in vitro against CMV, VZV, EBV, HHV-6, HPV, pox viruses (molluscum, vaccinia, smallpox), and HHV-8; less active against HSV (Exp Med Biol 1996;394:105). CMV strains resistant to ganciclovir with UL97 mutation are

usually sensitive to cidofovir. Cidofovir-resistant strains are usually resistant to ganciclovir and sensitive to foscarnet. HSV that is resistant to acyclovir is often sensitive to cidofovir.

INDICATIONS AND DOSE: *CMV retinitis* (Clin Opthalmol 2010;4:285) Cidofovir is recommended as an alternative to valganciclovir/ganciclovir for the treatment of CMV retinitis (2018 CDC OI guidelines); efficacy in other forms of CMV disease has not been established, but is expected (Arch Intern Med 1998;158:957). Topical use for *acyclovir-resistant HSV* (J Eur Acad Dermatol Venereol 2006;20:887). Cidofovir applied topically has been used to treat disfiguring HPV lesions (J Am Acad Dermatol 2006;55:533). A trial in 185 patients with HIV-associated PML failed (AIDS 2008;22:1759). There is a suggested but unproven role in HHV-8–associated primary effusion lymphoma (Clin Adv Hematol Oncol 2010;8:372; Clin Adv Hematol Oncol 2010;8:367).

Topical administration: Withdraw contents of IV vial (375 mg/5 mL) and mix with 33 g of Orabase gel with benzocaine.

Induction dose: 5 mg/kg IV over 1 hr weekly × 2 wks*.

Maintenance dose: 5 mg/kg IV over 1 hr every 2 wks*.

* Probenecid 2 g given 3 hrs prior to cidofovir and 1 g given at 2 and 8 hrs after infusion (total of 4 g). Patients must receive >1 L 0.95 *N* (normal) saline infused over 1–2 hrs immediately before cidofovir infusion.

NOTES ON ADMINISTRATION:

Cidofovir is diluted in 100 mL 0.9% saline.

Renal failure: Cidofovir is contraindicated in patients with preexisting renal failure (serum creatinine >1.5 mg/dL, creatinine clearance ≤55 mL/min or urine protein >100 mg/dL or 2 + proteinuria).

Co-administration of nephrotoxic drugs is contraindicated. There should be a 7-day "washout" following use of these drugs.

DOSE ADJUSTMENT FOR RENAL FAILURE DURING CIDOFOVIR TREATMENT:

Serum creatinine increase 0.3–0.4 mg/dL: Reduce dose to 3 mg/kg.

Serum creatinine increase ≥0.5 mg/dL or ≥3 + proteinuria: Discontinue therapy.

Gastrointestinal tolerability of probenecid may be improved with ingestion of food or an antiemetic prior to administration. Antihistamines or acetaminophen may be used for probenecid hypersensitivity reactions.

Cases of nephrotoxicity should be reported to Gilead Sciences, Inc.; 800-GILEAD-5, or to the FDA's Medwatch 800-FDA-1088.

CLINICAL TRIALS: Studies of the Ocular Complications of AIDS (SOCA) comparing cidofovir vs. deferred treatment of patients with CMV retinitis in the pre-HAART era demonstrated a median time to progression of 120 days in the treated group, compared with 22 days in the deferred group (Ann Intern Med 1997;126:257). Dose-limiting nephrotoxicity was noted in 24%, and dose-limiting toxicity to probenecid was noted in 7%.

PHARMACOLOGY:

Bioavailability: Requires IV administration; probenecid increases AUC by 40–60%, presumably by blocking tubular secretion. CSF levels are undetectable.

$T^{1/2}$: 17–65 hr.

Excretion: 70–85% excreted in urine.

SIDE EFFECTS: The major side effect is dose-dependent nephrotoxicity including Fanconi syndrome (JAC 2007;60:193). Proteinuria is an early indicator. IV saline and probenecid must be used to reduce nephrotoxicity. Monitor renal function with serum creatinine and urine protein within 48 hrs prior to each dose. About 25% will develop ≥2 + proteinuria or a serum creatinine >2–3 mg/dL, and these changes are reversible if treatment is discontinued (Ann Intern Med 1997;126:257,264).

Other side effects: Neutropenia in about 15% (monitor neutrophil count), Fanconi's syndrome with proteinuria, normoglycemic glycosuria, hypophosphatemia, hypouricemia, and decreased serum bicarbonate indicating renal tubule damage, ocular hypotony, anterior uveitis or iritis, and asthenia.

Probenecid causes side effects in about 50% of patients including fever, chills, headache, rash, or nausea, usually after 3–4 treatments. Side effects usually resolve within 12 hrs. Dose-limiting side effect is usually GI intolerance. Side effects may be reduced with antiemetics, antipyretics, antihistamines, or by eating before taking probenecid (Ann Intern Med 1997;126:257).

DRUG INTERACTIONS: Avoid concurrent use of potentially nephrotoxic drugs. Patients receiving these drugs should have a ≥7 day "washout" prior to treatment with cidofovir. Probenecid prolongs the half-life of acetaminophen, acyclovir, aminosalicylic acid, barbiturates, β-lactams, benzodiazepines, bumetanide, clofibrate, methotrexate, famotidine, furosemide, NSAIDs, theophylline, TDF, and AZT.

PREGNANCY: Category C. Embryotoxic and teratotoxic in rats and rabbits. Not recommended for humans.

Ciprofloxacin (and other fluoroquinolones)

TRADE NAME: Cipro (Bayer) and generic.

CLASS: Fluoroquinolone antibiotic.

FORMULATIONS, REGIMEN, AND COST: Tabs: 250 mg at $4.58, 500 mg at $5.36, 750 mg at $5.62; 500 mg XR at $10.56; 1,000 mg XR at $11.91. Vials for IV use: 400 mg at $3.34.

INDICATIONS AND DOSES:

Respiratory infections: 500–750 mg po bid × 7–14 days. *P. aeruginosa*: use 750 mg po bid or 400 mg IV q8h ≥15 days.

Gonorrhea: Ciprofloxacin not recommended, but gemifloxacin 320 mg plus azithromycin 2 g can be used as an alternative GC treatment in PCN allergic patients. (2015 CDC Guidelines for STDs).

M. avium: 500–750 mg po bid (alternative or third or fourth drug with serious disease).

Tuberculosis: 500–750 mg po bid (multidrug–resistant *M. tuberculosis* or liver disease). Preferred agent is moxifloxacin.

Salmonellosis: 500–750 mg po or 400 mg IV bid × 7–14 d for mild disease or 4–6 wks for CD4 <200 and/or bacteremia (preferred).

UTI: 250–500 mg po bid × 3–7 d (first line); uncomplicated UTI: ciprofloxacin XR 500 mg/d or ciprofloxacin 250 mg bid × 3 d.

Traveler's diarrhea: 500 mg po bid × 3 d (first line).

ACTIVITY: Active against most strains of Enterobacteriaceae, *P. aeruginosa*, *H. influenzae*, *Legionella*, *C. pneumoniae*, *M. pneumoniae*, *M. tuberculosis*, *M. avium* complex, most bacterial enteric pathogens other than *C. jejuni* and *C. difficile*. Somewhat less active against *S. pneumoniae* than levofloxacin and moxifloxacin. There is increasing and substantial resistance by *S. aureus* (primarily MRSA) (CID 2000;32:S114), *P. aeruginosa* (CID 2000;32:S146), *E. coli*, and *C. jejuni* (CID 2001;32:1201). There is also escalating concern about fluoroquinolone-resistant *N. gonorrhoeae* and *Salmonella*. Gemifloxacin (plus azithromycin) is the only fluoroquinolone recommended for gonococcal infections in PCN-allergic patients (2015 CDC Guidelines STD recommendations). Due to increasing fluoroquinolone-resistant *N. gonorrhoeae* (MMWR 2010;59:RR-12; Ann Intern Med 2007;147:81), test-of-cure is recommended at 1 wk (2015 CDC STD guidelines). Most strains of

Salmonella are fluoroquinolone-sensitive in HIV-infected patients (Trop Med Int Health 2010;15:697). For *tuberculosis* there is considerable enthusiasm for fluoroquinolone (moxifloxacin) use for resistant strains, and this is now in phase III testing at the FDA (Lancet 2010;10:621; Diacon AH et al., Lancet 2012). Replacing ethambutol or INH for moxifloxacin × 4 mos in a standard INH/rifampin/ethambutol/PZA regimen resulted in a faster initial decline in TB load, but was not as effective as standard of care (Gillespie SH et al., NEJM 2014).

PHARMACOLOGY:

Bioavailability: 60–70%.

$T^{1/2}$: 3.3 hrs.

Excretion: Metabolized and excreted (parent compound and metabolites) in urine.

Dose reduction in renal failure: CrCl>50 mL/min, 250–750 mg q12h; CrCl 10–50 mL/min, 250–500 mg q12h; CrCl<10 mL/min, 500 mg q24h.

SIDE EFFECTS: Usually well tolerated. Fluoroquinolones are now a major cause of *C. difficile*-associated colitis (Ann Intern Med 2006;145:758; NEJM 2005;353:2433; CID 2008;47:818; Infect Control Hosp Epidemiol 2009;30:264). All agents in the class are implicated; relative rates are unclear.

GI intolerance with nausea, 1.2%; diarrhea, 1.2%.

CNS toxicity: Malaise, drowsiness, insomnia, headache, dizziness, agitation, psychosis (rare), seizures (rare), hallucinations (rare).

Tendon rupture: About 100 cases reported involving fluoroquinolones, with ciprofloxacin accounting for 25% (CID 2003;36:1404). The incidence in a review of 46,776 courses was 0.1% with increased rates in older age and steroids as confounding risks (BMJ 2002;324:1306).

Torsades de pointes: Rates/10 million are: moxifloxacin, 0; ciprofloxacin, 0.3; levofloxacin, 5.4 (Pharmacother 2001;21:1468).

Candida vaginitis: Caution: Fluoroquinolones are relatively contraindicated in persons.

<18 yrs due to concern for arthropathy, which has been seen in beagles, but application to human disease is debated (Curr Opin Pediatr 2006;18:64). Some fluoroquinolones may cause false-positive urine screening tests for opiates (JAMA 2001;286:3115).

DRUG INTERACTIONS: Increased levels of theophylline, methotrexate, and caffeine; reduced absorption with cations (Al, Mg, Ca) in antacids, sucralfate, milk and dairy products, buffered ddI. Take fluoroquinolone 2 hr before cations.

PREGNANCY: Category C. Arthropathy in immature animals with erosions in joint cartilages; relevance to patients is not known, but fluoroquinolones are not FDA-approved for use in pregnancy or in children <18 yrs. Review of >400 first-trimester exposures showed no anomalies. Use is justified in severe MAC or multi-drug-resistant tuberculosis.

Clarithromycin

TRADE NAME: Biaxin (Abbott Laboratories) and generic.

CLASS: Macrolide antibiotic.

FORMULATIONS, REGIMEN, AND COST: Tabs: 250 mg at $4.52, 500 mg at $4.52, 500 mg XL at $5.00 (for qd dosing). Suspension: 250 mg/5 mL at $53.30 per 50 mL.

PATIENT ASSISTANCE PROGRAM: 800-659-9050.

ACTIVITY: *S. pneumoniae* (20–30% of strains and 40% of penicillin-resistant strains are resistant in most areas of the United States), good activity vs. most erythromycin-sensitive

S. pyogenes, M. catarrhalis, H. influenzae, M. pneumoniae, C. pneumoniae, Legionella, M. avium, T. gondii, C. trachomatis, and *U. urealyticum.* Activity against *H. influenzae* is often debated, although a metabolite shows better in vitro activity than the parent compound, and the FDA has approved clarithromycin for pneumonia caused by *H. influenzae.* There is concern about increasing rates of macrolide resistance by *S. pneumoniae* (JID 2000;182:1417; AAC 2001;45:2147; AAC 2002;46:265). Clinical trials show in vivo results are superior to in vitro activity, but excessive rates of breakthrough pneumococcal bacteremia have been reported when clarithromycin is used alone. Many authorities now prefer a β-lactam combined with a macrolide for serious pneumococcal infections, presumably due to the antiinflammatory effect of the macrolide (Drugs 2011;7:131; CID 2002;35:556).

CLINICAL TRIALS: Clarithromycin is highly effective in the treatment and prevention of *Mycobacterium avium* complex (MAC) disease (NEJM 1996;335:385; CID 1998;27:1278). Clarithromycin was superior to azithromycin in the treatment of MAC bacteremia in terms of median time to negative blood cultures 4.4 wks vs. >16 wks (CID 1998;27:1278). However, in a large prospective trial (*n* = 246) azithromycin dose of 600/d was equivalent to clarithromycin when combined with ethambutol. At 24 wk, culture clearance, relapse rates, clinical outcome, and mortality was not different between the groups (CID 2000;31:1254). There is no evidence that it is superior to azithromycin for MAC prophylaxis.

PHARMACOLOGY:

Bioavailability: 50–55%.

$T^{1/2}$: 4–7 hrs.

Elimination: Rapid first-pass hepatic metabolism plus renal clearance to 14-hydroxyclarithromycin.

TABLE 6.21 Fluoroquinolone summary

	Ciprofloxacin Cipro	Levofloxacin Levaquin	Moxifloxacin Avelox
Oral form	+	+	+
IV form	+	+	+
Price (AWP) oral formulation	$5.36 (500 mg), $10.72	$19.26 (500 mg tab)	$27.20 (400 mg tab)
T½	3.3 hrs	6.3 hrs	12 hrs
T½ renal failure	8 hrs	35 hrs	12 hrs
Oral bioavailability	65%	99%	90%
Activity in vitro[a]	+ + + (60–80%).	+ +	+
P. aeruginosa	+	+ +	+ +
S. pneumoniae	+ +	+ +	+ + +
Mycobacteria	—	+	+ +
Anaerobes			
Regimens (oral)	250–750 mg bid	500–750 mg/d	400 mg/d

[a] All fluoroquinolones are active against most Enterobacteriaceae, enteric bacterial pathogens (except *C. jejuni* and *C. difficile*), methicillin-sensitive S. aureus (generally not recommended), *Neisseria* spp., and pulmonary pathogens including *S. pneumoniae, H. influenzae, C. pneumoniae, Legionella,* and *M. pneumoniae*.

Major advantages of newer fluoroquinolones are once-daily dosing, good tolerability, and activity against S. pneumoniae, including >98% of penicillin-resistant strains (AAC 2002;46:265). The major newly recognized class side effect is Clostridium difficile- associated diarrhea or colitis (NEJM 2005;353:2433; NEJM 2005;353:2442, NEJM.

2005;353:2503). Other class side effects include prolongation of QT interval when given to persons predisposed primarily by concurrent medications (macrolides, class IA and III anti-arrhythmics), tendon rupture (risk with age and steroids), and CNS toxicity including seizures. All are contraindicated in persons <18 yrs and in pregnant women. Divalent and trivalent cations reduce absorption—avoid concurrent antacids with Mg^{++} or Al^{+++}, sucralfate, Fe^{++}, Zn^{++}, and buffered ddl; administer fluoronoquinolones 2 hrs before cations. The major concern is abuse and resistance, with particular concern for *P. aeruginosa*, Enterobacteriaceae, *S. pneumoniae, S. aureus, C. jejuni, N. gonorrhoeae, C. difficile,* and *Salmonella*.

TABLE 6.22 Clarithromycin indications and doses

Indication	Dose Regimen[a]
Pharyngitis, sinusitis, otitis, pneumonitis, skin and soft tissue infection [b]	250–500 mg po bid or 1 g (2XL tabs) qd
M. avium compex (MAC) prophylaxis [b]	500 mg po bid (2018 IDSA/ NIH/CDC Guidelines)
MAC treatment[b] plus EMB ± moxifloxacin or rifabutin	500 mg po bid (+ ethambutol 15 mg/kg po/d + rifabutin 300 mg po/d) (2018. IDSA/ NIH/CDC OI Guidelines)
Bartonella	500 mg po bid × ≥3 mos

[a] Doses of ≥2 g/d are associated with excessive mortality (CID 1999;29:125).
[b] FDA-approved for this indication.

TABLE 6.23 Clarithromycin interactions with antiretroviral agents

Agent	Clarithromycin	ARARTT Agent	Dose Recommendation Regimen
IDV	↑ 53%	↑ 29%	Standard—Reduce clarithromycin w/renal failure
RTV	↑ 77%	No data	Reduce clarithromycin dose by 50% if CrCl 30–60 mL/min, and by 75% if CrCl <30 mL/min
SQV	↑ 45%	↑ 177%	CrCl 30–60 mL/min: ↓50%; CrCl <30 mL/min: ↓75%. May ↑ risk of QTc prolongation. Consider azithromycin.
NFV	No data	No data	Reduce clarithromycin with renal failure

(continued)

TABLE 6.23 Continued

Agent	Clarithromycin	ARARTT Agent	Dose Recommendation Regimen
LPV/r	↑ 77%	↑	Reduce clarithromycin dose by 50% if CrCl 30–60 mL/min, and by 75% if CrCl <30 mL/min
NVP	↓ 30%	↑ 26%	Standard; monitor for efficacy or use azithromycin
EFV	↓ 39%	↑	Avoid if possible; consider azithromycin
ATV	↑ 94%	↑ 28%	Use half dose clarithromycin and decrease further with renal failure. Monitor for arrhythmia (QTc prolongation) or use azithromycin w/ESRD
DRV	↑ 57%	No change	Use half dose clarithromycin if CrCl 30–60 mL/min and reduce 75% if CrCl <30 mL/min
TPV	↑ 19%	↑ 66%	Use half dose clarithromycin if CrCl 30–60 mL/min and reduce 75% if CrCl <30 mL/min
FPV	No Change	↑ 18%	Standard doses w/FPV, but consider ↓ dose in renal failure w/boosted FPV
MVC	No change likely	Possible ↑	MVC dose is 150 mg bid
ETR	↓ 39%	↑ 42%	Consider azithromycin for MAC
RPV	No change likely	May increase RPV	May increase risk RPV and risk of QTc prolongation. Use azithromycin.

TABLE 6.23 Continued

Agent	Clarithromycin	ARARTT Agent	Dose Recommendation Regimen
COBI	May increase	May increase	Dose reduce clarithromycin in renal failure. Consider azithromycin
DTG	No change likely	May increase	Use usual dose
RAL	No change likely	No change likely	Use usual dose
EVG/c or/r	May increase	May increase	Use standard dose EVG. Dose reduce clarithromycin in renal failure. Consider azithromycin
BIC	No change likely	May increase	Use standard dose

Dose modification in renal failure: CrCl <30 mL/min half usual dose or double interval. Further dose reduction with PI/r,PI/c, or EVG/c co-administration.

SIDE EFFECTS: GI intolerance, 4% (vs. 17% with erythromycin); transaminase elevation, 1%; headache, 2%; PMC, rare. There are 38 cases of neurotoxicity reported (J Clin Neurosci 2011;18:313).

DRUG INTERACTIONS: Clarithromycin is a substrate and inhibitor of CYP3A4. It increases levels of rifabutin 56%, and levels of clarithromycin are decreased 50%. Consider using azithromycin. Clarithromycin should not be combined with rifampin, ergot alkaloid, carbamazepine (Tegretol), cisapride (Propulsid), or pimozide (Orap); increased levels of pimozide and cisapride may cause fatal arrhythmias. The same concern for QTc prolongation applies to concurrent use with atazanavir and saquinavir. (Use 50% clarithromycin dose or use azithromycin, which has no substantial interaction with these drugs.) May increase serum level CYP3A4 substrates. See Table 6.22 for interactions and dose adjustments for clarithromycin use with MVC, integrase inhibitors, NNRTIs, and PIs.

PREGNANCY: Category C; teratogenic in rats and mice, but not in rabbits or monkeys. Experience with >100 first-trimester exposures in women showed no defects. Acceptable to use for MAC if no alternatives.

Clindamycin

TRADE NAME: Cleocin (Pharmacia) and generic.

FORMULATIONS, REGIMEN, AND COST:

Clindamycin HCl caps: 75 mg, $0.60; 150 mg, $1.20; 300 mg at $3.72.

Clindamycin oral solution: 75 mg/5 mL (100 mL) at $62.03.

Clindamycin PO$_4$ with 150 mg/mL in 2, 4, and 6 mL vials: 600 mg vial at $4.21; 900 mg at $5.70.

INDICATIONS AND DOSES:

PCP: Clindamycin 600–900 mg q8h IV or 450 mg q6–h po + primaquine 15–30 mg (base) po qd.

Toxoplasmosis: Clindamycin 600 mg IV or po q6h + pyrimethamine 200 loading dose, then 50 mg (<60 kg) or 75 mg po (>60 kg) qd + leucovorin 10–20 mg/d (may be increased to 50 mg/d).

Other infections: 600 mg IV q8h or 300–450 mg po q6–8h.

ACTIVITY: Most gram-positive cocci are susceptible except *Enterococcus* and some community-acquired methicillin-resistant *Staphylococcus aureus* (MRSA). Most anaerobic bacteria are susceptible, but IDSA guidelines for intraabdominal sepsis (CID 2010;50:133) do not include clindamycin due to increasing resistance by *B. fragilis* (20–30%).

SIDE EFFECTS: GI, diarrhea in 10–30%. Up to 6% of patients develop *C. difficile*-associated diarrhea; may be severe (Ann Intern Med 2006;145:758); most respond well to discontinuation of the implicated antibiotic ± metronidazole (500 mg tid × 10 days) or oral vancomycin (125 mg qid × 10– d) (Infect Control Hosp Epidemiol 2010;31:431). Other GI side effects include nausea, vomiting, and anorexia. *Rash*: Generalized morbilliform rash is most common; less common is urticaria, pruritus, Stevens-Johnson syndrome.

DRUG INTERACTIONS: Loperamide (Imodium) or diphenoxylate/atropine (Lomotil and other antiperistaltic drugs such as narcotics) may increase risk of *C. difficile*-associated colitis and should not be used for therapy.

PREGNANCY: Category B.

Clotrimazole

TRADE NAMES: Lotrimin (Schering-Plough), Mycelex (Bayer), Gyne-Lotrimin (Schering-Plough), FemCare (Schering), and generic.

CLASS: Imidazole (related to miconazole).

FORMULATIONS, REGIMEN, AND COST:

Troche 10 mg at $3.21.
Topical cream (1%) 15 g at $5.98; 45 g at $12.00.
Topical solution/lotion (1%) 10 mL at $25.79.
Vaginal cream (1%) 45 g at $12.00.

INDICATIONS AND DOSES:

Thrush: 10 mg troche 5×/d; must be dissolved in the mouth. Clotrimazole troches are only slightly less effective than fluconazole for thrush but are sometimes preferred to avoid azole resistance (HIV Clin Trials 2000;1:47). The problem is the need for 5 doses/d, although treatment with lower doses is often successful. Recommended duration in 2018 IDSA/NIH/CDC Guidelines is 7–14 days.

Dermatophytic infections and cutaneous candidiasis: Topical application of 1% cream, lotion, or solution to affected area bid × 2–8 wks; if no improvement, reevaluate diagnosis.

Candidal vaginitis: Fluconazole 150 mg × 1 *or* Intravaginal, vaginal cream: One applicator (about 5 g) intravaginally hs. Recommended duration in 2018 IDSA/NIH/CDC Guidelines is 3–7 days and daily intravaginal or fluconazole 150 mg once weekly use for suppressive therapy in women with severe recurrent disease.

ACTIVITY: Active against *Candida* species and dermatophytes.

PHARMACOLOGY:

Bioavailability: Lozenge (troche) dissolves in 15–30 minutes; administration at 3-hr intervals maintains constant salivary concentrations above MIC of most *Candida* strains. Small amounts of drug are absorbed with oral, vaginal, or skin applications.

SIDE EFFECTS: Generally well tolerated. *Topical to skin (rare)*: Erythema, blistering, pruritus, pain, peeling, urticaria. *Topical to vagina (rare)*: Rash, pruritus, dyspareunia, dysuria, burning, erythema. *Lozenges*: Elevated AST (up to 15%; monitor LFTs); nausea and vomiting (5%).

PREGNANCY: Category C. May be used for oral or vaginal candidiasis.

Combivir—see Lamivudine; Zidovudine

Complera—see Rilpivirine; Emtricitabine, and Tenofovir

Crixivan—see Indinavir

Cytovene—see Ganciclovir

Cobicistat

TRADE NAME: Tybost.

FORMULATIONS, REGIME, AND COST: Trough CYP3A4 inhibition, cobicistat is indicated to enhance the pharmacokinetics of darunavir, atazanavir, and elvitegravir.

Cobicistat (Tybost): 150 mg oral tabs at $246.84/mo.

Elvitegravir: 150 mg, cobicistat 150 mg, tenofovir DF 300 mg, emtricitabine 200 mg tab (Stribild) at $3,707.99/mo.

Elvitegravir: 150 mg, cobicistat 150 mg, tenofovir alafenamie 10 mg, emtricitabine 200 mg tab (Genvoya) at $3,306.92/mo.

Darunavir: 800 mg/cobicistat 150 mg tab (Precobix) at $2,009.23/mo.

Atazanavir: 300 mg/cobicistat 150 mg tab (Evotaz) at $ 1,926.56/mo.

USUAL ADULT DOSING:

Dose when co-formulated with Elvitegravir, TDF, and FTC: Stribild 1 tablet (Elvitegravir [EVG] 150 mg, cobicistat [COBI] 150 mg, TDF 300 mg, FTC 200 mg) once-daily with food.

Dose when co-formulated with Elvitegravir, TAF, and FTC: Genvoya 1 tablet (Elvitegravir [EVG] 150 mg, cobicistat [COBI] 150 mg, TAF 10 mg, FTC 200 mg) once-daily with food.

With darunavir in treatment-naïve or treatment-experienced with no DRV mutations: DRV 800 mg/cobicistat 150 mg once-daily with food.

With atazanavir in treatment-naïve and treatment-experienced patients: Atazanavir 300 mg/cobicistat 150 mg once-daily with food.

RENAL DOSING:

EVG/COBI/TDF/FTC: CrCl >70 mL/min: use standard dose; avoid use in patient with CrCl <70 mL/min when combined with TDF.

EVG/COBI/TAF/FTC: CrCl >30 mL/min: use standard dose; avoid use in patient with CrCl <30 mL/min when combined with TDF. No renal dose adjustment needed with ATV/COBI or DRV/COBI.

CLINICAL TRIALS:
Study 114; Tybost FDA labeling: Treatment-naïve patients with CrCL >70 mL/min were randomized to ATV/COBI/TDF/FTC or ATV/r/TDF/FTC. Patients were well matched at baseline with 40% of patients with VL >100,000 copies/mL and a mean CD4 cell count of 352 cells/mm^3. At 48 wks, 85% and 87% of ATV/COBI/TDF/FTC- and ATV/r/TDF/FTC-treated patients had an undetectable VL, respectively. Both regimens were well tolerated with comparable discontinuation rate of 6–7%.

SIDE EFFECTS:
Generally well tolerated. In clinical trials with COBI-boosted EVG, only 3.7% of patients experienced ADR leading to EVG/COBI/TDF/FTC discontinuation compared to 5.1% of patients requiring discontinuation of EFV/TDF/FTC or ATV/rTDF/FTC.

- Nausea, diarrhea, vomiting, flatulence; nausea more common compared to EFV/TDF/FTC, but comparable to ATV/r TDF/FTC.
- COBI decreases tubular secretion of creatinine, resulting in increase in Scr and decrease in eGFR without change in measured GFR by iohexol clearance. Mean increase in Scr of 0.14 mg/dL (+ /− 0.13 µg/dL).

DOSING FOR DECREASED HEPATIC FUNCTION: Child-Pugh Class A and B: usual dose. Child-Pugh Class C: no data.

PHARMACOLOGY:
COBI has no anti-HIV activity, but increases CYP3A4 substrate drug concentrations (e.g., EVG, ATV, DRV). Relative to fasting conditions, light meal (~373 Kcal, 20% fat) and high-fat meal (~800 Kcal, 50% fat) increases EVG concentrations by 34% and 87%, respectively. COBI is metabolized by CYP3A and to a lesser extent CYP2D6. Approximately 86.2% of COBI is excreted predominantly in feces.

Protein binding: 97–98%.

$T^{1/2}$: 3.5 hrs.

Pharmacokinetics of COBI boosted DRV and ATV were bioequivalent to RTV boosted DRV and ATV.

DRUG INTERACTIONS:

COBI is a major substrate of CYP3A4, and minor substrate of CYP2D6.

COBI is inhibitor of CYP3A4, CYP2D6, and several transporters (P-gp, BCRP, OATP1B1, and OATP1B3). Substrates of these isoenzymes and transporters may be significantly increased.

COBI is modest inducer of CYP2C9; substrates of CYP2C9 may be decreased.

Contraindicated with the following drugs: Alfuzosin, rifampin, dronedarone, all ergot derivatives (e.g., dihydroergotamine, ergotamine, methylergonovine), cisapride, St. John's wort, lovastatin, simvastatin, pimozide, high dose sildenafil, triazolam, and oral midazolam.

The following drugs should be avoided with COBI: Ranolazine, flecainide, propafenone, bepridil, dofetilide, amiodarone, quinidine, dronedarone, fluticasone, salmeterol, eplerenone, lurasidone, ivabradine, flibanserin, fluticasone, silodosin, dospirenone (w/ ATV/c). Rivaroxaban, betrixaban, ticagrelor, and vorapaxar (may increase risk of bleed).

Dose adjustment needed with edoxaban, apixiban, and dabigatran based on renal function and indication.

Avoid co-administration with the following drugs: CYP 3A4 enzyme inducing anticonvulsants (carbamazepine, oxcarbazepine, phenobarbital, phenytoin), rifabutin, rifapentine.

No significant interaction with digoxin.

Cobicistat may increase concentrations of the following drugs:

Alfuzosin: Contraindicated. Consider doxazosin and terazosin for BPH (with close monitoring).

Amiodarone: Use with caution; monitor antiarrhythmic concentrations with dose adjustment.

Anticancer agents (e.g., dasatinib, nilotinib, vinblastine, vincristine): May require dose adjustment of dasatinib, nilotinib, vinblastine, vincristine with COBI co-administration. Monitor for therapeutic response and adverse drug reactions.

Astemizole: Contraindicated due to the potential for cardiac arrhythmia.

Atorvastatin: Start with low dose atorvastatin and titrate slowly. Avoid doses >40 mg/d.

Avanafil: Avoid co-administration of avanafil with COBI. Consider dose adjusted sildenafil, vardenafil, or tadalafil.

Bepridil: Use with caution; monitor antiarrhythmic concentrations with dose adjustment.

β-blocker (e.g., metoprolol, timolol, carvedilol); Concentrations of β-blocker that are CYP2D6 substrate may be increased. Use low-dose metoprolol, timolol, and carvedilol with slow titration. May consider atenolol.

Benzodiazepine (i.e., alprazolam, chlordiazepoxide, clonazepam, clorazepate, diazepam, estazolam, flurazepam, midazolam, triazolam). Oral midazolam contraindicated. Low dose IV midazolam can be considered with close clinical monitoring. Avoid triazolam co-administration. Other benzodiazepines that are CYP3A substrate may need dose adjustment. Consider lorazepam, temazepam, or oxazepam with COBI co-administration.

Bosentan: May significantly increase bosentan serum concentrations. No data. Recommendation based on RTV co-administration. Co-administer bosentan only after COBI dosing has reached steady-state. In patients on COBI (with DRV or ATV) for at least 10 days: start bosentan at 62.5 mg once-daily or every other day. In patients already on bosentan: discontinue bosentan for ≥36 hrs prior to initiation of cobicistat and restart bosentan at 62.5 mg once-daily or every other day after cobicistat (plus DRV or ATV) have reached steady-state (after 10 days). Consider ambrisentan for pulmonary HTN.

Buprenorphine: Monitor for possible increased sedation.

Buspirone: Buspirone dose may need to be decreased. Monitor for ADR (i.e., dizziness, drowsiness).

Calcium channel blockers (e.g., amlodipine, diltiazem, felodipine, nifedipine, verapamil, and nicardipine): Use with close monitoring. Consider decreasing calcium channel blockers dose by 50%, then titrate to effect.

Cisapride: Contraindicated due to potential for QTc prolongation and cardiac arrhythmia.

Clarithromycin: Clarithromycin and COBI may be increased. Dose: adjust clarithromycin dose according to renal function. CrCl >60 mL/min, use standard dose; CrCl <50–60 mL/min, 50% of clarithromycin dose. Avoid with QTc prolongation. Consider alternative (e.g., azithromycin).

Colchicine: No data. Recommendation based on RTV data. In patients with normal renal and hepatic function: Colchicine 0.6 mg × 1, followed by 0.3 mg 1 hr later for acute gout flare. Dose may be repeated no earlier than 3 days. For gout prophylaxis, use 25% of the original dose. Monitor closely for bone marrow suppression.

Cyclosporine: Use with dose adjustment and close monitoring of cyclosporine serum concentrations.

Disopyramide: Use with caution; monitor antiarrhythmic concentrations with dose adjustment.

Dronedarone: May significantly increase dronedarone concentrations. Contraindicated.

Efavirenz: Efavirenz concentrations decreased 7%. EFV may decrease COBI, DRV, and ATV with co-administration. DRV/COBI plus EFV not recommended. ATV 400 mg plus COBI 150 mg once-daily recommended in treatment-naïve patients only.

Etravirine: May decrease COBI and ATV concentrations. Co-administration of DRV/COBI or ATV/COBI with ETR is not recommended.

Ergot alkaloid (e.g., dihydroergotamine, ergotamine, methyle rgonovine): Contraindicated due to the potential for acute ergotism.

Erythromycin: Erythromycin, COBI, ATV, DRV, and EVG may be increased. Consider alternative (e.g., azithromycin). Avoid with QTc prolongation.

Everolimus: Monitor everolimus serum concentrations closely with proper dose adjustments.

Ethosuximide: Use with close monitoring.

Fentanyl: COBI may significantly increase fentanyl concentrations. Avoid or use low-dose fentanyl with close monitoring for adverse effects (including potential for respiratory depression).

Flecainide: Use with caution; monitor antiarrhythmic concentrations with dose adjustment.

HCV antivirals: Co-administration not recommended with boceprevir, simeprevir, grazoprevir, elbasvir, dasabuvir, ombitasvir, paritaprevir. Usual dose with sofosbuvir, velpatasvir. Daclastavir 60 mg/d with DRV/COBI. Dose not established with ledipasvir co-administration (use ATV/r or DRV/r).

HMG-CoA reductase inhibitors (e.g., pravastatin, atorvastatin, and rosuvastatin): Atorvastatin concentrations may be increased with COBI co-administration. Rosuvastatin concentrations increased 38%. Simvastatin and lovastatin contraindicated. Start with the lowest dose statins (rosuvastatin, atorvastatin) and titrate to effect. Interaction unlikely with pitavastatin and fluvastatin.

Inhaled and intranasal steroid (e.g., fluticasone, budesonide): Avoid co-administration if possible. Concurrent use of fluticasone or budesonide and COBI might lead to increased fluticasone plasma concentrations resulting in Cushing's syndrome. Consider beclomethasone.

Indinavir: When co-administered with ATV/COBI, both indinavir and atazanavir can significantly increase indirect bilirubin. Contraindicated.

Irinotecan: When co-administered with ATV/COBI, irinotecan concentrations may be significantly increased. Contraindicated with ATV/COBI co-administration.

Itraconazole: Monitor itraconazole serum with co-administration. Titrate itraconazole dose to target concentration of >1–2 µg/mL.

Ketoconazole: COBI and ketoconazole may be increased Alternative antifungal can be considered (e.g., fluconazole).

Lidocaine (systemic): Use with caution; monitor antiarrhythmic concentrations with dose adjustment.

Lovastatin: Contraindicated. Consider alternative statin (pravastatin, atorvastatin, and rosuvastatin, pitavastatin) with close monitoring.

Methadone: May increase methadone exposure. No data. Monitor for increased sedation.

Mexiletine: Use with caution; monitor antiarrhythmic concentrations with dose adjustment.

Midazolam (oral): Contraindicated with PO midazolam due to potential for increased sedation. Use IV midazolam with very close monitoring. Consider lorazepam.

Maraviroc: With DRV/COBI or ATV/COBI, decrease maraviroc to 150 mg twice-daily recommended. With EVG + COBI co-administration, consider MVC 150 mg twice-daily.

Neuroleptics (perphenazine, risperidone, thioridazine, haloperidol, aripiprazole, fluphenazine, quetiapine, ziprasidone): May need a lower dose of the neuroleptic. Monitor for ADR.

Nevirapine: With ATV/COBI co-administration, ATV concentrations may be decreased and NVP concentrations may be increased resulting in NVP-associated toxicity. Contraindicated.

Oral contraceptives (e.g., Norgestimate/ethinyl estradiol): With EVG/COBI co-administration, norgestimate AUC increased

126%. Ethinyl estradiol AUC decreased 22% and 30%with ATV/COBI and DRV/COBI co-administration, respectively. An additional or alternative barrier form of contraception should be considered.

Phenobarbital: May significantly decrease COBI and co-administered ARV (EVG, ATV, DRV) concentrations. Avoid co-administration. Consider valproic acid or levetiracetam. If co-administration can't be avoided, monitor phenobarbital concentrations and virologic response closely.

Phenytoin: May significantly decrease COBI and co-administered ARV (EVG, ATV, DRV) concentrations. Avoid co-administration. Consider valproic acid or levetiracetam. If co-administration can't be avoided, monitor phenytoin concentrations and virologic response closely.

Pimozide: Contraindicated due to potential for QTc prolongation and cardiac arrhythmia.

Pravastatin: Pravastatin concentrations may be increased. No data. Consider starting with 10 mg once-daily and titrate slowly.

Prednisone and methylprednisolone: Concurrent use of prednisone and COBI may lead in increased prednisolone plasma concentrations. May require a lower prednisone dose with long-term co-administration.

Propafenone: Use with caution; monitor antiarrhythmic concentrations with dose adjustment.

Proton pump inhibitor (e.g., omeprazole): Concentrations of ATV may be decreased with ATV/COBI coadministration. Avoid ATV/COBI co-administration with PPIs in treatment-experienced patients. Although separating omeprazole 20 mg and ATV/COBI administration time by 12 hrs can be considered in treatment-naïve patients, the author recommends using an alternative PI/COBI (e.g., DRV/COBI).

Quinidine: Use with caution; monitor antiarrhythmic concentrations with dose adjustment.

Ranolazine: Avoid co-administration.

Ribavirin: Use standard dose.

Rifabutin: EVG AUC and Cmin decreased by 21% and 67%, respectively. Rifabutin AUC decreased by 8%, but rifabutin active metabolite (25-O-desacetyl rifabutin) AUC increased 6.25-fold. Rifabutin 150 mg every other day recommended with COBI co-administration. Effects on ATV and DRV concentration are unknown; monitor closely for virologic response. Monitor rifabutin concentrations and potential adverse reactions (e.g., uveitis and neutropenia).

Rilpivirine: Usual dose recommended when RPV is co-administered with DRV/COBI or ATV/COBI. Consider monitoring QTc in patients at risk for QTc prolongation.

Rivaroxaban: Avoid co-administration due to potential increased risk of bleed.

Rosuvastatin: Rosuvastatin AUC increased 38% with EVG/COBI. No change in EVG concentrations. Initiate with low dose rosuvastatin (5 mg) with co-administration.

Salmeterol: Avoid co-administration due to potential QTc prolongation. Consider formoterol.

Selective serotonin reuptake inhibitors (SSRIs; e.g., paroxetine): COBI may affect SSRI concentrations. Start with low dose then titrate SSRI to therapeutic effect.

Sildenafil: COBI may significantly increase sildenafil concentrations. Use of high-dose sildenafil for treatment of pulmonary hypertension is contraindicated with COBI (consider dose adjusted tadalafil). Do not exceed sildenafil 25 mg in 48 hr when used for erectile dysfunction.

Simvastatin: Contraindicated. Consider alternative statin (pravastatin, atorvastatin, rosuvastatin, pitavastatin) with close monitoring.

Sirolimus: Avoid or use with dose adjustment and close monitoring of sirolimus serum concentrations.

Tacrolimus: Use with dose adjustment and close monitoring of tacrolimus serum concentration.

Tadalafil: Dose recommendation based on RTV co-administration data. Consider dose adjustment for ED: tadalafil 10 mg q72h. *For pulmonary HTN:* Once COBI is at steady-state (1 wk), administer tadalafil 20 mg/d once-daily, then titrate to 40 mg/d.

Telithromycin: Telithromycin, EVG, DRV, ATV, and COBI concentrations may be increased. Consider alternative antibiotic (e.g., azithromycin, fluoroquinolone). Monitor for hepatitis.

Tenofovir: No pharmacokinetic interactions. Monitor urine glucose, urine protein, Scr, and serum phosphate in patients at risk for renal impairment.

Terfenadine: Contraindicated due to potential for cardiac arrhythmia.

Tipranavir (TPV): COBI AUC decreased by 95%. TPV AUC decreased 54% with cobicistat compared to TVP/r. Avoid co-administration.

Trazodone: Use with dose adjustment and close monitoring. SSRI preferred due to better safety profile.

Tricyclic antidepressants (e.g., desipramine, amitriptyline, imipramine, nortriptyline, bupropion): Desipramine AUC increased 65%. Other TCAs concentrations may also be increased. Start with low-dose TCA and monitor for ADRs. SSRI preferred due to better safety profile.

Triazolam: Contraindicated due to potential for increased sedation. Consider lorazepam.

Vardenafil: COBI may significantly increase vardenafil concentrations. Avoid high-dose vardenafil. Dose adjustment: vardenafil 2.5 mg q72h.

Zolpidem: Zolpidem dose may need to be decreased.

Cobicistat concentrations may be decreased with the following drugs:

Carbamazepine and oxcarbazepine: Avoid co-administration. Consider valproic acid or levetiracetam. If co-administration can't be avoided, monitor carbamazepine concentrations and antiretroviral efficacy closely.

Dexamethasone: Dexamethasone (at steady-state) may decrease COBI (and co-administered ARV e.g., ATV, DRV and EVG) concentrations. Consider alternative corticosteroid (e.g., prednisone or methylprednisolone).

Rifampin: Rifampin may significantly decrease COBI, EVG, ATV, DRV concentrations. Contraindicated. Consider alternative antimycobacterial agent (e.g., fluoroquinolone, rifabutin).

Rifapentine: Rifapentine may significantly decrease COBI, ATV, DRV, and EVG concentrations. Avoid co-administration. Consider alternative antimycobacterial agent (e.g., fluoroquinolone, rifabutin).

St. John's wort: May significantly decrease ATV, DRV, COBI and EVG serum concentration. Contraindicated.

Enzalutamide and mitotane- May significantly decrease COBI. Avoid

Therapeutic drug monitoring recommended with the following drugs:

Voriconazole: COBI may increase or decrease Voriconazole serum concentration due to CYP3A4 inhibition and CYP2C9 potential induction. Co-administration is recommended only if the benefit outweigh risk. Monitor voriconazole serum concentration (target Cmin >2 µg/mL) with co-administration.

Warfarin: Warfarin concentrations may be increased or decreased due to CYP3A inhibition and potential CYP2C9 induction. Use with close INR monitoring.

Trimethoprim: Similar to COBI, high-dose trimethoprim may inhibit tubular secretion of creatinine resulting in an additive increase in Scr. Co-administration may result in an additive increase in Scr. Unless direct measurement of GFR (i.e., iohexol) can be performed, discontinuation is recommended with a Scr elevation of >0.4 mg/dL.

PREGNANCY: Category B. Not teratogenic in animal studies. Limited human data. Ritonavir is the preferred boosting agent for ATV and DRV in pregnancy (2018 Perinatal DHHS guidelines).

Dapsone

TRADE NAME: Generic.

CLASS: Synthetic sulfone that inhibits folic acid synthesis.

FORMULATIONS, REGIMEN, AND COST: Tabs: 25 mg at $1.06, 100 mg at $1.30.

COMPARISON PRICES FOR PCP PROPHYLAXIS:

Dapsone (100 mg/d): $39.00/mo.

TMP-SMX (1 DS/d): $39.60/mo.

Aerosolized pentamidine: $154.06/mo (plus administration costs).

Atovaquone (1500 mg/d): $2085.60/mo.

EFFICACY: A review of 40 published studies found dapsone (100 mg/d) to be slightly less effective than TMP-SMX for PCP prophylaxis, but comparable with aerosolized pentamidine and highly cost-effective (CID 1998;27:191). For PCP

TABLE 6.24 Dapsone indications and dose regimens

Indication	Dose Regimen
PCP prophylaxis	100 mg po qd
PCP treatment (mild to moderately severe)	100 mg po qd (plus trimethoprim 15 mg/kg/d po, in 3 doses) × 3 wks
PCP + toxoplasmosis prophylaxis	50 mg po qd (plus pyrimethamine 50 mg/wk plus folinic acid 25 mg/wk) or dapsone 200 mg (+ pyrimethamine 75 mg + leucovorin 25 mg) once weekly

treatment, dapsone/trimethoprim is as effective as TMP-SMX for patients with mild or moderately severe disease (Ann Intern Med 1996;124:792) and is a recommended alternative for regimen for mild to moderate PCP (2018 OI guidelines).

PHARMACOLOGY:

Bioavailability: Nearly completely absorbed except with gastric achlorhydria (dapsone is insoluble at neutral pH).

$T^{1/2}$: 10–56 hrs (average 28 hrs).

Elimination: Hepatic concentration, enterohepatic circulation, maintains tissue levels 3 wks after treatment is discontinued.

Dose modification in renal failure: None.

SIDE EFFECTS:

Most common in AIDS patients: Rash, pruritus, hepatitis, and hemolytic anemia in up to 20–40% receiving dapsone prophylaxis for PCP at a dose of 100 mg/d.

Most serious reaction: Dose-dependent hemolytic anemia, with or without glucose-6 phosphate dehydrogenase (G6PD) deficiency, and methemoglobinemia; rare cases of agranulocytosis (0.2–0.4%) and aplastic anemia. Suggested monitoring includes screening for G6PD deficiency prior to treatment in high-risk patients. The defect is not always a contraindication to high-risk drugs since most patients with positive tests tolerate these drugs (see below). An exception is patients with the high-risk variant of G6PD deficiency. A review of G6PD deficiency prevalence in 1,172 HIV-infected patients in Houston showed deficiency in 75 (6.8%): Blacks 66/699 (9.7%); Hispanics 5/253 (2.0%), and whites 1/153 (0.7%) (J Infect 2010;61:399). During follow-up, 40 patients with deficiency given TMP-SMX or dapsone; 5 (7%)

developed hemolytic anemia (the trigger was TMP/SMX in 4 cases). This study did not define the degree of G6PD deficiency. Other studies have shown hemolysis, and Heinz body formation is exaggerated in patients with G6PD deficiency, methemoglobin reductase deficiency, or hemoglobin M.

Asymptomatic methemoglobinemia independent of G6PD deficiency has been found in up to two-thirds of patients receiving dapsone 100 mg/d plus trimethoprim (NEJM 1990;373:776). Acute *methemoglobinemia* is uncommon, but the usual features are dyspnea, fatigue, cyanosis, deceptively high pulse oximetry, and chocolate-colored blood (JAIDS 1996;12:477). Methemoglobin levels are related to the dose and duration of dapsone therapy; TMP increases dapsone levels, so TMP may precipitate methemoglobinemia. Methemoglobin levels are usually <25%, which is generally tolerated except in patients with lung disease. Patients with glutathione or G6PD deficiency are at increased risk. The usual laboratory findings are increased indirect bilirubin, haptoglobin <25 mg/dL, elevated LDH, and a smear showing spherocytes and fragmented red blood cells (RBCs). Treatment for severe hemolysis consists of oxygen supplementation, transfusion for anemia, and discontinuation of the implicated drug. This is usually adequate if the methemoglobin level is <30%. Activated charcoal (20 g qid) may be given to reduce dapsone levels. Treatment for severe cases in the absence of G6PD deficiency is IV methylene blue (1–2 mg/kg by slow IV infusion). In less emergent situations, methylene blue may be given orally (3–5 mg/kg q4–6h); methylene blue should not be given with G6PD deficiency because methylene blue reduction requires G6PD; hemodialysis also enhances elimination.

GI intolerance: Common; may reduce by taking with meals.

Infrequent ADRs: Headache, dizziness, peripheral neuropathy. Rare side effect is "sulfone syndrome" after 1–4 wks of treatment, consisting of fever, malaise, exfoliative dermatitis, hepatic necrosis, lymphadenopathy, and anemia with methemoglobinemia (Arch Dermatol 1981;117:38).

DRUG INTERACTIONS: *Decreased dapsone absorption*: H$_2$ blockers, antacids, omeprazole, and other proton pump inhibitors. Dapsone levels decreased 7- to 10-fold by rifampin; use alternative. *Coumadin*, increased hypoprothrombinemia; *pyrimethamine*, increased marrow toxicity (monitor CBC); *probenecid*, increases dapsone levels; *primaquine*, hemolysis due to G6PD deficiency. *Trimethoprim*, increases levels of both drugs; monitor for methemoglobinemia.

RELATIVE CONTRAINDICATIONS: *G6PD deficiency*: Monitor hematocrit and methemoglobin levels if anemia develops.

PREGNANCY: Category C. No data in animals; limited experience in pregnant patients with Hansen's disease shows no toxicity. Can be used for PCP prophylaxis in pregnant women. Hemolytic anemia with passage in breast milk reported (CID 1995;21[suppl 1]:S24).

Daraprim—see Pyrimethamine

Darunavir (DRV)

TRADE NAME: Prezista (Janssen); Prezcobix (co-formulated with cobicistat).

CLASS: Protease inhibitor.

FORMULATIONS, REGIMEN, COST: 75 mg, 150 mg, 600 mg; 800 mg tablets; 100 mg/mL suspension (200 mL); Co-formulations: DRV/COBI 800-100 mg tablet; DRV/COBI/TAF/FTC 800-150-10-200 mg tablet

DRV/r 800/100 mg/d or DRV/r 600/100 mg bid ($1,757.77/mo plus RTV cost); DRV/COBI 800–150 mg ($2,009.23/mo); DRV/COBI/TAF/FTC 800-150-10-200 mg tablet ($4178/month)

PATIENT ASSISTANCE AND INFORMATION: 866-836-0114 (toll-free in US).

Treatment-naïve: DRV/r 800/100 mg/d or DRV/COBI 800/150 mg/d. Treatment-experienced with no DRV-associated resistance mutations (11I, 32I, 33F, 47V, 50V, 54M, 74P, 84V, 89V): DRV/r 800/100 mg/d or DRV/COBI 800/150 mg/d with food.

Treatment-experienced with 1 or more DRV resistance mutation (listed above): DRV/r 600/100 mg twice-daily with food.

Food: Take with food.

Renal failure: No dose adjustment, but with CrCL <70 mL/min avoid co-administration of DRV/COBI and TDF.

Hepatic failure: No dose adjustments for mild to moderate hepatic impairment; not recommended for severe hepatic impairment.

Storage: 15–30°C (59–86°F).

ACTIVITY: Median EC_{50} against clinical and lab strains, range 0.7–5 ng/mL; activity includes group M (A-G), O, and HIV-2.

ADVANTAGES: Potent anti-HIV activity; excellent activity against HIV strains that are resistant to other PIs; relatively good tolerability and less lipid effects than LPV/r; as effective with less discontinuation due to adverse events compared to ATV/r for treatment-naïve patients; cobicistat co-formulation and once-daily dosing in treatment-naïve patients and treatment-experienced patients with no DRV resistance mutations; good CNS penetration; resistance relatively uncommon with DRV/r-based ART. When combined with TDF/FTC or TAF/FTC, DRV/r can be recommended for patients in certain clinical scenarios.

DISADVANTAGES: Food requirement, RTV or cobicistat requirement, relatively high rate of rash reactions.

CLINICAL TRIALS:

TREATMENT-NAÏVE: *ARTEMIS Trial (Table 5-21A)*: DRV/r vs. LPV/r in treatment-naïve patients with a VL >5000 c/mL and any CD4 count. Participants were randomized to DRV/r (800/100 mg/d) or LPV/r (400/100 mg bid or 800/200 mg/d in combination with TDF/FTC). All patients received TDF/FTC (AIDS 2008;22:1389).

TABLE 6.25 ARTEMIS Trial—DRV/r vs. LPV/r in treatment-naïve patients: 96-wk results

	DRV/r[a] 800/100 qd n = 343	LPV/r[a] 400/100 bid or 800/200 qd n = 346
Baseline		
Viral load (median) (c/mL)	70,800	62,100
CD4 count (median) (cells/mm^3)	228	218
VL >100,000 c/mL	36%	36%
Results (96 wk)		
VL <50 c/mL	79%	71%[b]
Baseline >100,000	76%	63%[b]
CD4 change (cells/mm^3)	+ 171	+ 188
Adverse drug reactions (ADR)		
Discontinuations for ADRs	4%	9%[b]
Diarrhea	4%	11%[b]
Gr 2-4 ↑ Total cholesterol	18%	28%[b]
Triglyceride (median) (mg/dL)	+ 18	+ 56[b]

From AIDS 2009;23:1679.

[a] All patients received TDF/FTC.
[b] p <0.05.

DRV/r was equivalent to LPV/r in virologic response, showed better tolerability, and had a better lipid profile (AIDS 2009;23:1679). A post-hoc analysis found suboptimal adherence had minimal effect on virologic outcome with DRV/r but a much greater effect on LPV/r (76% vs. 53%; p <0.01) (JAC 2010;65:1505). Only 6 of the 31 virologic failures were associated with PI resistance mutations (AIDS 2009;23:1829).

TREATMENT EXPERIENCED: *TITAN Trial (Early virologic failure)*: DRV/r (600/100 mg bid) + optimized background regimen (OBR) vs. LPV/r (400/100 mg bid) + OBR in patients who had failed prior therapy and were naïve to LPV/r (Lancet 2007;370:49).

TABLE 6.26 TITAN trial comparing DRV/r- and LPV/r-based ART in patient with virologic failure on PI-based ART at 48 wks

	DRV/r n = 286	LPV/r. n = 293
Baseline		
Viral load ($\log_{10}$ median)	4.3	4.3
CD4 count (median) (cells/mm³)	235	230
Prior PI therapy ≥ 2 agents	32%	30%
Outcome at 48 wks		
Virologic failure (VL >400 c/mL)	10%	22%[a]
No. with primary PI resistance mutations	6	20
No. with NRTI resistance mutations	4	15
CD4 count (median) (cells/mm³)	+ 97	+ 102
Discontinuations due to adverse reactions	7%	7%

From AIDS 2009;23:1829.
[a] P = <0.05.

At 48 wks, DRV/r was superior to LPV/r in virologic outcome, although statistically significant superiority was not maintained when patients with baseline LPV resistance were excluded (AIDS 2009;23:1829). At 96 wks, VL was <50 c/mL in 60% of DRV/r recipients compared with 55% of LPV/r recipients. The frequency of diarrhea was significantly greater in LPV/r recipients (15% vs. 8%, $p = 0.01$); lipid changes were similar in the two groups, and more of the virologic failures in the LPV/r arm had PI resistance mutations (AIDS 2009;23:1829).

DUET-1 and -2: These two trials examined the potential benefit of ETR in patients starting DRV/r as part of a salvage regimen. Criteria for enrollment were virologic failure with ≥1 NNRTI mutations, ≥3 primary PI mutations and a VL >5,000 c/mL. All patients received DRV/r + an optimized background regimen (OBR).

The 24-wk results were reported for DUET-1 (Lancet 2007;370:29) and DUET-2 (Lancet 2007;370:39). Table 6.27 presents pooled 48-wk results of the two trials (AIDS 2009;23:2289; Expert Opin Pharmacother 2010;11:1433). Viral suppression to <50 c/mL was achieved in 57% of the ETR recipients vs. 36% of the controls, the mean CD4 count increases were 128 vs. 86/mm³, respectively, and rash was more common in the ETR group (21% vs. 12%) (Antiviral Ther 2010;15:1045). At 96 wks, viral suppression to <50 c/mL was maintained in all but 3% of those who had viral suppression at 48 wks (57% vs. 60%) (Antivir Ther 2010;15:1045).

TABLE 6.27 DUET-1 and -2: DRV/r + ETR + OBR vs. DRV/r + OBR: 48 wk results with pooled data for both trials

	DRV/r + ETR + OBR n = 599	DRV/r + Placebo + OBR n = 604
Baseline (median)		
HIV VL $\log_{10}$ c/mL	4.8	4.9
CD4 count (cells/mm³)	99	109
Results (48 wks)		
VL <50 c/mL	61%	40%[a]
CD4 count ↑ (cells/mm³)	+ 98	+ 73[b]
Active OBR agents with DRV FC <10		
1	46%	6%
2	63%	32%
3	78%	67%
Resistance mutations with failure		
Major PI	1/28	0/29
184V	5	7
ADR—rash	19%	11%[b]

From AIDS 2009;23:2289.

[a] P = <0.0001/.
[b] P = 0.0006.

POWER-1 and -2 (Lancet 2007;369:1169) were phase IIb trials that compared DRV/r plus an OBR (≥2 NRTIs ± ENF) to comparator PI (CPI) + OBR in patients with VL >1,000 c/mL, prior treatment with PI-based ART, and at least one primary PI resistance mutation (30N, 46I/L, 48V, 50L/V, 82A/F/S/T, I84V, or 90M). The OBR included LPV/r (36%), FPV (34%), SQV (35%), and ATV (17%); 47% received ENF. DRV was superior to alternative regimens available at that time (Table 6.28). Combined 96-wk data for POWER-1 and -2 (*n* = 467) showed virologic suppression to <50 of 39% for DRV/r vs. 9% for CPI (Antiviral Ther 2009;14:859). See Tables 6.28, 6.29, and 6.30.

ODIN: A phase III open-labeled trial in which treatment-experienced patients with no DRV resistance mutations were randomized to DRV/r (600/100 mg bid) vs. DRV/r (800/100 mg/d). The 48-wk results with 490 participants showed nearly

TABLE 6.28 POWER-1 and -2: DRV/r + OBR vs. OBR: results at 48 wks

	DRV/r + OBR *n* = 131	Comparator PI + OBR *n* = 124
Baseline		
VL (log$_{10}$ c/mL median)	4.6	4.5
CD4 count (mean) (cells/mm^3)	153	163
≥3 primary PI mutations	54%	62%
Outcome at 48 wks		
VL <50 c/mL	67 (45%)[a]	12 (10%)
CD4 count D (median) (cells/mm^3)	+ 102[a]	+ 19
Discontinue for ADR	7%	5%
Resistance correlates		
1 active drug in OBR	17/34 (50%)	1/40 (5%)
≥2 active drugs	27/48 (56%)	10/60 (17%)

From Lancet 2007;369:1169.
[a]P = <0.05.

TABLE 6.29 DRV mutation score and outcome: POWER and DUET trials

No. Mutations	POWER (24 wks)		DUET (24 wks)	
	N	VL <50 c/mL	N	VL <50 c/mL
0	76	62%	67	64%
1	115	57%	94	50%
2	134	46%	113	42%
3	65	25%	58	22%
4	58	16%	41	10%

identical results for VL <50 c/mL (72.1% for once-daily dosing vs. 70.9% for twice-daily dosing) (Lathouwers E. ICAAC 2010;Abstr. H1811). The analysis also showed no difference based on baseline viral load, number of PI resistance mutations at baseline, the number of active NRTIs in the OBR, TLOVR results, number who developed DRV resistance (1 among 102 treatment failures), or the number who developed PI resistance mutations (12% vs. 10%).

TRIO: This is a Phase II, noncomparative multicenter trial involving 103 patients with multidrug resistant HIV defined as (1) >3 NRTI resistance mutations; (2) >3 PI resistance mutations

TABLE 6.30 Correlation between baseline phenotypic DRV resistance test results and virologic response (POWER)

Phenotype -Fold Change	N	VL <50 c/mL at 24 wks
0–2	136	60%
2–7	85	47%
7–30	63	24%
>30	56	18%

with <3 primary DRV mutations (11I, 32I, 33F, 47V, 50V, 54 L/M, 73S, 76V, 84V, 89V); (3) virologic failure on an NNRTI with <3 ETR mutations; and (4) VL >1,000 c/mL. Treatment consisted of RAL, ETR, and DRV/r with or without ENF and NRTIs. Participants had baseline resistance patterns showing a median of four primary PI mutations, one NNRTI mutation, and six NRTI mutations. At 48 wks, 89 (86%) had VL <50 c/mL (CID 2009;49:1441). At 96 wks, all patients with VL <50 c/mL at 48 wks had VL <400 c/mL on the TRIO regimen (Fagard C. 2011 CROI:Abstr. 549). Pharmacology studies demonstrated that ETR increases trough levels of DRV and RAL, but the PK was variable (AIDS 2010;24:2581).

MONET: A total of 256 patients who had viral suppression (<50 c/mL) for >24 wks with PI-based ART (57%) or NNRTI-based ART (43%) and a median baseline CD4 of 574/mm^3 were randomized to DRV/r monotherapy (800/100 mg/d) or DRV/r once-daily plus two NRTIs (AIDS 2010;24:223). At 48 wks, DRV/r monotherapy was noninferior to standard therapy (AIDS 2010;24:223) (Table 6.31). One PI resistance mutation emerged in each group (Antivir Ther 2011;16:59).

MONOI: This is another study of DRV/r monotherapy (600/100 mg bid) after viral suppression, which enrolled treatment-experienced patients with no prior history of PI failure. Virologic suppression was comparable at 48 wks (92% vs. 88%) (AIDS 2010;24:2365). At 96 wks, VL was <50 c/mL in 91/97 (94%) of the DRV/r (monotherapy) arm and 87/96 (90%) of the DRV/r + 2NRTI arm (Marc-Antoine V. 2011 CROI:Abstr. 534).

TABLE 6.31 MONET trial: DRV/r vs. DRV/r + 2 NRTIs: 48-wk results

	DRV/r *n = 127*	*DRV/r + 2 NRTIs* *n = 127*
HIV VL <50 c/mL	86.2%	87.8%
Intent-to-treat[a]	84.3%	85.3%

From AIDS 2010;24:223.
[a] Intent-to-treat with switch = failure.

NRTI-SPARING: *A5262: DRV/r + RAL*: The trial was a single-arm open-label study with 112 treatment-naïve patients given DRV/r (800/100 mg/d) + RAL (400 mg bid). At wk 48 there were 28 virologic failures including 11 who rebounded. Of the 28 failures, 13 (46%) had VL 50–200 c/mL. Higher failure rates correlated with low baseline CD4 count and VL >100,000 c/mL. Resistance testing showed five with RAL resistance mutations and no PI resistance mutations (Taiwo B., AIDS. 2011;25:2113.551).

DRV/r + EFV: In a pharmacokinetic study, DRV/r 900/100 mg/d was given for 10 days, followed by addition of EFV 600 mg/d (AAC 2010;54:2775). There was a 57% decrease in DRV trough levels and an increase in EFV AUC, but the results suggested adequate drug levels for treatment-naïve patients.

DRV/r + MVC: A pharmacokinetic trial of MVC 300 mg/d + DRV/r 800/100 qd demonstrated therapeutic MVC levels suggesting potential for further once-daily study (Taylor A. 2011 CROI:Abstr. 636). However, once-daily MVC when combined with DRV/r was inferior to DRV/r + TDF/FTC (Stellbrink et al., AIDS. 2016;30(8): 1229–1238).

RESISTANCE: No single PI mutation results in complete loss of DRV activity. Resistance is best determined by the cumulative number of resistance mutations ("DRV score") or by phenotypic resistance testing. Reduced in vitro and in vivo activity is seen with the following protease gene mutations: 11I, 32I, 33F, 47V, 50V, 54L/M, 73S, 74P, 76V, 84V, and 89V. The most common DRV resistance mutations are 33F, 32I, and 54L (AAC 2010;54:3018). Correlation was seen between the mutation score and virologic outcome in POWER and DUET trials and for baseline phenotype resistance test. Genotypic Interpretation Systems (GIS) performed well for predicting resistance phenotype in an analysis of 100 resistant HIV strains (AAC 2010;54:2473). As with other PI/r-based regimens, most virologic failures on DRV/r were not associated with PI or NRTI mutations (AIDS 2004;23:1829).

PHARMACOLOGY:

Renal failure: Pharmacology is not changed in persons with CrCl 30–60 mL/min; there are no data for patients CrCl <30 mL/min, but drug levels are unlikely to be affected.

Hepatic disease: Pharmacokinetics are not significantly altered by mild or moderate liver disease (Clin Pharmacokinet 2010;49:343). There are no data for severe hepatic failure; use with caution or the manufacturer suggest avoiding.

Bioavailability: 37% without RTV, 82% with RTV. RTV increases DRV exposure 14-fold. Food increases C_{max} and AUC 30%. DRV should always be given with RTV and food.

Single daily dose: A PK substudy from ARTEMIS showed a median DRV trough level at 24 hrs post dose (800/100 mg) of >1,000 ng/mL (median 3,300 ng/mL)—well above the EC_{50} of HIV, which is 55ng/mL for wild-type. A randomized trial with 590 treatment-naïve patients compared once-daily DRV/r (800/100 mg/d) to twice-daily DRV/r (600/100 mg bid), each combined with 2 NRTIs. Results at 48 wks showed 72% (qd) and 70% (bid) had VL <50 c/mL (AIDS 2011;25:929).

T½: 15 hrs when given with RTV.

CNS Penetration: 9.4%. Exceeded the CI_{50} of wild-type by 20-fold and scored highest in CNS penetration among PIs (JAIDS 2009;52:56). On the four-category CNS penetration scoring system, DRV ranks in category 3 (Neurology 2011;76:693) (see pg. 550t).

Excretion: Metabolized extensively by CYP3A; 80% recovered in stool, 4% in urine.

SIDE EFFECTS:

Hepatotoxicity: Drug-induced hepatitis is reported in 0.5% of patients given DRV/r; this includes serious fatal cases which are more common in patients with preexisting liver disease.

Rash: The manufacturer issued a warning on skin reactions to DRV in August 2009. Phase 3 studies showed Grade ≥2 rashes in 9%, Grade 3–4 in 1.3%; the drug was discontinued in 2%. Severe rashes including Stevens-Johnson syndrome and erythema multiforme have been reported (JAIDS 2010;53:614) but occurred in <0.1%. Rashes usually occur in the second week and resolve in 1–2 wks with continued treatment. Rash reactions are unusual after 4 wks of treatment. DRV should be stopped immediately if the rash is severe or accompanied by fever, malaise, fatigue, muscle or joint aches, blisters, oral lesions, facial edema, conjunctivitis, hepatitis, or eosinophilia. LFTs should be monitored. DRV contains a sulfonamide moiety and should be avoided in patients with severe sulfonamide allergy.

Metabolic effects: Glucose intolerance, fat redistribution, and lipodystrophy. Hyperglycemia (blood glucose ≥161 mg/dL) in 2–6%, triglycerides >400 mg/dL in 25%.

Transaminase elevations: >2.5 ULN in 10%.

GI intolerance: Diarrhea, vomiting, and/or abdominal pain in 2–3%.

Headache: 1–4%.

DRUG INTERACTIONS:

Drugs not recommended for concurrent use with DRV/r or DRV/ COBI: astemizole, cisapride, dexamethasone (at steady-state), dofetilide, ergot derivative, eplerenone, fentanyl, fluticasone, flibanserin, ivabradine, lurasidone, midazolam, triazolam, pimozide, terfenadine, triazolam, alfuzosin, bepridil, flecainide, propafenone, amiodarone, quinidine, dronedarone, ranolazine, salmeterol, simvastatin, lovastatin, rifampin, rifapentine, fluticasone, lidocaine, rifampin, rifapentine, phenobarbital, phenytoin, high dose sildenafil, St. John's wort, simvastatin, lovastatin, rivaroxaban, betrixaban, ticagrelor, vorapaxar, silodosin, enzalutamide, mitotane,

OTHER CAUTIONS:

Anticoagulant-edoxaban, apixiban, and dabigatran: may increase anticoagulant. Dose adjustment needed based on renal function and indication.

Antifungals—Ketoconazole and itraconazole: Increased levels of both azoles and DRV. *Voriconazole* AUC decreased 40%

by RTV 200 mg/d; use with caution, or avoid and monitor voriconazole trough.

Rifabutin: Use rifabutin 150 mg q24h. Consider rifabutin TDM.

Calcium channel blockers (felodipine, nifedipine, amlodipine, diltiazem, nicardipine): concentrations increased; monitor.

Steroids (dexamethasone, fluticasone): Dexamethasone may decrease levels of DRV; systemic steroid levels increased with inhaled fluticasone; consider alternatives, especially for long-term use.

Statins: Atorvastatin: AUC increased 4-fold; start with 10–20 mg and titrate up (max. 40 mg/d). *Pravastatin* AUC level increased by a mean of 81%, but 5-fold in some patients. Use lowest doses and monitor. Consider pitavastatin, no significant change in levels.

Immunosuppressants (cyclosporine, tacrolimus, sirolimus): Levels increased; reduce dose and monitor immunosuppressant levels closely.

Methadone: DRV/r decreases R-methadone 16%; monitor for withdrawal.

Oral contraceptives: Ethinyl estradiol levels decreased 44%; use alternative or additional birth control method.

PDE5 inhibitors (sildenafil, vardenafil, tadalafil): Do not exceed 25 mg sildenafil q48h, 2.5 mg vardenafil q72h, or 10 mg tadalafil q72h.

SSRIs (sertraline, paroxetine): AUC decreased 49% and 39%, respectively; monitor antidepressant response.

Clarithromycin: Levels of clarithromycin increased 59%; reduce dose 50% if CrCl 30–60 mL/min, 75% if CrCl <30 mL/min.

Warfarin: S-warfarin AUC decreased 21%. Monitor INR.

Trazodone: Levels and side effects (nausea, dizziness, hypotension) of trazodone may increase. Use lower dose or use with caution.

ddI: Should be taken 1 hr before or 2 hrs after DRV.

Antiarrhythmics: Bepridil, lidocaine, quinidine, amiodarone may increase levels; avoid.

Buprenorphine: Norbuprenorphine AUC increased 46%; no dose adjustment but monitor for sedation. *Carbamazepine*: DRV serum concentration unchanged, carbamazepine serum concentrations increased 45%. Monitor carbamazepine concentrations with co-administration.

Colchicine: DRV/r increases colchicine level, dose reduction required. After DRV/r has reached steady-state (10–14 days), colchicine 0.6 mg × 1, then 0.3 mg 1 hr later.

Concurrent use with other ARVs: The combination of DRV/r and EFV is of interest as a potential NRTI-sparing regimen. A pharmacokinetic study showed that EFV substantially reduced DRV trough levels (ratio 0.45), AUC (0.86), and half-life (0.56). Nevertheless, DRV levels were well above the EC_{50} for wild-type virus. The investigators suggested a daily regimen of DRV/r 900/100 mg + EFV 600 mg for an NRTI-sparing regimen in treatment-naïve patients (AAC 2010;54:2775). This study was performed before the 400 mg formulation of DRV was available; standard once-daily dose of 800/100 mg may be adequate.

PREGNANCY: Category C. DRV/r 600/100 mg po bid in combination with ABC/3TC or TDF/FTCis a preferred ARV regimen in pregnancy (2018 DHHS Perinatal HIV Guidelines). No evidence of human teratogenicity with 9 birth defects out of 425 first-trimester exposure (2.21%) (Antiretroviral Pregnancy Registry; July 2017). Case reports indicate low levels of DRV in pregnancy (Antiviral Ther 2010; AIDS 2009;23:1923; Antiviral Ther 2008;13:839; Antiviral Ther 2010;15:677), but all seven of these cases successfully prevented vertical transmission. A more recent report using once-daily dosing with DRV/r 800/100 mg showed trough levels >1,400 ng/mL in the second and third trimesters (AIDS 2010;24:1083), but the DHHS Perinatal HIV Guidelines recommend against DRV/r once-daily dosing.

TABLE 6.32 Dose adjustments for concurrent use of DRV with other antiretrovirals

Drug	Effect on Co-admin Drug	Effect on DRV AUC	Dose
RAL	—[a]	C_{min} ↓36%	Clinical significance unknown. Use standard dose DRV/r or DRV/cobi—good virologic suppression
DTG	DTG AUC decreased 22%	—	DTG 50 mg once-daily plus DRV/r standard dose.
EVG	DRV AUC ↓11%	EVG AUC 10%. (NS)	EVG 150 mg/d plus DRV/r 600/100 mg bid
BIC	BIC may ↑	—	Dose not established. Usual DRV/r dose likely.
ddI	—	—	ddI requires empty stomach so separate dosing; take ddI 1 hr before or 2 hrs after DRV/r
TDF	AUC ↑22%	—	No dose adjustment
EFV	AUC ↑21%	C_{min} ↓31%	DRV/r 600/100 po bid or consider DRV/r. 800–950/100 mg/d (PI-naïve patients)
NVP	AUC ↑27%	—	Standard doses both drugs
ATV/r	—	—	Standard DRV/r + ATV 300 mg/d yields comparable AUC to ATV/r when administered alone
IDV/r	↑23%	↑24%	Dose not established; avoid

TABLE 6.32 Continued

Drug	Effect on Co-admin Drug	Effect on DRV AUC	Dose
LPV/r	AUC↑37%	AUC ↓50%	Dose not established; avoid
SQV/r	—	AUC ↓25%	Dose not established; avoid
FPV, NFV, TPV	?	?	Not studied; Avoid co-administration
RTV	—	↑14-fold	Standard regimen: DRV/r 600/100 mg bid or DRV/r 800/100 mg/d
ETR	AUC ↓37%	—	Combination is well established with DRV/r 600/100 mg BID plus ETR 200 mg BID.
RPV	RPV AUC ↑130%	–	DRV/r 800/100 mg/d plus RPV 150 mg/d. Monitor QTc in patients at risk for prolongation.
MVC	↑4x	—	MVC 150 mg bid

[a] Indicates no clinically significant effect.

Daunorubicin Citrate Liposome Injection

TRADE NAME: DaunoXome (Gilead Sciences).

CLASS: Daunorubicin encapsulated within lipid vesicles or liposomes.

FORMULATIONS, REGIMEN, AND COST: Vials containing equivalent of 50 mg daunorubicin at $1,380/50 mg vial.

INDICATIONS AND DOSES: *Note*: Liposomal doxorubicin (Doxil), 20 mg/M^2 every 2–3 wks, is equally as effective.

FDA labeling: First-line cytotoxic therapy for advanced HIV-associated Kaposi's sarcoma (KS). Pegylated liposomal doxorubicin plus ART is often considered the preferred treatment for moderate to advanced KS (AIDS 2004;20:1737). Indications and treatment options. Administer IV over 60 minutes in dose of 40 mg/M^2; repeat every 2 wks. CBC should be obtained before each infusion and therapy withheld if absolute leukocyte count is <750/mL. Treatment is continued until there is evidence of tumor progression with new visceral lesions, progressive visceral disease, >10 new cutaneous lesions, or 25% increase in the number of lesions compared with baseline.

Dose adjustment for hepatic impairment: Bilirubin 1.2–3 mg/dL: 3/4 of a normal dose; bilirubin >3 mg/dL: 1/2 of normal dose.

CLINICAL TRIALS: Controlled trials comparing liposomal doxorubicin (Doxil) or liposomal daunorubicin vs. chemotherapy show better response and less toxicity with Doxil and DaunoXome, which are considered equivalent (Oncologist 2007;12:114–23; J Clin Oncol 1996;14:2353; J Clin Oncol 1998;16:2445; J Clin Oncol 1998;16:683). A randomized trial of pegylated liposomal doxorubicin vs. paclitaxel in 73 patients with advanced Kaposi's sarcoma showed similar response rates (56% vs. 46%) and similar 2-yr survival rates (79% vs. 78%) (Cancer 2010;116:3969).

PHARMACOLOGY: Mechanism of selectively targeting tumor cells is unknown. Once at the tumor, daunorubicin is released over time.

SIDE EFFECTS:

Granulocytopenia and mucositis are the most common toxicities requiring monitoring of the CBC (Clin Cancer Res 2001;7:3040).

Cardiotoxicity with decreased ejection fraction and congestive failure is the most serious side effect. It is most common in patients who have previously received anthracyclines or who have preexisting heart disease. Cardiac function (history and physical examination) should be evaluated before each infusion, and LVEF should be monitored when the total dose is 320 mg/M^2, 480 mg/M^2, and every 160 mg/m^2 thereafter.

The triad of back pain, flushing, and chest tightness is reported in 14%; this usually occurs in the first 5 minutes of treatment, resolves with discontinuation of the infusion, and does not recur with resumption of infusion at a slower rate.

Other: Alopecia, foot-hand syndrome (painful desquamating dermatitis of hands and feet), erythrodysesthesia and hyperpigmented lesions on mucous membranes of the mouth, and lines on nails (Dermatol Online 2008;14:18).

Care should be exercised to avoid drug extravasation, which can cause tissue necrosis.

DRUG INTERACTIONS: Additive bone marrow suppression with AZT, ganciclovir, sulfamethoxazole/trimethoprim, and pyrimethamine; monitor closely with co-administration.

PREGNANCY: Category D. Studies in rats showed severe maternal toxicity, embryo lethality, fetal malformations, and embryotoxicity.

ddl—see Didanosine

d4T—see Stavudine

Desyrel—see Trazodone

Didanosine

TRADE NAMES: Videx and Videx EC (Bristol-Myers Squibb) and generic.

CLASS: Nucleoside analog reverse transcriptase inhibitor (NRTI).

FORMULATIONS, REGIMEN, AND COST:

Enteric coated caps (Videx EC): 125, 200, 250, and 400 mg.
Generic ddI EC: 125, 200, 250, and 400 mg.

Pediatric powder: 2 g (4 oz) and 4 g (8 oz).

Regimen: Weight <60 kg, 250 mg/d. With TDF*, ddI 200 mg/d. Weight >60 kg, 400 mg/d. With TDF*, ddI 250 mg/d. *Combination is not recommended; see warnings.

Take 30 min before a meal or >2 hrs after a meal.

AWP: For 400 mg/d, $515.84 (brand)/mo or $368.72 (generic)/mo. Note: Pharmacy purchase price of generic is much lower than AWP.

COMBINATIONS:

ddI + d4T: Avoid co-administration. Increased risk of mitochondrial toxicity with increased rates of lactic acidosis, pancreatitis, and peripheral neuropathy (AIDS 2007;21:2455; JAIDS 2006;43:556; AIDS 2003;17:2045).

ddI + ABC: Avoid co-administration. Excessive rates of virologic failure, possibly due to selection of K65R mutation by both drugs.

ddI + TDF + NNRTI: High rates of virologic failure and blunted CD4 response. Avoid combination (CID 2005;41:901; AIDS 2004;18:459; Antivir Ther 2005;10:171).

TDF increases intracellular levels of ddI, risking ddI toxicity and poor immune recovery with a blunted CD4 response (AIDS 2005;19:1987). This is reduced with proper dose adjustment of ddI, but even the modified dose has been associated with excessive rates of virologic failure, best documented when combined with NNRTIs (see drug interactions) (AIDS 2005;19:213; CID 2005;41:901). As a consequence, the 2018 DHHS Guidelines have recommended avoidance of ddI + TDF + NNRTI. The European Agency for Evaluation of Medicinal Products recommends avoiding TDF + ddI completely (www.mmhiv.com/link/EAEMA-ddi-TDF).

FOOD EFFECT: Food decreases ddI EC levels 55%; must take >30 min before or ≥2 hr after meal.

HEPATIC FAILURE: Standard dose.

PATIENT ASSISTANCE PROGRAM: 800-272-4878 (8 AM–5 PM CST Mon.–Fri.).

ADVANTAGES: Once-daily therapy; extensive experience and, active against some AZT- and d4T-resistant strains depending on the number of TAMs.

DISADVANTAGES: Need for empty stomach; toxicity profile including pancreatitis, neuropathy, and other mitochondrial toxicities; restricted use with TDF and d4T, and contraindicated with ribavirin. Limited data in regimens not including AZT or d4T. Potential for cross-resistance with TDF and ABC. Possible association with noncirrhotic portal hypertension.

CLINICAL TRIALS: ddI has been included in numerous trials in combination with 3TC, d4T, FTC, and AZT.

ACTG 384 compared AZT/3TC vs. ddI + d4T, each in combination with NFV or EFV, in 908 participants (NEJM 2003;349:2293). At a median follow-up of 2.3 yrs, virologic outcomes were superior with EFV + AZT/3TC compared with EFV + ddI + d4T or to either NRTI combination with NFV. Treatment-limiting toxicity, especially peripheral neuropathy, was significantly greater with ddI + d4T. ddI should not be paired with d4T based on this and other studies demonstrating excessive rates of peripheral neuropathy, lactic acidosis, and pancreatitis (BMS warning letter to providers, January 5, 2001).

Jaguar: ddI intensification after virologic failure resulted in a median decrease in VL of 0.5 $\log_{10}$ c/mL at week 4 (JID 2005;191:840). The extent of decrease in VL correlated with TAMs: 0–1 TAMs, 0.8–1.0 $\log_{10}$ c/mL; 2 TAMs, 0.7 $\log_{10}$ c/mL; ≥3 TAMs, no significant response. The L74V mutation also predicted failure to respond. Clinical cutoffs were defined in this study using the PhenoSense assay. Those with a fold-change (FC) ≤1.3 had the best response to addition of ddI; those with FC between 1.3 and 2.2 had an intermediate response; and those with FC ≥2.2 had minimal response (JID 2005;191:840).

FTC-301A: Participants taking ddI + FTC with EFV experienced potent virologic suppression (78% had VL <50 c/mL at 48 wks) (JAMA 2004;292:180).

GESIDA 3903: This trial compared ddI + 3TC with AZT/3TC (in combination with EFV). At 48 wks, ddI + 3TC was noninferior to AZT/3TC (70% and 63% had VL <50 c/mL, respectively) (CID 2008;47:1083).

ACTG 5175 (PEARLS trial): This multinational randomized trial compared 3 treatment regimens in 1,571 treatment-naïve patients randomized to AZT/3TC + EFV or ddI + FTC + ATV, or TDF/FTC + EFV. The ddI + FTC + AFV arm was stopped by the DSMB due to an excessive rate of virologic failure at week 72. Among the remaining 1,045 participants on AZT/3TC vs. TDF/FTC, CD4 increase and virologic response were comparable at 184 wks, but there were fewer serious ADRs with TDF/FTC (Campbell TB. PLoS Med. 2012;9(8):e1001290).

NUCREST: This study examined the relative efficacy of recycling NRTIs in 719 patients with virologic failure and at least one NRTI resistance mutation. The overall response rate with recycling was 65% and was highest with ddI + 3TC (HIV Clin Trials 2010;11:294).

RESISTANCE: L74V and K65R are the most important resistance mutations. The L74V mutation results in cross-resistance to ABC, and the K65R mutation causes cross-resistance with ABC and TDF. Susceptibility to ddI is decreased with the accumulation of multiple TAMs: NRTI resistance is associated with the presence of ≥3 of the following: 41L, 67N, 210W, 215Y/F, and 219Q/E. M184V reduced phenotypic susceptibility but does not cause clinically significant resistance unless combined with other mutations.

PHARMACOLOGY:

Bioavailability: Tablet, 40%; powder, 30%; food decreases bioavailability by 47% with buffered ddI, 27% with ddI EC. Take all formulations on an empty stomach. They scored "0" for CNS penetration in the comparative merits of ART agents (JAIDS 2009;52:56): Class 2 in the four-class CNS penetration scoring system (Neurology 2011;76:693).

$T^{1/2}$: 1.5 hr.

Intracellular $T^{1/2}$: 25–40 hr.

TABLE 6.33 Dose adjustment for ddI with renal failure

Wt	CrCl (mL/min)			
	>60	30–59	10–29	<10
>60 kg	400 mg/d	200 mg/d	150 mg/d	100 mg/d
<60 kg	250 mg/d	150 mg/d	100 mg/d	75 mg/d

CNS penetration: CSF levels are ~20% of serum levels (CSF-to-plasma ratio, 0.16:0.19).

Elimination: Renal excretion: 50% unchanged in urine.

SIDE EFFECTS:

BLACK BOX WARNINGS: *(1) Pancreatitis, (2) lactic acidosis, and (3) fatal lactic acidosis* with ddI/d4T. Note that the relative risk of mitochondrial toxicity is correlated with affinity for mitochondrial DNA polymerase-γ. The rank order is ddI >d4T >AZT (ABC, TDF, TAF, 3TC, and FTC have minimal risk) (HIV Clin Trials 2009;10:306; Top HIV Med 2008;16:127; J Biol Chem 2001;276:40847).

Pancreatitis (Black box FDA warning): Reported in 1–9% (7–9% in the pre-HAART era; <1% in the HAART era). ddI-associated pancreatitis is fatal in 6% (JID 1997;175:255). The frequency of pancreatitis is dose-related. Risk factors for ddI-associated pancreatitis include renal failure, alcohol abuse, morbid obesity, history of pancreatitis, hypertriglyceridemia, cholelithiasis, endoscopic retrograde cholangio-pancreatography (ERCP), and concurrent use of ribavirin, d4T, 3TC, TMP-SMX, anti-TB agents, allopurinol, or pentamidine (Int J STD AIDS 2008;19:19). A review of pancreatitis in the EuroSIDA cohort with 9,678 patients failed to show a pancreatitis risk associated with ddI unless it was combined with d4T (AIDS 2008;22:47). Pancreatitis has been reported with ddI in the absence of d4T, but this side effect with ddI alone or d4T alone is less frequent.

Peripheral neuropathy with pain, numbness, and/or paresthesias in extremities. Frequency is 5–12%; it is increased significantly when ddI is given with d4T, hydroxyurea, or both (AIDS 2000;14:273). Onset usually occurs at 2–6 mos of ddI therapy and may be persistent and debilitating if ddI is continued despite symptoms.

GI intolerance with buffered powder are common. The EC formulation is preferred because it causes fewer GI side effects. An alternative to buffered ddI is ddI pediatric powder reconstituted with 200 mL water and mixed with 200 mL Mylanta DS or Maalox extra strength with anti-gas suspension in patient's choice of flavor. The final concentration is 10 mg/mL.

Cardiovascular risk: A review of NRTIs for risk of myocardial infarction by D:A:D showed recent ddI use was associated with a relative risk of 1.41 (JID 2010;201:318). ddI is also associated with significant elevations in LDL-cholesterol levels (AIDS 2011;25:185). The D:A:D analysis found a strong association between ddI treatment and cardiovascular events (JID 2010;201:318). The mechanism is unclear.

Hepatitis with increased transaminase levels. A study of liver stiffness evaluated by elastography showed the highest rates (16%) were associated with ddI therapy (Antiviral Ther 2010;15:753).

Noncirrhotic portal HTN resulting in esophageal variceal bleeding, liver failure, and death. Causal association not clearly established.

Miscellaneous: Rash, bone marrow suppression, hyperuricemia, hypokalemia, hypocalcemia, hypomagnesemia, optic neuritis, and retinal changes.

Class adverse effect: Lactic acidosis and severe hepatomegaly with hepatic steatosis caused by mitochondrial toxicity. The most frequent cause is ddI + d4T which should be avoided, especially in pregnancy (black box FDA warning) based on reports of at least two fatal cases. Didanosine can cause lipoatrophy, which is also believed to be mediated by mitochondrial toxicity.

DRUG INTERACTIONS:

Tenofovir: ddI + TDF co-administration is not recommended by the authors. DHHS and IAS-USA guidelines recommends avoiding ddI-TDF + NNRTI combination. Concurrent use of TDF and ddI results in a 48–64% increase in the ddI AUC (Curr Med Chem 2006;13:2789), and this results in an increased risk of ddI-associated side effects, including lactic acidosis and pancreatitis. The recommendation is to reduce the ddI dose, but this has been complicated by suspiciously high failure rates, especially when used in NNRTI-based ART (Antivir Ther 2005;10:171). A second concern is high risk for selection of K65R and high rates of virologic failure with selection of K65R (AIDS 2005;19:1695; AIDS 2005;19:1183; Antiviral Ther 2005;10:171). A third concern has been raised by several reports of blunted CD4 response with this combination when the ddI dose is not adjusted (AIDS 2005;19:569; AIDS 2005;19:1107; AIDS 2005;19:695).

Drugs that cause peripheral neuropathy should be used with caution or avoided: d4T, EMB, INH, vincristine, gold, disulfiram, or cisplatin.

Atazanavir: Food with ATV + ddI EC results in reduced ddI exposure and requires separate administration. Poor virologic efficacy in ACTG 5175. This was a trial comparing EFV + AZT/3TV, ATV + ddI + FTC, and EFV/TDF/FTC that was stopped prematurely by the DSMB due to excessive failure rates with ATV + ddI + FTC (NIAID Bulletin May 27, 2008).

Tipranavir: Separate administration by 2 hrs.

Methadone reduces AUC of buffered ddI by 41%; use ddI EC which is not effected (JAIDS 2000;24:241).

Allopurinol increases ddI concentrations. This combination is contraindicated (FDA warning June 19, 2009).

Oral ganciclovir increases ddI AUC by 100% when administered 2 hrs after ddI or concurrently. Monitor for ddI toxicity and consider dose reduction.

Ribavirin increases intracellular levels of ddI and may cause serious toxicity; avoid combination (Antiviral Ther 2004;9:133). This combination is contraindicated (FDA warning June 19, 2009).

Buffered formulation (powder): BIC, DTG, EVG, RPV, IDV, TPVATV, NFV, ketoconazole, tetracyclines, fluoroquinolones give >2 hrs. before cation antacid and ddI (buffered formulation). Avoid RAL co-administration.

CAUTION: FDA warning for ddI + ribavirin based on 23 cases of pancreatitis and/or lactic acidosis (with some fatalities); this combination is contraindicated. TDF increases levels of ddI; dose reduction to 250 mg/d (for >60 kg) or 200 mg/d (for <60 kg); this combination is not recommended. d4T + ddI is contraindicated in pregnant women and should be avoided in all patients.

PREGNANCY: Category B. The 2018 DHHS Guidelines for Antiretroviral Drugs in Pregnant Women no longer recommend ddI as an "alternative" to ABC/3TC or TDF/FTC. Relevant studies have shown no harm in rodent teratogen and carcinogenicity studies; placental passage in humans shows newborn-to-maternal drug ratio of 0.5 and pharmacokinetics are not altered in pregnancy (JID 1999;180:1536). The combination of ddI and d4T is contraindicated in pregnancy due to excessive rates of lactic acidosis and hepatic steatosis (Sex Transm Infect 2002;78:58). The Pregnancy Registry showed birth defects in 20/427 (4.68%) first-trimester exposures for reporting through July 31, 2017. This exceeds the expected rate of 2.7%, but it is not statistically significant and no consistent pattern was observed.

Diflucan—see Fluconazole

Dolutegravir (Tivicay)

TRADE NAME: Tivicay.

CLASS: Integrase inhibitor.

FORMULATIONS, REGIMEN, AND COST:.
Dolutegravir 50 mg tablet at $1,842.82/mo for 50 mg/d and $3,685.64/mo for 50 mg bid).
   CO-FORMULATIONS:

   Triumeq: DTG/ABC/3TC 50/600/300 mg tablet at $2,648.84/mo.
   Juluca: DTG/RPV 50/25 mg tablet at $3,094.80/mo.

REGIMENS:

For ARV-naïve patients or ARV-experienced integrase strand transfer inhibitor (INSTI)-naïve patients:
Dolutegravir (DTG) 50 mg once-daily with or without food.
DTG/ABC/3TC 50/600/300 mg (Triumeq) 1 tablet with or without food daily.

For INSTI-experienced patients with certain INSTI-associated resistance substitutions or clinically suspected INSTI resistance: DTG 50 mg twice-daily. Consider taking with food to maximize absorption.

For virologically suppressed patients with no known resistance mutations to DTG or RPV: DTG/RPV 50/25 mg/d with food.

Co-administration with EFV, FPV/r, TPV/r, rifampin: increase DTG dose to 50 mg twice-daily. Consider taking with food to maximize absorption.

Co-administration with DRV/r, ATV/r, NRTIs: Standard dose.

PHARMACOLOGY: DTG inhibits integrase, an essential enzyme responsible for catalyzing the insertion of HIV DNA into the host genome.

Absorption: Low, moderate, and high fat meals increase DTG AUC 33%, 41%, and 66%, respectively, can be taken with or without food.

Elimination: Eliminated mainly by metabolism via a UGT141-meditated glucuronidation pathway with some contribution from CYP3A. In vitro DTG is a P-gp substrate. 53% excreted as unchanged drug and 25.5% excreted as DTG metabolites in feces. <1% excreted in urine.

Protein binding: High protein binding >98.9%.

Half-life: 14 hrs.

RENAL DOSING: Usual dose, but in patients with CrCL<30 mL/min, DTG AUC is decreased by 40%. Although the clinical significance is unknown, INSTI-experienced patients with INSTI resistance mutation may be at increased risk for virologic breakthrough. Use with close monitoring.

DOSING FOR DECREASED HEPATIC FUNCTION: No dosage adjustment necessary for patients with mild to moderate hepatic impairment (Child-Pugh Score A or B). For severe hepatic impairment (Child-Pugh Score C); no data; avoid. Increased risk of hepatitis observed in patients with HBV BCV co-infection.

CLINICAL STUDIES:

FLAMINGO: DTG vs. DRV/r plus TDF/FTC or ABC/3TC in ARV-naïve patients (Clotet B et al., Lancet 2014;383:2222). Open-label, randomize comparison of once-daily DTG and DRV/r 800/100 mg plus TDF/FTC or ABC/3TC (two-thirds of patients received TDF/FTC) in ARV-naïve patients. At 48 wks, virologic suppression was achieved in 90% of DTG group and 83% of the DRV/r group. This established superiority of DTG (p = 0.025), but the difference was driven by higher discontinuation due to ADRs in the DRV/r-treated group.

DTG/ABC/3TC vs. EFT/TDF/FTC in treatment-naïve patients (Walmsley et al., NEJM 2013;369:180). Treatment-naïve patients (n = 833) were randomized to DTG/ABC/3TC or EFV/TDF/FTC. Patients were well matched at baseline. At week 48, 88% of DTG-treated patients vs. 81% of EFV-treated patients achieved virologic suppression (adjusted difference 7.4% [95% CI, 2.5%, 12.3%]). The difference in outcome was driven by a higher drop out rate due to rash and CNS ADRs in the EFV-treated patients (2% vs. 10%).

SPRING-2 -DTG vs. RAL in treatment-naïve patients (Raffi et al., Lancet 2013;381:735). Randomized study that compared DTG (n = 411) an RAL (n-411) combined with ABC/3TC or TDF/FTC in treatment-naïve patients. At 48 wks, 88% of DTG treated patients vs. 85% of RAL treated patients achieved virologic suppression (p = NS). Both regimens were well tolerated with only 2% discontinuation rates. Only 1 RAL-treated and none of the DTG-treated patients developed integrase inhibitor resistant mutations.

SAILING-DTG vs. RAL plus OBT in treatment-experience patients (Cahn P et al., Lancet 2013;382:700). Randomized study that compared DTG 50 mg bid (n = 400) to RAL 400 mg bid (n = 361) plus

OBT in treatment experienced patients, integrase inhibitor-naïve patients. At week 48, 71% of patients on DTG vs. 64% of patients on RAL had an undetectable VL (difference 7.4%, 95% CI, 0.7 to 14.2). There were fewer treatment-emergent integrase inhibitor resistance on DTG (4 vs. 17 patients; p = 0.003).

RESISTANCE: Resistance Q148H and G140S with mutations 74I/M, 92Q, 97A, 138 A/K, 140A, and 155H is associated with DTG resistance.

Other major mutation: 121Y.

Virologic response rate with the following baseline genotype:

N155H without Q148 mutation: 80%; Y143C/H/R without Q148: 56%; Q148H/R plus G140A/S: 56%.

Q148H substitution plus 2 or more of the following mutations L741/M, E138A/D/KT, G140A/S, Y143H/R, E157Q, G163E/K/Q/R/S, or G193 E/R: only 18%.

SIDE EFFECTS: Generally well tolerated. In comparative trials, more patients discontinued EFV-based regimen due to rash and CNS side effects, and more patients discontinued DRV/r due to adverse events or withdrawal of consent. Other adverse effects comparable to RAL- and EFV-based regimen. About 2–3% of patient discontinued DTG-based regimen due to adverse drug reaction.

LFT elevation (2%). Patients co-infected with hepatitis B or C may be at increased risk for worsening or development of transaminase elevations, CK elevation (3–4%), neutropenia (2%), diarrhea (1%), headache, nausea.

Pseudo CrCl decrease is due to inhibition of tubular secretion of creatinine. No significant change in GFR observed when measured by iohexol clearance.

Other uncommon ADRs: Abdominal pain, vomiting, fatigue, myositis, pruritus, dizziness, insomnia, hypersensitivity reaction (<1%) characterized by rash, constitutional findings (fever, malaise, fatigue, muscle or joint aches, blisters, conjunctivitis, facial edema, hepatitis, eosinophilia, angioedema), and sometimes organ dysfunction, including liver injury. Must discontinue if hypersensitivity reactions develop.

DRUG INTERACTIONS: DTG is a substrate of UGT1A1-mediated glucuronidation pathway and to a lesser extent CYP3A. DTG does not induce or inhibit CYP450 isoenzymes. DTG inhibits OCT2 transporter. Increased concentrations of OCT2 substrates can occur. In addition to increased concentrations of dofetilide and metformin, other OCT2 substrates (i.e., amantadine, cimetidine, cisplatin, and ranitidine) may also be increased.

Efavirenz: 57% decrease in DTG plasma concentration. EFV concentrations not affected (compared to historical control). Dose: DTG to 50 mg twice-daily in ARV-naïve patients or ARV-experienced INSTI-naïve patients.

Etravirine: 71% decrease in DTG plasma concentration. ETR concentrations not affected (compared to historical control). DTG should not be used with ETR without co-administration of ATV/r, DRV/r, or LPV/r.

Nevirapine: No data. May decrease DTG concentrations. Avoid co-administration.

Rilpivirine: No significant change in RPV concentrations. DTG AUC increase 12%. Use standard dose.

Tenofovir: Tenofovir AUC increased 12%. No significant change in DTG plasma concentrations. Use standard dose.

Fosamprenavir/r: 35% decrease in DTG plasma concentration. Amprenavir concentrations not affected (compared to historical control). Dose: DTG to 50 mg twice-daily in ARV-naïve patients or ARV-experienced with no INSTI-associated resistant mutations.

Tipranavir/r: 59% decrease in DTG plasma concentration. TPV concentrations not affected (compared to historical control). Dose: DTG to 50 mg twice-daily in ARV-naïve patients or ARV-experienced INSTI-naïve patients.

Lopinavir/r: No significant change in DTG plasma concentrations. LPV concentrations not affected (compared to historical control) Use standard dose.

Darunavir/r: DTG AUC decreased 22% DRV concentrations not affected (compared to historical control). Use standard dose.

Atazanavir/r: DTG AUC increased 62% and 91% with ATV/r and ATV co-administration, respectively. No significant. Use standard dose.

Maraviroc: Interaction unlikely. Use standard dose.

Metformin: May increase metformin concentration; monitor closely when starting or stopping DTG and metformin together. Metformin dose adjustment may be needed. Use with caution or avoid with renal insufficiency.

Dofetilide: May significantly increase dofetilide serum concentrations and increase risk of cardiac arrhythmias. Contraindicated; do not co-administer with dofetilide.

Polyvalent cation-containing agents (e.g., Mg Al, Fe, or Ca) in antacids, laxatives, sucralfate, oral calcium supplements, buffered medications (e.g., ddl buffered powder): 74% decrease in DTG concentration. Avoid co-administration. Take DTG 2 hr before or 6 hr after taking medications containing polyvalent cations.

Carbamazepine, oxcarbazepine, phenobarbital, phenytoin, St. John's Wort: May decrease DTG concentrations. Avoid co-administration.

No significant interactions with methadone, midazolam oral contraceptives (norgestimate and ethinyl estradiol), prednisone, rifabutin, omeprazole. Use standard dose.

PREGNANCY: Pregnancy category B. No human data. Animal studies have revealed no evidence of impaired fertility or harm to the fetus. There is insufficient data to be recommended by the DHHS perinatal guidelines. Recently, a report from Botswana noted four cases of neural tube defects in women who conceived while taking DTG (Tsepamo Study, 22nd International AIDS Conference, Amsterdam, 2018, TUSY15). Causality has not been established and data collection is ongoing. DHHS and WHO guidelines recommend using alternative ART in women who desire to get pregnant or are of childbearing potential but not on effective contraception (https://aidsinfo.nih.gov/news/2109/recommendations-regarding-the-use-of-dolutegravir-in-adults-and-adolescents-with-hiv-who-are-pregnant-or-of-childbearing-potential and http://www.who.int/hiv/pub/guidelines/ARV2018update/en/). RAL is the preferred INSTI in pregnancy.

Doxycycline

TRADE NAMES: Vibramycin (Pfizer), Doryx, and generic.

CLASS: Tetracycline antibiotic.

FORMULATIONS, REGIMEN, AND COST: 50 mg, 75 mg, 100 mg, 150 mg cap and tab at $2.36 per 100 mg. Suspension 25 mg/5 mL (60mL) $33.62.

> INDICATIONS AND DOSE: 100 mg po bid.
> *C. trachomatis*: 100 mg po bid × 7 days.
> *Bacillary angiomatosis*: 100 mg po bid × ≥3 mos; lifelong with relapse.
> *Syphilis (primary, secondary, and early latent) in patients with contraindication to penicillin*: 100 mg bid × 14 days + close monitoring.
> *Respiratory tract infections (sinusitis, pneumonia, otitis)*: 100 mg bid × 7-14 days.

PHARMACOLOGY:

> *Bioavailability*: 93%. Complexes with polyvalent cations (Ca^{++}, Mg^{++}, Fe^{++}, Al^{+++}, etc.), so milk, mineral preparations, cathartics, and antacids with metal salts should not be given concurrently. Administer doxycycline 2 hrs before cations.
> $T^{1/2}$: 18 hrs.
> *Elimination*: Excreted in stool as chelated inactive agent independent of renal and hepatic function.
> *Dose modification with renal or hepatic failure*: None.

SIDE EFFECTS: GI intolerance (10% and dose-related, reduced with food), diarrhea; deposited in developing teeth, so contraindicated from mid-pregnancy to term and in children <8 yrs of age (Committee on Drugs, American Academy of Pediatrics); photosensitivity (exaggerated sunburn); *Candida* vaginitis; "black tongue"; rash; esophageal irritation.

DRUG INTERACTIONS: Chelation with cations to reduce oral absorption (administer doxycycline 2 hrs before cations); half-life of doxycycline decreased by carbamazepine, cimetidine, phenytoin, barbiturates; may interfere with oral contraceptives; potentiates oral hypoglycemics, digoxin, and lithium.

PREGNANCY: Category D. Use in pregnant women and infants risks hepatotoxicity and may cause retardation of skeletal development and bone growth; tetracyclines localizes in dentin and enamel of developing teeth to cause enamel hypoplasia and yellow-brown discoloration. Tetracyclines should be avoided in pregnant women.

Dronabinol

TRADE NAME: Marinol (United Pharmaceuticals).

CLASS: Psychoactive component of marijuana.

FORMULATIONS, REGIMEN, AND COST: Gel-caps: 2.5 mg at $5.89, 5 mg at $12.26, 10 mg at $22.52.

> INDICATION AND DOSE: For anorexia associated with weight loss (also used in higher doses as antiemetic in cancer patients). Long-term therapy with dronabinol has led to significant improvement in appetite but no significant weight gain in three controlled trials (J Pain Sympt Manage 1995;10:89; AIDS Res Hum Retroviruses 1997;13:305; Psychopharmacology 2010;212:675). The latter study with a crossover design also showed improvement in sleeping and

mood. Another randomized trial showed smoked cannabis reduced chronic pain (p = 0.3) (Neurology 2007;68L515). It should be noted that the beneficial effects often required higher than the recommended doses of dronabinol, and, when weight gain is achieved, it is primarily due to an increase in body fat (J Pain Symptom Manage 1997;14:7; AIDS 1992;:127). The need for high maintenance doses is more likely in patients who are chronic marijuana users (Psychopharmacology 2010;212:675).

RECOMMENDATIONS FOR MANAGEMENT:

Standard dose: 2.5 mg bid (before lunch and before dinner).

CNS symptoms (dose-related mood high, confusion, dizziness, somnolence) usually resolve in 1–3 days with continued use. If these symptoms are severe or persist, reduce dose to 2.5 mg before dinner and/or administer at bedtime.

Dose escalation: If tolerated and additional therapeutic effect desired, increase dose to 5 mg bid.

High dose: 10 mg bid is occasionally required, especially for control of nausea.

PHARMACOLOGY:

Bioavailability: 90–95%.

$T^{1/2}$: 25–36 hr.

Elimination: First-pass hepatic metabolism and biliary excretion; 10–15% in urine.

Biologic effects post-dose: Onset of action: 0.5–1.0 hr, peak 24 hr.

Duration of psychoactive effect: 4–6 hr; appetite effect: $\geq$24 hrs.

SIDE EFFECTS (dose-related):

3–10%: CNS with "high" (euphoria), somnolence, dizziness, paranoia, GI intolerance, anxiety, emotional liability, confusion.

Low doses (10–20 mg/d) are well tolerated; 30 mg/d is poorly tolerated. There is minimal effect on cognitive function (Psychopharmacology 2005;181:170).

Others: Depersonalization, confusion, visual difficulties, central sympathomimetic effects, hypotension, palpitations, vasodilation, tachycardia, and asthenia.

BLACK BOX WARNINGS: None.

DRUG INTERACTIONS: Sympathomimetic agents (amphetamines, cocaine)—increased hypertension and tachycardia; anticholinergic drugs (atropine, scopolamine), amitriptyline, amoxapine, and other tricyclic antidepressants—tachycardia, drowsiness. There is no effect on PI levels (Ann Intern Med 2003;139:258), but PI/c and COBI may increase dronabinol concentrations. Drug–drug interactions with NRTI, NNRTIs, integrase inhibitors are unlikely.

WARNINGS: Dronabinol is a psychoactive component of *Cannabis sativa* (marijuana).

Schedule III (CIII): Potential for abuse. Use with caution in patients with psychiatric illness (mania, depression, schizophrenia), with cardiac disorder (hypotension), and in elderly patients. Caution should also be exercised in patients concurrently receiving sedatives and/or hypnotics and in patients with history of or current substance abuse.

WARN PATIENT OF THE FOLLOWING:

CNS depression with concurrent use of alcohol, benzodiazepines, barbiturates.

Avoid driving, operating machinery, etc. until safety and tolerance is established.

Mood and behavior changes.

Food increases AUC 28%. Avoid meals with >40–60 g fat, especially during the first 2–4 wks, which is the time of the greatest CNS effect.

PREGNANCY: Category C.

Elvitegravir (EVG)

TRADE NAME: Vitekta (Gilead).

CLASS: Integrase inhibitor: EVG inhibits integrase, an essential enzyme responsible for catalyzing insertion of HIV DNA into the host genome.

FORMULATIONS, REGIMEN, AND COST:.

Elvitegravir (Vitekta) 85 mg and 150 mg tablet at $45.07/tab ($1,352/mo).

CO-FORMULATIONS:

Genvoya: Elvitegravir/cobicistat/tenofovir alafenamide/ emtricitabine(EVG/COBI/TAF/FTC) 150/150/10/200 mg tablet at $3,306.92/mo.

Stribild: Elvitegravir/cobicistat/tenofovir DF/emtricitabine (EVG/COBI/TDF/FTC) 150/150/300/200 mg tablet at $3,707.99/mo).

DOSING REGIMENS:

EVG 85 mg/d with ATV/r 300/100 mg/d or LPV/r 400/100 mg bid co-administration.
EVG 150 mg/d with DRV/r 600/100 mg bid, FPV/r 700/100 mg bid, or TPV/r 500/200 mg bid co-administration.
Stribild 1 tablet (Elvitegravir (EVG) 150 mg, cobicistat (COBI) 150 mg, TDF 300 mg, FTC 200 mg) once-daily with food.
Genvoya 1 tablet (Elvitegravir (EVG) 150 mg, cobicistat (COBI) 150 mg, TAF 10 mg, FTC 200 mg) once-daily with food.

RENAL DOSING:

EVG: no dose adjustment required.
Stribild: CrCl >70 mL/min: use standard does; avoid use in patient with CrCl <70 mL/min at the start of treatment. D/C if CrCL <50 mL/min.

Genvoya: CrCl >30 mL/min: use standard does; avoid use in patient with CrCl <30 mL/min.

DOSING FOR DECREASED HEPATIC FUNCTION: Child-Pugh Class A and B: usual dose. Child-Pugh Class C: no data.

CLINICAL STUDIES:

EVG/COBI + TDF/FTC vs. ATV/r + TDF/FTC (DeJesus E et al., Lancet 2012;379:2429). This randomized, double-blind, phase III, noninferiority trial compared EVG/cobi + TDF/FTC with ATV/r + TDF/FTC. 708 ARV-naïve patients were randomized to receive EVG/cobi/FTC/TDF (n = 353) or ATV/r + FTC/TDF (n = 355). Patients were well matched at baseline with median CD count of ~350–360 cells/µL and mean VL of 4.8 log10 copies/mL (~40% with >100,000 c/mL). EVG/cobi/FTC/TDF was noninferior to ATV/FTC/TDF. An undetectable (VL <50 copies/mL) was achieved in 316 patients [89.5%] vs. 308 patients [86.8%], (adjusted difference 3.0%, 95% CI –1.9% to 7.8%). No difference in virologic response was observed when stratified by baseline VL </= 100,000 c/mL compared to >100,000 c/mL. Both regimens were well-tolerated with 13 (3.7%) and 18 (5.1%) patients discontinuing EVG/cobi + TDF/FTC and ATV/r + TDF/FTC, respectively. Fewer patients receiving EVG/cobi/FTC/TDF had elevated ALT than did those receiving ATV/r + FTC/TDF (15.3% vs. 21.6%) and had smaller median increases in triglyceride (90 µmol/L vs. 260 µmol/L). However, EVG/cobi/FTC/TDF had a greater median decline in eGFR (–12.7 mL/min vs. –9.5 mL/min).

EVG/COBI/TDF/FTC vs. EFV/TDF/FTC (Sax PE et al., Lancet 2012;379:2439). This prospective study randomized 700 ARV-naïve patients to EVG/COBI/FTC/TDF (n = 348) or EFV/FTC/TDF (n = 352), once-daily. Patients were well matched at baseline with median CD4 count of ~380 cells/uL and one-third of patients with VL >100K c/mL. EVG/COBI/FTC/TDF was noninferior to EFV/FTC/TDF; 305/348 (87.6%) vs. 296/352 (84.1%) of patients had HIV RNA <50 copies per mL at week 48, respectively (difference 3.6%, 95% CI, –1.6% to 8.8%). Discontinuation due to adverse events was comparable between the two groups. EVG-treated patients experience lower incidence of lipid elevation, rash, and CNS side effects compared to EFV-treated patients.

RESISTANCE:

The sequential use of EVG and RAL is not recommended due to the potential of cross-resistance.

Major EVG mutations: 66I/A/K, 92Q/G, 97A, 121Y, 147G, 148R/H/K, 155H.

Primary EVG mutations: TT66I, E92Q, Q148R, and N155H. Compared to wild-type, these primary mutations resulted in median 44-fold decrease in susceptibility to EVG. Of these mutations, E92Q, Q148R, and 155H confer >5-fold reduced susceptibility to RAL. T66I confers <3-fold decreased susceptibility to RAL.

Secondary EVG mutations: H51Y, L68I/V, G140C. S153A, E157Q, V165I, and H183P.

In a pooled analysis of patients with virologic failure and genotypic/phenotypic data available (23/669), NRTI mutations were the most common with M184V/I (12 of 23) and K65R (4 of 23). Eleven of 23 patients also developed integrase inhibitor mutations.

PHARMACOLOGY:

Relative to fasting conditions, high-fat meal increases EVG concentrations 87%.

EVG Cmax= 1.7 + /- 0.4 µg/mL; AUC = 23 =/-7.5 µg/mL; Cmin =0.45 =/-0.26 µg/mL (Cmin ~11-fold above IC95 of 45 ng/mL).

EVG is metabolized via CYP3A4 and to a lesser extent glucuronidation (UGT1A1/3). 94.8% of EVG excreted predominantly in feces, respectively.

EVG: 98–99%; no data on CNS penetration.

$T^{1/2}$: ~9.5 hrs (with COBI boosting).

SIDE EFFECTS:

Generally well-tolerated. In clinical trials, 3.7% of patients experienced serious ADR leading to EVG/COBI/TDF/FTC discontinuation compared to 5.1% of patients requiring discontinuation of EFV/ TDF/FTC or ATV/rTDF/FTC.

Nausea (16%), diarrhea (12%), vomiting, flatulence (2%). Nausea more common compared to EFV/TDF/FTC, but comparable to ATV/rTDF/FTC.

RENAL EFFECTS:

COBI decreases tubular secretion of creatinine, resulting in increase in Scr and decreases in eGFR without change in measured GFR by iohexol clearance. Mean increase in Scr of 0.14 mg/dL (+ /– 0.13 µg/dL).

With TDF/FTC co-administration, numerically more patients (8 of 701) discontinued EVG/COBI/TDF/FTC due to renal adverse events compared to ATV/r + TDF/FTC and EFC/TDF/FTC arm. However, TAF/FTC is associated with less renal adverse events.

EVG/COBI/TDF/FTC may cause proximal tubular dysfunction (hypophosphatemia, proteinuria, and/or normoglycemic glycosuria).

With TDF/FTC or TAF/FTC co-formulation: Acute exacerbation of hepatitis B with discontinuation.

Rash (3%): Less common compared to EFV/TDF/FTC (15%) and ATV/r + TDF/FTC (6%).

CNS: Somnolence (1%), headache (7%), dizziness (3%), insomnia (3%), abnormal dreams (9%), CNS ADR lower compared to EFV/TDF/FTC and comparable to ATV/r + TDF/FTC.

No effect on cholesterol and lower triglyceride elevation compared to ATV/r + TDF/FTC.

Decreased bone mineral density: However, DXA results and bone fracture are not significantly different between EVG/ COBI/TDF/FTC and ATV/r + TDF/FTC or EFV/TDF/FTC. Improvement in BMD observed when switching from TDF/ FTC to TAF/FTC co-formulations.

Lactic acidosis and hepatic steatosis: Although listed as black box warning with all NRTIs, casual relationship with TDF and TAF is not established. In vitro, TDF is one of the NRTI's least associated with mitochondrial toxicity.

DRUG INTERACTIONS:

EVG is substrate of CYP3A4. Any CYP3A4 inhibitor and inducer may increase or decrease EVG serum concentrations, respectively.

Drug–drug interactions with COBI and RTV needs to be considered since EVG requires boosting with COBI or RTV.

> *Contraindicated with the following drugs*: Alfuzosin, rifampin, all ergot derivatives, cisapride, St. John's wort, lovastatin, simvastatin, pimozide, high does sildenafil, triazolam, and oral midazolam.

> *The following drugs should be avoided with EVG/c and EVG/r*: Ranolazine, flecainide, propafenone, bepridil, dofetilide, amiodarone, quinidine, dronedarone, fluticasone, salmeterol, eplerenone, lurasidone, ivabradine, flibanserin, fluticasone. silodosin, rivaroxaban, betrixaban, ticagrelor, vorapaxar (may increase oral anticoagulation, avoid.)

> Dose adjustment needed with edoxaban, apixiban, and dabigatran based on renal function and indication.

> *Avoid co-administration with the following drugs*: CYP 3A4 enzyme inducing anticonvulsants (carbamazepine, oxcarbazepine, phenobarbital, phenytoin), rifabutin, rifapentine, dexamethasone (at steady-state), enzalutamide, and mitotane.

> *ATV/r*: EVG 85 mg/d + ATV/r 300/100 mg/d.

> *DRV/r*: EVG 150 mg/d + DRV/r 600/100 mg bid.

> Avoid once-daily DRV/COBI + EVG due to decreased EVG concentrations.

> *FPV/r*: EVG 150 mg/d + FPV/r 700/100 mg bid.

> *IDV*: No data; avoid.

> *LPV/r*: EVG 85 mg/d + LPV 400/100 mg bid.

> *NFV*: No data; avoid.

> *SQV/r*: No data; avoid.

> *TPV/r*: EVG 150 mg/d + TPV/r 500/200 mg bid; avoid EVG/COBI.

> *NRTIs*: Usual dose.

> *MVC*: MVC 150 mg bid with EVG/c or EVG/r.

EFV: No data; avoid.

ETR: Avoid EVG/COBI; EVG + PI/r (dose above) plus ETR 200 mg bid.

NVP: May decrease EVG; avoid.

RPV: May increase RPV; avoid with EVG/COBI; monitor QTc with EVG/r.

Ibalizumab-uiyk: Interaction unlikely; use standard dose.

T-20: Interaction unlikely; use standard dose.

PREGNANCY: Category B. Not teratogenic in animal studies. No human teratogenicity data. Inadequate concentrations of both EVG and COBI in second and third trimesters, with reports of virologic breakthroughs. Continue EVG-based regimens with close monitoring only in patients who are virologically suppressed (DHHS Perinatal Guidelines 2018).

Efavirenz (EFV)

TRADE NAME: Sustiva (Bristol-Myers Squibb), Stocrin (Merck).

CLASS: NNRTI.

FORMULATIONS, REGIMEN, AND COST:

Forms: Caps 50 and 200 mg; tabs 600 mg. Combination tab: Atripla. (EFV/TDF/FTC 600/300/200 mg); Symfi (EFV/TDF/3TC 600/300/300 mg); Symfi Lo (EFV/TDF/3TC 400/300/300 mg)

Regimens: 600 mg/d or Atripla, preferably in the evening on an empty stomach. Administration on empty stomach may reduce CNS side effects.

AWP: Sustiva $1,176.74/mo, Atripla $3,057.89/mo, Symfi and Symfi Lo $1961/month. Some studies have found that lower doses (200 or 400 mg/d) can improve tolerance without loss of potency by screening for genetic changes that prolong the half-life (JID 2011;203:246) or by therapeutic monitoring (Antivir Ther 2011;16:189). However, testing for polymorphisms at codon 516 of the CYP2B6 gene is not routinely available.

FOOD EFFECT: Take on empty stomach or with a low-fat meal; a concurrent meal with 40–60 g of fat increases AUC >30% and peak level 40–50%, which may increase side effects. The recommendation to take on an empty stomach applies primarily to the initial weeks of treatment, when CNS side effects are greatest.

RENAL FAILURE: Standard dose (EFV).

HEPATIC FAILURE: No recommendations; use with caution.

PATIENT ASSISTANCE PROGRAM: 800-861-0048 (7 AM–7 PM) CST Mon.– Fri.).

INDICATIONS AND DOSE: EFV-based ART is an alternative regimen in certain clinical situations for treatment-naïve patients. The standard dose is 600 mg/d, usually in combination with TDF/FTC or TAF/FTC, taken in the evening to reduce the CNS side effects that are common in the first 2–3 wks.

DISCONTINUATION: To reduce risk of NNRTI resistance, the recommendations for planned discontinuation of EFV-based ART are to stop EFV and continue two NRTs for 1–2 wks ("staggered discontinuation") or to substitute PI-based ART for 1 mo ("substituted discontinuation").

TIMING: EFV is usually taken in the evening so that major CNS effects go unnoticed during sleep. However, morning dosing is safe, effective, and preferred by some patients due to sleep disturbances (Scand J Infect Dis 2006;38:1089).

CNS PENETRATION: Levels in CSF are 0.26–1.2% plasma levels. On the four-class ranking system for CNS penetration EFV ranks category 3 (Letendre. 17th CROI 2010: Abstr. 172).

ADVANTAGES: Sustained activity with over 5-yr follow-up; once-daily therapy; low pill burden; co-formulation available as a one-pill daily dose.

DISADVANTAGES: High rate of CNS effects in first 2–3 wks; higher rate of discontinuation compared to integrase inhibitor-based regimen; single mutation confers high-level EFV resistance and does not impair fitness resulting in persistence of K103N mutation; potential for teratogenicity if used in the first 8 wks of pregnancy; long and variable half-life complicates discontinuation with risk of resistance.

DURABILITY: Retrospective analysis of 3,565 patients given various ART regimens (this analysis did not include integrase inhibitor-based regimen) found that EFV was the most likely to show sustained viral suppression (JID 2005;192:1387).

CLINICAL TRIALS:
ACTG 5142: A seminal study that compared EFV-based vs. LPV/r- based ART in treatment-naïve patients. Entry criteria were VL >2000 c/mL and any CD4 count. Results are summarized in Table 6.35 (NEJM 2008;358:2095). Conclusions from this study were that (1) EFV-based ART was virologically superior to LPV/r-based ART, (2) LPV/r was superior with respect to drug options lost due to resistance after failure and in the magnitude of the CD4 count increase, (3) EFV/thymidine analogues were associated with more lipoatrophy, and (4) triglyceride elevation was greater with EFV + LPV/r than when combined with a thymidine analog NRTI.

COMPARISON WITH NVP: *2NN*: This trial randomized 1147 treatment-naïve patients to receive EFV, NVP qd, NVP bid, or EFV + NVP, each in combination with 3TC + d4T (Lancet 2004;363:1253). By ITT analysis at 48 wks, the frequency of virologic suppression to <50 c/mL was EFV, 70%; NVP bid, 65.4%; NVP once-daily, 70%; and NVP/EFV, 62.7%. EFV and NVP were comparable, but NVP did not meet FDA criteria for noninferiority to EFV (Lancet 2004;363:1253). The only significant difference in virologic outcome was between EFV and EFV + NVP. The median increase in CD4 count was 150–170/mm³ in all four groups. NVP therapy was implicated in two drug- related deaths. A Cochrane Database Review compared EFV and NVP when combined with two NRTIs and concluded they were equivalent in antiviral activity but had different side effects (Cochrane Database Syst Rev 2010;12:CD004246).

ACTG 364 enrolled 195 patients who failed treatment with NRTIs but were naïve to PIs and NNRTIs. Participants received one to two NRTIs + NFV, EFV, or NFV/EFV. VL was <50 c/mL in 22%, 44%, and 67%, respectively at 40–48 wks. The superior results with EFV vs. NFV were statistically significant (NEJM 2001;345:398).

COMPARISON WITH INTEGRASE INHIBITOR-BASED REGIMEN: *STARTMRK*: Randomized trial of ART-naïve patients (*n* = 198) comparing RAL (100, 200, 400, 600 mg twice-daily) to EFV, both in combination with TDF/FTC. The groups were well matched at baseline with VL 4.6–4.8 log and CD4 271–314. VL <50 c/mL achieved in 85–88% of patients across all arms at 48 wks. At 96 wks, RAL arm continued to be effective with VL suppression (<50 c/mL) observed in 83% and 84% of RAL- and EFV-treated patients, respectively. A more rapid virologic suppression (4 vs. 8 wks) was observed in the RAL treated group. As expected, CNS adverse events were more common in the EFV arm compared to RAL arm (Sax PE et al., Lancet 2012;379:2439).

Randomized trial of 700 ARV-naïve patients compared EVG/cobi/TDF/FTC (*n* = 348) to EFV/TDF/FTC (*n* = 352) once-daily. The groups were well matched at baseline with median CD4 count of ~380 cell/uL and one-third of patients with VL >100K c/mL. EVG/cobi/TDF/FTC was noninferior to EFV/TDF/FTC; 305/348 (87.6%) vs. 296/352 (84.1%) of patients were virologically suppressed (VL<50 c/mL) at 48 wks. EVG-treated patients experienced lower incidence of CNS side effects, lipid elevation, and rash compared to EFV-treated patients. The development of integrase inhibitor mutation up to week 144 was infrequent (White KL et al., Antiviral Ther 2015;20:317).

FOTO: Sixty patients with durable viral suppression on TDF/FTC/EFV were randomized to continue this regimen or to take it for 5 consecutive days (Monday–Friday) followed by a 2-day

TABLE 6.34 Comparative trials of EFV-based ART in treatment-naïve patients

Study	Comparison	N	Dur (wk)	VL <50	VL <200–400
DuPont 006 (NEJM1999; 341:1865)	EFV + AZT/3TC	154	48	64%[a]	70%
	IDV + AZT/3TC	148		43%	48%
	IDV + EFV	148		47%	53%
ACTG 384 (NEJM 2003; 349:2293)	EFV + AZT/3TC	155	48	—	88%[a]
	EFV + ddI + d4T	155		—	63%
	NFV + AZT/3TC	155		—	67%
	NFV + ddI + d4T	155		—	68%
	NFV + EFV + AZT/3TC	182		—	84%
	NFV + EFV + ddI + d4T	178		—	81%
GS-903 (JAMA 2004;292:191)	EFV + TDF + 3TC	299	48	78%	82% (68%)
	EFV + d4T + 3TC	301	144	74%	79% (62%)
CLASS (JAIDS 2006;43:284)	APV/r + ABC/3TC	96	48	59%	75%
	d4T + ABC/3TC	98		60%	81%
	EFV + ABC/3TC	97		72%	80%
2NN (Lancet 2004;363:1253)	EFV + 3TC + d4T	400	48	70%	—
	NVP + 3TC + d4T	387		65%	—
GS-FTC 301A (JAMA 2004;292:180)	EFV + FTC + ddI	286	60	78%[a]	81%
	EFV + d4T + ddI	285		59%	68%
INITIO (Lancet 2006;368;287)	EFV + ddI + d4T	288	192	74%[a]	—
	NFV + ddI + d4T	805		62%	—
	EFV + NFV + ddI + d4T	280		62%	—
ACTG 5095 (NEJM 2004;350:1850)	EFV + AZT/3TC ± ABC	765	32	83%[a]	89%
	AZT/ABC/3TC	382		61%	74%
BMS 034 (JAIDS 2004;36:1011)	ATV + AZT/3TC	286	98	32%[aa]	70%
	EFV + AZT/3TC	280		37%[aa]	64%

(continued)

TABLE 6.34 Continued

Study	Comparison	N	Dur (wk)	VL <50	VL <200–400
GS-934 (NEJM 2006;354:251)	TDF/FTC + EFV	255	48	80%[a]	84% (71%)[a]
	AZT/3TC + EFV	254	144	70%	73% (58%)
ESS 30009 (JID 2005;192:1921)	ABC/3TC + TDF	102	12[b]	___	[b]
	ABC/3TC + EFV	169	48	71%	75%
CNA 30024 (CID 2004;39:1038)	EFV + AZT/3TC	325	48	69%	71%
	EFV + ABC/3TC	324		70%	74%
EFV 30021 (CID 2004;39:411)	EFV + AZT/3TC bid	378	48	63%	65%
	EFV + AZT bid + 3TC qd	276		61%	67%
CAN 30021 (JAIDS 2005;38:417)	EFV + ABC/3TC bid	386	48	68%	___
	EFV + ABC/3TC qd	384		66%	___
ACTG 5142 (NEJM 2008;358:2095	LPV/r + 3TC + (d4T or AZT)	250	96	77%	86%
	EFV + 3TC + (d4T or AZT)	253		89%[a]	93%
	LPV/r (533/133 mg bid) + EFV	253		83%	92%
MERIT (JID 2010;201:797)	EFV + 2 NRTIs	361	48	65%	73%
	MVC + 2 NRTIs	360		69%c 84	71%
STARTMRK (JAIDS 2009;52:350)	EFV + TDF/FTC	282	96	78%	___
	RAL + TDF/FTC			84%	___
Lancet 2013;379:2439	EFV/TDF/FTC	352	48	84%	
	EVG/cobi/TDF/FTC			88%	
ECHO/THRIVE (IAC 2010:LBPE17	EFV + 2 NRTIs	682	48	82%	___
	RPV + 2 NRTIs	686		83%	___

TABLE 6.34 Continued

Study	Comparison	N	Dur (wk)	VL <50	VL <200–400
ACTG 5202 (Ann Intern Med 201;154:445)	ATV/r + (TDF/ FTC or ABC/ 3TC)	702	96	____	83%
	EFV + (TDF/FTC or ABC/3TC)	698		____	85%

[a]Superior to comparator arm (P<0.05).
[aa]Low value compared to other studies attributed to failure to use optimal transport medium.
[b]Arm terminated early due to high failure rate when analysis at >8 wks of treatment showed virologic non-response in 49% of the TDF group vs. 5% of the EFV group.
[c]Post-hoc analysis showed equivalence of regimens when adjusted for MVC recipients who acquired X4 virus between screening and treatment initiation.

interruption (Saturday and Sunday) (Five On, Two Off, or "FOTO"). At 24 wks, there were no virologic failures (VL >50 c/mL) among 25 patients in the FOTO arm. At that time the control arm receiving daily therapy was switched to the FOTO regimen. At 48 wks, virologic response was good with (1) no blips associated with FOTO, (2) strong patient preference for the FOTO regimen, and (3) EFV levels <1,000 ng/mL at a mean of 60 hrs after dosing in 52% in the FOTO arm vs. 10% in the standard treatment arm (not associated with virologic failure) (HIV Clin Trials 2007;8:19; Chen C. 5th IAS 2009;Abstr. MOPEB063).

ECHO and THRIVE: See rilpivirine.

MERIT: This study compared bid MVC vs. EFV, each combined with AZT/3TC, in 721 treatment-naïve patients. At 48 wks, the MVC regimen was "not inferior," but this was due to more adverse reactions requiring discontinuation in the EFV arm (13.6% vs. 4.2%) and more virologic failures in the MVC arm (11.9% vs. 4.2%)

(JID 2010;201:803). A subsequent reanalysis of the MERIT results (MERIT ES) excluded patients who had R5-tropic virus at baseline using the original Trofile assay but who were subsequently found to have dual/mixed-tropic virus by the enhanced sensitivity assay (Trofile ES) (HIV Clin Trials 2010;11:125–32). In this analysis, virologic results were similar with superior tolerability and CD4 increases in the MVC arm, leading to the approval of MVC for treatment-naïve patients.

SWITCH STUDIES: *SWITCH-EE trial*: Participants were receiving EFV + 2 NRTIs, with tolerance of the regimen and VL <50 c/mL. At entry, the patients were randomized to receive continued EFV or switch to ETR, and then at 6 wks were switched to the alternative, an NNRTI with continuation of the NRTI backbone. The analysis of patient preference showed those who continued EFV preferred that agent (15/21, 71%) and those who started with ETR preferred ETR (16/17, 94% (*p* <0.0001). The ETR recipients had lower total cholesterol and LDL cholesterol levels (*p* = <0.000) (AIDS 201;25:57).

DMP 049 was a study of patients who were responding well to PI-based ART regimens with VL <50 c/mL and were randomized to continue the PI-based regimen or switched to EFV (JAIDS.

2002;29[suppl 1]: S19). At 48 wks, VL was <50 c/mL in 97% of the EFV arm and 85% of the PI continuation arm.

ALIZE-ANRS-099 was a randomized trial of switch to EFV + FTC + ddI qd vs. continued PI-based ART in patients with viral suppression. At 12 mos, outcomes were comparable among the 355 patients for viral suppression (JID 2005;191:830). At 4 yrs, 68% remain on the regimen and 57% had VL <50 c/mL.

AI266073 queried patient's preference when randomized to switch to TDF/FTC/EFV or continue the original regimen after achieving viral suppression on a PI-based regimen: 80% preferred the TDF/FTC/EFV regimen (AIDS Patient Care STDS 2010;24:87).

Toxicity: Multiple studies address the issue of lipodystrophy complicating PI-based ART to determine the effect of changing to EFV-based ART vs. continuation of the original regimen. A review of 14 such studies with 910 patients (Topics HIV Med 2002;10:47) showed virologic failure in only 6 patients who switched to

EFV-based ART. Effects on triglycerides and cholesterol were variable, and lipodystrophy was rarely reversed. One report found that adding pravastatin was a more effective strategy than switching ART (AIDS 2005;19:1051).

ACTG 5142R: The NRTI-sparing combination most extensively studied is LPV/r 533/133 mg bid + EFV 600 mg/d, in ACTG 5142 (see Table 6.35). Intent-to-treat analysis found that 83% of LPV/r/EFV recipients had VL <50 c/mL at 96 wks. Recommendations for the dose adjustment with the tablet formulation is uncertain because the studies were done using the capsule formulation of LPV/r 533/133 bid (AAC 2003;47:350). With the tablet formulation, most recommend 6 tabs/d (600/150 mg bid) in patients with PI resistance, but standard dose (400/100 bid; 4 tabs/d) in patients with no PI resistance.

A5116 was a randomized, open-label switch study of LPV/r (533 mg/133 mg bid) + EFV (600 mg/d) vs. EFV + 2 NRTI in subjects who received at least 18 mos of a three- or four-drug PI- or NNRTI-based regimen as a first regimen; they had plasma VL <200 c/mL and no documented phenotypic resistance. Among 236 participants, EFV + 2 NRTIs was superior in terms of viral suppression (14 vs. 7) and tolerability (20 vs. 6 discontinuations) (*p* <0.0015) (AIDS 2007;21:325).

Other NRTI-sparing regimens containing EFV include EFV 600 mg/d + FPV/r 1,400/300 mg/d (PI-naïve only) or EFV 600 mg/d + FPV/r 700/100 mg bid. EFV combined with ATV is more complicated because the unboosted ATV AUC is reduced 74% with EFV. The recommended regimen is EFV 600 mg/d on an empty stomach and ATV/r 400/100 mg/d on a full stomach.

RESISTANCE: The K103N mutation is most common and causes high-level resistance to EFV as well as NVP and DLV. This may be present as a "minority quasispecies" at baseline that is detected only with allele-specific PCR and can lead to rapid virologic failure (CID 2009;48:239). In one study of clinical samples, K103N was detected with conventional genotypic testing in 10.5% and by allele-specific PCR only) in 14%. A systematic review of the literature

TABLE 6.35 ACTG 5142: EFV + 2 NRTIs vs. LPV/r + 2 NRTIs vs. EFV + LPV/r in treatment-naïve patients

96-Wk Results	EFV	LPV/r	EFV + LPV/r[c]
	n = 253	n = 250	n = 253
VL <50 c/mL	89%[a]	77%	83%
Not failed wk 96	76	67	73
CD4 count (median)	241	285[a]	268
Resistance [b]			
NNRTI	18/33 (48%)	2/52 (4%)[a]	27/39 (69%)
PI (major)	0	0[a]	2/39 (6%)
NRTI – 184V	8/33 (24%)	7/54 (14%)	1/39 (3%)
Metabolic study			
Triglyceride (>750 mg/dL)	6%	16%	34%
Total cholesterol (mg/dL)	+ 33	+ 33	+ 33
LDL Cholesterol (mg/dL)	+ 21	+ 26	+ 26
Lipoatrophy	32%	18%[a]	18%[a]

From NEJM 2008;358:2095.

[a] P = <0.5: EFV superior to LPV/r for virologic failure; LPV/r superior to EFV for CD4 increase, resistance mutations and lipoatrophy.

[b] Resistance reported for no. resistance mutation/no. strains tested in patients with virologic failure.

[c] LPV/r dose = 533/133 mg.

(1974–December 2010) found the most common low-frequency resistance mutations were 103N and 181C, and these were associated with significantly higher rates of virologic failure with EFV-based regimens (JAMA 2011;305:1327; J Med Virol 2009;81:1983). The K103N mutation does not reduce HIV fitness, so there is no benefit with continuation of EFV, and there is possible harm since continuation is likely to select for more NNRTI mutations that could reduce effectiveness of ETR. Other major RT mutations associated with reduced susceptibility are RT codon mutations 181C/I, 188L, 190S/A, and 225H. The 181C/I mutation is not selected by EFV, but it contributes to low-level EFV resistance. Detection of this mutation as a minority variant using allele-specific PCR found that a minority 181C mutation was associated with a 3-fold risk of EFV failure in ACTG 5095 (AIDS 2008;22:2107; AIDS 2007;21:813).

PHARMACOLOGY:

Oral bioavailability: Not known. High-fat meals increase absorption of both capsule and tablet forms by 39% and 79%, respectively, and should be avoided in patients who are experiencing CNS side effects. Serum levels are highly variable likely due to CYP2B6 polymorphisms, and this variation explains some of the variations in virologic response and CNS side effects (AAC 2004;48:979).

T1/2: 36–100 hr depending on the CYP2B6 genotype of the host (CID 2007;45:1230).

Distribution: Highly protein-bound (>99%); CSF levels are 0.25–1.2% plasma levels, which is above the IC_{95} for wild-type HIV (JID 1999;180:862). Virologic failure correlates with levels <1.1 mg/L (12th CROI, Boston, Feb. 2005;Abstr. 80). EFV is category 2 in the four-category CNS penetration score (Neurology 2011;76:693).

Elimination: Metabolized by the cytochrome P450 metabolic pathway, primarily CYP2B6 and, to a lesser extent, CYP3A4. Studies of polymorphisms at codon 516 of the CYP2B6 gene have shown significant differences that correlate with half-life, drug levels, and CNS toxicity (CID 2006;42:401; CID 2007;45:1230). Depending on these genetic differences in the plasma half-life of EFV, the duration of therapeutic levels vs. wild-type HIV (>46 ng/mL) varies from 5.8 days to 14 days, the frequency of therapeutic levels lasting >21 days ranged from 5% to 29%, and median plasma levels of EFV at 24 hrs ranged from a median of about 3,000 ng/mL with the GG genotype at codon 516 to >9,000 ng/mL with the TT genotype (CID 2006;42:401; CID 2007;45:1230). Prolonged half-life and high levels are more common in African Americans due to higher prevalence of the TT genotype (AAC 2003;47:130). The substantial variations in EFV levels shown by these data complicate drug discontinuation and correlate with CNS side effects. One group has used these (CY2B6 polymorphism) data to reduce standard EFV dosing to 200–400 mg/d with substantial reduction CNS toxicity in 10 of 14 patients (CID 2007;45:1230). The drug induces its own metabolism so that duration of treatment will affect serum concentrations.

Dose modification with renal or hepatic disease: No dose modification (AIDS 2000;14:618; AIDS 2000;14:1062). More frequent monitoring is advocated when given with hepatic disease.

SIDE EFFECTS:

Switch in patients with NVP-induced rash or hepatotoxicity: A meta-analysis of 13 reports with 239 patients found that 30 (13%) developed a recurrence of the rash when switched to EFV (Lancet Infect Dis 2007;7:722). Review of 11 patients with NVP-induced hepatoxicity found no recurrences (Lancet Infect Dis 2007;7:733).

Rash: Approximately 15–27% of EFV recipients develop a rash, which is usually morbilliform and does not require discontinuation of the drug. More serious rash reactions that require discontinuation are blistering and desquamating rashes, noted in about 1–2% of patients, and Stevens-Johnson syndrome, which has been reported in 1 of 2,200 EFV recipients. The median time to onset of the rash is 11 days, and the duration with continued treatment is 14 days. The frequency with which discontinuation is required is 1.7% compared with 7% given NVP, 4.3% given DLV, and 2% given ETR.

CNS side effects have been noted in up to 52% of patients but are sufficiently severe to require discontinuation in only 2–5%. Symptoms are noted on day 1 and usually resolve after 2–4 wks. They include confusion, abnormal thinking, abnormal dreams, impaired concentration, depersonalization, and dizziness. Other side effects include somnolence, insomnia, amnesia, hallucinations, and euphoria. Patients need to be warned of these side effects before starting therapy and should also be told that symptoms improve with continued dosing and infrequently persist longer than 2–4 wks.

A substudy of *ACTG A5097* provided periodic neuropsychiatric testing of 170 EFV recipients for 184 wks (HIV Clin Trials 2009;10:343). CNS side effects declined to baseline levels at 4 wks, and long-term follow-up found that the majority had no residual neuropsychologic deficits, although a small number had high scores for stress, anxiety, and unusual dreams. There is evidence that the CNS toxicity is *dose related* (JAIDS 2009;52:240; CID 2007;45:1230) based on correlation with serum levels and response to dose reduction, although some studies do not support this correlation (Antiviral Ther 2005;10:489; Antiviral Ther 2009;14:75). It is recommended that the drug be given in the evening on an empty stomach during the initial weeks of treatment because a high-fat meal increases absorption by up to 80%. There is a potential additive effect with alcohol or other psychoactive drugs. Patients need to be cautioned to avoid driving or other potentially dangerous activities if they experience these symptoms. Two studies with extensive neurocognitive analyses showed no evidence that EFV was associated with an increase in serious mental health problems (Ann Intern Med 2005;143:714; CID 2006;42:1790), although serious disorders have been reported including severe depression in 2.4% (Bristol-Myers Squibb letter to providers, March 2005), and another cohort study showed the odds ratio for cognitive impairment with EFV was 4.0 ($p = 0.008$) (Neurology 2011;76:1403). A review of 843 patients given EFV in EuroSIDA found that 138 (16%) stopped the drug due to CNS toxicity (Antiviral Ther 2009;14:75).

In a retrospective review of ACTG 5095, 9% of patients intolerant of EFV were switched to NVP with resolution of EFV-associated reactions (CID 2010;51:365). One report indicated safety and effectiveness if switching from EFV to NVP in patients with CNS toxicity; 41 of 47 experienced resolution of CNS symptoms (46th ICAAC 2008;Abstr. 1236). Switching from EFV to ETR is another within-class change that has been successful in a randomized trial (AIDS 2011;25:65). Another option is dose reduction of EFV (600–400 mg) based on plasma concentrations (JAIDS 2009;52:240; CID 2007;45:1230) or based on genetic analysis for variants that determine EFV metabolism, half-life, and risk of CNS toxicity (CYP3A4, CYP2A6, and CYP2B6) (JID 2011;203:246). Compared to LPV, long-term use of EFV was associated with worse speed of information processing, executive functioning, verbal fluency, and working memory (Ma Q et al., J Neurovirol 2016;22:170–178).

Hyperlipidemia: The D:A:D study found that EFV is associated with increased triglyceride and total cholesterol levels; these effects were greater for EFV compared to NVP (JID 2004;189:1056). D:A:D did not find a risk of cardiovascular disease associated with NNRTI use (NEJM 2007;356:1723). ACTG 5142, a large trial comparing EFV and LPV/r-based ART in treatment-naïve patients, found similar changes in lipids (LDL cholesterol and triglyceride changes), but lipid levels were greatest in those given both agents (NEJM 2008;358:2095). Lipid levels were more favorable with ATV/r than EFV in ACTG 5202 (Ann Intern Med 2011;154:445–456). Lipids levels were also more favorable with EVG/cobi/TDF/FTC than EFV/TDF/FTC (Lancet 2012;379:2439).

False-positive urine cannabinoid (marijuana) test: This occurs with the screening test only and only with the Microgenic's CEDIA DAU Multilevel THC assay. Confirmatory tests are negative (World 1999;96:7).

False-positive benzodiazepine test: (Triage 8, Drug Screen Multi 5).

Increased transaminase levels: Levels >5 × ULN in 2–8% (Hepatology 2002;35:182; HIV Clin Trials 2003;4:115). Frequency is increased with hepatitis C or with use of concurrent hepatotoxic drugs. Hepatotoxicity is less frequent and less severe than seen with NVP; grades 3–4 in 12% given NVP vs. 4% given EFV in one study of 298 patients (HIV Clin Trials 2003;4:115). The mechanism is unknown. Discontinuation of EFV is recommended if hepatotoxicity is symptomatic (infrequent) or ascribed to hypersensitivity, or if the transaminase levels are >10× ULN in the absence of other causes (grade 4) (Clin Liver Dis 2003;7:475).

Vitamin D deficiency: This is a possible association from the SUN study with an OR of 2.0 (CID 2011;52:396). Consequences are unclear.

BLACK BOX WARNINGS: None.

TABLE 6.36 EFV–PI interactions and dose recommendations

PI	AUC Co-admin. Drug	EFV AUC	Recommendation
IDV	↓31%	No change	IDV 1,000 mg q8h + EFV 600 mg qhs or. IDV 800 mg bid + RTV 200 mg bid + EFV 600 mg qhs
NFV	↑20%	No change	NFV 1250 mg bid + EFV 600 mg qhs
SQV	↓62%	↓12%	Consider SQV/r 1,000/100 mg bid
SQV/RTV	↓60%	No change	SQV/r 1,000/100 bid + EFV 600 mg qhs
LPV/r	↓19%[a]	No change	LPV/r 500/125 bid or 400/100 bid (treatment-naïve); LPV/r 600/150 bid (treatment experienced)
ATV	↓74%	No change	ATV/r 400/100 mg/d + EFV 600 mg/d; unboosted ATV not recommended; ATV/r + EFV not recommended in ARV-experienced patients.
FPV	C_{min} ↓. 36%	No change	FPV/r 700/100 mg bid + EFV 600 mg/d or FPV/r. 1400/300 mg/d + EFV 600 mg qhs
TPV	↓31%	No change	TPV/r 750/200 mg bid + EFV 600 mg/d
DRV	↓13%	↑21%	Limited data; consider DRV/r 600/100 mg bid + EFV. 600 mg qhs; consider TDM
RTV	↑20%	↑20%	Standard doses
MVC	↓45%	No change	MVC 600 mg bid; EFV 600 mg qhs
RAL	↓36%	No change	Standard dose
DTG	↓57%	No change	DTG 50 mg bid + EFV 600 mg qhs (use only if no INSTI resistance)
EVG	May ↓↓	May ↑	Avoid co-administration
BIC	May ↓	—	Dose not established. Avoid

[a] Compared to standard dose LPV/r.

DRUG INTERACTIONS: EFV both induces and, to a lesser extent, inhibits the cytochrome P450 CYP3A4 enzymes in vitro. Enzyme induction has been observed in the majority of PK studies.

Contraindicated drugs for concurrent use: Astemizole, terfenadine, rifapentine, cisapride, pimozide, ergot alkaloids, St. John's wort, and bepridil.

Other drugs with significant interactions: EFV may reduce concentrations of *phenobarbital, phenytoin, and carbamazepine;* monitor levels of anticonvulsant. *Rifampin* decreases EFV levels by 25%; rifampin levels are unchanged: some advocate higher doses of EFV (800 mg/d for persons >60 kg); a pharmacologic study found that concurrent use in patients with HIV and TB resulted in highly variable EFV levels but good clinical outcomes (JAC 2006;58:1299). However, most studies have suggested that the standard 600 mg dose is adequate, including the N2R trial designed to examine this issue (CID 2009;48:1752). Another option is to take EFV with a 40–60 g fat meal, which will substantially increase EFV AUC. *Rifabutin* has no effect on EFV levels, but EFV reduces levels of rifabutin by 35%; with concurrent use, the recommended dose of rifabutin is 450 mg/d or 600 mg 3×/wk plus the standard EFV dose (MMWR 2002;51[RR-7]:48). *Rifampin* preferred with EFV co-administration. Concurrent use with *ethinyl estradiol* no effect or slightly increased. *Levonorgestrel* AUC increases 56% with EFV. The FDA recommends a second form of contraception, but the current 2018 Perinatal Guidelines do not include a restriction of use of EFV in pregnant women or in women planning to become pregnant.

EFV reduces *methadone* levels by 52%; titrate methadone dose to avoid opiate withdrawal. EFV also decreases levels of *buprenorphine* by 50% but, due to buprenorphine's high opiate receptor binding affinity, it may be preferred to methadone in opiate-dependent patients since no withdrawal symptoms were observed (J Phar Biomed Anal 2007;44:188). EFV decreases *simvastatin* AUC by 58%, *atorvastatin* AUC by 43%, and *pravastatin* AUC by 44%. An increase in statin dose may be needed, but do not exceed the maximum dose (JAIDS 2005;39:307). *Atorvastatin, pravastatin,* or *rosuvastatin* may be preferred. Monitor carefully when using *warfarin* with EFV. There is a 46%

incidence of rash reactions when combining EFV and *clarithromycin*, and levels of clarithromycin are decreased 39%; consider azithromycin. *Voriconazole. Diltiazem* AUC decreased 69%. Titrate to effect. *Sertraline* AUC decreased 39%. Titrate to effect. *Bupropion* AUC decreased 55%. Titrate to effect. *Atovaquone/proguanil*: Atovaquone AUC decreased 75% and proguanil AUC decreased 43%. Consider alternative for malaria and PCP prophylaxis.

PREGNANCY: Category D. This drug caused birth defects (anencephaly, anophthalmia, and microphthalmia) in 3 of 20 gravid cynomolgus monkeys, but this has not been borne out in human studies. There have been seven reports of neural tube defects in infants born to women with first-trimester exposures to EFV (Arch Intern Med 2002;162:355; AIDS 2002;16:299; Ely. 15th CROI 2008;Abstr. 624; Bristol-Myers Squibb letter to providers, March 2005). The Antiretroviral Pregnancy Registry (through July 2015) showed birth defects in 22/990 (2.22%) live births with first-trimester exposures. These include one case each of sacral aplasia, meningomyelocele, hydrocephalus, facial clefts, and anophthalmia. A review of 344 women who conceived on EFV-based ART in West Africa found no congenital malformations (JAIDS 2011;56:183). Analysis of more than 2,000 live births did not show a teratogenicity risk with efavirenz exposure (Perinatal Guidelines 2018). The 2018 DHHS Guidelines for Use of Antiretroviral Drugs in Pregnancy do not restrict the use of EFV in pregnant women or in women planning to become pregnant. This recommendation consistent with both the British HIV Association and WHO guidelines. Women treated with an EFV-based regimen who become pregnant should continue current regimen if virologically suppressed. The 2018 DHHS Guideline pregnancy statement recommends efavirenz as an alternative to DRV/r-, ATV/r-, RAL-based regimen in patients not eligible for preferred regimens. Pregnant women exposed to EFV should be registered at www.APRegistry.com (Antiretroviral Pregnancy Registry), or call 800-258-4263 (8:30 AM–5:30 PM EST, Mon.–Fri.).

Emtricitabine (FTC)

TRADE NAME: Emtriva (Gilead Sciences).

CLASS: NRTI.

FORMULATIONS, REGIMEN, AND COST:

Forms: FTC (Emtriva): Caps 200 mg; oral solution 170 mL bottle with 10 mg/mL; Co-formulations: TDF/FTC (Truvada): Tab 300/200 mg; TAF/FTC (Descovy); EFV/TDF/FTC (Atripla)— tab 600/300/200 mg; RPV/TDF/FTC (Complera) tab 25/ 300/200 mg; RPV/TAF/FTC (Odefsey) tab 25/25/200 mg; EVG/COBI/TDF/FTC (Stribild) tab150/150/300/200 mg; EVG/COBI/TAF/FTC (Genvoya) tab 150/150/10/200 mg; BIC/TAF/FTC (Biktarvy) tab 50/25/200 mg; DRV/COBI/ TAF/FTC (Symtuza) tab 800/150/10/200 mg.

Regimens: FTC, 200 mg/d or 240 mg oral solution qd; Truvada, 1 tab qd; Atripla, 1 tab qhs on empty stomach; Complera, 1 tab qd with a meal; Odefsey 1 tab qd with a meal; Stribild 1 tab qd with food; Genvoya 1 tab qd with food; Biktarvy 1 tab qd with or without food.

AWP: FTC (Emtriva) at $643.82/mo; Co-formulations: Truvada, $ 1,881.14/mo; Atripla,

$2658.24/mo; Complera, $ $3,216.92/mo; Odefsey at $3,009.29; Stribild at $3,707.99/mo; Genvoya at $3,306.92; Biktarvy at $3,534.78/mo; Symtuza at $4178/mo.

FOOD EFFECTS: None.

RENAL IMPAIRMENT: Dose adjustment for CrCl: 30–49 mL/ min, 200 mg q48h; 15–29 mL/min, 200 mg q72h; <15 mL/ min or dialysis, 200 mg q96h.

Adjust Truvada CrCl 30–49 mL/min; 1 tab q48h (consider switch to TAF-based regimen); Avoid other TDF/FTC co-formulations (Atripla, Stribild, Complera) with CrCl <50 mL/min.

Avoid TAF/FTC co-formulations (Descovy, Odefsey, Genvoya, Biktarvy, Symtuza) with CrCL <30 mL/min.

HEPATIC FAILURE: No dose adjustment.

PATIENT ASSISTANCE: 1-800-226-2056 (9 AM–8 PM EST, Mon.–Fri.).

ADVANTAGES: Potent antiretroviral activity, well tolerated, no food effect, longer intracellular half-life than 3TC, once-daily dosing, multiple coformulations. No risk of accumulating additional mutations after 184V with continued use. Delays TAMs. Possible decreased risk of K65R with TDF/FTC vs. TDF/3TC and decreased risk of M184V with TDF/FTC vs. AZT/3TC. Active against HBV. May be less prone to the 184V resistance mutation compared to 3TC (HIV Clin Trials 2011;12:61).

DISADVANTAGES: Rapid selection of 184V RT mutation in nonsuppressive regimen with substantial loss of activity. Activity against HBV sometimes complicates HIV treatment decisions. Associated with skin hyperpigmentation (uncommon).

3TC COMPARISON: Similar to 3TC in activity against HIV, loss of most activity and rapid selection of M184V mutation, prolonged intracellular half-life and activity against HBV (AAC 2004;48:3702; CID 2006;42:126). May be less likely to select for M184V mutation than 3TC, and emergence of K65R with TDF/FTC may be less likely than with TDF + 3TC.

CLINICAL TRIALS:

GS-301A was the FDA registration trial using FTC (200 mg/d) vs. d4T, each in combination with ddI + EFV in 571 treatment-naïve patients. At 60 wks, VL <50 c/mL was achieved in 76% of FTC recipients compared to 54% in the d4T group (P <0.001), and the CD4 count at 48 wks was greater with FTC, a mean of 153/mm^3 vs. 120/mm^3 (P = 0.02) (JAMA 2004;292:180).

GS-303 was a 3TC equivalence open label trial in which 440 patients receiving 3TC as a part of ART were randomized to continue bid 3TC or to switch to FTC. At 48 wks, virologic failure occurred in 7% of FTC recipients and 8% of 3TC recipients (AIDS 2004;18:2269).

Protocol 350, a continuation study, found equivalent rates of viral suppression for GS-303 participants for an additional median follow-up of 152 wks (AIDS 2004;18:2269).

ALIZE-ANRS-099: Switch study in 355 patients randomized to continue PI-based ART or switch to FTC + ddI + EFV once-daily. At 48 wks, 87% and 79% had a VL <50 c/mL with EFV vs. PI/r-based ART, respectively (p <0.05) (JID 2005;191:830).

GS-903: A randomized, double-blind study in which 602 treatment-naïve patients received either TDF or d4T in combination with 3TC + EFV. Virologic suppression (<50 c/mL) was equivalent through 144 wks. K65R emerged in 8 and 2 patients in the TDF and d4T arms, respectively. Lipid levels were more favorable in TDF arm and lipoatrophy more common with d4T. Renal safety profile similar between arms (JAMA 2004;292:191–201).

GS-934: 517 treatment-naïve patients were randomized to receive EFV + AZT/3TC or EFV + TDF/FTC. At 144 wks, more patients experienced virologic suppression in the TDF/FTC arm by ITT analysis, 71% vs. 58% <400 c/mL. The difference was explained primarily by the higher proportion of discontinuations due to adverse events in the AZT/3TC arm (9% vs. 4%), most of which were due to anemia (NEJM 2006;354:251). No K65R mutations were observed, and M184V was less common with TDF/FTC than with AZT/3TC (JAIDS 2006;43:535).

Hepatitis B: FTC is considered equivalent to 3TC for activity against HBV (AIDS 2011;25:73; CID 2010;51:1201) and is approved for that indication. One study found that resistance by YMDD mutants was delayed with FTC compared to 3TC (AIDS 2005;19:221). Another study found no detectable HBV DNA levels with FTC monotherapy in 65% of patients at 24 wks (AAC 2006;50:1642). Current recommendations are that TDF/FTC or TDF/3TC-based ART be used in co-infected patients who require treatment of HBV, regardless of the need for HIV treatment. If the decision is to treat HBV without treating HIV, the agents used to treat HBV should be one that is inactive against HIV: interferon, adefovir, or telbivudine (2015 DHHS HIV Treatment Guidelines; CID 2006;43:904).

RESISTANCE: Nonsuppressive therapy with FTC results in the rapid selection of the M184V mutation, which confers high-level resistance to 3TC and FTC, modest decreases in susceptibility to ABC and ddI, and increased susceptibility to TDF, AZT, and d4T. K65R or multiple TAMs reduce activity of FTC 3- to 7-fold. With maximum selective pressure, the TDF/FTC combination produces mutants with the K65R and M184V genotype in vitro (AAC 2006;50:4087); although K65R has not been observed in clinical trials (GS-934 and Abbott 418) using this combination. All of these changes apply to 3TC as well. A comparison of results for resistance in three trials showed the frequency of the 184V mutation with viral failure was greater with 3TC compared to FTC (36% vs. 19%) (HIV Clin Trials 2011;12:61).

PHARMACOLOGY:

Bioavailability: 93% for the capsule and 75% for the solution; not altered by meals.

Levels: C_{max} 1.8 ± 0.7 µg/mL; C_{min} 0.09 µg/mL.

Distribution: Protein-binding <4%, concentrated in semen.

$T^{1}/2$: plasma, 10 hr; intracellular, 39 hr (AAC 2004;48:1300).

Elimination: 13% metabolized to sulfadioxide and glucuronide metabolites. Unchanged drug and metabolites are renally eliminated.

SIDE EFFECTS:

BLACK BOX WARNINGS: Lactic acidosis: Rare and only when used with other NRTI, usually a thymidine analogue.

Flare of HBV when FTC is discontinued in co-infected patients.

Generally well tolerated with minimal toxicity. Occasionally, patients note nausea, diarrhea, headache, asthenia, or rash; about 1% discontinue the drug due to adverse effects. *Lactic acidosis and hepatic steatosis,* including fatal cases, have been reported with nucleosides. Rare patients who do not tolerate FTC will tolerate 3TC (JAC 2006;58:227). *Skin hyperpigmentation* has been noted primarily on palms and soles in 3% and almost exclusively in Africans and African Americans. FTC is active against HBV, so discontinuation may result in *HBV exacerbation*.

DRUG INTERACTIONS: None of clinical consequence are known.

PREGNANCY: Category B. The 2018 DHHS Guidelines on Use of Antiretroviral Drugs in Pregnancy list FTC as one of the preferred NRTI to be used in combination with TDF as the NRTI backbone.

Pharmacokinetic studies in pregnancy show FTC levels are modestly lower (Best, 15th CROI;Abstr. 629). The data for birth defects with FTC exposure in the Pregnancy Registry are 60/2,614 (2.3%) which compares to 2.72% without ART exposure (last updated July 31, 2017).

Enfuvirtide (ENF, T20)

TRADE NAME: Fuzeon (Hoffmann-La Roche).

FORMULATIONS, REGIMEN, AND COST: Single-dose vials with 108 mg ENF as lyophilized powder (sufficient for 90 mg dose) to be reconstituted with 1.1 mL sterile water. ENF is packaged in a 30-day kit containing 60 single-use vials of ENF, 60 vials of sterile water for injection, 60 reconstitution syringes (3 cc), 60 administration syringes (1 cc), and alcohol wipes.

> ADULT DOSE: 90 mg (1mL) SC q12h into upper arm, anterior thigh, or abdomen with each injection given at a site different from the preceding injection site.
>
> STORAGE: The kit can be stored at room temperature. However, once ENF powder has been reconstituted, it must be refrigerated at 36–46°F (2–8°C) and used within 24 hrs.
>
> COST: $3,759.60/mo or $45,115.2/yr (AWP). Cost-effective analysis is estimated at $69,500/life-yr saved (JAIDS 2005;39:69).
>
> PATIENT ASSISTANCE: 800-282-7780.

ADVANTAGE: Novel mechanism of action, potent antiviral activity, virtually no resistance in patients not previously treated with this drug, well-studied with well-documented in vivo activity in heavily treatment-experienced patients.

DISADVANTAGES: Requirement for twice-daily subcutaneous injections, local reactions at injection sites, expense, and rapid development of resistance with virologic failure. The main concern is the effect on quality of life.

MECHANISM OF ACTION: ENF binds to HR1 site in the gp41 subunit of the viral envelope glycoprotein and prevents conformational change required for viral fusion and entry into cells. Discontinuation of ENF in 25 patients with ENF resistance resulted in an increase in VL with decrease in resistance; retreatment with ENF led to undetectable virus by week 16 (JID 2007;195:387).

CLINICAL TRIALS:

TORO-1 (North America and Brazil) and TORO-2 (Australia and Europe): Pooled data presented to the FDA were from 2 randomized, controlled, open-label studies involving 995 treatment-experienced patients with virologic failure (NEJM 2003;348:2175; NEJM

TABLE 6.37 TORO-1 and -2: 48- and 96-wk results

	Results	*ENF/OBR*	*OBR*
48 Wks		*n = 661*	*n = 334*
NEJM 2003;348:2175 and JAIDS 2005;40:404	VL <400 c/mL VL <50 c/mL CD4 count (mean)	34%[a] 18% + 91 cells/mm^3	12% 8% + 45 cells/mm^3
96 wks		*n = 368*	—
(AIDS Pat Care STDs 2007;21:533)	<400 c/mL <50 c/mL CD4 count	27% 18% + 166	— — —

[a] P <0.001 compared to results in control arm.

2003;348:2186) (Table 6.37). ENF plus an optimized background regimen (OBR) was superior to an OBR alone. Patients had a baseline VL of 5.2 $\log_{10}$ c/mL, a mean of 12 prior antiretroviral agents, and 80–90% had ≥5 resistance mutations to NRTIs, NNRTIs, or PIs. The VL change from baseline to week 24 was –1.52 $\log_{10}$ c/mL for patients in the ENF arm compared to –0.73 $\log_{10}$ for patient receiving only the OBR (P <0.0001). As expected, patients with two or more active antiretrovirals, based on history and genotype or phenotype resistance testing, were more likely to achieve a VL <400 c/mL.

Other salvage studies: ENF has shown to increase efficacy of other salvage regimens.

ENF switch: EASIER-ANRS-138 was a randomized trial comparing continuation of ENF-based ART with substitution of RAL for ENF (N = 170). At 24 wks, switch to RAL was associated with significant improvements in pain, social functioning, and physical activity scores (HIV Clin Trials 2010;11:283).

RESISTANCE AND CROSS-RESISTANCE: Resistance to ENF occurs rapidly with nonsuppressive therapy and is associated with

TABLE 6.38 Summary of salvage trials with and without ENF[a]

Trial	Agent	N	Control	Study Agent	Study Agent + ENF
RESIST (Lancet 2006;368:466)	TPV/r	1,483	10%	23%	36%
POWER (Lancet 2007;369:1169)	DRV/r	255	15%	44%	58%
MOTIVATE (NEJM 2008;359:1442)	MVC	1,048	19%	42%	63%
BENCHMRK (NEJM 2008;359:339)	RAL	521	34%	57%	80%

[a] Results are % with VL <50–400 c/mL at 48 wks.

mutations in the HR1 region of gp41 at codons 36, 37, 38, 39, 40, 42, and 43 (J Virol 2005;79:4991). These mutations reduce fusion efficiency, resulting in reduced fitness; mutations at codons 36 and 38 emerge rapidly (AIDS 2006;20:2075; JAIDS 2006;43:60), usually within 2 wks with incomplete viral suppression. Mutations in gp41 codons 36–43 were noted in 98% of patients with virologic failure in TORO-1 and -2 (AIDS Res Human Retroviruses 2006;22:375). These mutations do not cause cross-resistance with other entry inhibitors such as CCR5 inhibitors. Discontinuation of ENF in patients with ENF-resistant strains results in a moderate increase in VL and disappearance of ENF mutations within 16 wks (JAIDS 2006;43:60; JID 2007;195:387). A case report showed selection of ENF-resistant HIV-1 in CSF led to loss of viral suppression in plasma (CID 2010;50:387).

CURRENT STATUS: The introduction of new antiretroviral agents in 2005-18 (DRV, TPV, ETR, RAL, MVC, DTG, EVG, BIC) largely supplanted the need for ENF, and many receiving ENF were switched to alternative agents for improved quality of life. Thus, the demand for ENF has decreased substantially (HIV Clin Trials 2010;11:283; HIV Clin Trials 2009;10:432; JAC 2009;64:1341; JAIDS 2009;52:382). A potential contemporary use in patients with drug-susceptible HIV infection is the need for parenteral therapy.

PHARMACOLOGY:

> *Absorption*: Well absorbed from subcutaneous (SC) site with an absolute bioavailability of 84.3%. Following 90 mg SC, the mean C_{max} was 5.0 µg/mL, C_{min} was 3.3 µg/mL, and AUC was 48.7 µg/mL/hr. Virologic failure is associated with C_{trough} levels <2.2 µg/mL (JAC 2008;62:384).
>
> *Distribution*: Vd = 5.5L. Levels in CSF are nil (Antiviral Ther 2008;13:369; Neurology 2011;76:693).
>
> *Protein binding*: 92%.
>
> *Metabolism*: After SC injection, the drug is completely absorbed and largely catabolized, but about 17% is converted to an

active deaminated form. Metabolism is not influenced by cytochrome P450 (Clin Pharmacokinet 2005;44:175).

$T^{1/2}$: 3.8 hr.

Dosing with renal failure: No dose adjustment (CID 2004;39:119).

Dosing with hepatic insufficiency: No data; usual dose.

DRUG INTERACTIONS: None. In vitro, enfuvirtide did not inhibit or induce the metabolism of CYP3A4, CYP2D6, CYP1A2, CYP2C19, or CYP2E1 substrates. Does not interact with TPV/r, DRV/r, RAL, ETR, MVC, SQV/r, RTV, or rifampin (JID 2006;194:1319).

SIDE EFFECTS:

Injections site reactions: A review by the FDA of 663 ENF recipients found the injection site reactions occurred in 98%, including pain (96%; severe pain in 11%), induration (90%; severe in 57%), erythema (91%), nodules or cysts (80%), and/or pruritus (65%). Duration of the reaction was >3 days in 41% and >7 days in 24%. Treatment was discontinued in 7% due to these reactions (Gibbs N. 12th CROI, Boston, Feb. 2005:Abstr.837). Successful desensitization has been reported (CID 2004;39:110). Injection site reactions can be managed by rotating sites and massaging the area after injection. Excisional biopsies of these lesions show inflammation resembling granuloma annulare, with most of the inflammatory and collagen changes in areas where ENF was injected. These changes were noted even when there was no clinical reaction, which suggests a hypersensitivity reaction (Am Acad Dermatol 2003;49:826). A randomized study to evaluate 3 delivery systems (27 gauge needle, 31 gauge needle or needle-free injection device). At week 12, 85% of participants selected to use the needle-free device (Antiviral Ther 2008;13:449).

Occasional ADRs: Bacterial pneumonia (event rate per 100 patient-years in trials was 4.68 in the treatment arm vs. 0.61 in controls). Relationship to ENF is unclear (JAC 2010;65:138).

Rare ADRs: Hypersensitivity with rash, nausea, vomiting, chills, fever, hypotension, elevated transaminase, glomerulonephritis, thrombocytopenia, neutropenia, eosinophilia, fever, hyperglycemia,

Guillain Barré syndrome, sixth-nerve palsy, elevation in amylase and lipase (for rare ADRs, a causal relationship is not established).

BLACK BOX WARNING: None.

PREGNANCY: Category B. Not teratogenic in animal studies. There are no data concerning safety or pharmacokinetics in pregnancy. Does not cross the placenta (limited data) (AIDS 2006;20:297). Breastfeeding not recommended. The 2018 DHHS Guidelines for Anti-Retroviral Treatment in Pregnancy do not recommend ENF in treatment-naïve due to inadequate data.

Entecavir

TRADE NAME: Baraclude.

FORMULATIONS, REGIMEN, AND COST: 0.5 mg and 1.0 mg tabs at $44.43, 0.05 mg/mL solution (210 mL) at $1,036.80.

INDICATION: Chronic HBV infection with evidence of active disease. One study found that switching from 3TC to entecavir in monoinfected patients resulted in an increase in HBV

TABLE 6.39 Response of chronic HBV to entecavir treatment

| | A1463022 HBeAg Pos | | A1463027 HBeAg Neg | |
	Entecavir	3TC	Entecavir	3TC
Dose/d	0.5 mg	100 mg	0.5	100 mg
Sample size	314	314	296	287
Histologic Improvement	72%[a]	62%	70%[a]	61%
Undetectable HBV DNA	67%[a]	36%	90%[a]	72%

[a] Superior to treatment with 3TC (*P* <0.05) (package insert; NEJM 2006; 354:1011; NEJM 2006;354:1001).

suppression and no evidence of HBV resistance (Hepatol Int 2010;4:594). See Table 6.39.e.

Regimen: NRT-naïve patients, 0.5 mg po qd on empty stomach (2 hrs before or after food). For 3TC-refractory patients, 1 mg po qd on empty stomach.

Use in HIV/HBV co-infection: Entecavir is generally considered one of the best drugs for HBV infection (CID 2010;51:1201). A 2010 meta-analysis of 20 studies of outcome at 1 yr from clinical trials of HBV infection found that TDF and entecavir are the most effective agents for initial treatment (Gastroenterology 2010;139:1218), but the use of entecavir in HBV/HIV co-infected patients is complicated because it has in vitro and in vivo activity against HIV as well as HBV. Use in co-infected patients has been associated with a significant decrease in HIV viral load and emergence of the 184V RT resistance mutation (NEJM 2007;356:2614; AIDS 2007;21:2365). It should not be used in HIV/HBV co-infected patients unless it is part of a fully suppressive ART regimen.

RESISTANCE: In vitro tests show that 3TC-resistant strains are 8- to 30- fold less sensitive to entecavir (see Table 6.40). Resistance to entecavir can emerge during treatment but is infrequent and requires additional RT mutations (AAC 2004;48:3498). HBV strains from patients who failed entecavir are resistant to 3TC but sensitive to adefovir. One trial of entecavir in HIV/HBV co-infected patients with HBV rebound showed a good response to entecavir with a mean decrease of 3.5 $\log_{10}$ c/mL in HBV DNA levels (AIDS 2008;22:1779).

PHARMACOLOGY:

Bioavailability: 100% for both oral solution and tablet forms when taken on an empty stomach. If taken with a fatty meal, the C_{max} is decreased 45% and AUC is decreased 18–20%.

$T^{1/2}$: 24 hr (J Clin Pharmacol 2006;46:1250); intracellular: 15 hrs.

Elimination: Entecavir does not induce or inhibit the CYP450 metabolic pathway. It is eliminated predominantly by renal clearance.

SIDE EFFECTS:

Similar to 3TC in comparative trials for 48 wks.

Rare, major severe reaction is lactic acidosis with steatosis, including fatalities (class effect, causal relationship with entecavir unknown).

Exacerbation of HBV when entecavir is discontinued.

DRUG INTERACTIONS: ARV drug-drug interaction unlikely.

PREGNANCY: Category C; not recommended for co-infected patients unless entecavir is given with a fully suppressive ARV regimen since it is active vs. both HIV and HBV. Report exposures during pregnancy to www.apregistry.com/.

TABLE 6.40 Entecavir vs. 3TC-resistant HBV

	3TC-Refractory Cases	
	Entecavir n = 124	3TC n = 116
Histologic improvement	55%[a]	28%
Ishak fibrosis score improved	34%[a]	16%
HBV DNA Undectectable. (<300 c/mL)	19%[a]	1%
Mean Viral load change. ($\log_{10}$ c/mL)	−5.1%[a]	−0.5
ALT normal (<1 × ULN)	61%[a]	15%
HBeAg seroconversion	8%	3%

[a] Superior to treatment with 3TC (P <0.05) (package insert; NEJM 2006;354:1011; NEJM 2006;354:1001).

Epivir—see Lamivudine

EPO—see Erythropoietin

Epzicom—see Abacavir and Lamivudine

Erythropoietin (EPO)

TRADE NAME: Epogen; Procrit (Ortho Biotech).

FORMULATIONS, REGIMEN, AND COST: Vials with 2,000, 3,000, 4,000, 10,000, 20,000, and 40,000 units. Standard dose of 40,000 U/wk costs $729.36 (Epogen); $1,070.88 (Procrit).

PATIENT ASSISTANCE PROGRAM: 800-553-3851.

PRODUCT INFORMATION: Recombinant human erythropoietin (rHU EPO) is a hormone produced by recombinant DNA technology. It has the same amino acid sequence and biologic effects as endogenous erythropoietin, which is produced primarily by the kidneys in response to hypoxia and anemia. It acts by stimulating the proliferation of marrow RBC progenitor cells.

INDICATIONS: Serum erythropoietin level <500 milliunits/mL plus anemia ascribed to HIV infection, or to medications, including AZT (Ann Intern Med 1992;117:739; JAIDS 1992;5:847).

DOSE RECOMMENDATIONS: Although the FDA-approved dose for initial therapy is 10,000 units 3×/wk, the standard starting dose used in clinical practice is 40,000 units/wk, and trials investigating every-other-week dosing demonstrated good clinical efficacy (CID 2004;38:1447). Dosing for patient with ESRD on HD: 50–100 units/kg 3×/wk. Onset of action is within 1–2 wks, reticulocytosis is noted at 7–10 days, increases in hematocrit are noted in 2–6 wks, and desired hematocrit is usually attained in 8–12 wks. Response is dependent on the degree of initial anemia, baseline EPO level, dose, and available iron stores. Transferrin saturation should be ≥20%; serum ferritin should be ≥100 ng/mL. If levels are suboptimal, supplement with iron. (Some experts advocate routine iron supplementation in all patients taking EPO.) If after 4 wks of therapy the Hb rise is <1 g/dL, dose may be increased to 60,000 units SQ weekly. After an additional 4 wks, if Hgb does not increase by at least 1 g/dL from baseline value, discontinue EPO therapy. After achieving the desired response (i.e., increased Hgb or Hct level or reduction in transfusion requirements), titrate the dose for maintenance. Target Hb is 10–11.3 g/dL. When dosed to target a Hgb level of 13.5 g/dL there is a significant risk of cardiovascular complications compared to a target of 11.3 g/dL (NEJM 2006;355:2085 and 2144; FDA warning, November 22, 2006)—death 7.3% vs. 5% ($p = 0.07$) and congestive heart failure 9% vs. 6.6% ($p = 0.07$). Keep dose steady or reduce by 25% when Hb >12 g/dL. Reduce dose by 25% if Hgb increases >1 g/dL in any 2-wk period and hold if Hgb is >13 g/dL or Hct >40%, and reinitiate with a 25% reduction when Hgb is less than 11 g/dL. With failure to respond or suboptimal response, consider iron deficiency, occult blood loss, folic acid or B_{12} deficiency, or hemolysis.

EFFICACY: A trial using EPO in 1,943 HIV-infected patients with HCT <30% used an initial dose of 4,000 units SQ 6 d/wk, and mean weekly doses ranged from 22,700–32,500 units/wk (340–490 units/kg/wk). Response to treatment, defined as an increase in baseline HCT by 6 percentage points (i.e., 30–36%) with no transfusions within 28 days, was achieved in 44%. Transfusion requirements were significantly reduced from 40–18% at 24 wks and the average hematocrit increased from 28–35% at 1 yr. Subset analysis demonstrated that this response was independent of AZT administration (Int J Antimicrob Ag 1997;8:189). In one study anemia was a risk factor for death, and this risk was decreased with EPO (CID 1999;29:44).

PHARMACOLOGY:

Bioavailability: EPO is a 165-amino acid glycoprotein that is not absorbed with oral administration. IV or SC administration is required; SC is preferred.

$T^{1/2}$: 4–16 hr.

Elimination: Poorly understood but minimally affected by renal failure.

Dose adjustment in renal or hepatic failure: None.

SIDE EFFECTS: Increased risk of cardiovascular complications when targeting a Hgb level of 13.5 g/dL compared to 11.3 g/dL (NEJM 2006;355:2085). The 2007 FDA black box warning recommends EPO dose adjustment to the lowest level that avoids the requirement for transfusions and not to exceed a hemoglobin of 12 g/dL (FDA Advisory, March 9, 2007). Other side effects are infrequent and not severe. Headache and arthralgias are most common; less common are flu-like symptoms, GI intolerance, diarrhea, edema, and fatigue. Hypertension is an uncommon complication that has been noted more frequently in patients with renal failure. EPO is contraindicated in patients with hypertension that is uncontrolled. The most common reactions noted in the therapeutic trial with 1,943 AIDS patients were rash, injection site reaction, nausea, hypertension, and seizures.

PREGNANCY: Category C. Teratogenic in animals; no studies in humans.

Ethambutol (EMB)

TRADE NAME: Myambutol (Lederle) and generic.

FORMULATIONS, REGIMEN, AND COST: 100 and 400 mg tab; 100 mg tabs at $0.57/tab and 400 mg tabs at $1.56.

PATIENT ASSISTANT PROGRAM: 800-859-8586.

INDICATIONS AND DOSE: Active tuberculosis or infections with *M. avium* complex (MAC) or *M. kansasii* (see

Table 6.41). *Ethambutol dosing for MAC*: 15 mg/kg/d + macrolide.

PHARMACOLOGY:

Bioavailability: 77%.
$T^{1/2}$: 3.1 hr.
Elimination: Renal.

Dose modification in renal failure: CrCl >50 mL/min – 15–25 mg/kg q24h; CrCl 10–50 mL/min – 15–25 mg/kg q24h-q36h; CrCl <10 mL/min – 15–25 mg/kg q48h.

SIDE EFFECTS: Dose and duration-related ocular toxicity (decreased acuity, restricted fields, scotomata, and loss of color discrimination) with 25 mg/kg dose (0.8%), hypersensitivity (0.1%), peripheral neuropathy (rare), GI intolerance (Drug Saf 2008;31:127; Expert Opin Drug Saf 2006;5:615). Ocular toxicity usually improves when the drug is discontinued, but recovery is often partial (Brit J Ophthal 2007;91:895).

WARNINGS: Patients to receive EMB in doses of 25 mg/kg or higher should undergo a baseline screening for visual acuity and red-green color perception; this examination should be repeated at monthly intervals during treatment (MMWR 1998;47[RR-20]:31).

TABLE 6.41 Ethambutol dosing for tuberculosis

Dosing Interval	Weight		
	40–55 kg	56–75 kg	76- >90 kg
Daily	800 mg	1200 mg	1600 mg
2×/wk	2000 mg	2800 mg	4000 mg
3×/wk	1200 mg	2000 mg	2400 mg

From 2017 IDSA/NIH/CDC Guideline for Prevention and Treatment of HIV Associated Opportunistic Infections.

DRUG INTERACTIONS: Aluminum-containing antacids may decrease absorption.

PREGNANCY: Category C. Teratogenic at high doses in animals; no reported adverse effects in women with >320 case observations. Avoid in first trimester if possible.

Etravirine (ETR)

TRADE NAME: Intelence (Janssen Pharmaceuticals).

CLASS: Second generation non-nucleoside reverse transcriptase inhibitor.

FORMULATIONS, REGIMEN, AND COST:

Formulations: 25 mg, 100 mg and 200 mg tabs.
Dose: 200 mg po bid with food.
AWP: $1,411.42/mo.
Storage: Room temperature.
PATIENT ASSISTANCE: 1-800-652-6227.
Once-daily ETR: A pharmacokinetic trial found that once-daily administration produced a lower C_{min}, but was >50-fold higher than the IC_{50} of wild-type HIV with or without concurrent DRV (AIDS 2009;23:2289; Antivir Ther 2010;15:711).
DRUG INTERACTION WARNING: ETR should not be given in combination with any other NNRTI, unboosted PI, DRV/c, ATV/c, TPV/r, FPV/r, or ATV/r (clinical significance against ATV/r co-administration unclear).
FOOD EFFECT: Take with food; type of food is not relevant.
RENAL FAILURE: No data; standard dose likely appropriate since renal excretion is minimal. Minimal removal with dialysis (AIDS 2009;23:740).
HEPATIC FAILURE: Child-Pugh Class A and B: Standard dose; class C: One report of a very high ETR level (3,257 ng/mL)

and prolonged half-life (237 hrs) in a patient with decompensated liver disease (AIDS 209;23:1293).

ADVANTAGES: Activity against most HIV strains that are resistant to first-generation NNRTIs (EFV and NVP), pharmacologic barrier to resistances compared to EFV. Some advantages compared to EFV; reduced CNS toxicity.

DISADVANTAGES: Recommended regimen is bid dosing with food (although PK allows once-daily dosing); high incidence of rash (9%). Concurrent use of TPV, ATV, and FPV are not recommended; reduced activity with poor ETR mutation score.

RESISTANCE: ETR is active against most but not all EFV or NVP-resistant virus. Resistance to ETR can be determined by phenotype or by genotype analysis using one of two weighted scoring systems.

The *Tibotec system* predicted virologic response in the DUET trials (AIDS 2010;24:503):

3 points: 181I/V.

2.5 points: 101P, 100I, 181C, 230L.

1.5 points: 138A, 106I, 190S, 179F.

1 point: 90I, 179D, 101E, 101H, 98G, 179T, 190A.

0–2 points predicts a 74% response,

2.5–3–5 points predicts a 52% response, and.

>4 points predicts a 38% response.

The *Monogram scoring system* predicts phenotypic susceptibility:

4 points: 100I, 101P, 181C/I.

3 points: 138A/G, 179E, 190Q, 230L, 238N.

2 points: 101E, 106A, 138K, 179L, 188L.

1 point: 90I, 101H, 106M, 138Q, 179D/F/M, 181F, 190E/T, 221Y, 225H, 238T.

A score of >4 is associated with reduced susceptibility.

Note: The FDA also included other IAS-USA mutations, but clinical significance is unclear compared to other NNRTIs.

CLINICAL TRIALS:

DUET-1 & -2: ETR + DRV/r + OBR vs. placebo + DRV/r + OBR (N = 1203). Enrollment requirements were virologic failure on current ART regimen with VL >5,000 c/mL + genotypic resistance to first-generation NNRTIs and at least three primary PI mutations. At 48 wks, outcome was superior with ETR vs. placebo for viral suppression to <50 c/mL by ITT analysis (61% vs. 39%) (Table 6.42) (Lancet 2007;370:29). At 96 wks, VL was <50 c/mL in 57% of 599 patients in the ETR arm and 36% of the 604 patients in the placebo arm (p <0.0001) (Antiviral Ther 2010;15:1045). The mean increase in CD4 count was 128 cells/mm³ in ETR recipients vs. 86 cells/mm³ in placebo recipients. A subset analysis of patients with virologic failure suggested that ETR protected against DRV resistance (AIDS 2010;24:921).

ANRS-139 (TRIO): Criteria for entry were VL >1,000 c/mL, treatment-naïve to DRV, RAL, and ETR, and the following: >3 PI resistance mutations, virologic failure with NNRTIs, treatment susceptibility to DRV, and <3 of the following DRV mutations: 11I, 32I, 33F, 47V, 50V, 54L/M, 73S, 76V, 84V, and 89V. Treatment was with RAL 400 mg bid, ETR 200 mg bid, and DRV/r 600/100 bid with or without ENF and NRTIs. At 48 wks, 86% of 100 participants had a VL <50 c/mL; the median CD4 count increase was 108 cells/mm³. Grade 3–4 adverse reactions were reported in 15 (15%) (CID 2009;49:1441). Among 14 virologic failures, 3 had ETR resistance mutations (AIDS 2010;24:2651). A pharmacokinetic study of TRIO participants found that the addition of ETR increased trough levels of DRV by 71% and RAL by 34% (JAIDS 2010;24:2581).

EFV to ETR SWITCH for CNS TOXICITY: This phase IV, double-blind, placebo-controlled trial randomized patients with grade 2–4 CNS toxicity plus VL <50 c/mL to ETR-based ART or continued EFV-based ART (Waters L. 2010 IAS, Vienna; Abstr. LBPE19). At 12 wks, all 38 participants maintained viral control and ETR-recipients experienced a significant reduction of grade 2–4 CNS toxicity, especially abnormal dreams and insomnia. Lipids also improved.

SENSE: Randomized trial of 157 treatment-naïve patients given ETR or EFV, each with 2 NRTIs. The 12-wk results showed virologic suppression to <400 c/mL was achieved in 87.9% of ETR recipients compared to 93% with EFV (*p* = NS) and CD4 count increases were similar (146 vs. 121/mm^3). Drug-related adverse events were much more common with EFV (17% vs. 46%, *p* <0.001) (AIDS 2011;25:335).

SWITCH EFV → ETR (SWITCH-EE): Pharmacokinetic studies indicate that this switch does not require dose adjustment of ETR (JAIDS 2009;52:222). See SWITCH-EE trial (EFV → ETR and ETR → EFV).

PHARMACOLOGY:

Absorption: Bioavailability is unknown. Fasting decreases exposure by 50%; ETR should be taken with food but the content of the meal does not appear to be important. Median trough 275 ng/mL (range is 81–2980).

Distribution: Protein binding, 99%. ETR CNS penetration effectiveness score is 2 (Neurology 2011;76:693).

Metabolism: Metabolized by CYP3A4, CYP2C9, and CYP2C19. ETR does not induce or inhibit its own metabolism.

Elimination: Primarily stool, with <1.2% recovered in urine. Clearance is reduced with HCV or HBV co-infection but no dose adjustment is recommended. Standard dose is recommended for Child Pugh Score A & B, and there is inadequate data for category C.

$T^{1/2}$: 41±20 hrs. No difference is noted in pharmacokinetics based on gender, race or age (18–77 yrs).

SIDE EFFECTS:

Severe side effects: Contact Tibotec (1-877-732-2488) and/or FDA 1-800-FDA-1088 or www.fda.gov/medwatch.

Most serious: Severe cutaneous reactions including Stevens-Johnson syndrome and erythema multiforme (These are rare).

Most common: Rash and nausea.

Number of discontinued treatments due to ADR in clinical trials: 2%.

Rash: Rate in registration trials was 9% vs. 3% in controls. Rash was noted in 19% of participants in DUET-1 and -2 (21% vs. 12% in ETR vs. placebo recipients) and was the most common adverse event prompting discontinuation (JAIDS 2010;53:614). This included two cases of Stevens-Johnson syndrome. The early access experience and most controlled trials report discontinuation due to rash in 1.3–2%. Rashes are most common in women, most common at week 2 and infrequent after week 4. Patients with rash due to EFV or NVP generally tolerated ETR, and most rashes resolved in 1–2 wks with continuation of ETR.

GI Intolerance: Rates of nausea, vomiting, diarrhea, and abdominal pain in registration trials was 2–5% for each GI side effect and not different from controls.

Hepatoxicity: Grade ≥ 3 hepatotoxicity (ALT or AST >5 × ULN) in 2–3% in registration trials, but rates were 4 × higher with HBV or HCV co-infection. Data from DUET-1 and -2 showed no increase in hepatotoxicity rates in patients with HBV or HCV coinfection (JAC 2010;65:2450).

Lipids: Grade ≥ 3 LDL-C (>190 mg/dL) and triglyceride >750 mg/dL were noted in 5–7% in registration trials.

Psychiatric: Grade ≥3–0.2%; significantly less than EFV.

DRUG INTERACTIONS: See Tables 6.42 and 6.43.

ETR is a substrate for CYP3A4, 2C19, and 2C9 and undergoes glucuronidation in vitro; it is an inducer of CYP3A4, 2B6, and Phase II enzyme and an inhibitor of 2C9 and 2C19.

Switches from EFV to ETR are anticipated due to resistance or intolerance. This switch has potential pharmacologic complications due to the long half-life of EFV and its prominent impact on hepatic cytochrome CYP450 enzymes, especially CYP3A4. A trial of co-administration found significantly lower ETR levels, with ETR ratios of AUC-0.71, C_{max} 0.78, C_{trough} 0.67. The authors concluded that the CYP3A4 induction effect of EFV lasted at least 2 wks after discontinuation, but the decrease in ETR levels was probably not clinically significant (JAIDS 2009;52:222).

An extensive drug interaction report from the sponsor reports the following drug interactions (Clin Phamacokinet 2011;50:25):

Drugs with no clinically significant effect on ETR: Atorvastatin, clarithromycin, methadone, omeprazole, oral contraceptives, paroxetine, ranitidine, and sildenafil.

Drugs that have no clinically significant interactions: Azithromycin and ribavirin.

Caution advised with: Digoxin (follow levels), *Warfarin* (levels may be increased), *rifabutin* in presence of some *PI/r*, clarithromycin (decreased, use azithromycin for MAC), *clopidogrel* (may decrease efficacy), *diazepam* (lower diazepam dose or alternative), *dexamethasone* (at steady-state, may decrease ETR use with caution or alternative), *cyclosporine* (may decrease cyclosporine levels).

Not recommended: Carbamazepine, phenytoin, rifampin, rifapentine, St. John's wort (may significantly decrease ETR levels).

PREGNANCY: Category B. Studies of ETR in pregnant women are inadequate to recommend use or dose although preliminary data suggest pharmacokinetics are 1.2- to 1.6-fold increased with ETR exposure during pregnancy. Moderate to high placental transfer (0.19–4.25). The 2015 DHHS Guidelines on Antiretroviral Agents for Pregnant Women classify ETR as "not recommended in treatment-naïve-patients.".

(continued)

TABLE 6.42 ETR drug interactions with ART (AUC)

Co-agent	AUC. ETR	Co-admin ARV (AUC)	Recommendation
TDF	↓ 19%	↑ 15% (NS)	Standard dose
TAF	—	—	No data. Interaction unlikely
EFV	↓ 41%	May ↓	Avoid
NVP	↓ 55%	May ↓	Avoid
MVC	↓ 36%	↓ 53%	MVC 600 mg bid (if not co-administered w/ a PI)
MVC + DRV/r	↓	↑ 110%	Decrease MVC 150 mg bid
NFV	↓	May ↑	No data—avoid
ATV	↑ 50%	↓ 17%	Avoid
ATV/r	↑ 30%	↓ 14%	Avoid, but clinical significance unclear
ATV/c	May ↑	May ↓	No data. Avoid
FPV/r	NC	↑ 69%	Avoid, but clinical significance unclear
DRV/r	↓ 37%	↑ 15%	Standard doses DRV/r 600/100 mg bid; extensive data
DRV/c	May ↑	May ↓	No data. Avoid
LPV/r	↓ 30–45%	↓ 18%	Standard doses
TPV/r	↓ 76%	↑ 18%	Avoid
SQV + LPV/r		NC	Standard doses
RTV (high dose)	↓ 46%		Avoid
IDV	↑ 50%	↓ 46%	Avoid
RAL	↑ 10%	↓ 10%	RAL 400 mg bid. Avoid RAL HD once-daily dosing.

TABLE 6.42 Continued

Co-agent	AUC. ETR	Co-admin ARV (AUC)	Recommendation
DTG	—	↓ 71%. ↓ 25% (w/ DRV/r)	Must be given with boosted PI (DRV/r). DTG 50 mg/d + ETR 200 mg bid + PI/r
EVG/c	—	EVG may↓	Avoid. Use RTV to boost EVG
EVG/r	↔	↔	Dose w/ETR: EVG85 mg + ATV/r300/100 mg/d or EVG150 mg + DRV/r600/100 mg bid
BIC		May ↓	No data. Avoid

NC, No significant change.

TABLE 6.43 ETR drug interactions with other drugs

Class	Agent	Effect on Co-administered Drug or ETR
	Atorvastatin	↓AUC statin 37%; use standard dose and monitor response
	Lovastatin	Statin may be ↓
	Simvastatin	Statin may be ↓
	Rosuvastatin	Considered preferred; standard dose; no interaction
	Pravastatin	Considered preferred; standard dose; no interaction
	Pitavastatin	Considered preferred; Standard dose; no interaction

(continued)

TABLE 6.43 Continued

Class	Agent	Effect on Co-administered Drug or ETR
Anti-mycobacterial agents	Rifampin Rifabutin	Significant ↓ ETR-avoid Rifabutin AUC ↓17%; ETR ↓37% Rifabutin 300 mg/d and ETR standard dose if no PI/r used. If DRV/r, SQV/r, LPV/r used with ETR, do not co-administer rifabutin.
Gastric agents	Omeprazole Ranitidine	ETR AUC ↑ 41%; standard dose ETR AUC ↓ 14%; standard dose
Antibiotics	Clarithromycin	ETR AUC ↑ 42%; Clarithromycin AUC ↓ 39% MAC, but active metabolite increased—use azithromycin S. pneumonia—use azithromycin
Methadone	Methadone	No change; standard doses
Anti-arrhythmia drugs	See comment	Amiodarone, bepridil, disopyramide, flecainide, lidocaine, mexiletine, propafenone, quinidine—may ↓ with ETR co-administration; use with caution
Anticonvulsants	Phenobarbital, Phenytoin, Carbamazepine, Oxcarbazepine	ETR levels ↓↓– avoid Anticonvulsant levels may ↓ also. Consider levetiracetam.
Erectile dysfunction	Sildenafil	Sildenafil AUC ↓ 57%; titrate to effect
	Vardenafil; Tadalafil	May decrease PDE-5 inhibitors; titrate to effect.
Oral contraceptive	Ethinyl Estradiol/ Norethindrone	Ethinyl estradiol AUC ↑ 22%, No change in norethindrone significance unclear; Use standard dose.

TABLE 6.43 Continued

Class	Agent	Effect on Co-administered Drug or ETR
Steroids	Dexamethasone	↓ ETR levels may ↓ – consider alternative steroid
Antifungal	Azoles (See pg. 208)	ETR AUC ↑ 86% with fluconazole. ETR AUC ↑ 36% with voriconazole. ETR levels may ↑ with other azoles. Standard dose with caution—voriconazole, fluconazole and posaconazole. Itraconazole levels may ↓ and voriconazole levels ↑14%; monitor levels and consider dose adjustment
Antidepressants	St. John's wort	May significantly ↓ ETR—Avoid
	Paroxetine	No change. Standard dose.
Immuno suppressants	Cyclosporin, Tacrolimus, Sirolimus	May ↓ immunosuppressants; Monitor levels closely
Antiplatelet	Clopidogrel	May ↓ the efficacy of clopidogrel. Avoid
Anticoagulation	Warfarin	May increase or decrese INR; Monitor closely

Famciclovir—see Acyclovir

Fenofibrate—see also Gemfibrozil

TRADE NAME: Tricor (Abbott Laboratories), Antara (Reliant), Lofibra (Gate), Triglide (Sciele Pharmaceutical, Inc.).

CLASS: Fibrate.

FORMULATIONS, REGIMEN, AND COST: Tricor tabs, 48 and 145 mg; Lofibra caps 67 mg, 134 mg, 200 mg, Antara caps, 30 and 90 mg, Fenofibrate micronized cap 43, 67, 130, 134, 200 mg; Fenofibrate cap 50 mg, 150 mg.

COST: 48 mg tab at $2.95, 145 mg tab at $8.86.

INDICATIONS AND DOSES: Fibrates have documented evidence of reducing risk of cardiovascular disease in patients who have dyslipidemia without HIV infection, and they have documented benefit for reducing triglycerides and increasing HDL in HIV-infected patients (Expert Opin Drug Metab Toxicol 2010;6:995). The usual indication is hypertriglyceridemia, especially levels of >500–700 mg/dL. Starting dose Tricor 48 mg/d then increase if necessary at 4–8 wk intervals; maximum dose, 145 mg/d; some authorities consider this the usual dose (CID 2006;43:645). Take as a single daily dose with meal. Fenofibrate is by far the most prescribed fibrate in the United States with 73% of the market (JAMA 2011;305:1221) Gemfibrozil is second with 11%.

MONITORING: Triglyceride levels: Discontinue use if ineffective after 2 mos at 145 mg/d (maximum dose). Warn patients to report symptoms of myositis and obtain CPK if there is muscle tenderness, pain, or weakness. Monitor AST + ALT; discontinue if there is an otherwise unexplained CPK increase to ≥3× ULN.

PRECAUTIONS: Avoid or use with caution with gallbladder disease, hepatic disease, or renal failure with CrCl <50 mL/min.

CLINICAL TRIALS: *ACTG 5087* compared fenofibrate 200 mg/d and pravastatin 40 mg/d in 194 HIV-infected patients with dyslipidemia. At 48 wks most patients required the addition of the alternative agent. Both drugs were well tolerated, and the combination produced substantial benefit, but <10% of patients achieved the goals set by the National Cholesterol Education Program (NCEP) at 1 yr (AIDS Res Human Retroviruses 2005;21:757).

Another trial compared fenofibrate to pioglitazone in patients with metabolic syndrome attributed to PI-based ART (CID 2005;40:745). Pioglitazone improved insulin resistance, reduced triglyceride levels, and increased levels of HDL cholesterol, and fenofibrate did not significantly alter lipids or insulin resistance (CID 2005;40:745). Other studies have found that fenofibrate has a significant benefit in reducing triglyceride levels in patients with ART-associated hyperlipidemia (Am J Med Sci 2004;327:315; CID 2006;43:645).

PHARMACOLOGY:

Bioavailability: Good, improved 35% with food.

$T^{1/2}$: 20 hr.

Elimination: Renal, 60%; fecal, 25%.

Renal failure: 54 mg/d; increase with caution due to risk of myopathy and monitor CPK.

SIDE EFFECTS:

Hepatic: Dose-related hepatotoxicity with increased transaminase levels to >3× ULN in 6% receiving doses of 134–201 mg/d; most had return to normal levels with drug discontinuation or with continued treatment.

Influenza-like syndrome.

Rash, pruritus, and/or urticaria in 1–3%.

Myositis: Warn patient about symptoms of muscle pain, tenderness, and/or weakness, especially with fever or malaise. Measure CPK and discontinue if significantly typical symptoms occur.

Rare: Pancreatitis, agranulocytosis, cholecystitis, eczema, thrombocytopenia.

DRUG INTERACTIONS:

Oral anticoagulant: Potentiates warfarin activity. Cholestyramine and colestipol bind fenofibrate; take fenofibrate >1 hr before or 4–6 hrs after bile acid binding agent; Statins may increase risk of rhabdomyolysis with renal failure.

PREGNANCY: Category C.

Fentanyl

TRADE NAME: Duragesic patch (Janssen), Fentanyl Oralet (Abbott Laboratories), and generic.

CLASS: Opiate; Schedule II controlled substance.

FORMULATIONS, REGIMEN, AND COST:
Injection-fentanyl citrate, 50 µg/mL/2/mL vial at $0.48 å Buccal (transmucosal) lozenge – 200, 300, 400 µg, 600 µg, 800 µg, 1,200 µg, 1,600 µg.
Transdermal:

  12 µg/hr Duragesic 12: $20.30.
  25 µg/hr (10 cm²) Duragesic 25: $14.43.
  50 µg/hr (20 cm²) Duragesic 50: $26.38.
  75 µg/hr (30 cm²) Duragesic 75: $40.24.
  100 µg/hr (40 cm²) Duragesic 100: $53.41.

INDICATIONS: Chronic pain requiring opiate analgesia.

DOSING RECOMMENDATIONS: Dose depends on desired therapeutic effect, patient weight, PIs, cobicistat (avoid co-administration) interactions and most importantly, existing opiate tolerance. The initial dose in opiate-naïve patients is a system delivering 12 µg/hr to 25 µg/hr. Cachectic patients should not receive a higher initial dose unless they have been receiving the equivalent of 135 mg of oral morphine.

MAINTENANCE: Most patients are maintained with patch applications at 72-hr intervals. Adequacy of analgesia should be evaluated at 72 hrs. The dose should be increased to maintain the 72-hr interval if possible, but application every 48 hrs is another option. Supplemental opiates may be required with initial use to control pain and to determine optimal fentanyl dose. The suggested conversion ratio is 90 mg of oral morphine/24 hrs to each 25 μg/hr labeled delivery.

APPLICATION INSTRUCTIONS: The protective liner-cover should be peeled just prior to use. Apply is to a dry, nonirritated, flat surface of the upper torso by firm pressure for 30 seconds. Hair should be clipped, not shaven, and the skin cleansed with water (not soaps or alcohol that could irritate skin) prior to application. Avoid external heat to the site because absorption is temperature-dependent. Rotate sites with sequential use. After removal, the used system should be folded so the adhesive side adheres to itself and flushed in the toilet.

Note: Buccal (transmucosal) form should be used only with monitoring in the hospital (OR, ICU, EW) due to life-threatening respiratory depression. Use in AIDS is primarily restricted to management of chronic pain in late-stage disease using the transdermal form. This drug should not be used for the management of acute pain.

PHARMACOLOGY: Transdermal fentanyl systems deliver an average of 25 μg/hr/10 cm^2 at a constant rate. Serum levels increase slowly, plateau at 12–24 hrs, and then remain constant for up to

TABLE 6.44 Fentanyl dose conversion chart

Generic Name	Equianalgesic Dose (mg)	
	Parenteral	Oral
Codeine	120	200
Fentanyl	0.1	NA
Hydrocodone	NA	20
Hydromorphone	1.5	6–7.5
Meperidine	75–100	300
Morphine	10	30–40
Oxycodone	NA	15–30

TABLE 6.45 Equivalence of fentanyl patches and oral morphine sulfate

Oral MS/d	Fentanyl (µg/hr)	Oral MS/d	Fentanyl (µg/hr)
45–134 mg	25	495–584 mg	150
135–224 mg	50	675–764 mg	200
225–314 mg	75	855–994 mg	250
315–404 mg	100	1035–1124 mg	300

72 hrs. The labeling indicates the amount of fentanyl delivered per hour. Peak serum levels for the different systems are the following: Fentanyl, 25: 0.3–1.2 ng/mL; 50: 0.6–1.8 ng/mL; 75: 1.1–2.6 ng/mL; and 100: 1.9–3.8 ng/mL. After discontinuation, serum levels decline with a mean half-life of 17 hrs. Absorption depends on skin temperature and theoretically increases by one-third when the body temperature is 40°C. In acute pain models, the 100 µg/hr form provided analgesia equivalent to 60 mg of morphine IM.

SIDE EFFECTS:

Respiratory depression with hypoventilation. This occurs throughout the therapeutic range of fentanyl concentration but increases at concentrations >2 ng/mL in opiate-naïve patients and in patients with pulmonary disease.

CNS depression is seen with concentrations >3 ng/mL in opiate-naïve patients. At levels of 10–20 ng/mL there is anesthesia and profound respiratory depression.

Tolerance occurs with extended courses, but there is considerable individual variation.

Local effects include erythema, papules, pruritus, and edema at the site of application.

Drug interactions include increased fentanyl levels with all CYP3A4 inhibitors (cobicistat and PIs) given concurrently. The drug is metabolized by cytochrome P450 isoenzyme 3A4, so strong inhibitors of CYP 3A4 will increase fentanyl and risk respiratory arrest. This includes all PIs and especially ritonavir- and cobicistat-boosted PIs. Consider morphine with concurrent use with cobicistat PIs. EFV, NVP, ETR may decrease fentanyl levels. Interaction unlikely with MVC, BIC, DTG, RPV, RAL, ENF, and NRTIs.

PREGNANCY: Category C.

Filgrastim—see G-CSF

Fluconazole

TRADE NAME: Diflucan (Pfizer) and generic.

CLASS: Triazole related to other imidazoles: ketoconazole, clotrimazole, miconazole; triazoles (fluconazole and itraconazole) have three nitrogens in the azole ring.

FORMULATIONS, REGIMEN, AND COST: Tabs: 50 mg at $5.57, 100 mg at $8.75, 150 mg at $13.93, 200 mg at $14.32. IV vials: 200 mg at $14.51, and 400 mg at $15.24; oral solution 10 mg/mL (35 mL bottle) at $35.80, 40 mg/mL (35 mL bottle) at $130.40.

PATIENT ASSISTANCE PROGRAM: 800-869-9979.

ACTIVITY: *Candida*: Active vs. 95% of all strains in fluconazole-naïve patients except *C. krusei*, many *C. glabrata*, and some *C. tropicalis* and *C. parapsilosis*. Also active against: Blastomyces, Coccidioidomyces, Histoplasma, Paracoccidioidomyces, Sporothrix, and Cryptococcus. Not active against Aspergillus, Phycomyces, *P. boydii*, and Zygomyces.

FUNGUS-SPECIFIC USES: See *Candida*, cryptococcosis, and histoplasmosis.

RESISTANCE: Fluconazole is the preferred azole for systemic treatment of candidiasis, but a major concern with long-term use is azole-resistant candidiasis, which correlates with amount of azole exposure and CD4 count <50/mm^3 (JID 1996;173:219). All oral systemically active azoles predispose to resistance. Some cases involve evolution of resistance by *C. albicans*, and others reflect substitution with non-albicans species such as *C. glabrata* or *C. krusei* (AAC 2002;46:1723). Resistance is uncommon when fluconazole is used to treat vaginitis (CID 2001;33:1069; Med Mycol 2005;43:647). Fluconazole-resistant strains of *Candida* can often be treated with caspofungin (AAC 2002;46:1723), micafungin (CID 2004;39:842) or amphotericin and possibly itraconazole, voriconazole (CID 2001;33:1447), or posaconazole. Resistance does not appear to be an issue with cryptococcal infections (but reports of reduced efficacy with MIC μg/mL) with the possible exception *C. gatti* (AAC 2009;53:309; J Med Microbiol 2011;60:961), which is a regional risk in the Pacific Northwest US, British Columbia, and South America (MMWR 2010;59:865).

CLINICAL TRIALS: Cochrane Library review of 38 trials of treatment of oropharyngeal candidiasis in HIV-infected patients found that (1) fluconazole had a higher cure rate to topical agents (OR = 1:1.7), (2) cure rates for fluconazole and itraconazole were similar (OR = 1.05), (3) mycological cure rates were significantly better with fluconazole and itraconazole than with clotrimazole (OR = 1:1.5 and 1:2.2), and (4) continuous fluconazole was superior to intermittent fluconazole for preventing recurrence of thrush (OR = 0.04) (Cochrane Database Syst Rev 2006; CD 003940), but this is generally not recommended due to risk of resistance. The efficacy of fluconazole for the treatment of cryptococcal meningitis appears to be dose related, with doses of 1,200–2,000 mg/d in one study (CID 2008;47:1556).

PHARMACOLOGY:

> *Bioavailability*: >90%.
> *CSF levels*: 50–94% of serum levels.
> $T^{1/2}$: 30 hr.
> *Elimination*: Renal; 60–80% of administered dose excreted unchanged in the urine.

TABLE 6.46 Dose recommendations for fluconazole[b]

Indications	Dose Regimen	Comment
Candidiasis		
Thrush		
Acute[a]	100 mg po qd × 7-14 d	Response rate 80% to 100%, usually within 5 days; may need up to 400–800 mg/d. Maintenance therapy often required in late-stage disease without immune reconstitution. Topical therapy (e.g., clotrimazole) can be considered before systemic therapy. Chronic treatment: Indication is severe or frequent recurrence. Options are topical agent prn or chronic suppressive oral fluconazole. Risk of fluconazole resistance is increased
Secondary Prevention[a]	100 mg po 3 ×/wk or qd	
Esophagitis		
Acute	100–200 mg po qd or IV up to 400 mg/d × 14-21 d	Relapse rate is 85–90%. Relapse rate is >80% within 1 yr in absence of maintenance therapy and immue reconstitution. Maintenance may be required for recurrent esophagitis but increases risk of resistance. Discontinue when CD4 >200
Maintenance	100–200 mg po qd	

(*continued*)

TABLE 6.46 Continued

Indications	Dose Regimen	Comment
Vaginitis		
Treatment	150 mg po × 1	Response rate 90% to 100% in absence of
Prevention[a]	Multiple recurrences: 150 mg po qw	HIV infection
		Topical azoles generally preferred.
Cryptococcosis		
Non-meningeal, acute; focal pulmonary d	400 mg/d po × 12 mos	Fluconazole 400 mg × 6–12 mos is recommended by the IDSA as the preferred treatment for mild to moderate cryptococcal pneumonia. For more severe pulmonary disease with cryptococcemia treat as CNS disease.
Meningitis and disseminated disease		
Acute (alternative)	1200 mg/d (up to 2000 mg/d) po ×10-12 wks or 1200 mg/d x 2 weeks + flucytosine, then flucon 800mg/d x 10 weeks followed by maintenance or 1200 mg/d + 5FC ×6 wks, then consolidation and maintenance.	Acute treatment with Lipid amphotericin B + 5-FC ≥ 2 wks is preferred
Consolidation (after ampho induction)[a]	400 mg po qd × ≥8 wks, followed by maintenance	Continue maintenance until immune reconstitution with CD4 ≥100/mm³ × >3 mos and VL <50.
Maintenance	200 mg po qd	
Coccidioidomycosis		

TABLE 6.46 Continued

Indications	Dose Regimen	Comment
Meningitis[a]	400–800 mg IV or po	Preferred for meningeal form.
Non-meningeal		
Acute	400–800 mg po qd	Ampho B or lipid Ampho usually preferred for severe disease, except with mild focal pulmonary disease.[a]
Maintenance[a]	400 mg po qd	Itraconazole considered equally effective.
Histoplasmosis		
Treatment (alternative)	800 mg/d	Amphotericin B and itraconazole preferred.

[a] Preferred agent (2018 CDC/IDSA/NIH OI Guidelines).
[b] From CID 2005;41:1217; CID 2010;50:291;2015 IDSA/NIH/CDC Guidelines for Treatment and Prevention of Opportunistic Infections; and American Thoracic Society (Am J Respir Crit Care Med 2011;183:96).

Dose modification in renal failure: CrCl >50 mL/min, usual dose; 10–50 mL/min, half dose; CrCl <10 mL/min, quarter dose; hemo- dialysis, standard dose (200–400 mg) after each dialysis.

SIDE EFFECTS: Generally well tolerated. Headache, nausea, and abdominal pain, the most common side effects, are dose-related and most common with >400 mg/d (JAC 2006;57:384). GI intolerance (1.5–8%, usually does not require discontinuation), rash (5%), transient increases in hepatic enzymes (5%), increases of ALT or AST to >8× upper limit of normal requires discontinuation (1%), dizziness, hypokalemia, and headache (2%). Reversible alopecia in 10–20%

receiving ≥400 mg/d at median time of 3 mos after starting treatment (Ann Intern Med 1995;123:354).

DRUG INTERACTIONS: Inhibits cytochrome P450 (2C8/9/19 and 3A4) hepatic enzymes resulting in increased levels of atovaquone, some benzodiazepines, alprazolam, diazepam, midazolam, triazolam, clarithromycin, fentanyl, glyburide, glipizide, phenytoin, warfarin, SQV, rifabutin, cyclosporine, simvastatin, lovastatin, tacrolimus, and sirolimus; cisapride, terfenadine, and astemizole may cause life- threatening arrhythmias. Fluconazole levels are reduced with rifampin; with rifabutin there is no effect on fluconazole levels, but rifabutin AUC increases 80%; consider rifabutin TDM. Unlike ketoconazole, voriconazole, and itraconazole, fluconazole can be used without dose modification with PIs and NNRTIs except with NVP, which increases with NVP levels—monitor for hepatotoxicity and rash or avoid this combination. Fluconazole increases TPV AUC by 50%; do not exceed fluconazole 200 mg. Use standard dose with other PI/r. ETR AUC increased 86% with fluconazole co-administration. Fluconazole increases AZT AUC 74% due to decreased AZT glucuronidation; monitor for AZT toxicity. Use standard dose with other NRTIs. Fluconazole may decrease efficacy of clopidogrel; may increase RPV concentrations (monitor QTc with co-administration). Significant drug interaction unlikely with BIC, RAL and DTG. With MVC: use standard dose.

PREGNANCY: Category C. Animal studies show reduced maternal weight gain and embryo lethality with dose >20× comparable to doses in humans; skeletal and craniofacial abnormalities noted in infants born to four women given fluconazole in pregnancy. Single dose considered safe for candida vaginitis; topical treatment preferred. Amphotericin B preferred for systemic fungal infection in first trimester, if efficacy expected.

Flucytosine (5-FC)

TRADE NAME: Ancobon (ICN Pharmaceuticals) and generic.

CLASS: Structurally related to fluorouracil.

FORMULATIONS, REGIMEN, AND COST: Caps: 250 mg at $82.07, 500 mg at $158.81.

INDICATIONS AND DOSE: Used with amphotericin B or fluconazole to treat serious cryptococcosis. IDSA guidelines (OI guidelines 2018) and ATS Guidelines (Am J Respir Crit Care 2011;183:96) recommend treating cryptococcal meningitis with amphotericin B + flucytosine 100 mg/kg/d in 4 doses for ≥2 wks based on several studies showing benefit of this treatment (reduced rate of relapse and more rapid sterilization of CSF) compared with amphotericin B alone (CID 2010;50:345; NEJM 1997;337:15; NEJM 1992;326:83; Ann Intern Med 1990;113:183; JID 1992;165:960; CID 1999;28:291). The combination of amphotericin and flucytosine is synergistic against *Cryptococcus* in vitro and in vivo (AAC 2006;50:113). The combination of fluconazole + 5-FC is also effective, but toxicity at higher 5-FC doses may limit use of 5-FC (CID 1994;19:741; JID 1992;165:960). Fluconazole (1200 mg/d) + 5-FC (100 mg/kg/d) × 2 wks, followed by fluconazole 800 mg/d resulted in fewer deaths at 2 wks (10% vs. 37%) compared to fluconazole (800 mg) alone (CID 2010;50:338). 5-FC (150 mg/kg/d) with fluconazole has been studied for treatment of nonmeningeal cryptococcosis (CID 2000;30:710). Neutropenia and thrombocytopenia are relative contraindications to flucytosine. Multiple trials suggest amphotericin B + 5-FC for 14 days is the most effective induction regimen in patients with a high fungal burden at baseline (CID 2008;3:e2870). Flucytosine is concentrated in urine and can be used for *Candida* UTIs (CID 2011;52 Suppl 6:S457).

Dose: 25 mg/kg po q6h (100 mg/kg/d).

RESISTANCE: MIC ≥32 mg/mL may be considered resistant.

PHARMACOLOGY:

Bioavailability: >80%.
$T^{1/2}$: 2.4–4.8 hr.
Elimination: 63–84% unchanged in urine.
CNS penetration: 80% of serum levels.

Dose modification in renal failure: CrCl >40 mL/min, 25.0 mg/kg q6h; 20–40 mL/min, 25 mg/kg q12h; 10–20 mL/min, 25 mg/kg q24h; <10 mL/min, 25 mg/kg q48h (use with close monitoring of CBC and 5-FC serum level).

Therapeutic monitoring: Measure serum concentration 2 hrs post-oral dose with goal of peak level of 30–80 µg/mL after 3–5 days.

SIDE EFFECTS: Dose-related leukopenia and thrombocytopenia, especially with levels >100 µg/mL and concurrent use of other marrow-suppressing agents and in patients with renal insufficiency, which can occur secondary to concurrent amphotericin B therapy; GI intolerance; rash; hepatitis; peripheral neuropathy.

DRUG INTERACTIONS: Drugs that cause bone marrow suppression (e.g., AZT, ganciclovir, pyrimethamine, interferon). Avoid or use with caution.

PREGNANCY: Category C; teratogenic in animal studies. First-trimester exposures to doses 400–800 mg/d may be associated with rare and distinctive birth defects. Avoid during pregnancy.

Fluoroquinolones—see Ciprofloxacin

Fluoxetine

TRADE NAME: Prozac and Prozac Weekly (Eli Lilly) and generic.

CLASS: Selective serotonin reuptake inhibitors (SSRI) antidepressant. Other drugs in this class include Paxil, Zoloft, Celexa, and Lexapro.

FORMULATIONS, REGIMEN, AND COST: Caps: 10 mg at $2.60, 20 mg at $2.67, 40 mg at $5.33; 60 mg tab at $6.86. Solution 20 mg/5 mL (120 mL bottle) $118.; 90 mg delayed release cap at $39.20.

INDICATIONS AND DOSE:

Major depression: 10–40 mg/d usually given once-daily in the morning. Onset of response requires 2–6 wks. Doses of 5–10 mg/d may be adequate in debilitated patients. Prozac weekly: 90 mg/wk.

Obsessive-compulsive disorder: 20–80 mg/d.

PHARMACOLOGY:

Bioavailability: 60–80%.

$T^{1/2}$: 7–9 days for norfluoxetine (active metabolite).

Elimination: Metabolized by liver to norfluoxetine; fluoxetine eliminated in urine.

Dose modification in renal failure: None.

Dose modification in cirrhosis: Half-life prolonged; reduce dose.

SIDE EFFECTS: Toxicity may not be apparent for 2–6 wks. GI intolerance (anorexia, weight loss, nausea) in 20%; anxiety, agitation, insomnia, sexual dysfunction in 20%; less common are headache, tremor, drowsiness, dry mouth, sweating, diarrhea, acute dystonia, akathisia (sensation of motor restlessness).

Note: Case reports have suggested an association with suicidal ideation; reanalysis of data showed no significant difference compared with treatment with other antidepressants or placebo (J Clin Psychopharmacol 1991;11:166). Nevertheless, the FDA required manufacturers of SSRIs to add a warning label concerning increased risk of suicide with antidepressant initiation.

DRUG INTERACTIONS:

MAO inhibitors: Avoid initiation of fluoxetine until ≥14 days after discontinuing MAO inhibitor; avoid starting MAO inhibitor until ≥5 wks after discontinuing fluoxetine (risk is "serotonergic syndrome").

Inhibits 2D6 >2C9; 1A2 >3A4); Substrate 2C9, 2D6: May increase levels of tricyclic agents (desipramine, nortriptyline, etc.), phenytoin, digoxin, Coumadin, terfenadine (ventricular arrhythmias; avoid), SQV, astemizole (avoid), theophylline, thioridazine (contraindicated), mesoridazine (avoid), haloperidol, carbamazepine, and pimozide (avoid).

Ritonavir: Serotonin syndrome has been reported (AIDS 2001;15:1281).

Linezolid: Avoid co-administration. May increase risk of serotonin syndrome. Discontinue fluoxetine or other SSRI 14 days before starting linezolid (CID 2006;42:1578), but some advocate a shorter washout period (CID 2006;43:180).

PREGNANCY: Category C.

Flurazepam—see Benzodiazepines

Fosamprenavir (FPV)

TRADE NAME: Lexiva (ViiV Healthcare/GlaxoSmithKline); in Europe, Telzir (ViiV Healthcare/GlaxoSmithKline).

CLASS: Protease inhibitor (pro-drug of amprenavir).

FORMULATIONS, REGIMEN, AND COST:

> *Form*: 700 mg tab at $20.07; 50 mg/mL solution (225 mL) at $184.54.
>
> *Regimen*: Four regimens are FDA-approved.
>
> FPV 1400 mg bid (without ritonavir, Pl-naïve only); FPV/r preferred.
>
> FPV/r 1400/100 mg/d (PI-naïve only) with food.
>
> FPV/r 1400/200 mg/d (PI-naïve only) with food (FPV/r 1400/ 100 mg/d preferred).
>
> FPV/r 700/100 mg bid (PI-naïve or experienced) with food.
>
> *AWP*: $2408.86/mo for 1,400 mg bid regimen.
>
> PATIENT ASSISTANCE PROGRAM: 877-844-8872.
>
> FOOD EFFECT: Not significant except with RTV boosting.
>
> EFV: With EFV, use RTV-boosted regimens. If using once-daily regimen, increase RTV dose to 300 mg/d (FPV/r 1400/300

mg/d). If using twice-daily regimen, use standard dose (FPV/r 700/100 mg bid).

No data with cobicistat boosting.

RENAL FAILURE: Standard dose.

HEPATIC FAILURE: Child-Pugh score: 5–8, FPV 700 mg bid without RTV boosting; >8, avoid FPV.

STORAGE: Room temperature, up to 25°C (77°F).

WARNINGS: Hepatic disease; dose modification.

ADVANTAGES: (1) Potency comparable to LPV/r (Lancet 2006:368:476) and ATV/r in treatment-naïve patients, (2) no food requirement (except suspension that needs to be taken with food), (3) may be given once-daily with RTV 100 mg (treatment-naïve only), and (4) no significant PI resistance when FPV/r is used in treatment-naïve patients.

DISADVANTAGES: (1) Once-daily therapy not recommended for PI-experienced patients; (2) no advantage over coformulated LPV/r, DRV/c, ATV/c when given at 700/100 mg bid in terms of efficacy, tolerability, or lipid effects; and (3) once-daily FPV/r (1,400/100 mg) is not as extensively studied as once-daily DRV/r or ATV/r; (4) cross-resistance with DRV/r with certain APV mutations.

CLINICAL TRIALS: See Table 6.47. The *KLEAN* trial (Lancet 2006;368:476) was the major comparative clinical trial in treatment-naïve patients. Comparison of FPV/r bid vs. LPV/r bid found nearly identical results at 48 wks in all important endpoints, including viral suppression to <50 c/mL (66% vs. 65%), CD4 count increase, treatment discontinuation due to adverse events (12% vs. 10%), effect of treatment on lipids, and frequency of treatment-emergent drug resistance. (Note: LPV/r formulation used in this trial was the gel capsule formulation.).

In the *SOLO* trial, FPV/r 1400/200 qd (with ABC/3TC) was noninferior at 48 wks to NFV + ABC/3TC in treatment-naïve patients (AIDS 2004;18:1529). Patients who completed SOLO and had viral suppression (<400 c/mL) on FPV/r were followed for up to 142 wks. At 142 wks, VL was <400 c/mL in 159/211 (75%) and

TABLE 6.47 Clinical trials of FPV in treatment-naïve and PI-experienced patients

Trial	Regimen	N	Wks	VL (c/mL) <400	<50
SOLO Treatment-naïve (AIDS 2004;18:1529)	FPV/r 1400/200 mg/d + ABC/3TC	322	48	69%	55%
	NFV 1250 mg bid + ABC/3TC	327		68%	53%
NEAT Treatment-naïve (JAIDS 2004;35:22)	FPV 1400 mg bid + ABC/3TC	166	48	[b] 66%	[b] 57%
	NFV 1250 mg bid + ABC/3TC	83		52%	42%
CONTEXT Failure 1-2 PI regimens (6th CROI 2003, Abstr. 178)	FPV/r 700/100 mg bid + 2 NRTIs	107	48	58%	[c] 46%
	FPV/r 1400/200 mg/d + 2 NRTIs[a]	105			37%
	LPV/r 400/100 mg bid + 2 NRTIs	103		61%	50% [b]
TRIAD Failure >PI regimens (JAC 2009;64:398)	FPV/r 700/100 mg bid	24	24		21%
	FPV/r 1400/100 mg bid	24			24%
	FPV 1400 mg bid + LPV/r 533/133 mg bid	20			20%
KLEAN Treatment-naïve (Lancet 2006;368:476)	FPV/r 700/100 mg bid + ABC/3TC qd	434	48	73%	66%
	LPV/r 400/100 mg bid + ABC/3TC qd	444		71%	65%
COL100758 Treatment-naïve (AIDS Res Hum Retroviruses 2009;25:395)	FPV/r 1400/200 mg/d	57	96	53%	53%
	FPV/r 1400/100 mg/d	58		[b] 78%	66%

TABLE 6.47 Continued

Trial	Regimen	N	Wks	VL (c/mL)	
				<400	<50
ALERT Treatment-naïve (AIDS Res Ther 2008;5:5)	FPV/r 1400/ 100 mg/d + TDF/FTC qd	45	48	79%	75%
	ATV/r 300/ 100 mg/d + TDF/FTC qd	49		87%	83%

[a] The once-daily regimen in the CONTEXT trial was dropped due to virologic inferiority.
[b] Superior to comparator (P <0.05).
[c] FPV/r did not meet the FDA criteria for "noninferiority" criteria compared to LPV/r.

<50 c/mL in 139/211 (66%). The median increase in CD4 cell count was 292/mm³. Resistance tests in 14 virologic failures showed no PI resistance mutations. The most common adverse reactions were diarrhea (10%), nausea (8%), and increased triglycerides (7%) (Clin Ther 2006;28:745).

COL100758 Trial: This was an open-label trial in which 115 treatment-naïve patients were randomized to receive FPV/r 1400/ 200 mg/d vs. FPV/r 1400/100 mg/d. At 96 wks, patients receiving RTV 100 mg/d had greater viral suppression to <400 c/mL (78% vs. 53%; p <0.006), lower triglyceride elevations (+27 vs. +48 mg/dL), fewer premature discontinuations for adverse reactions (12 vs. 24), and fewer virologic failures (5 vs. 8). None of the 8 with virologic failures had PI resistance mutations (AIDS Res Hum Retroviruses 2009;25:395).

LESS Trial: This was another trial comparing FPV/r 1400/100 vs. FPV/r 1400/200 mg, but in this case the randomization came after achieving virologic suppression (<400 c/mL) on FPV/r 1400/ 200 mg once-daily. At 24 wks, VL was <50 c/mL in 92% and 94% for the daily RTV dose of 100 mg or 200 mg/d, respectively. Again, the lower dose of RTV was associated with lower triglyceride levels (HIV Clin Trials 2010;11:239).

The *NEAT Trial* found unboosted FPV to be superior to NFV (JAIDS 2004;35:22). In a long-term follow-up analysis at 120 wks in a subset of 211 patients who continued FPV/r qd in a open label single-arm study, 139 (66%) still had VL <50 c/mL (Clin Ther 2006;28:745).

ALERT Trial: This was a trial comparing once-daily FPV/r (1400/100 mg) vs. ATV/r (300/100 mg), each in combination with TDF/FTC in 106 randomized treatment-naïve patients. At baseline the median VL was 4.9 $\log_{10}$ c/mL in each arm, and baseline CD4 counts were 176 and 205 cells/mm^3. At 48 wks, VL was <50 c/mL in 40/53 (75%) of FPV/r recipients and 44/53 (83%) of ATV/r recipients by ITT analysis (p = 0.34). Changes in lipids were similar (AIDS Res Ther 2008;5:5), but median triglyceride levels were higher with FPV/r (150 vs. 131 mg/dL). A subsequent report indicated that 4 FPV and ATV virologic failures had archived resistance strains (AIDS Res Hum Retroviruses 2010;26:407).

RESISTANCE: In trials of FPV in PI-naïve patients, the predominant mutations in patients experiencing virologic failure were 32I, 46I/L, 47V, 50V, 54L/M, and 84V, all mutations that cause minimal cross-resistance with other PIs except for DRV. The primary PI mutation is I50V, which decreases susceptibility to LPV and DRV, and I84V, a multi-PI resistance mutation. Patients failing FPV/r in the SOLO trial had no PI mutations.

PHARMACOLOGY:

Absorption: Not affected by food; bioavailability not established.
Elimination: APV is an inhibitor, substrate, and likely an inducer of P450 3A4 at steady-state.
$T^{1/2}$: 7.7 hr.
CNS penetration: Effectiveness score is 2 in a four-class system (Neurology 2011;76:693).

TABLE 6.48 Combination of FPV with other PIs and with NNRTIs

Drug	Co-admin. Drug	FPV	Comment
NVP	↑13%	↑ 29%	Avoid unboosted FPV. Dose FPV/r. 700/100 bid with NVP standard. Limited data (historical comparison AAC 2006;50:315)
EFV	↓ 30%	C_{min} ↓ 36%	Increase RTV dose to 300 mg/d (FPV/r 1400/300 QD) with once-daily dosing or use 700/100 mg bid
ATV	↓ 20%	↑ 78%	Avoid; inadequate data
IDV	No data	↑33%	Dose regimens not established
LPV/r	Trough ↓ 53%	Trough ↓ 64%	Avoid since doses are not established
DRV	No data	No data	No data; avoid
SQV	No data	↓ 32%	Avoid; inadequate data
ETR	No data	↑ 70%	Avoid; clinical significance unclear
MVC	May ↑	No change likely	MVC 150 mg bid
TPV	No data	↓ 41%	Avoid
NFV	No data	↑ 150%	Avoid; inadequate data
RTV	No data	↑ 100%	1400/200 mg or 1400/100 mg/d or 700/100 mg bid
DLV	↓ 61%	↑ 130%	Avoid co-administration
RAL	No change likely	No change likely	Usual dose
RPV	May ↑	No change likely	Usual dose. Monitor QTc in patients at risk for QTc prolongation.
DTG	DTG Cmin ↓ 49%	No change likely	DTG 50 mg twice-daily. Use only if no DTG resistant mutations.
EVG	No change	No change	Dose: EVG 150 mg/d + FPV/r 700/100 mg bid
BIC	May ↑ or ↓		No data. Avoid

SIDE EFFECTS: The most common causes for drug discontinuation for adverse reactions (6% in registration trials) are GI intolerance, transaminase elevations and rash.

Skin rash: The common adverse reaction is skin rash, seen in 12–33% of patients (package insert); rash is sufficiently severe to result in discontinuation in <1%. FPV contains a sulfa moiety, so caution is advised with use in patients with a history of severe sulfa allergy, but no increase in rates of rashes was noted in such patients in the registration trials.

> *Cardiovascular disease*: A case control trial (*ANRS-04*) found that FPV treatment was associated with an increased risk of myocardial infarction with an odds ratio of 1.52 (Arch Intern Med 2010;170:1228). This risk was also noted in the D:A:D review. As a result of these reports, the supplier sent a safety advisory in 2009 concerning the potential risk of FPV for acute myocardial infarction and increased cholesterol and triglycerides (December 3, 2009).
>
> *GI intolerance* is most common and includes nausea, vomiting, diarrhea, and/or abdominal pain, which are reported in up to 40%, but is severe in only 5–10%; diarrhea is less frequent than with NFV (NEAT and SOLO trials). GI side effects with FPV/r were similar to those of LPV/r in the KLEAN trial.
>
> *Hepatotoxicity*: ALT levels are increased >5x ULN in 6–8%.
>
> *Lipodystrophy*: Observed with FPV.

BLACK BOX WARNING: None.

DRUG INTERACTIONS:

The following drugs should be avoided: Alfuzosin, amiodarone, astemizole, bepridil, cisapride, eplerenone, ergotamine derivatives, dexamethasone (at steady-state), dofetilide, dronedarone, ergotamine, flibanserin, fentanyl, flecainide, fluticasone, ivabradine, lovastatin, lurasidone, midazolam, pimozide, propafenone, quinidine, salmeterol, ranolazine, rifampin, rifapentine, rivaroxaban, betrixaban, ticagrelor, vorapaxar (may increase oral anticoagulation, avoid.), silodosin, enzalutamide, mitotane. high-dose sildenafil, St. John's wort, simvastatin, terfenadine, and triazolam.

The following drugs should be given concurrently with caution:

Anticoagulant: may increase edoxaban, apixiban, and dabigatran concentrations. Dose adjustment required based on renal function and indication.

Antacids: Decrease FPV 18%: Give 2 hrs before, 1 hr after or simultaneously with FPV; no data for FPV/r; (PPIs, no effect).

Phenobarbital, phenytoin, oxcarbazepine, and *carbamazepine* have potential to decrease APV levels and various effects on anticonvulsant levels; monitor anticonvulsant levels and use FPV/r or use alternative anticonvulsant.

Ethinyl estradiol/norethindrone decreases APV levels 22%; avoid co-administration.

R-methadone (active) levels decrease by 13%, and APV AUC is decreased by 25%; no withdrawal symptoms observed.

Paroxetine AUC ↓55% w/FPV/r; titrate to effect.

Alprazolam **concentrations may be incrased. Alprazolam** should be given with caution.

Rifampin decreases APV AUC by 82% and should not be used concurrently.

Rifabutin decreases APV AUC by 15% and FPV increases rifabutin AUC by 193%; use standard FPV dose and rifabutin at 150 mg/d or 300 mg 3×/wk. For the treatment of TB, most experts recommend 150 mg/d or 300 mg 3×/wk with FPV/r. Consider rifabutin TDM.

Clarithromycin increases APV AUC by 18%; use standard doses, reduce clarithromycin dose with renal failure.

Voriconazole: No data but voriconazole level may be decreased with FPV/r. Use TDM

Ketoconazole increased APV AUC by 32% and ketoconazole AUC increases 44%; use standard doses of FPV and do not exceed 200/mg/d ketoconazole. Use TDM

Atorvastatin levels increased 150%; maximum daily dose of 10 mg.

Sildenafil: FPV increases *sildenafil* AUC by 2–11×; do not exceed 25 mg/48 hrs.

Vardenafil AUC may also be increased; limit dosage to 2.5 mg/24 hrs (2.5 mg/72 hrs with FPV/r).

Fluticasone: Avoid; consider beclomethasone.

Pitavastatin, rosuvastatin: no interaction.

Colchicine: FPV increases colchicine levels; dose reduction needed.

PREGNANCY: Category C. Animal studies showed no embryo-fetal developmental abnormalities. Low placenta transfer. There are inadequate data on safety to routinely recommended in pregnancy. With RTV boosting, adequate APV pharmacokinetics in the third trimester, but inadequate data to recommend (2018 DHHS Perinatal HIV Guidelines).

Foscarnet

TRADE NAME: Foscavir; generic foscarnet (Hospira Worldwide).

FORMULATIONS, REGIMEN, AND COST: Vials: 6,000 mg (250 mL) at $390.37 and 12,000 mg (500 mL).

PATIENT ASSISTANCE PROGRAM: 877-946-7747.

INDICATIONS AND ACTIVITY: Active against herpes viruses including CMV, HSV-1, HSV-2, EBV (oral hairy leukoplakia), VZV, HHV-6, HHV-8 (KS-related herpes virus), most ganciclovir-resistant CMV, and most acyclovir-resistant HSV and VZV. Also active against HIV-1 and HIV-2 in vitro and in vivo and has been used for HIV salvage (Antiviral Ther 2006;11:561; J Clin Virol 2008;43:212; J Clin Virol 2010;47:79). The frequency of CMV resistance in vitro is 20–30% after 6–12 mos of foscarnet treatment (JID 1998;177:770). Clinical effectiveness for CMV retinitis is equivalent to that of ganciclovir (NEJM 1992;326:213; Ophthalmology 1994;101:1250) but has more treatment-limiting side effects. In vitro activity against HHV-8 is good, but results with foscarnet treatment of KS are variable; if KS is a true neoplasm, this treatment is of doubtful utility once malignant transformation has occurred (Science 1998;282:1837).

ADMINISTRATION: Controlled IV infusion using ≤24 mg/mL (undiluted) by central venous catheter or <12 mg/mL (diluted in 5% dextrose or saline) via a peripheral line. No other drug is to be given concurrently via the same catheter. Induction dose of 90 mg/kg q12h is given over ≥2 hr via infusion pump with adequate hydration. Maintenance treatment with 90–120 mg/kg/d is given over ≥2 hrs by infusion pump with adequate hydration. Many use 90 mg/kg/d for initial maintenance and 120 mg/kg/d for maintenance after re-induction for a relapse. See Tables 6.49, 6.50 and 6.51 for doses and dose adjustments in renal failure.

PHARMACOLOGY:

Bioavailability: 5–8% absorption with oral administration, but poorly tolerated.

$T^{1/2}$: 3 hr.

CSF levels: 15–70% of plasma levels.

Elimination: Renal exclusively.

Intravitreal foscarnet: 2.4 mg × 1 to 4 doses over 7–10 days in combination with systemic anti-CMV therapy for vision-threatening lesion.

SIDE EFFECTS:

Dose-related renal impairment: 37% treated for CMV retinitis have serum creatinine increase to ≥2 mg/dL; most common in second week of induction and usually reversible with recovery of renal function within 1 wk of discontinuation.

TABLE 6.49 Dose recommendations for foscarnet

Indication	Dose Regimen
CMV retinitis	Induction: 60 mg/kg IV q8h or 90 mg/kg IV q12h × 14–21 days. Maintenance: 90–120 mg/kg IV qd[a]
CMV (other sites)	60 mg/kg IV q8h or 90 mg/kg IV q12h × 14–21 days, indications for maintenance treatment are unclear, but can be considered with relapse.
Acyclovir-resistant HSV	40 mg/kg IV q8h or 60 mg/kg q12h × 3 wks
Acyclovir-resistant VZV	40 mg/kg IV q8h or 60 mg/kg q12h × 3 wks

[a] Survival and time to relapse may be significantly prolonged with maintenance dose of 120 mg/d vs. 90 mg/d (JID 1993;168:444).

Monitor creatinine 2–3×/wk with induction and every 1–2 wks during maintenance. Modify dose for creatinine clearance changes. Foscarnet should be stopped for creatinine clearance <0.4 mL/min/kg.

TABLE 6.50 Foscarnet dose adjustment in renal failure for HSV and CMV infection (in mg/kg)

CrCl. (mL/min/kg)	HSV: Equivalent to 60 mg/kg q12h or. 40 mg/kg q8h	CMV: Equivalent to (60 mg/kg q8h)	(90 mg/kg q12h)
>1.4	40 q8h	60 q8h	90 q12h
>1.0–1.4	30 q8h	45 q8h	70 q12h
>0.8–1.0	35 q12h	50 q12h	50 q12h
>0.6–0.8	25 q12h	40 q12h	80 q24h
>0.5–0.6	40 q24h	60 q24h	60 q24h
=0.4–0.5	35 q24h	50 q24h	50 q24h
<0.4	Not recommended [b]	Not recommended [b]	Not recommended [b]

TABLE 6.51 Foscarnet maintenance dose recommendations

Adjusted dose based on recommendations with normal renal function

CrCl (mL/min/kg)	90 mg/kg/d. (once-daily)	120 mg/kg/d. (once-daily)
>1.4[a]	90 q24h	120 q24h
>1.0–1.4[a]	70 q24h	90 q24h
>0.8–1.0[a]	50 q24h	65 q24h
>0.6–0.8[a]	80 q48h	105 q48h
>0.5–0.6	60 mg q48h	80 q48h
>0.4–0.5	50 mg q48h	65 q48h
<0.4	Not recommended	Not recommended

[a] Low dose for initial therapy, high dose for relapse.
[b] 38% removal with HD; consider 60 mg/kg post HD (JID 1991;64:785).

Changes in serum electrolytes including hypocalcemia (15%), hypophosphatemia (8%), hypomagnesemia (15%), and hypokalemia (16%). Patients should be warned to report symptoms of hypokalemia (perioral paresthesias, extremity paresthesias, and numbness). Monitor serum calcium, magnesium, potassium, phosphate, and creatinine, usually ≥2×/wk during induction and 1×/wk during maintenance. If paresthesias develop with normal electrolytes, measure ionized calcium at start and end of infusion.

Seizures: related to renal failure and hypocalcemia.

Penile ulcers.

Miscellaneous: Nausea, vomiting, headache, rash, fever, hepatitis, marrow suppression.

DRUG INTERACTIONS: Concurrent administration with IV pentamidine may cause severe hypocalcemia. Avoid concurrent use of potentially nephrotoxic drugs such as amphotericin B, aminoglycosides, and pentamidine. Possible increase in seizures with imipenem.

PREGNANCY: Category C. Teratogenic in rodents. Recommend as alternative treatment of life- and site-threatening CMV infections.

Foscavir—see Foscarnet

Fungizone—see also Amphotericin B

Ganciclovir and Valganciclovir

TRADE NAME (IV AND ORAL FORMS): Ganciclovir: Cytovene, IV (Roche) and generic; Vitrasert, ocular implant has been discontinued; Zirgan 0.15% ophthalmic gel (Bausch & Lomb).
  Valganciclovir: Valcyte, PO (Roche).

CLASS: Synthetic purine nucleoside analog of guanine.

FORMULATIONS, REGIMEN, AND COST: Ganciclovir: 500 mg vial at $86.40; valganciclovir: 450 mg tab at $64.40; 0.15% gel (5g) at $334.70.

> DOSE RECOMMENDATIONS: Ganciclovir, 5 mg/kg IV q12h × 2 wk (induction), then 5 mg/kg IV qd (maintenance); valganciclovir, 900 mg po q12h × 3 wk (induction), then 900 mg/d (maintenance). Valganciclovir is the preferred oral formulation because it provides blood levels of ganciclovir comparable with those achieved with recommended doses of IV ganciclovir (NEJM 2002;346:1119). Oral ganciclovir should no longer be used, and IV ganciclovir is reserved primarily for seriously ill patients and those who are unable to take oral medications.
>
> *For vision-threatening CMV*: Administer intravitreal ganciclovir 2 mg × 1–4 doses over 7–10 days in combination with systemic anti-CMV treatment.
>
> *Herpetic keratitis*: 1 drop in affected eye 5×/d until corneal ulcer heals, then apply 1 drop 3×/d for 7 days.

TABLE 6.52 Mean AUC with valganciclovir compared with IV ganciclovir in standard doses

	Valganciclovir	IV Ganciclovir
Induction AUC (µg/hr/mL)	32.8	28.6
Maintenance (µg/hr/mL)	34.9	30.7

From NEJM 2002;346:1119.

PATIENT ASSISTANCE PROGRAM: 800-282-7780.

ACTIVITY: Active against herpes viruses including CMV, HSV-1, HSV-2, EBV, VZV, HHV-6, and HHV-8 (KSHV). About 10% of patients given ganciclovir ≥3 mos for CMV will have resistant strains that are sensitive to foscarnet (JID 1991;163:716; JID 1991;163:1348). The frequency of ganciclovir resistance at 9 mos in patients receiving maintenance IV ganciclovir

TABLE 6.53 Ganciclovir and valganciclovir dose modification in renal failure (induction dose)

Ganciclovir (IV Form)		Valganciclovir[b] (Oral Form)	
CrCl	Dose	CrCl	Dose
>80 mL/min	5 mg/kg q12h	>60 mL/min	900 mg bid
50–79 mL/min	2.5 mg/kg q12h	40–59 mL/min	450 mg bid
25–49 mL/min	2.5 mg/kg q24h	25–39 mL/min	450 mg/d
10–24 mL/min	1.25 mg/kg q24h	10–24 mL/min	450 mg qod (induction); 450 2×/wk (maintenance)
<10 mL/min[a]	1.25 mg/kg 3×/wk	<10 mL/min	Not recommended

[a] Hemodialysis: 1.25 mg/kg 3×/wk; give post-dialysis.
[b] Maintenance dose = 50% of induction dose.

therapy for CMV show progressive retinitis is 26% (JID 1998;177:770). Ganciclovir is active in vitro against HHV-8, but the clinical experience with ganciclovir treatment of KS is variable. A preliminary trial targeting the HHV-8 ORF 36 and ORF 21 lytic genes using high dose AZT (600 mg qid) and valganciclovir (900 mg bid) showed impressive results in 14 patients with Castleman disease (Blood 2011;117:6977).

INDICATIONS AND DOSE REGIMEN:

CMV retinitis: A controlled trial of 141 patients randomized to receive IV ganciclovir (5 mg/kg/bid × 3 wks followed by 5 mg/kg qd) vs. oral valganciclovir (900 mg bid × 3 wks followed by 900 mg/d) showed comparable response rates (77% vs. 72% at 4 wks) and median time to progression (125 vs. 160 days) (NEJM 2002;346:1119). Oral valganciclovir is now the standard treatment. Multiple trials show that IV ganciclovir, IV foscarnet, IV cidofovir, oral valganciclovir, and the ganciclovir implant are all effective. The most effective systemic treatment in terms of efficacy, convenience, and avoidance of toxicity is valganciclovir (Clin Ophth 2010;4:111). The preferred contemporary approach is ART used in combination with valganciclovir to prevent systemic CMV disease and contralateral retinitis (NEJM 1997;337:83;337:105; Am J Ophthalmol 1999;127:329). Selected patients, especially those with zone 1 vision-threatening retinitis, should receive 2 mg intravitreal injection of ganciclovir 1 to 4 doses over 7–10 days. Current guidelines for initial management of CMV retinitis are summarized on pg. 711 (Clin Ophthalol 2010;4:285.).

Discontinuation of maintenance therapy can be considered in the setting of immune reconstitution with a CD4 count >100/mm^3 for 3–6 mos (JAMA 1999;282:1633). The 2018 CDC/NIH/IDSA Opportunistic Infections Guidelines recommendation is to make this decision in consultation with an ophthalmologist based on magnitude and duration of the CD4 response, anatomic location of the lesion, vision in the other eye, and feasibility of ophthalmologic monitoring. Every 3 months ophthalmology follow-up required.

Other forms of disseminated CMV: Ganciclovir or foscarnet are the standard agents to treat CMV esophagitis, colitis, pneumonitis, and neurologic disease (AIDS 2000;14:517; CID 2002;34:101). Recommendations for suspending maintenance therapy with immune reconstitution are unclear for non-ocular CMV, but most will follow the guidelines for CMV retinitis using a CD4 threshold of 100 cells/mm^3 × ≥3 mos (AIDS 2001;15:F1). Failures ascribed to lack of CMV-specific CD4 responses with recurrent CMV retinitis have been reported (JID 2001;183:1285).

PHARMACOLOGY:

Bioavailability: Valganciclovir, 60% absorption with food vs. 6–9% for oral ganciclovir. The valganciclovir formulation is rapidly hydrolyzed to ganciclovir after absorption.

Serum level: Mean peak concentration with IV induction doses is 11.5 µg/mL (MIC$_{50}$ of CMV is 0.1–2.75 µg/mL).

CSF concentrations: 24–70% of plasma levels; *intravitreal concentrations*: 10–15% of plasma levels – 0.96 µg/mL (JID 1993;168:1506).

T$^{1/2}$: 2.5–3.6 hr with IV administration; 3–7 hr with oral administration. Intracellular T$^{1/2}$: 18 hr.

Elimination: IV form: 90–99% excreted unchanged in urine. Oral form: 86% in stool and 5% recovered in urine.

Renal failure: Hemodialysis removes 50% of ganciclovir (Clin Pharmacol Ther 2002;72:142).

SIDE EFFECTS, IV FORM:

Neutropenia with ANC <500/mm^3 (25–40%) requires discontinuation of drug or G-CSF in 20%. Discontinuation or reduced dose will result in increased ANC in 3–7 days. Monitor CBC 2–3×/wk and discontinue if ANC <500/mm^3 or platelet count <25,000/mm^3.

Thrombocytopenia in 2–8%.

CNS toxicity in 10–15% with headaches, seizures, confusion.

Hepatotoxicity in 2–3%.

GI intolerance 2% (diarrhea).

Note: Neutropenia (ANC <500/mm^3) or thrombocytopenia (<25,000/dL) are contraindications to initial use.

SIDE EFFECTS, ORAL FORM: Of 212 patients with CMV retinitis followed for a median of 272 days, 10% developed neutropenia with ANC <500/mm^3, hemoglobin <8 g/dL in 12%, diarrhea in 35%, nausea in 23%, and fever in 18% (JAIDS 2002;30:392). This is similar to the side effects with oral or IV ganciclovir.

DRUG INTERACTIONS: AZT increases the risk of neutropenia, and concomitant use is not recommended. Other marrow-toxic drugs include interferon, sulfadiazine, hydroxyurea, pyrimethamine, TMP- SMX, flucytosine, and cytotoxic agents (vincristine, vinblastine, and doxorubicin). Oral and IV ganciclovir increase AUC of ddI by 111% and 50–70%, respectively; avoid or monitor for adverse effect of ddI (MMWR 1999;48[RR-10]:48). Probenecid increases ganciclovir levels by 50%. Additive or synergistic activity with foscarnet in vitro against CMV and HSV.

PREGNANCY: Category C. Teratogenic in animals in concentrations comparable to those achieved in humans; should be avoided unless need justifies the risk.

G-CSF (Filgrastim)

TRADE NAME: Neupogen (Amgen); Granix (Teva).

FORMULATIONS, REGIMEN, AND COST: 300 µg vial and prefilled syringe at $345.70; 480 µg vial and prefilled syringe at $550.45.

REIMBURSEMENT ASSISTANCE/APPEAL: 800-272-9376.

Note: 300 µg vial and 480 µg vial with leftover drug may be reused. Pharmacists commonly instruct patients to discard unused portion; the cost-effective alternative is to retain the unused portion in refrigerated syringes for later use. For example, a 75 µg dose = 1 immediate dose and 3 syringes with subsequent doses.

PATIENT INSTRUCTIONS: Subcutaneous injections are usually self-administered into the abdomen or upper thighs or in the back of upper arms if injected by someone else. Injection sites should be rotated. The drug should be stored in a refrigerator at 36–46°F.

PRODUCT INFORMATION: A 20-kilodalton glycoprotein produced by recombinant technique that stimulates granulocyte precursors.

INDICATIONS: AIDS patients may tolerate low ANC levels better than cancer patients do in terms of infectious complications (Arch Intern Med 1995;155:1965; Infect Control Hosp Epidemiol 1991;12:429). G-CSF is "not routinely indicated" for neutropenic patients with HIV infection, according to the guidelines of USPHS/IDSA (MMWR 1999;48[RR-10]; CID 2000;30[suppl 1]:S29). Nevertheless, the incidence of bacterial infections appears to be increased 2- to 3-fold in patients with an ANC <500/mL (Lancet 1989;2:91; Arch Intern Med 1995;155:1965), and most HIV-infected patients respond to G-CSF. A therapeutic trial in 258 HIV-infected patients with ANC of 750–1,000/mm^3 found that G-CSF recipients had 31% fewer bacterial infections, 54% fewer severe bacterial infections, and 45% fewer hospital days for these infections, but no mortality benefit (AIDS 1998;12:65).

Dose: Initial dose of G-CSF is 5 µg/kg/d subcutaneously (based on lean body weight). For practical purposes, the dose can be a convenient approximation of the calculated dose using a volume of 1 cc (300 µg), 0.5 cc (150 µg), 0.25 cc (75 µg), or 0.2 cc (60 µg). This may be increased by 1 µg/kg/d after 5–7 days up to 10 µg/kg/d or decreased 50%/wk and given either daily, every other day, or 2–3×/wk. Monitor CBC 2×/wk and keep ANC >1,000–2,000/mL (NEJM 1987;317:593). If unresponsive after 7 days at 10 µg/kg/d, treatment should be discontinued. Usual maintenance dose is 150–300 µg given 3–7×/wk.

PHARMACOLOGY:

Absorption: Not absorbed with oral administration. G-CSF must be given IV or SQ; SQ is usually preferred.

$T^{1/2}$: 3.5 hr (SQ injection).

Elimination: Renal.

SIDE EFFECTS: Medullary bone pain is the only important side effect, noted in 10–20%, and is usually manageable with acetaminophen.

Rare side effects: Mild dysuria, reversible abnormal liver function tests, increased uric acid, and increased LDH.

DRUG INTERACTIONS: Should not be given within 24 hrs of cancer chemotherapy. Lithium may ↑ leukocytosis. Vincristine ↑ peripheral neuropathy (J Clin Oncol 1996;14:935).

PREGNANCY: Category C. Caused abortion and embryo lethality in animals at 2–10× dose in humans; no studies in humans.

Gemfibrozil—see also Fenofibrate

TRADE NAME: Lopid (Pfizer) and generic.

CLASS: Antihyperlipidemic; fibric acid derivative (like clofibrate).

FORMULATIONS, REGIMEN, AND COST: 600 mg tab at $1.55/ tab.

INDICATIONS AND DOSE: Elevated serum triglycerides; may increase LDL cholesterol and cholesterol levels. 600 mg bid po >30 minutes before meal. Meta-analysis found that fibrates decrease total cholesterol by 8% and triglycerides by 30% (Am J Ther 2010;17:e182).

MONITORING: Blood lipids, especially fasting triglycerides and LDL cholesterol; if marked increases in LDL cholesterol, discontinue gemfibrozil and expect return of LDL cholesterol to pretreatment levels in 6–8 wks. Gemfibrozil should be discontinued if there is no decrease in triglyceride or cholesterol level at 3 mos. Obtain liver function tests and CBC at baseline, at 3–6 mos, and then yearly. Discontinue gemfibrozil for otherwise unexplained abnormal liver function tests.

PHARMACOLOGY:

Bioavailability: 97%.

$T^{1/2}$: 1.3 hr.

Elimination: renal – 70%, fecal – 6%.

Hepatic failure: Reduce dosage; use with caution.

Renal failure: Consider reducing dose.

Precautions: Contraindicated with gallbladder disease, primary biliary cirrhosis, and severe renal failure.

SIDE EFFECTS:

Blood lipids: May increase LDL cholesterol and total cholesterol by a mechanism that is poorly understood.

Gallbladder: Gemfibrozil is similar to clofibrate and may cause gallstones and cholecystitis ascribed to increased biliary excretion of cholesterol.

Miscellaneous: GI intolerance, decreased hematocrit and/or WBC (rare).

DRUG INTERACTIONS:

Gemfibrozil and statins have resulted in rhabdomyolysis and renal failure; possible increased risk of myositis when used with statins; monitor closely for evidence of myositis with concurrent use (JAIDS 2009;52:235; Ann Intern

Med 2009;150:301). Rosuvastatin AUC increased 90%; use fenofibrate instead.

Oral anticoagulants: May potentiate activity of warfarin.

PREGNANCY: Category C.

Halcion—see Benzodiazepines

Humatin—see Paromomycin

Ibalizumab-Uiyk

TRADE NAME: Trogarzo.

CLASS: CD4-directed post-attachment HIV-inhibitor.

FORMULATIONS, REGIMEN, AND COST: Available in a 200 mg (13.3 mL) IV vial, under aseptic technique withdraw 13.3 mL from vial then transfer into a 250 mL 0.9% saline IV bag (after reconstitution store at room temperature for ≤4 hrs or refrigerated for ≤24hrs). Infuse first bolus dose over 30 minutes, and then subsequent dose can be infused over 15 minutes.

   AWC: $118,000/yr.
   Dose: 2,000 mg IV × 1 (loading dose), then 800 mg IV q2 week.
   Dosing in renal impairment: No data. Usual dose likely.
   Dosing in hepatic impairment: No data. Usual dose likely.

CLINICAL TRIALS:
TMB-301 was a single arm, multicenter study involving 40 heavily treatment-experienced HIV-infected with documented resistance to NRTI, NNRTI, and PI class. At baseline, patients enrolled had a median VL of 35,350 copies/mL and CD4 of 73 cells/mm³. In addition to NRTI, NNRTI, and PI resistant mutations, patients were previously treated with INSTIs (78%), T-20 (30%), and MVC (20%).

Patients were started on an optimized ART regimen (with at least one other active ARV) 1 wk after Ibalizumab-uiyk infusion. At week 25, 43% of patients achieved VL <50 copies. Patients had a mean CD4 count increase of 44 cells/mm3.

RESISTANCE: In patients experiencing virologic failure, phenotypic changes in the HIV-1 envelope with a loss of N-link glycosylation sites in the V5 loop of pgp120 has been associated with decreased susceptibility of Ibalizumab-uiyk. No cross-resistance between Ibalizumab-uiyk and currently available ARVs.

PHARMACOLOGY: Ibalizumab-uiyk binds to domain 2 of CD4 and interferes with post-attachment steps required for HIV-1 entry. In combination with an optimized background regimen, ibalizumab-uiyk is FDA indicated for the treatment of multidrug resistant HIV-1 in highly treatment-experienced patients. Steady-state concentrations of 30 µg/mL achieved after the first 800 mg maintenance dose. Dose dependent half-life of 2.7–64 hrs between the dosing range of 0.3–25 mg/kg (Vd = 4.8L).

SIDE EFFECTS: In heavily treatment-experienced patients (n = 40), most common ADRs reported were: diarrhea (8%), dizziness (8%), nausea (5%), and rash (5%). The majority (90%) of reported ADRs were mild or moderate in severity with only two patients required study drug discontinuation (IRIS and severe rash).

Reported laboratory abnormalities in heavily treatment experienced patients (unclear association with Ibalizumab-uiyk) were *bilirubin elevation* ($\geq$ 2.6 × ULN), 5%; any direct bilirubin elevation, 3%; Scr (>1.5× baseline or >1.8 ULN), 10%; hyperglycemia (>250 mg/dL), 3%; elevated lipase (>3× ULN), 5%, uric acid (>12 mg/dL); anemia (Hgb <8.5 g/dL), 3%; thrombocytopenia (platelets <50K/mm³), 3%; leukopenia (<1,500 cells/mm³), 5%; neutropenia (ANC <600 cells/mm³), 5%.

DRUG INTERACTIONS: No known drug interactions. ARV drug–drug interactions unlikely.

PREGNANCY: No human or animal data. Use only if benefits outweigh potential risk.

Indinavir (IDV)

TRADE NAME: Crixivan (Merck).

CLASS: Protease inhibitor.

FORMULATIONS, REGIMEN, COST:

Forms: IDV caps 200and 400 mg.

Regimens: IDV 800 mg q8h; IDV/r, 800/100 mg bid.

AWP: $548/mo (IDV 800 q8h).

FOOD EFFECT: Unboosted, take 1 hr before or 2 hrs after meal, or take with light, low-fat meal. No food restrictions for IDV/r.

FLUIDS: Must take ≥1.5 L/d to minimize the risk of kidney stones.

RENAL FAILURE: No restrictions but should hydrate well.

STORAGE: Room temperature, 15–30°C (59–86°F); protect from moisture.

PATIENT ASSISTANCE PROGRAM: 800-850-3430.

INDICATIONS AND DOSE: This drug played a central role in the early HAART era with extraordinary results in ACTG 320 and Merck Trial 035 (NEJM 1997;337:725 & 734). IDV has now been largely replaced by alternative PIs that are more potent, more convenient, and less toxic. When used, the standard regimens are IDV/r 800/100 mg bid or 800/200 mg bid (increased risk of renal calculi).

ADVANTAGES: Extensive experience with long-term follow-up; extensive experience in pregnancy.

DISADVANTAGES: Need for q8h dosing on an empty stomach if used without RTV boosting; risk of nephrolithiasis and need for large fluid intake with or without RTV boosting; dermatologic side effects, including dry skin, alopecia, and paronychia; inferior virologic efficacy compared to multiple alternative regimens; IDV and IDV/r are not recommended as first-line therapy by the 2018 DHHS or the 2017 IAS-USA guidelines.

RESISTANCE: Mutations 10I/R/V, 20M/R, 24I, 32I, 36I, 54V, 71V/T, 73S/A, 77I, 82A/F/T, 84V, and 90M correlate with reduced in vitro activity (AAC 1998;42:2775; Topics HIV Med 2006;14:125). Substitutions at codons 46, 82, and 84 are major mutations that predict resistance but are not necessarily the first mutations. In general, at least three mutations are necessary to produce phenotypic resistance. The overlap with other PIs is not extensive, but multiple mutations contribute to class resistance (Nature 1995;374:569).

PHARMACOLOGY:

Bioavailability: Absorption is 65% in fasting state or with only a light, nonfat meal. Full meal decreases IDV levels 77%; give 1 hr before or 2 hrs after meal, with light meal, or with RTV. Food has minimal effect on IDV when it is co-administered with RTV. CNS penetration is relatively good compared to other PIs (CNS Drugs 2002;16:595).

$T^{1/2}$: 1.5–2.0 hr (serum).

C_{max}: Peak levels correlate with nephrotoxicity, and trough levels correlate with efficacy, but levels seem somewhat unpredictable even when IDV is boosted with RTV (JAIDS 2002;29:374). Penetration into CSF is moderate (CSF-to-serum = 0.06:0.16) but is superior to that of other PIs and adequate to inhibit IDV-sensitive strains (AAC 2000;44:2173), since levels achieved are above the IC_{95} for most HIV isolates (AIDS 1999;13:1227). In ranking CNS penetration; effectiveness is the highest in a four-class system (Neurology 2011;76:693).

Elimination: Metabolized via CY3A4. Inhibits CYP3A4 and glucuronidation. Urine shows 5–12% unchanged drug and glucuronide and oxidative metabolites.

TABLE 6.54 Clinical trials of IDV in treatment-naïve patients

Trial	Regimen	No.	Dur (wks)	VL <50	VL <200-500
ACTG 320 (NEJM 1997;337:725)	IDV 800 mg q8h + AZT/3TC	577	24		60%[a]
	AZT/3TC	579			9%
Merck 035 (NEJM 1997;337:734)	IDV + AZT/3TC	32	52	80%	90%[a]
	IDV	28		0	43%
	AZT/3TC	31		0	0
Dupont 006 (NEJM 1999;341:1865)	EFV + AZT/3TC	154	48	64%[a]	70%[a]
	IDV + AZT/3TC	148		43%	48%
	IDV + EFV	148		47%	53%
Merck 060 (AIDS 2000;14:367)	IDV + AZT/3TC	52	52		60%[a]
	AZT/3TC	50			46%
Atlantic (AIDS 2003;17:987)	IDV + ddI + d4T	417	48	55%	57%
	NVP + ddI + d4T	394		54%	58%
	3TC + ddI + d4T	396		46%	59%
CNAAB 3005 (JAMA 2001;285:1155)	ABC/AZT/3TC	282	48	40%	51%
	IDV + AZT/3TC	280		46%	51%
CNA 3014 (Curr Med Res J 2004;20:103)	ABC/AZT/3TC	169	48	60%	66%[a]
	IDV + AZT/3TC	173		50%	50%
START-1 (AIDS 2000;14:1481)	IDV + 3TC + d4T	101	48	49%	53%
	IDV + AZT/3TC	103		47%	52%

[a] Superior to comparator (P <0.05).

Dose in renal failure: Standard dose. This also applies to hemodialysis and peritoneal dialysis (Nephrol Dial Transplant 2000;15:1102).

SIDE EFFECTS:

Asymptomatic increase in indirect bilirubin to ≥2.5 mg/dL without an increase in transaminases noted in 10–15% of patients.

Clinically inconsequential, and rarely associated with jaundice or scleral icterus.

Mucocutaneous: Paronychia and ingrown toenails, alopecia, dry skin, mouth, and eyes (common).

Class adverse effects: Insulin-resistant hyperglycemia, lipodystrophy, hyperlipidemia (increased triglyceride, cholesterol, LDL levels), and possible increased bleeding with hemophilia (AIDS 2001;15:11). IDV use is associated with a substantial increased risk (RR 1.12/yr) of cardiovascular disease that is presumably due to its effect on plasma lipids and documented in the D:A:D review (JID 2010;201:318). Use of IDV is generally not recommended in patients with hemophilia due to the availability of many alternative PIs.

Nephrolithiasis ± hematuria in 10–28%, depending on duration of treatment, age, RTV boosting, and fluid prophylaxis (J Urol 2000;164:1895). The cause is crystallization of the drug with high serum levels and/or dehydration; IDV crystals can be detected in urine of up to 60% of IDV recipients. The frequency of nephrolithiasis with renal colic, flank pain, hematuria, and/or renal insufficiency in the ATHENA cohort with 1219 IDV recipients was 8.3/100 patient-years; risk factors included low weight, low mean body mass, regimens with >1,000 mg IDV, and warm climate (Arch Intern Med 2002;162:1493). Factors that do not appear to influence risk are CD4 cell count and urine pH. Patients should drink 48 oz of fluid daily to maintain urine output at ≥150 mL/hr during the 3 hrs after ingestion; stones are crystals of IDV ± calcium (Ann Intern Med 1997;349:1294). Nephrolithiasis usually reflects peak plasma concentrations >10 µg/mL (AIDS 1999;13:473). This is most likely with IDV in standard doses or ritonavir-boosted IDV regimens, with the 800/100 mg bid or 800/200 mg bid (JAIDS 2002;29:374).

Nephrotoxicity: A retrospective review of renal failure in the ANRS-C03 cohort showed the RR with IDV/r was 2.3 (HIV Med 2010;11:308). In a prospective study of 184 IDV recipients, routine urinalysis indicated pyuria in 35%; this was often accompanied by proteinuria, hematuria, and IDV crystals (JAIDS 2003;32:135). About 25% with persistent pyuria developed elevated serum creatinine that persisted ≥3 mos after IDV was discontinued. Interstitial nephritis with pyuria and renal insufficiency was previously reported in about 2% of IDV recipients (CID 2002;34:1033). Acute renal failure due to IDV is reported, but rare (AIDS 1998;12:954). However, a long term study of 1281 patients given ART on average of 7 yrs showed IDV was the only antiretroviral agent associated with long term renal dysfunction (CID 2009;49:1950).

Alopecia: May involve all hair-bearing areas (NEJM 1999;341:618).

GI intolerance: Primarily nausea, with occasional vomiting, epigastric distress.

Less common: Increased transaminase levels, headache, diarrhea, metallic taste, fatigue, insomnia, blurred vision, dizziness, rash, and thrombocytopenia. Rare cases of fulminant hepatic failure and death. Fulminant hepatitis has been associated with steatosis and an eosinophilic infiltrate, suggesting a drug-related injury (Lancet 1997;349:924). Gynecomastia has been reported (CID 1998;27:1539).

BLACK BOX WARNING: None.

DRUG INTERACTIONS: IDV is a substrate and inhibitor of CYP4503A4. Avoid co-administration of cisapride, astemizole, eplerenone, fentanyl, midazolam, triazolam, ergotamines, dexamethasone (at steady-state), alprazolam, amiodarone, terfenadine pimozide, bepridil, dofetilide, lurasidone, quinidine, alfuzosin, ivabrandine, flibanserin, irinotecan, salmeterol, flecainide and propafenone, atazanavir, fluticasone, lovastatin, lurasidone, ranolazine, rifampin, rifapentine, simvastatin, rivaroxaban, betrixaban, ticagrelor, vorapaxar, silodosin, enzalutamide, and mitotane.

high-dose sildenafil, and St. John's wort.

Dose adjustment needed with edoxaban, apixiban, and dabigatran based on renal function and indication.

Dose modification: Rifabutin: IDV levels decreased 32% and rifabutin levels increased 2×; reduce rifabutin dose to 150 mg/d or 300 mg 3×/wk and increase IDV dose to 1,000 mg tid with IDV/r; use standard PI dose and rifabutin 150 mg q24h. Consider rifabutin TDM.

Azoles: Clarithromycin levels increase 53%; no dose change; consider decreasing clarithromycin with renal impairment. *Grapefruit juice* reduces IDV levels 26%. *Oral contraceptives*: Norethindrone levels increase 26% and ethinylestradiol levels increase 24%; no change. *Carbamazepine* markedly decreases IDV levels. *Phenytoin, oxcarbazepine, and phenobarbital* may decrease IDV levels; avoid or use with close monitoring of IDV levels with IDV/r. IDV increased *sildenafil* AUC 340% (AIDS 1999;13:F10). The maximum recommended dose is 25 mg/48 hrs. *Vardenafil* AUC increased 16×; IDV AUC decreases 30%; dose should be limited to 2.5 mg/d or use alternative; with IDV/r it should be limited to 2.5 mg/3 days. *Tadalafil* AUC increased; use 5 mg initially and do not exceed 10 mg/72 hrs. *Methadone*: no change in methadone levels. *St. John's wort* reduces IDV AUC by 57%; avoid (Lancet 2000;355:547). *Vitamin C* (>1 g/d): decreases IDV C_{min} 32%. *Amlodipine* AUC increased 90%; use with close monitoring. *Colchicine*: IDV increases colchicine levels.

PREGNANCY: Category C. Negative rodent teratogenic assays; minimal placental transfer. No evidence of teratogenicity in case reports to the antiretroviral pregnancy registry. Pharmacokinetic studies in PACTG 358 showed that mean levels at 30–32 wks gestation were 74% lower than at 6 wks postpartum with unboosted IDV. There is concern for this low IDV level and a theoretical concern for the associated hyperbilirubinemia. Boosted IDV (400/100 mg bid) provided low serum concentrations, but no alternative IDV-boosted dosing regimens have been studied in pregnancy. The 2018 DHHS Guidelines on Antiretroviral Drugs in Pregnant Women do not recommended IDV/r in pregnancy.

Data from the Pregnancy Registry through July 2017 showed birth defects in 7/289 (2.42%) IDV recipients, which is comparable to the 2.7% risk noted in the absence of ART.

TABLE 6.55 Recommendations for IDV in combination with other PIs or with NNRTIs

Agent	AUC	Concurrent Use Regimen
RTV[a]	IDV ↑ 2-5×	RTV 100 mg bid + IDV 800 mg bid
SQV	SQV ↑4-7×; IDV no effect	Limited data; possible in vitro antagonism (JID. 1997;176:265); avoid
NFV	NFV ↑80%; IDV ↑50%	IDV 1200 mg bid + NFV 1250 mg bid (limited data)
NVP	NVP no effect; IDV ↓28%	IDV 1,000 mg q8h or IDV/r + NVP standard
DLV	DLV no effect; IDV ↑40%	DLV 400 mg tid + IDV 600 mg q8h
EFV	EFV no effect; IDV ↓31%	EFV 600 mg qhs + IDV 1,000 mg q8h or. IDV/r 800/200 mg bid + EFV 600 mg qhs
LPV/r	LPV no change; IDV ↑3×	IDV 600 mg bid + LPV/r 400/100 mg bid
ATV	Combination contraindicated, because both drugs cause indirect hyperbilirubinemia	
FPV	APV↑33%	Regimen not established
TPV	No data	No data; avoid
MVC	May ↑ MVC	MVC 150 mg bid + IDV standard
ETR	No data; may ↓ IDV	Inadequate data; avoid
RPV	No data; may ↑ RPV	Monitor QTc in patients at risk for QTc prolongation
RAL	No data; may ↑ RAL	Standard dose likely
DTG	No data; may ↑ DTG	Standard dose likely
EVG	No data	Avoid
BIC	No data; may ↑ BIC	Standard dose likely

Invirase—see Saquinavir

Isoniazid (INH)

TRADE NAMES: Nydrazid, Laniazid, Teebaconin, and generic; combination with rifampin, Rifamate; combination with rifampin and pyrazinamide, Rifater (Aventis).

FORMULATIONS, REGIMEN, AND COST: 50, 100, and 300 mg tabs; $0.40 per 300 mg tab.

Hydrazid IV: Injections 100 mg/mL 10 mL vial $352.06; INH liquid 50 mg/5 mL (473 mL) $173.90.

Rifamate: $6.37/tab.

Rifater: $4.71/tab.

COMBINATIONS: Caps with rifampin: 150 mg INH + 300 mg rifampin (Rifamate) and tabs with 50 mg INH + 120 mg rifampin and 300 mg PZA (Rifater).

INDICATIONS AND DOSES: Prophylaxis and treatment of tuberculosis is based on 2017 CDC/NIH/IDSA Guidelines for Opportunistic Infections.

Treatment of latent tuberculosis: INH once-daily or twice weekly for 9 mos (if there is no evidence of active TB and no history of treatment for active or latent tuberculosis). The estimated efficacy of INH prophylaxis is a 64% reduction in active TB cases (Lancet Infect Dis 2010;10:489). A Cochrane Library review of 12 controlled trials concluded that the treatment of latent TB in patients with HIV reduces the risk of active TB, especially in those with a positive skin test (Cochrane Database Syst Rev 2010;20:CD000171).

Treatment of active TB: A multidrug regimen should be started immediately and include INH, RIF or rifabutin, PZA, and EMB. Based on a review from tuberculosis authorities at the NIH (Bethesda), the Institute of Infectious Diseases and Molecular Medicine (Cape Town), and the MRC (London) (Lancet 2011 doi:10. 1016/j.physletb. 2003.10.071).

The efficacy of INH prophylaxis is well-established in persons with a positive skin test and HIV infection.

The protection is about 60%, but the duration is limited.

INH prophylaxis in HIV-infected patients is more effective if given 36 mos vs. 6 mos. The benefit in the trial summarized in the Cochrane Review (above) showed an OR of 0.57 for TB with INH prophylaxis; benefit was limited to patients with a positive skin test, and the risk of drug induced hepatitis or resistance was low. There was increased mortality in the group with INH for 36 mos and negative skin tests that was unexplained and appeared unrelated to drug toxicity.

COMPLIANCE: Adherence concerns have resulted in a preference for DOT in all patients treated for active tuberculosis and for treatment of latent TB with HIV co-infection.

PHARMACOLOGY:

Bioavailability: 90%.

$T^{1/2}$: 1–4 hr; 1 hr in rapid acetylators.

Elimination: Metabolized and eliminated in urine. Rate of acetylation is genetically determined. Slow inactivation reflects deficiency of hepatic enzyme N-acetyltransferase and is found in about 50% of whites and African Americans. Rate of acetylation does not affect efficacy of standard daily or DOT regimens.

Dose modification in renal failure: Half dose with creatinine clearance <10 mL/min in slow acetylators.

SIDE EFFECTS: A review of 24,221 patients given INH prophylaxis showed adverse events in 132 (0.54%) including rash in 61 (0.25%), peripheral neuropathy in 50 (0.21%), clinical hepatotoxicity in 17 (0.07%) (AIDS 2010;24 Suppl 5:S29).

Hepatitis: ALT elevations are noted in 10–20%, clinical hepatitis in 0.6%, and fatal hepatitis in 0.02% (Am J Respir Crit Care Med 2003;167:603). The risk of hepatitis increases with increased age, alcoholism, prior liver disease, pregnancy, and concurrent rifampin.

One report showed hepatotoxicity rates (defined as an ALT >5 ULN) of 0.15% in 11,141 patients treated for latent TB. It was 1% in those receiving multiple antituberculosis drugs for active TB (JAMA 1999;281:1014). 2016 CDC/ATS/IDSA Guidelines for Management of TB in patients with HIV co-infection in the US recommend monitoring for clinical evidence of hepatitis by requiring monthly INH prescriptions contingent on this review. LFTs should be obtained if there are symptoms suggesting hepatitis. If INH is taken for latent TB it should be stopped if the ALT is >3× ULN with symptoms or >5× ULN without symptoms.

> *Peripheral neuropathy* due to increased excretion of pyridoxine, which is dose-related and rare (0.2%) with usual doses. It is prevented by use of concurrent pyridoxine (10–50 mg/d), which is recommended for patients with HIV co-infection. Overdose of INH may require high doses of pyridoxine (Pharmacotherapy 2006;26:529).
>
> *Miscellaneous reactions*: Rash, fever, adenopathy, GI intolerance.
>
> *Rare reactions*: Psychosis, arthralgias, optic neuropathy, marrow suppression.

DRUG INTERACTIONS:

> Increased effects of *warfarin, benzodiazepines (midazolam, triazolam), carbamazepine, cycloserine, ethionamide* (may increase INH levels; monitor for INH toxicity), *phenytoin*, and *theophylline*.
>
> *INH absorption* decreased with aluminum-containing antacids.
>
> *Ketoconazole*: Decrease ketoconazole levels (based on case reports).
>
> *Food*: Decreases absorption.

Tyramine reaction (cheese, wine, some fish): Rare patients develop palpitations, sweating, urticaria, headache, and vomiting.

PREGNANCY: Category C. Not teratogenic in animals. Possible increased risk of hepatotoxicity; monitor transaminase levels monthly during pregnancy and post-partum. This recommendation also applies to treatment of latent TB. Should give pyridoxine to prevent neurotoxicity and vitamin K to prevent hemorrhagic disease.

Itraconazole

TRADE NAME: Sporanox (Janssen) and generic.

CLASS: Triazole (like fluconazole) with three nitrogens in the azole ring; other imidazoles have two nitrogens.

FORMULATIONS, REGIMEN, AND COST: 100 mg caps at $9.28; oral solution with 10 mg/mL (150 mL) at $322.98.

PATIENT ASSISTANCE PROGRAM: 800-652-6227.

ACTIVITY AND PERSPECTIVE: In vitro activity against H. capsulatum, *B. dermatitidis, Aspergillus, Cryptococcus, Candida* spp. Strains of *Candida* that are resistant to fluconazole may be sensitive to itraconazole (AAC 1994;38:1530). Compared with fluconazole, itraconazole appears to be equivalent for non-meningeal coccidioidomycosis (Ann Intern Med 2000;133:676), superior for penicilliosis (Am J Med 1997;103:223), inferior for cryptococcosis (CID 1999;28:291), and equivalent for most candidiasis (HIV Clin Trials 2000;1:47). Major concerns are somewhat erratic absorption, multiple drug interactions, and cardiotoxicity with congestive heart failure (FDA Health Advisory, 5/09/02).

PHARMACOLOGY:

Bioavailability: Caps require gastric acid for absorption; average bioavailability is 55% and improved when taken with food and/or acidic drinks such as colas and orange juice (AAC 1995;39:1671). PPIs, H2 blockers, and antacids should be avoided. Follow serum levels to ensure absorption. The usual therapeutic level anticipated with a standard dose is 1–10 µg/mL. The liquid formulation is better absorbed and should be taken on an empty stomach. Some consider the liquid formulation to be preferred for all oral itraconazole therapy. The 2011 ATS Guidelines on treatment of fungal infections favor the liquid form due to the widespread use of PPIs, H2 blockers, and antacids (Am J Resp Crit Care Med 2011;183:96). However, nearly all studies were performed using the capsule formulation, and bioavailability studies have shown substantial variation. Based on these concerns, some authorities prefer the liquid formulation only for thrush—where its topical effect may improve efficacy—for patients with known achlorhydria and for patients with inadequate serum levels.

Reference laboratories for serum levels: Dr. Michael Rinaldi, Dept. of Pathology, Mail Code 7750, University of Texas Health Science Center, 7703 Floyd Curl Drive, San Antonio, TX 78229-3900; telephone 210-567-4131. Cost is $59. Specimen should be 2–4 mL serum or plasma obtained 2 hrs post dose after day 5 of treatment sent in frozen state. Results are available in 3 days. Goal is level of ≥1 µg/mL.

$T^{1/2}$: 64 hr.

Elimination: CYP 3A4 inhibitor and substrate; metabolites include hydroxy itraconazole, which is active in vitro against many fungi. Renal excretion is 0.03% of parent drug and 40% of metabolites.

Dose modification with renal failure: None.

Dose modification with liver disease: No data. Use with caution. Manufacturer suggests monitoring serum levels.

SIDE EFFECTS:

Cardiotoxicity: The negative inotropic effect was noted in animal toxicity studies, and in clinical trials an additional 58 cases with CHF reported to the FDA "Drug Watch," (an anecdotal

TABLE 6.56 Itraconazole dose regimens[a]

Usual Doses

    Loading dose: 200 mg tid × 3 days for serious infections
    Capsules: 100–200 mg po qd or bid with food (200–400 mg/d)
    Oral liquid: Preferred oral form 100 mg po qd or bid on empty stomach
    (100–200 mg/d)

    IV: 200 mg IV bid × 6 (loading), then 200–400 mg/d po (IV not available in US)

Pathogen	Dose (oral)	Comment
Aspergillosis	(Not recommended)	Voriconazole preferred
Blastomycosis	200 mg/d or bid (caps)	
Candidiasis Thrush	200 mg/d (liquid) swish & swallow (S&S)	As effective as fluconazole, but absorption more erratic and there are more drug interactions (HIV Clin Trials 2000;1:47)
Esophagitis	200 mg/d (liquid) S&S	
Vaginitis	200 mg/d × 3 days or 200 mg bid × 1 (caps)	For fluconazole-resistant *Candida*, options include itraconazole, voriconazole (po or IV), caspofungin (IV), posaconazole po, anidulafungin IV, micafungin IV or amphotericin (IV). Voriconazole is the most predictably active triazole.
Coccidioidomycosis	Acute non-meningeal, mild: 200 po tid × 3 days then 200 mg po bid Chronic suppressive treatment: itraconazole 200 mg po bid	Non-meningeal form For meningeal form, fluconazole 400–800 mg/d is preferred.
Cryptococcosis	200 mg/d (caps) tid × 3 days, then bid × 8 wks, then 200 mg/d maintenance	For patients with meningeal form who cannot tolerate fluconazole during maintenance therapy and for non-meningeal cryptococcosis Fluconazole and amphotericin preferred

TABLE 6.56 Continued

Dermatophyte	200 mg/d (caps)	*Tinea corporis* and *T. cruris*: 15 days *T. pedis, T. manum*: 30 days *T. capitis*: 4 to 8 wks (monitor LFTs)
Histoplasmosis	Acute: 200 mg tid × 3 days, then bid Continuation: 200 mg bid × 12–24 mos. or Maintenance: 200 mg po	Preferred azole Amphotericin B preferred for 1-2 wks for initial treatment of severe disseminated histoplasmosis; then itra 200 mg/d × 12 mos. Itraconazole is appropriate for acute phase treatment of those with mild illness
Onychomycosis Fingernails Toenails	200 mg/d (caps) 1 wk/mo × 2 mos 1 wk/mo × 4 mos.	Warn patients of and monitor for cardiotoxicity and hepatotoxicity.
Penicilliosis	Acute, severe disease: amphotericin B 0.7 mg/kg/d × 2 wks, followed by itraconazole 200 mg bid × 10 wks Mild disease: 200 mg po bid × 8 wks, followed by 200 mg/d	Preferred azole
Sporotrichosis	200 mg bid	

[a] From The 2018 IDSA/NIH/CDC Guidelines for Treatment and Prevention of Opportunistic Infections in HIV-infected Adults and Adolescents and 2011 ATS Guidelines for Treatment of Fundal Pulmonary Infections (Am J Respir Crit Care Med 2011;183:96).

series of cases reported to the FDA and reported by that agency through May, 2001) (Drug Saf 2006;29:567).

Hepatoxicity: Elevation of hepatic enzymes in 4%, but clinically significant hepatitis is uncommon (Lancet 1992;340:251). Hepatic enzymes should be monitored in patients with prior hepatic disease, and patients should be warned to report symptoms of hepatitis.

Other: Most common side effects are *GI intolerance* (3–10%) and *rash* (1–9% and most common in immunosuppressed patients).

Rare: Infrequent dose-related toxicities include hypokalemia, adrenal insufficiency, impotence, gynecomastia (at doses >600 mg/d), hypertension, and edema. Ventricular fibrillation due to hypokalemia has been reported (JID 1993;26:348).

DRUG INTERACTIONS: Impaired absorption of caps with *H2 blockers, proton pump inhibitors, antacids, or sucralfate.* Itraconazole is a potent CYP3A4 inhibitor and substrate, resulting in bidirectional inhibition with increased levels of itraconazole and the following interacting drugs: *clarithromycin, erythromycin, DLV, RPV, and PIs, especially RTV-boosted PIs. Colchicine* level may be increased. Reduce IDV dose to 600 mg q8h and do not exceed 400 mg/d of itraconazole. NVP and ETR may decrease itraconazole levels; monitor levels. With DRV/r, TPV/r, and LPV/r, do not exceed itraconazole 200 mg/d. With all PIs, monitor for toxicity. MVC: Use 150 mg bid. Should not be given concurrently with eplerenone, terfenadine, cisapride, pimozide, quinidine, bepridil, flecainide, propafenone, fentanyl, dofetilide, amiodarone, dronedarone, astemizole, alfuzosin, oral midazolam, lurasidone, ivadradine, flibanserin, triazolam, lovastatin, lurasidone, ranolazine, simvastatin, rifampin, rifabutin, phenytoin, carbamazepine, phenobarbital, rivaroxaban, betrixaban, ticagrelor, vorapaxar, silodosin, enzalutamide, mitotane, or ergotamine. Itraconazole increases levels of cyclosporine, sirolimus, tacrolimus, oral hypoglycemics, calcium channel blockers, and digoxin. Itraconazole decreases clopidogrel efficacy; avoid. Dose adjustment needed with edoxaban, apixiban, and dabigatran based on renal function and indication.

Note: Rifabutin: use with caution (increases rifabutin, decreases itraconazole levels by 75%. *Phenytoin, oxcarbazepine, carbamazepine, phenobarbital,* and *rifapentine may significantly* decrease itraconazole level; monitor itraconazole level.

PREGNANCY: Category C. Teratogenic to rats in high doses. Generally not recommended in pregnancy, but some studies have found it to be safe (Am J Obstet Gynecol 2000;183:617).

Kaletra—see Lopinavir/Ritonavir

Lamivudine (3TC)

TRADE NAME: Epivir (ViiV Healthcare/GlaxoSmithKline).

CLASS: Nucleoside analog reverse transcriptase inhibitor (NRTI).

FORMULATIONS, REGIMEN, AND COST:

Epivir 3TC: 150 mg and 300 mg tabs; 10 mg/mL solution (240 mL.
bottle).
> *Regimen*: 150 mg bid or 300 mg/d.
> *AWP*: $324.33/mo.
Combivir AZT/3TC: 300/150 mg.
> Regimen: 1 bid.
> AWP: $931.61/mo.
Trizivir AZT/3TC/ABC: 300/150/300 mg.
> *Regimen*: 1 bid.
> *AWP*: $1,738.46/mo.
Epzicom 3TC/ABC: 300/600 mg.
> Regimen: 1 qd.
> AWP: $1,395/mo.

TABLE 6.57 3TC dosing in renal failure

CrCl	Dose
>50 mL/min	150 mg bid or 300 mg/d
30–49 mL/min	150 mg/d
15–29 mL/min	150 mg, then 100 mg/d
5–14 mL/min	150 mg, then 50 mg/d[a]
<5 mL/min or dialysis	150 mg × 1 then 25 mg/d[a]

[a]Some experts recommend higher than FDA recommended dosing in ESRD in patients unable to use liquid 3TC.

Epivir HBV 100 mg tab at $17.90/tab; Epivir HBV 5 mg/mL solution.

(240 mL) at $214.81.

FOOD: No effect.

Triumeq: DTG/ABC/3TC (50/600/300 mg tab).

    Regimen: 1 tab qd with or without food.

Triumeq: DTG/ABC/3TC 50/600/300 mg tablet at $3118.62/mo.

Symfi: EFV/TDF/3TC (600/300/300 mg tab);

Symfi Lo: EFV/TDF/3TC (400/300/300 mg tab).

Regimen: 1 tab qd without food.

Symfi and Symfi Lo tablets at $1961/mo.

Combinations to avoid: 3TC/FTC, TDF/3TC/ABC, and TDF/3TC/ddI.

HEPATIC FAILURE: No recommendation; usual dose likely.

HEPATITIS B: Standard dose is 100 mg/d; co-infected patients should receive the HIV dose of 300 mg/d (or FTC 200 mg/d) + a second agent active against HBV such as TDF or TAF in a fully-suppressive HIV regimen regardless of CD4 count if HBV treatment is indicated.

PATIENT ASSISTANCE: 800-722-9294.

INDICATIONS AND DOSES:

HIV: 3TC or FTC are recommended as components of all initial regimens in the 2018 DHHS Guidelines, the 2017 IAS-USA guidelines, and virtually all other guidelines. The standard dose is 150 mg bid or 300 mg/d without regard for meals. 3TC is co-formulated as Combivir, Trizivir, and Epzicom, which improves convenience and reduces co-pays.

Hepatitis B: 3TC is a potent inhibitor of HBV replication (NEJM 2004;350:1118). Several studies have verified activity with HBeAg seroconversion in 22–29%, undetectable HBV DNA in 40–87% of patients coinfected with HBV and HIV (JID 1999;180:607; Hepatology 1999;30:1302; CID 2001;32:963; CID 2006;43:904), and improved hepatic histology (NEJM 1998;339:61; Ann Pharamacother 2010;44:1271; CID 2010;51:1201). Mutations on the YMDD polymerase gene confer 3TC resistance with HIV co-infection at a rate of 15–20% in year 1 and 70–90% by year 4 (AIDS 2006;20:863). These mutations result in HBV virologic failure and, in some cases, a hepatitis flare (J Clin Virol 2002;24:173; Lancet 1997;349:20; CID 1999;28:1032).

A second anti-HBV agent should be given to protect against resistance; TDF is a preferred agent if there is no baseline resistance (CID 2010;51:201). There are four distinct mechanisms of HBV flares with HBV treatment and HIV co-infection: (1) 3TC-resistant HBV, (2) 3TC (or FTC) discontinuation, (3) IRIS, or (4) hepatotoxicity of antiretroviral agents. Note that some experts conclude that the preferred drugs for HBV in monoinfected patients are TDF and entecavir (Clin Gastroenterol Hepatol 2008;6:1315; CID 2010;51:201; AntivirL Ther 2010;15:487). See below for guidance in treating HBV-HIV co-infection (CID 2006;43:904).

Treatment of HBV only: With HIV co-infection, TDF can be used only with a fully suppressive HIV regimen; entecavir can also be used only with full suppression of HIV due to the weak activity of entecavir vs. HIV causing the 184V resistance mutation.

Treatment of HIV and HBV: Use TDF + 3TC or TDF/FTC or TAF/FTC as the backbone for a fully HIV suppressive regimen.

ADVANTAGES: Potent activity against HIV, well tolerated, no food effect, may be taken once-daily, co-formulated with AZT (Combivir), AZT/ABC (Trizivir), and ABC (Epzicom); active against HBV. 3TC resistance by HIV (M184V) increases susceptibility to AZT, d4T, and TDF and delays accumulation of TAMs, and may partially reverse their effects. M184V reduces VL by about 0.5 $\log_{10}$ c/mL as a single agent in patients who have drug-resistant virus. Continued administration of 3TC (or FTC) with the M184V resistance mutation results in modest antiretroviral activity and does not select for additional NRTI resistance mutations.

DISADVANTAGES: Single resistance mutation (M184V) occurs early with virologic failure and causes high-level resistance to 3TC and FTC; use in HBV co-infection requires additional agents active against both HIV and HBV. Dose adjustment required with renal failure. May be more likely to select for M184V than FTC; combination of TDF + 3TC may select for more K65R than TDF/FTC.

CLINICAL TRIALS: There is extensive experience with 3TC combined with AZT, TDF, d4T, and ddI, confirming antiviral potency, excellent long and short-term tolerability, but also early acquisition of the M184V resistance mutation if viral suppression incomplete.

ACTG 384 found that AZT/3TC + EFV was superior to ddI + d4T + EFV in virologic suppression and tolerability (NEJM 2003;349:2298).

GS-903 compared TDF vs. d4T, each in combination with 3TC and EFV, for initial therapy. Results at 144 wks were similar, with 62% and 68% in the d4T and TDF group, respectively, achieving VL <400 c/mL by ITT (M = F) analysis (JAMA 2004;292:194).

CNA 30024 compared ABC/3TC vs. AZT/3TC, each with EFV, in 699 treatment-naïve patients. At 48 wks, VL was <50 c/mL in 69% and 70%, respectively, by ITT analysis (CID

2004;39:1038). This paved the way to coformulation as Epzicom.

ESS 30008 compared ABC/3TC twice-daily vs. once-daily in patients who had viral suppression with ABC/3TC twice-daily combined with a PI or NNRTI (NEJM 2004;350:1850).

Triple nucleoside regimens: ACTG 5095 compared AZT/3TC/ABC vs. EFV/3TC/AZT ± ABC.

RESISTANCE: Monotherapy with 3TC or nonsuppressive therapy with 3TC-containing regimens results in the rapid selection of the M184V mutation, which confers resistance to 3TC and FTC. Strains with the M184V mutation have enhanced susceptibility to AZT, d4T, and TDF and a modest decrease in susceptibility to ABC and ddI that is not clinically relevant in the absence of other NRTI mutations. The M184V mutation appears to be associated with persistent anti-HIV activity (mean of 0.5 $\log_{10}$ c/mL) (JID 2005;192:1537), presumably due to reduced viral fitness (New Microbiol 2004;27 Suppl 2:31; Expert Rev Anti Infect Ther 2004;2:147). K65R and multiple TAMs reduce activity of 3TC 3- to 9-fold. The Q151M complex and the T69 insertion mutation are associated with 3TC resistance, as well as with broad multinucleoside resistance. All of these changes are also found with FTC (JAIDS 2006;43:567).

PHARMACOLOGY:

Bioavailability: 86%.

$T^{1/2}$: 5–7 hr; Intracellular $T^{1/2}$: 18–22 hr.

CNS penetration: 13% (CSF-to-plasma ratio = 0.11). These levels exceed the IC_{50} and have been shown to clear HIV RNA from CSF (Lancet 1998;351:1547). The CNS penetration score is 2 in a four-class system (Neurology 2011;76:693).

Elimination: Renal excretion accounts for 71% of administered dose.

SIDE EFFECTS: Experience with more than 25,000 patients given 3TC through the expanded access program and >8,000 participants in clinical trials has demonstrated minimal toxicity. Infrequent complications include headache, nausea, diarrhea, abdominal pain, and insomnia. Comparison of side effects in 251 patients given 3TC/AZT and 230 patients given AZT alone in four trials (A3001, A3002, B3001, and B3002) indicated no clinical or laboratory complications uniquely associated with 3TC. Pancreatitis has been noted in some pediatric patients given 3TC.

    Class side effect: Lactic acidosis and steatosis are listed as toxicities associated with the NRTI class, though it is unlikely that these occur as a result of 3TC therapy (CID 2002;34:838).

    Hepatitis B: In HIV-infected patients with HBV co-infection, discontinuation of 3TC may cause fulminant hepatic deterioration with increases in HBV DNA levels and ALT (FDA black box warning). Monitor hepatic function and clinical course carefully for several months when 3TC is discontinued in patients with HIV/HBV co-infection. Immune reconstitution and development of HBV resistance may also cause a hepatitis B flare.

BLACK BOX WARNINGS: (1) Lactic acidosis (rare), (2) hepatic failure with chronic HBV infection with immune reconstitution, development of HBV resistance to 3TC, or discontinuation of an agent with activity vs. HBV (TDF, 3TC, or FTC). Note that lactic acidosis and mitochondrial toxicity is listed in the black box warning but are very rare, and this drug along with TDF are used as substitutes with NRTI-induced mitochondrial toxicity as shown in the STACCATO trial (JAC 2008;61:1340; AIDS 2003;17:2495).

DRUG INTERACTIONS: TMP-SMX (1 DS daily) increases levels of 3TC; however, no dose adjustment is necessary due to the safety profile of 3TC.

PREGNANCY: Category C. Recommended (with ABC, or TDF) as the preferred NRTI backbone in the 2018 DHHS Guidelines for

Antiretroviral Drugs in Pregnant HIV Infected Women. Special consideration is needed with HBV co-infection. Negative carcinogenicity and teratogenicity studies in rodents; placental passage studies in humans show newborn-to-maternal drug ratio of 1.0. Studies in pregnant women show that 3TC is well-tolerated and has pharmacokinetic properties similar to those of non-pregnant women (JID 1998;178:1327; MMWR 1998;47[RR-2]:6). Use in pregnancy is extensive; safety is well-established, and, when historically combined with AZT, efficacy in preventing perinatal transmission is also well-established (Lancet 2002;359:1178). The Pregnancy Registry shows birth defects in 149/4880 (3.05%) first-trimester exposures, a rate similar to 2.7% for women without RT exposure (www.apregistry.com, accessed 7/31/17).

HBV co-infection in pregnancy: The risk of HBV transmission is greatest in the third trimester and correlates with HBV viral load. 3TC, FTC, and TDF are the best drugs to prevent perinatal HBV transmission (Curr Hepat Res 2010;9:147).

Leucovorin (Folinic Acid)

TRADE NAME: Generic.

CLASS: Calcium salt of folinic acid.

FORMULATIONS, REGIMEN, AND COST:

Oral tabs: 5, 10, 15, and 25 mg tabs; 5 mg tab, $2.80.
Parenteral: 50, 100, 200, 350, 500 mg; 3 mg/mL; 100 mg, $24.00.
INDICATIONS: Antidote for folic acid antagonists.
Note: Protozoa are unable to utilize leucovorin because they require *p*-aminobenzoic acid as a cofactor. It does not interfere with antimicrobial activity of trimethoprim, or pyrimethamine. Usual use in HIV-infected patients is to prevent hematologic toxicity of pyrimethamine. Therapy is

usually oral but should be parenteral if there is vomiting or NPO status.

Toxoplasmosis treatment: Pyrimethamine 200 mg ×1, then 50–75 mg/d + leucovorin 10–25 mg/d × 6 wks; maintenance pyrimethamine 25–50 mg/d + leucovorin 10–25 mg/d (in combination with sulfadiazine or clindamycin).

Toxoplasmosis prophylaxis: Leucovorin, 25 mg/wk (with dapsone 50 mg/d + pyrimethamine 50 mg/wk).

PHARMACOLOGY: Normal folate levels are 0.005–0.015 µg/mL, levels <0.005 indicate folate deficiency and levels <0.002 cause megaloblastic anemia. Oral doses of 15 mg/d result in C_{max} of 0.268 µg/mL.

SIDE EFFECTS: Nontoxic in therapeutic doses. Rare hypersensitivity reactions.

PREGNANCY: Category C.

Lopinavir/Ritonavir (LPV/r)

TRADE NAME: Kaletra (Abbott Laboratories).

CLASS: Protease inhibitor (boosted with co-formulated ritonavir).

FORMULATIONS, REGIMEN, AND COST:

Forms: LPV/r 100/25 and LPV/r 200/50 mg tabs at $ $1,160.50/mo; LPV/r oral solution, 80/20 mg/mL (160 mL) at $ $1,087.97/mo.

Regimens: 400/100 mg bid or 800/200 mg/d (2 tabs bid or 4 tabs qd); oral solution 5 cc bid or 10 cc qd. Oral solution is sometimes preferred where there is GI intolerance; contains 42% alcohol. Once-daily therapy of 800/200 mg was found therapeutically equivalent to standard bid therapy in *treatment-naïve* patients, but recommended only for patients with <3 LPV mutations. Once-daily dosing is associated with lower and more variable trough levels (JID 2004;189:265), so bid dosing FDA labeled for *treatment-experienced* patients; however, most experts recommend DRV/r in PI-experienced patients with or without PI mutations. The recommended dose regimen in *pregnancy* is LPV/r 400/100 mg (600/150 mg bid during the second and third trimesters). This is 2–3 200/50 mg tabs bid as an alternative regimen for patients who are unable to tolerate ATV/r or DRV/r (2018 DHHS Pregnancy and Perinatal Guidelines JAIDS 2010;54:381).

AWP: $1034.88/mo.

PATIENT ASSISTANCE: 800-659-9050.

FOOD: Take tabs with or without food. Take oral solution with food.

RENAL FAILURE: Standard dose.

HEPATIC FAILURE: No recommendation; use with caution.

STORAGE: Tablets are stable at room temperature. Oral solution is stable until date on label at 2–8°C, and for 2 mos at room temperature (<25°C[77°F]).

ADVANTAGES: Potent antiretroviral activity; durability demonstrated with 7-yr follow-up data (HIV Clin Trials 2009;9:1); minimal evidence of PI resistance with virologic failure when used as first PI; co-formulated with RTV; efficacy of once-daily therapy established; frequently more active against PI-resistant virus than some other approved PIs with the exception of TPV/r and DRV/r; no resistance with failure in patients without prior PI mutations (as with other boosted PIs); alternative PI-based regimen in pregnancy in patients who are unable to tolerate DRV/r or ATV-based regimens.

DISADVANTAGES: Need for bid dosing in patients with ≥3 LPV mutations; Higher rates of GI intolerance compared to ATV/r and DRV/r; hyperlipidemia and other PI-associated metabolic toxicities; need for 200 mg/d RTV (in contrast to ATV/r, DRV/r, and FPV/r). Possible association with increased risk of MI.

TABLE 6.58 Clinical trials of LPV/r in treatment-naïve patients

Trial		N	Dur (wks)	VL <50 c/ mL	VL <200– 400 c/mL
AB M98- 863 (NEJM 2002;346:2039)	d4T + 3TC + LPV/r	326	48	67%	75%[a]
	d4T + 3TC + NFV	327		53%	63%
KLEAN (Lancet 2006;368:476)	ABC/3TC + FPV/r	434	48	66%	73%
	ABC/3TC + LPV/r	444		65%	71%
AB M02- 418 (JAIDS 2006;43:153-60)	TDF/FTC + LPV/ r bid	75	48	64%	—
	TDF/FTC + LPV/ r qd	115		70%	—
ACTG 5142 (NEJM 2008;358:2095)	LPV/r + 3TC + (d4T or AZT)	250	96	77%	86%
	EFV + 3TC + (d4T or AZT)	253		89%[a]	93%
	LPV/r + EFV	250		83%	92%
GEMINI (JAIDS 2009;50:367)	LPV/r + TDF/FTC	135	48	64%	83%
	SQV/r + TDF/FTC	128		65%	80%
CASTLE (JAIDS 2010;53:323)	LPV/r + TDF/FTC	440	96	68%	—
	ATV/r + TDF/FTC	443		74%[a]	—
ARTEMIS (AIDS 2009;23:1679)	LPV/r + TDF/FTC	346	96	71%	—
	DRV/r + TDF/FTC	343		79%[a]	—
M05-730 (JAIDS 2009;50:474)	LPV/r 800/200 qd + TDF/FTC	333	48	77%	—
	LPV/r 400/100 bid + TDF/FTC	331		76%	—

[a] Significantly better than comparator (P <0.05).

CLINICAL TRIALS:

Long-term follow-up: A EuroSIDA review found that LPV/r had a better record for long-term durability than EFV based on discontinuation rates (HIV Med 2011;12:259).

Long-term follow-up: A 6-yr follow-up of 63 participants enrolled in a LPV/r trial found that 62 had persistent VL <50 c/mL and a continuing increase in CD4 cell counts with a mean total increase at week 312 of 528/mm^3 (CID 2007;44:749). The mean CD4 count in those with a baseline count <50/mm^3 was 553/mm^3. The importance of this long-term follow-up is the admittedly anecdotal demonstration of sustained antiviral activity and continuing immunologic recovery, even for patients who initiated therapy late in the disease course. In a 7-yr follow-up of 100 treatment-naïve patients randomized to LPV/r + d4T + 3TC, 59% remained on LPV/r-based ART with VL <50 c/mL. Of the 28 with resistance data, none had PI resistance mutations (HIV Clin Trials 2008;9:1).

Once-daily LPV/r: The M05-730 trial included 633 treatment-naïve patients randomized 3:2 to LPV/r 800/200 mg/d vs. 400/100 mg bid, each in combination with TDF/FTC. At 48 wks, efficacy was comparable for once- vs. twice-daily regimens in terms of viral suppression to 50 c/mL (77% vs. 76%), viral suppression in patients with baseline VL >100,000 and <100,000 c/mL (55% vs. 55%), and CD4 count increase (185 and 194 cells/mm^3) (AIDS Res Hum Retrovir 2007;23:1505). Lipid changes were similar. Diarrhea was more common with the once-daily regimen (17% vs. 5%) ($p = 0.01$) and was the most common severe adverse event. Adherence was monitored by MEMS and was better with once-daily therapy for prescribed doses taken (99.8% vs. 92.6%). The 96-wk results of M05-730 demonstrated that once-daily LPV/r and twice-daily LPV/r had comparable rates of viral suppression to VL <50 c/mL (65% vs. 69%, respectively; P = NS). There were similar increases in CD4 count, similar rates of adverse reactions, and no PI resistance mutations (AIDS Res Hum Retrovir 2010;26:841).

LPV/r monotherapy: LPV/r monotherapy has been studied in multiple small trials, including one using monotherapy as initial therapy (*MONARK*) and four induction-maintenance trials (*OK-04, M03-613, SHCS,* and *KalMO*) that were nearly identical: standard ART regimens were given for 6 mos, and patients who achieved a VL <50 c/mL at 6 mos were randomized to monotherapy on LPV/r or continued LPV/r-based ART.

Patients with LPV/r monotherapy in *M03-613* and *KalMO* had somewhat higher failure rates than controls on triple-drug regimens, but they rarely had resistance mutations and resuppressed when NRTIs were added back. Note that the need for reinduction was not classified as failure in these trials. In OK-04, the rate of reinduction was 12/100 (AIDS 2008;22:777).

TABLE 6.59 LPV/r monotherapy

Study	Criteria	Duration	LPV/r		LPV/r + 2 NRTIs	
			No	VL <50	No	VL <50
MONARK (AIDS 2008;22:385)	ART-naïve	48 wks	83	67%	53	75%
OK-04[a] (JAIDS 2009;51:147)	Induction maintenance	96 wks	100	87%	98	78%
M03-613 (JAC 2008;61:1359)	Induction maintenance	96 wks	78	50%	77	61%
KalMO (HIV Clin Trials 2009;10:368)	Induction maintenance	96 wks	30	80%	30	87%
SHCS (AIDS 2010;24:2347)	Induction maintenance	[b]	42	75%	18	100%
STAR (Bunupuradah. CROI 2011: Abstr. 584)	NNRTI failures (Thailand)	48 wks	100	65%	100	83%

[a] OK-04 was a trial of LPV/r + AZT/3TC vs. EFV/AZT/3TC.
[b] Study terminated when 6 patients in the monotherapy group had virologic failure.

The *MONARK* trial randomized treatment-naïve patients with VL <100,000 c/mL and CD4 counts >100/mm^3 to treatment initiated with LPV/r or LPV/r + AZT/3TC. At 48 wks, VL was <50 c/mL in 67% of the monotherapy arm and 75% of the triple therapy arm (Table 6.59) (AIDS 2008;22:385). At 96 wks, 39 of the 83 (47%) assigned to monotherapy had a VL <50 c/mL (HIV Med 2010;11:137). Only 3 of 83 actually had VL >400 c/mL, but many changed regimens for other reasons, and the investigators were concerned about low-level viremia with monotherapy. They stated that LPV/r monotherapy "cannot be systematically recommended".

The *STAR* trial included 200 Thais who failed NNRTI-based regimens and were randomized to receive LPV/r or LPV/r + TDF/FTC. At 48 wks, VL <50 c/mL was achieved in 64% of the monotherapy group compared to 84% in the triple therapy arm (P = <0.01) (Bunupuradah. 2011 CROI;Abstr. 584).

Swiss HIV Cohort Study: This study included patients with viral suppression randomized to LPV/r monotherapy (n = 62) or continued LPV/r-based ART. Six monotherapy patients failed within 24 wks. Five had lumbar punctures, and all had elevated levels of HIV RNA in the CSF (mean VL >10,000 c/mL). Of the 6 with virologic failure, 5 had symptoms and 4 had neurologic symptoms. The study was stopped and the investigators speculated that monotherapy might be associated with CNS compartment failure (AIDS 2010;24:2347).

A *review of 6 randomized trials* of LPV/r monotherapy concluded that the risk of virologic failure was higher compared to LPV/r + 2 NRTIs (32% vs. 23%) (P = 0.04), but the results were comparable when NRTIs were restarted (AIDS 2009;23:279). Other concerns have been the use of monotherapy before at least 9 mos of viral suppression, poor adherence (Antiviral Ther 2009;14:195), and persistence of high levels in CSF (AIDS 2010;24:2347).

TREATMENT-EXPERIENCED PATIENTS: *M98-957* was a salvage trial involving 57 patients who had failed at least two PI-containing regimens. The trial compared two doses of LPV/r (533/133 mg bid and 400/100 mg bid), each combined with EFV. At 72 wks, ITT analysis showed the VL was <400 and <50 c/mL in 67%

and 61%, respectively. Response was correlated with the number of LPV resistance mutations at baseline, with VL <400 c/mL in 91% of those with 0–5 mutations, 71% with 6–7 mutations, and 33% with 8–10 mutations (Antiviral Ther 2002;7:165).

M97-765 was a Phase II study in 70 NNRTI-naïve patients with a VL of 1,000–100,000 c/mL (median VL 10,000 c/mL and median CD4 349/mm³) on a PI regimen. Patients received LPV/r + NVP and 2 NRTIs. At 48 wks, 60% had VL <50 c/mL by ITT analysis (J Virol 2001;75:7462).

BMS 043 was an open-label randomized trial comparing unboosted atazanavir (ATV) with LPV/r, both in combination with two NRTIs selected by resistance testing, in 300 patients failing a PI-based regimen with HIV RNA ≥1,000 c/mL (Curr Med Res Opin 2005;21:1683). Virologic suppression was superior in the LPV/r arm at 24 wks (−2.11 vs. −1.57 $\log_{10}$ c/mL, p = 0.032). Virologic suppression to <50 c/mL was found in 54% of those taking LPV/r vs. 38% of those taking ATV by ITT analysis (p = 0.008). Differences between LPV/r and ATV were more pronounced in those with greater antiretroviral experience or resistance.

RESIST: Subset analysis of TPV/r vs. LPV/r in patients with 3-class failure showed a better virologic response (<400 c/mL) at 24 wks in patients randomized to TPV/r (116/293, 40%) vs. LPV/r (62/290, 21%) (Lancet 2006;368:46).

ACTG 5143: Randomized trial of patients with prior PI failure to determine if double-boosted PIs (LPV/r + FPV) would achieve viral suppression. The study was stopped prematurely due to lack of trends showing better viral suppression and low PI levels in the dual PI arm (HIV Clin Trials 2008;9:9).

SWITCHMRK: Patients with undetectable VL on LPV/r-based ART >3 mos were randomized to RAL vs. remaining on LPV/r. All participants received 2 NRTIs with the assigned "third drug." The analysis for 702 participants at 24 wks found that the RAL + 2 NRTI recipients had a better lipid profile, but the number with VL <50 c/mL was greater in the LPV/r arm (90% vs. 84%). Noninferiority was not established, and the study was stopped (Lancet 2010;375:396).

NRTI-SPARING REGIMENS: *ACTG 5142* compared the efficacy of LPV/r 533/133 mg bid + EFV 600 mg/d vs. EFV + 2 NRTIs vs. LPV/r + 2 NRTIs. The NRTI-sparing regimen was effective but associated with higher serum lipids than either of the standard regimens and also with high rates of NNRTI resistance with failure (JAIDS 2007;21:325).

A5116 was a randomized trial comparing LPV/r 533/133 mg bid + EFV 600 mg/d vs. EFV + 2 NRTIs in patients with VL <200 c/mL on ART for >18 mos. The latter regimen was superior to the NRTI-sparing regimen in terms of toxicity (17% vs. 5%; P <0.002), and there was a trend toward greater virologic failure in the NRTI-sparing arm (P = 0.09, ITT) (AIDS 2007;21:325). In patients with baseline VL >100,000 c/mL, there was a longer time to virologic failure in the EFV + 2 NRTIs compared to LPV/r + EFV and LPV/r + 2NRTI arm (p = 0.02) (NEJM 2008;358:2095).

PROGRESS: LPV/r + RAL vs. LPV/r + TDF/FTC in treatment-naïve patients (Reynes et al.,18th IAS 2010, Vienna; Abstr. MOABO101). At 48 wks, patients in the NRTI sparing arm had virolologic response rates (83% vs. 85% <50 c/mL by TLOVR analysis). Two in each group discontinued due to adverse events, and CD4 count increases were similar. Concerns with this study are low baseline VL (mean VL 18,000 c/mL) and small samples size (N = 206).

RESISTANCE: The presence of ≥6 of the following mutations are associated with decreased activity: 10F/I/R/V, 20M/R, 24I, 32I, 33F, 46I/L, 47V/A, 50V, 53L, 54V/L/A/M/T/S, 63P, 71V/T, 73S, 82A/F/T/S, 84V, and 90M. Major mutations include 32I, 47V/A 76V, and 82A/F/T/S (AAC 2002;46:2926; J Virol 2001;75:7462). Most patients who receive LPV/r as their first PI have no PI resistance mutations at virologic failure. Mutations 47A and 32I may be associated with high-level resistance (Topics HIV Med 2006;14:125). The I50V mutation selected by fosamprenavir causes significant loss of susceptibility to LPV. 63P is common without PI exposure; this mutation combined with other PI resistance mutations has been associated with LPV/r failure (Topics in HIV Med 2003;11:92).

PHARMACOLOGY:

Bioavailability: The tablet formulation shows no significant difference in AUC or C_{max} whether given in a fed or fasting state. With the oral solution, there is an AUC increase of 80% when given with a moderate-fat meal. The addition of RTV results in a significant increase in LPV concentrations, AUC, and $T^{1/2}$ due to inhibition of the cytochrome P450 CYP3A4 isoenzymes. The mean steady-state LPV plasma concentrations are 15- to 20-fold higher than those without RTV. Protein binding is extensive, but there is sufficient CNS penetration to exceed the IC_{50} (AIDS 2005;19:949). The CNS penetration score is 3 in a four-class system (Neurology 2011;76:693).

$T^{1/2}$: 5–6 hr.

Metabolism/excretion: Metabolized primarily by cytochrome P450 CYP3A4 isoenzymes. LPV/r inhibits CYP3A4 isoenzymes, but the effect is less than that of therapeutic doses of RTV, and similar to that of IDV. Based on PK data with APV, LPV/r may be an inducer of CYP3A4 at steady state. Less than 3% excreted unchanged in urine.

Renal failure: No data are available, but usual dose is recommended. LPV/r is not removed with hemodialysis (AIDS 2001;15:662); however, LPV trough is lower in HD. Use with caution in patients with PI resistant mutations.

Hepatic failure: No dose modification recommendations are available. Use with caution in end-stage liver disease.

SIDE EFFECTS: The drug is less well-tolerated compared to some other PIs (e.g., DRV/r, ATV/r), with 2% discontinuing therapy due to adverse drug reactions in Phase II and III clinical trials through 48 wks.

Diarrhea: The most common adverse reactions are gastrointestinal, with diarrhea of at least moderate severity in 15–25%.

Abdominal pain and nausea is also common and may improve with oral solution.

Transaminase levels: Laboratory abnormalities through 72 wks included transaminase increases (to >5× normal) in 10–12%.

PR and QTc interval prolongation: Affect on PR interval is similar for most PIs and effect on QT is minimal (JAIDS 2011;25:367).

Class adverse reactions: Insulin resistance, fat accumulation, and hyperlipidemia. Clinical trials show triglyceride increases to >750 mg/dL in 12–22%, and cholesterol increases to >300 mg/dL in 14–22% of treatment-naïve patients receiving LPV/r. In HIV-negative men given LPV/r for 10 days, the major effect was an increase in triglyceride levels averaging 83%; there was minimal effect on insulin sensitivity (AIDS 2004;18:641). Comparative trials with DRV/r (ARTEMIS) and with ATV/r (CASTLE) demonstrated that LPV/r is associated with significantly greater increases in triglycerides and total cholesterol levels (JAIDS 2010;53:323). The D:A:D analysis of 33,308 patients with 580 myocardial infarctions found a relative risk with LPV/r-based ART of 1.3/yr, with 150 events in 37,136 patient- years of LPV/r data (JID 2010;20:318). An analysis of 7,053 HIV-infected patients in Quebec showed LPV/r was associated with a RR of 1.93 for an AMI compared to age matched HIV negative persons (Durand. JAIDS 2011;57:175).

Report of 7 cases of renal or parotid lithiasis (AIDS 2004;18:705).

DRUG INTERACTIONS:

Antiretroviral agents: The major effect is due to the inhibition of CYP3A4 isoenzymes, which results in prolongation of the half-life of drugs metabolized by this route. It is likely an inducer of CYP3A4 and glucuronyl transferase at steady-state.

Avoid concurrent use: Eplerenone, rifampin, simvastatin, lovastatin, midazolam, triazolam, lurasidone, cisapride, pimozide, ergotamine derivatives and St. John's wort, astemizole, and terfenadine.

Avoid: Bepridil, alfuzosin, amiodarone, ivabradine, flibanserin, dexamethasone (at steady-state), dofetilide, lurasidone, fentanyl, flecainide, propafenone, fluticasone, salmeterol ranolazine, rifapentine, rivaroxaban, betrixaban, ticagrelor, vorapaxar, silodosin, enzalutamide, mitotane, high-dose sildenafil, and *quinidine*.

Drugs that require a modified dose: *Rifabutin* AUC increased 3-fold; with standard LPV dose, rifabutin dose to 150 mg q24h. Consider rifabutin TDM. Note that a pharmacokinetic trial of the FDA-recommended dose of rifabutin 150 mg q48h appeared to give inadequate rifabutin exposure with LPV/r (CID 2009;49:1305). *Clarithromycin* AUC increased 77%; reduce clarithromycin dose in renal failure; use 50% clarithromycin dose with CrCl 30–60 mL/min and 25% dose with CrCl <30 mL/min. *Methadone* AUC decreased by 53%; monitor for withdrawal (conflicting data on withdrawal symptoms). *Trazodone* AUC increased 240%. Avoid or use lowest trazodone dose with close monitoring. *Bosentan*: LPV/r increased bosentan 48-fold on day 4 and 5-fold on day 10 (at steady state). Bosentan 62.5 mg; co-administer only after >10 days of RTV-boosted PI. *Atorvastatin* AUC increased 5- to 6-fold; use lowest dose (10 mg/d) or use alternative, such as pitavastatin, pravastatin, or rosuvastatin (5 mg/d). *Pravastatin* levels increased 33%; no dose adjustment. *Ketoconazole* levels increased 3-fold; limit to ≤200 mg/d. *Voriconazole*: RTV 200 mg/d reduces voriconazole AUC 40%; avoid or consider TDM. *Itraconazole* levels increased; do not exceed 200 mg/d or monitor levels. May increase anticoagulant concentrations. Dose adjustment needed with edoxaban, apixiban, and dabigatran based on renal function and indication.

Oral contraceptives: Ethinyl estradiol AUC decreased by 42%; use additional or alternative methods.

Drugs for erectile dysfunction: Sildenafil level increase anticipated; start with 25 mg/48h; *vardenafil,* no data; start with 2.5 mg/72h; *tadalafil,* start with 5 mg and increase to 10 mg q72h as tolerated.

Disulfiram: Oral solution of LPV/r contains alcohol; avoid.

Fluticasone: May increase levels of fluticasone with decreased serum cortisol levels; avoid coadministration. Beclomethasone preferred.

Prednisone: May increase prednisone level; consider dose adjustment with long-term use.

Anticonvulsants: LPV and phenytoin levels decreased by 33% and 31%, respectively.

Carbamazepine and phenobarbital may decrease serum level of LPV. Consider TDM or use alternative anticonvulsants (i.e., valproic acid, lamotrigine, levetiracetam). *Valproic acid*: valproic acid concentrations were not significantly lower; LPV AUC increased 38%. *Lamotrigine*: LPV not affected, but lamotrigine AUC decreased 50%. Titrate to effect.

Atovaquone levels may be decreased, requiring dose adjustment.

TDF AUC increase 32%; clinical significance unknown; dose adjustment not recommended.

Tacrolimus half-life increased 10-fold (Clin Pharmacokinet 2007;46:941); *sirolimus and cyclosporine* $T^{1/2}$ may also be increased significantly. Dose reduction recommended based on TDM.

Digoxin AUC increased 81%; monitor closely.

Bupropion AUC decreased 46%; titrate to effect.

PREGNANCY: Category C. LPV is an alternative PI for pregnant women according to the 2018 DHHS Recommendations for Use of Antiretroviral Drugs for Pregnant HIV-1 Infected Women. Most of the pharmacology and clinical trials have used the 133/33 mg LPV/r capsules, which demonstrated decreased levels in the third trimester (AIDS 2006:20:1931). This led to the recommendation by some experts to use LPV/r 600/150 mg or 500/125 mg bid during the second and third trimesters especially in patients with PI-experienced patients in the 2018 recommendations. Pharmacokinetic studies with the tablet form found a median AUC of 72 μg*hr/mL in the second trimester, 97 μg*hr/mL with the increased dose in the third trimester, and 129 μg*hr/mL 2 wks postpartum (JAIDS 2010;54:381). The Pregnancy Registry reported birth defects in 30/1400 (2.14%) first-trimester exposures, which is less than the background rate without LPV exposure (07/31/2017).

TABLE 6.60 Dose adjustments for concurrent use of LPV/r with other antiretroviral agents

Drug	Effect on Co-administered Drug	Effect on LPV	Dose Recommendation
EFV	No change	↓36%	EFV 600 mg hs + LPV/r 400/100 mg or 500/125 mg bid (treatment-naïve) or 600/150 mg bid (treatment-experienced). LPV/r qd not recommended
IDV	C_{min} ↓45%	No change	IDV 600 mg bid + LPV/r 400/100 mg bid
ETR	↓17%	↓18%	Standard doses
NVP	No change	C_{min} ↓55%	NVP standard + LPV/r 400/100 mg bid (treatment-naïve) or 600/150 mg bid (treatment-experienced). LPV/r 500/125 mg bid can be considered. LPV/r qd not recommended
SQV	↑	↑	SQV 1,000 mg bid + LPV/r 400/100 mg bid[a]

TABLE 6.60 Continued

Drug	Effect on Co-administered Drug	Effect on LPV	Dose Recommendation
NFV	↑25%	↓27%	Data insufficient; avoid coadministration
ATV	C_{min} ↑45%	No change	Dose: ATV 300 mg/d + LPV/r 400/100 bid
FPV	C_{min} ↓4%	C_{min} ↓53%	No clear dose recommendation. Avoid or consider FPV 1400 mg bid + LPV/r 600/150 mg bid.
DRV	AUC ↓50%	AUC ↑53%	Avoid.
TPV	—	AUC ↓55%	Avoid.
MVC	↑4×	—	MVC dose 150 mg bid
RAL	Interaction unlikely	—	RAL 400 mg bid plus standard dose LPV/r
TDF	TDF AUC ↑32%	No change	Clinical significance unknown. Use standard dose.
RPV	May increase	No change likely	Use standard dose. Monitor QTc in patients at risk for QTc prolongation.
DTG	No change		DTG 50 mg/d + standard dose LPV/r
EVG	EVG AUC ↑75%		EVG 85 mg/d + LPV/r 400/100 mg bid
BIC	BIC may ↑	- No change likely	No data. Dose not established

[a] Shows synergy in vitro (AAC 2002;46:2249).

Lotrimin—see Clotrimazole

Maraviroc (MVC)

TRADE NAME: Selzentry (ViiV/GlaxoSmithKline; Celsentri).

CLASS: CCR5 antagonist entry inhibitor.

FORMULATIONS, REGIMEN, AND COST: 150 and 300 mg tabs, at $ $1,679.68/mo.

STANDARD DOSE: 300 mg po bid with or without food.

Note: Dose varies based on concurrent meds.

Strong CYP 3A4 inhibitors (which includes all PIs (except TPV/r) and cobicistat) + /– CYP3A4 inducer: MVC 150 mg bid. No dose adjustment based on concurrent use of drugs that are not strong inducers or inhibitors of CYP3A including BIC, DTG, ENF, NVP, RAL, RPV, TPV/r: MVC 300 mg bid. Strong CYP 3A4 inducers including EFV, ETR, and rifampin without use of PI or cobicistat; MVC 600 mg bid.

Renal failure: Renal excretion accounts for <25% of clearance. (1) CrCl <30 mL/min or HD, reduce dose to 150 mg bid if signs of postural hypotension and (2) CrCl <30 mL/min + co-administration of CYP3A inhibitor. Avoid.

Hepatic failure: Limited data show minimal effect. No dose adjustment.

STORAGE: Room temperature.

INDICATIONS: HIV-infected patients with (1) R5 virus only as shown by a co-receptor tropism assay and (2) virologic failure and resistance to multiple antiretroviral agents.

ADVANTAGES: (1) Active against R5-tropic HIV strains, including strains resistant to other antiretroviral agents, (2) established efficacy in patients with multiple drug exposure and treatment failure (MOTIVATE trials), (3) no food effect, and (4) overall outcome similar to EFV for treatment-naïve patients without EFV side effects (MERIT trial).

DISADVANTAGES: (1) Requirement for pretreatment screening with expensive co-receptor tropism assay; (2) twice-daily dosing; (3) need for caution with pre- existing liver disease, including chronic hepatitis B or C; (4) studied only with AZT/3TC for initial therapy and not a recommended initial ARV regimen; and (5) drug interactions requiring dose adjustment.

RESISTANCE: Failure occurs by two distinctive mechanisms:

Selection of preexisting X4 or dual/mixed (D/M) tropic HIV that escaped detection on baseline tropism screening (J Virol 2006;80:4909). These accounted for 60% of MVC failures using the original Trophile assay. The enhanced susceptibility tropism assay (Trofile ES) is more sensitive (99.7%) at detecting X4- or D/M-tropic virus present at low levels. R5 strains remain susceptible to MVC in this case. Prevalence of R5 virus is 80–90% in treatment-naïve patients (JID 2005;192:466; JID 2005;191:866) and 50–60% in treatment-experienced patients (JID 2006;194:926; CID 2007;44:591). Phenotypic tropism assay is preferred, but genotypic tropism assay should be considered as an alternative before initiating MVC and with virologic failure,

MVC resistance is attributed to mutations in the V3 loop of the HIV envelope (gp120), usually with mutations at multiple sites that result in a reduction in maximal percent inhibition rather than a fold increase in IC_{50} seen with other antiretroviral agents (Top HIV Med 2007;15:119). Polymorphisms 4L, 11R and 19S are associated with reduced response.

HIV strains resistant to MVC by these mechanisms do not show cross-resistance to ENF, which blocks HIV entry by a completely different mechanism (and should be additive or synergistic with MVC). There is no cross-resistance between MVC and other classes of antiretroviral agents (AAC 2005;49:4751). Analysis of R5-V3 sequences in 498 treatment-naïve HIV-infected patients demonstrated a baseline prevalence of resistance of <5% (JAC 2010;65:2502).

PHARMACOLOGY:

MVC binds the transmembrane co-receptor of R5-tropic virus to prevent its interaction with the V3 loop of gp120. This blocks viral entry (AIDS 2009;23:1931).

Absorption: 32%.

Food effect: Minimal.

$T^{1/2}$: 10 hrs.

Excretion: Stool (75%), urine (20%).

Pharmacokinetics: Substrate for CYP3A and Pgp (CID 2009;47:236).

CNS penetration: Score is 3 in a four-class system (Neurology 2011;76:693).

CLINICAL TRIALS: *MOTIVATE-1 and -2*: Phase III trials of MVC (300 mg/d or bid) plus optimized background therapy (OBT) vs. OBT in highly treatment experienced patients. Enrollment criteria: R5 virus, three-class exposure, and treatment failure with VL >5,000 c/mL. Randomization was 2:2:1 for MVC 300 mg bid, 300 mg/d, or OBR. Results at 48 wks for 1,049 randomized patients

TABLE 6.61 48-wk results of MOTIVATE-1 & -2 Comparing OBR vs. MVC + OBR (2-dose regimens)

	MVC qd n = 414	MVC Bid n = 426	OBR Alone n = 209
Baseline			
CD4 count (mean)	187/mm^3	196/mm^3	189/mm^3
HIV VL (mean log$_{10}$ c/mL	4.9	4.9	4.9
<2 active drugs OBR	66%	65%	70%
Results			
VL <50 c/mL	46%	43%	17%
VL <400 c/mL	52%	56%	23%
ADR with discontinuation	5%	5%	5%
AST >5× ULN	4%	4%	3%

TABLE 6.62 MERIT trial of MVC vs. EFV, each with AZT/3TC in treatment-naïve patients (post-hoc analysis) at 48 wks

	MVC n = 311	EFV n = 303
Baseline		
CD4 median (cells/mL)	254	236
Viral load ($\log_{10}$ c/mL)	4.88	4.85
Results (48 wks)		
Discontinuation due to lack of efficacy	29 (9.3%)	12 (4.0%)[a]
Adverse events	13 (4.2%)	43 (14.2%)[a]
CD4 count change (cells/mm³)	+ 212	+ 171

From JID 2010;201:803.
[a] P <0.05.

are summarized in Table 6.61 (NEJM 2008;359:1429). The 96-wk data showed VL <50 c/mL in 39% and 41% of patients treated with MVC once- or twice-daily, respectively (JAIDS 2010;55:558). Among those with VL< 50 c/mL at 48 wks, virologic suppression (<50 c/mL) was maintained in 81% of those randomized to receive once-daily MVC and 87% of those receiving twice-daily MVC.

MERIT: MVC vs. EFV in treatment-naïve patients. Participants had R5-tropic virus at baseline and were randomized to receive MVC or EFV, each in combination with 2 NRTIs. Of 1,277 participants 895 began therapy with either MVC + AZT/3TC or EFV + AZT/3TC. Results are summarized in Table 6.62 based on the post hoc analysis (MERIT ES) that corrected for erroneous Trophile assays at baseline (JID 2010;201:803). In the 96-wk follow-up of MERIT, virologic suppression (<50 c/mL) was maintained in 63% of the EFV arm and 59% of the MVC arm; time to loss of virologic response (TLOVR) in responders was 61% with EFV and 61% with MVC; median CD4 count increase (cells/mm³) was 171 with EFV and 212 with MVC; and discontinuations for adverse events were 16% with EFV and 6% with MVC (HIV Clin Trials 2010;11:125). These results showed

EFV-based ART had somewhat better virologic outcomes (that was not statistically significant) and MVC showed better tolerance (HIV Clin Trials 2011;12:24).

Dual/Mixed-Tropic Virus Study (A4001029): This was an exploratory, randomized, blinded, placebo-controlled trial to determine the safety and efficacy of MVC treatment in patients with D/M-tropic HIV. Entry criteria were the same as for MOTIVATE-1 and -2, and participants were randomized 1:1:1 to receive MVC twice-daily + OBR or MVC once-daily + OBR or OBR alone (JID 2009;199:1638). Although MVC was not virologically effective in this population, there was no decline in CD4 count. These results suggest that the switch to X4 virus is a consequence of disease progression rather than a cause (JID 2011;203:237).

NRTI-SPARING: *A4001078 - MVC 150 mg/d + ATV/r 300/100 mg/d vs. ATV + TDF/FTC:* A pilot trial of a NRTI-sparing regimen in 120 treatment-naïve patients with a mean baseline CD4 count of 351 cells/mm^3 and median VL 4.6 log$_{10}$ c/mL (Mills A. 2010 IAS, Vienna; Abstr. THLBB203). At 24 wks, the MCV + ATV/r arm had a numerically lower response rate (80 vs. 89%; *p* = NS) and more treatment-limiting side effects (16% vs. 8%).

MVC/RAL/ETR: A prospective study of 28 triple-class failure patients given RAL 400 mg bid, MVC 600 mg bid, and ETR 200 mg bid, 26 (92%) had VL <50 c/mL at 48 wks (AIDS 2010;24:924).

INTENSIFICATION: The goal was to determine the potential value of the immunomodulary properties of MVC. Patients (*n* = 45) with CD4 counts <350 cells/mm^3 and VL <48 c/mL (PloS One 2010;5:e13188) were randomized to add MVC or placebo. MVC increased activation of T cells in the gut and blood but had no effect on the CD4 count (Hunt P. CROI 2011:Abstr.153LB). Treatment intensification also failed to reduce CSF viral load (JAIDS 2010;55:590).

PHARMACOLOGY: See JAIDS 2006;42:183; Nat Med 2005;11:1170; JAIDS 2006;42:183.

> *CNS penetration* shows a CSF-to-plasma ratio of 0.09, and CSF showed no detectable HIV in all 9 patients with VL <40 c/mL (JAIDS 2010;55:606).

Bioavailability: 25–35%, no dose adjustment with or without food.

$T^{1/2}$: 14–18 hrs.

Excretion: 25% metabolized by CYP3A4 and 11% hydroxylated. Unchanged drug and metabolites are excreted via the GI tract accounting for 76%. About 25% is renally excreted. MVC with a CYP3A4 inhibitor is not recommended in patients with CrCl <30 mL/min. Renal clearance accounts for <25% of total clearance.

SIDE EFFECTS: The drug is usually well-tolerated. The most common ADRs are GI intolerance with diarrhea (22%), nausea (18%), headache (14%), and fatigue (12%), but many of these reactions were noted in a comparable number of placebo recipients. The most important ADR in trials has been postural hypotension, which may occur more frequently in those without dose adjustment with concurrent use of a CYP3A4 inhibitor and those with renal failure or with initial dosing using higher doses (e.g., 600 mg twice-daily) before enzyme induction has occurred. Consider dose escalation. Grade 3–4 hepatotoxicity has been reported in 3–5% and sometimes follows a pruritic rash with eosinophilia. This was an early concern with MVC, but an analysis of 2,350 recipients found only 2 cases of severe hepatotoxicity, and both were confounded by other factors (AIDS 2010;24:2743). In clinical trials, there was a significant increase in URIs in MVC recipients (5% vs. 2%), but other infections do not appear to be increased. There was concern that decreased immune surveillance due to CCR5 blockade would promote lymphomas, but that has not been the experience to date. The 96-wk data from the MOTIVATE-1 & -2 and MERIT trials with 1499 MVC recipients showed no increase in cancer rates (Walmsley, 2010 IAS;Abstr. TUPE0157). The CCR5 receptor plays a role in the pathophysiology of West Nile Virus infection, so there a theoretical possibility that MVC could increase this risk (JID 2010;201:178), but this has not been seen clinically. The first CCR5 antagonist (aplaviroc) was withdrawn due to severe hepatotoxicity, which has not been a subsequent concern with MVC as noted above (AIDS 2010;24:2473). The same applies to malignancy (Eur J Med Res 2007;12:409). MVC

TABLE 6.63 Maraviroc ART drug interactions

Drug	Effect of Interaction	Recommendations/ Comments
NVP	MVC serum concentration is not significantly affected	MVC 300 mg bid + SD NVP if no PI is used
EFV	MVC AUC decreased by 45%	MVC 600 mg bid if no PI is used
ATV	MVC AUC increased 3.6× with ATV/r; MVC increased 5×	MVC 150 mg bid with ATV or ATV/r
TDF	No significant change in MVC concentrations	MVC 300 mg bid
SQV/r	MVC AUC increased 877%	MVC 150 mg bid
SQV/r + EFV	MVC AUC increased 400%	MVC 150 mg bid
LPV/r	MVC AUC increased 295%	MVC 150 mg bid
ATV/r or ATV/c	MVC AUC increased 388%	MVC 150 mg bid
TPV/r	No significant interaction	MVC 300 mg bid
LPV/r + EFV	MVC AUC 2.5×	MVC 150 mg bid
ETR	MVC AUC decreased 53%	MVC 600 mg bid
DRV/r or DRV/c	MVC AUC likely increase	MVC 150 mg bid
ETR + DRV/r	MVC AUC increased 210%	MVC 150 mg bid
FPV, FPV/r, IDV, DLV	Unknown. Anticipate MVC AUC increase	MVC 150 mg bid
RTV	MVC AUC increases 2.6× with RTV 200 mg/d	MVC 150 mg bid
DRV/r	MVC AUC increased 305% with co-administration	MVC 150 mg bid
RPV	Interaction unlikely	MVC 300 mg bid + RPV 25 mg/d
DTG	Interaction unlikely	MVC 300 mg bid + DTG 50 mg/d
EVG/cobi or EVG/r	Cobicistat or RTV may significantly increase MVC	MVC 150 mg bid + SD EVG
RAL	MVC AUC decreased 14%	MVC 300 mg bid
BIC	Interaction unlikely	MVC 300 mg bid

TABLE 6.64 Maraviroc non-ART drug interactions

Drug	Effect of Interaction	Recommendations/ Comments
Carbamazepine	MVC AUC may significantly decrease with carbamazepine	MVC 600 mg bid, or consider alternative anticonvulsant (i.e., valproic acid or levetiracetam)
Clarithromycin	May increase MVC serum concentrations	MVC 150 mg bid
Erythromycin	May increase MVC serum concentrations	MVC 150 mg bid
Ethinylestradiol	No significant interaction	MVC 300 mg bid. Consider additional barrier contraception.
Itraconazole	May increase MVC serum concentrations	MVC 150 mg bid
Ketoconazole	MVC AUC increased 5-fold with co-administration.	MVC 150 mg bid
Levonorgestrel	No significant interaction	MVC 300 mg bid. Consider an additional barrier contraception
Nefazodone	May increase MVC serum concentrations	MVC 150 mg bid
Phenobarbital	MVC AUC may significantly decrease with phenobarbital co-administration	MVC 600 mg bid, or consider alternative anticonvulsant (i.e., valproic acid or levetiracetam)
Phenytoin	MVC AUC may significantly decrease with phenytoin co-administration	MVC 600 mg bid, or consider alternative anticonvulsant (i.e., valproic acid or levetiracetam).
Rifabutin	Modest impact on MVC serum concentrations	MVC 300 mg bid (No data)
Rifampin	MVC AUC decreased 66% with co-administration	MVC 600 mg bid- (Limited clinical data)
Sulfamethoxazole-trimethoprim	MVC AUC increased 10%	MVC 300 mg bid

appears to be "lipid neutral" and may reduce levels of immune activation better than EFV according to a substudy of MERIT (PLoS One 2010;5:e13188).

BLACK BOX WARNINGS: Severe hepatotoxicity that may be preceded by a pruritic rash and eosinophilia suggesting a systemic allergic reaction.

DRUG INTERACTIONS: See Tables 6.63 and 6.64:
MVC does not inhibit or induce CYP3A4 so it does not alter levels or require dose changes of concurrent agents that use the P450 metabolic pathway.

Concurrent use of drugs that induce CYP3A4 include EFV which decreases MVC AUC by 45%, rifampin which decreases the AUC by 63%, and ETR which decreases MVC 53%. The dose of MVC to compensate for this difference is 600 mg bid. Other CYP3A4 inducers include barbiturates, carbamazepine, phenytoin, primidone, and St. John's wort; avoid or increase MVC dose (600 mg bid).

Concurrent use of drugs that inhibit CYP3A4, including all boosted PIs other than TPV/r, which increases MVC AUC 2- to 8-fold; the dose of MVC should be 150 mg bid. Other drugs that inhibit CYP3A4 include cobicistat, azoles (ketoconazole, itraconazole), erythromycin, clarithromycin, and nefazodone; reduce dose (MVC 150 mg bid). Some SSRIs, diltiazem, verapamil, amiodarone, cimetidine, and fluvoxamine may also increase MVC levels, but there are no dose recommendations. Consider standard dose in patients with normal renal function. If potent inducers are used with potent inhibitors, use MVC at 150 mg bid (e.g., EFV + ATV/r + MVC dosed 150 mg bid).

PREGNANCY: Category B. Not teratogenic in animal studies, but experience in humans is very limited. Limited placental transfer. PK study found a 21% decreased in MVC concentrations during the third trimester. Insufficient data to recommended in pregnancy by the 2018 DHHS Guidelines for Pregnant Women with HIV Infection because safety has not been established.

Marinol—see Dronabinol

Megace—see Megestrol Acetate

Megestrol Acetate

TRADE NAME: Megace (Bristol-Myers Squibb) and generic.

CLASS: Synthetic progestin related to progesterone.

FORMULATIONS, REGIMEN, AND COST: Tabs: 20 mg at $0.69, 40 mg at $1.23. Oral suspension: 40 mg/mL at $180.54/240 mL; 625 mg/5mL (150mL) at $998.46.

PATIENT ASSISTANCE: 800-272-4878.

INDICATIONS: Appetite stimulant to promote weight gain in patients with HIV infection or neoplastic disease.

USUAL REGIMEN:

Oral suspension: 400 mg/d, up to 800 mg/d.

Tablets: 400–800 mg/d (suspension usually preferred).

EFFICACY: A controlled trial of 271 patients with HIV-associated wasting found that those given megestrol 800 mg/d gained a mean of 4 kg more than placebo recipients. (Ann Intern Med 1994;121:393). However, most of the weight gain was fat. Another study showed that the increase in caloric intake was not sustained after 8 wks (Ann Intern Med 1994;121:400). Published data for use in HIV infection are available only for men. A review of appetite stimulants for patients with cystic fibrosis came to no clear conclusions but provided the best supportive data for megestrol compared to dronabinol, mirtazapine, and cyproheptadine (J Hum Nutr Diet 2007;20:526). Megestrol can cause hypogonadism, so it may require discontinuation or a replacement dose of testosterone in men (200 mg q2wk) or anabolic steroids and resistance exercises (NEJM 1999;340:1740).

PHARMACOLOGY:

Bioavailability: >90%.

$T^{1/2}$: 30 hr.

Elimination: 60–80% excreted in urine; 7–30% excreted in feces.

SIDE EFFECTS:

Most serious are hypogonadism (which may exacerbate wasting), diabetes, and adrenal insufficiency.

Most common are diarrhea, impotence, rash, flatulence, asthenia, and hyperglycemia (5%).

Less common or rare include carpal tunnel syndrome, thrombosis, nausea, vomiting, edema, vaginal bleeding, and alopecia. High doses (400–1,600 mg/d): hyperpnea, chest pressure, mild increase in blood pressure, dyspnea, congestive heart failure.

A review of FDA reports of adverse drug reactions with megestrol included 5 cases of Cushing syndrome, 12 cases of new-onset diabetes, and 17 cases of possible adrenal insufficiency (Arch Intern Med 1997;157:1651). One report suggested a 6-fold increase in the risk of deep venous thrombosis (J Am Med Dir Assoc 2003;4:255). Another review reported an association with osteonecrosis (JAIDS 2000;25:19).

DRUG INTERACTIONS: Not a substrate of CYP3A4. No significant drug–drug interactions.

PREGNANCY: Category D. Progestational drugs are associated with genital abnormalities in male and female fetuses exposed during first 4 mos of pregnancy.

Mepron—see Atovaquone

Methadone

TRADE NAME: Dolophine (Roxane) and generic.

CLASS: Opiate schedule II. The FDA restricts physician prescribing for methadone maintenance to those licensed to provide this service and those attached to methadone maintenance programs. However, licensed physicians can prescribe methadone for pain control.

FORMULATIONS, REGIMEN, AND COST: Tabs: 5 mg at $0.32, 10 mg at $0.44. Oral solution 10 mg/mL (30 mL) at $25.35. IV injection 10 mg/mL (20 mL) at $247.30. Usual yearly cost of medication for methadone maintenance averages $180.

INDICATIONS AND DOSES:

Detoxification for substantial opiate abstinence symptoms: Initial dose is based on opiate tolerance, usually 15–20 mg; additional doses may be necessary. Daily dose at 40 mg usually stabilizes patient; when stable 2–3 days, decrease dose 20% per day. Must complete detoxification in <180 days or consider maintenance.

Maintenance as oral substitute for heroin or other morphine-like drugs: Initial dose 15–30 mg depending on extent of prior use, up to 40 mg/d. Subsequent doses depend on response. Usual maintenance dose is 40–100 mg/d, but higher doses are sometimes required. Most states limit the maximum daily dose to 80–120 mg/d, but doses may be increased due to drug–drug interactions (especially with EFV and NVP).

Note: During first 3 mos, and for all patients receiving >100 mg/d, observation is required 6 days/wk. With good adherence and rehabilitation, clinic attendance may be reduced for observed ingestion 3 days/wk with maximum 2-day supply for home administration. After 2 yrs, clinic visits may be reduced to 2×/wk with 3-day drug supplies. After 3 yrs, visits may be reduced to weekly with a 6-day supply. In a trial of Directly Administered Antiretroviral Therapy (DAART) with observed ART at the time methadone was given, adherence with supervised doses was strongly associated with virologic success (AIDS Patient Care STDs 2007;21:564).

Pain control: 2.5–10.0 mg po q3–4h or 5–20 mg po q6–8h for severe chronic pain in terminally ill patients.

TABLE 6.65 Drug interactions with methadone

Drug	Effect on Methadone	Effect on Co-administered Drug	Comment
NRTIs			
ABC	Clearance ↑22%	↓ Peak	Dose adjustment unlikely
AZT	None	AUC ↑43%	Monitor for AZT toxicity
3TC	No effect	—	Standard doses
ddI	None	ddI EC – no change	ddI EC preferred
d4T	None	AUC ↓23%	No dose adjustment
TDF	No effect	No effect	Standard doses
DLV	No data; may ↑	No effect	Use standard DLV dose; monitor for methadone toxicity
NNRTIs			
EFV	AUC ↓52%	No data	Likely to need ↑ methadone dose
NVP	AUC ↓41%	No effect	Withdrawal common. Increase methadone based on symptoms of withdrawal.
ETR	None	No effect	No dose adjustment; monitor for withdrawal
RPV	AUC decreased 16%	No effect likely	Usual dose. Monitor for withdrawal and titrate dose
PIs			
DRV/r	AUC ↓16%	↓	Monitor for withdrawal
FPV/r	AUC ↓16%	↓25%	Monitor for withdrawal
SQV/r	↓10–20% with. SQV/r	No effect	Dose SQV/r 1,000/100 bid

TABLE 6.65 Continued

Drug	Effect on Methadone	Effect on Co-administered Drug	Comment
ATV	No effect	No effect	ATV: No empiric dose adjustment ATV/r: No data; monitor
TPV/r	↓48%	No effect	Empiric dose adjustment; monitor, may need methadone increase
IDV	No effect	No effect	Standard doses
LPV/r	AUC ↓25–50%	↓	Monitor dose increase (conflicting data)
NFV	AUC ↓40%	No effect	Monitor. Withdrawal rare
Other			
MVC	No data	No data	Interaction unlikely
RAL	No effect	No effect	Usual dose
DTG	No effect	No change likely	Usual dose
EVG/COBI	No effect	No change likely	Usual dose
BIC	–	–	Interaction unlikely. Use usual dose
Fluconazole	↑30%	No effect	Monitor for methadone toxicity
Rifampin	↓↓	No effect	Need ↑ methadone dose
Rifabutin	No effect	No effect	No dose adjustment
Rifapentine	↓↓	No effect likely	Need ↑ methadone dose
Phenytoin, carbamazepine, phenobarbital	↓↓	No effect	May need ↑ methadone dose

See Review: Curr HIV/AIDS 2010;7:152.

PHARMACOLOGY:

Bioavailability: >90% absorbed.

$T^{1/2}$: 25 hr. Duration of action with repeated administration is 24–48 hr, but analgesic $T^{1/2}$ is shorter.

Elimination: Metabolized by liver via CYP450 2B6>2C19>3A4. Parent compound excreted in urine with increased rate in acidic urine; metabolites excreted in urine and gut.

SIDE EFFECTS:

Acute toxicity: CNS depression (stupor or coma), respiratory depression, flaccid muscles, cold skin, bradycardia, hypotension. *Treatment*: Respiratory support ± gastric lavage (even hours after ingestion due to pylorospasm) ± naloxone (respiratory depression may last longer than naloxone duration of action; repeated dosing may be needed; may precipitate acute withdrawal syndrome).

Chronic toxicity: Tolerance/physical dependence with abstinence syndrome following withdrawal; onset at 3–4 days after last dose of weakness, anxiety, anorexia, insomnia, abdominal pain, headache, sweating, and hot-cold flashes. *Treatment*: Detoxification.

QTc prolongation (dose related).

DRUG INTERACTIONS: See Table 6.65.

PREGNANCY: Category C. Avoid during first 3 mos and use sparingly, in small doses, during last 6 mos.

Mycelex—see Clotrimazole

Mycobutin—see Rifabutin

Mycostatin—see Nystatin

Nebupent—see Pentamidine

Nelfinavir (NFV)

TRADE NAME: Viracept (ViiV Healthcare).

CLASS: Protease inhibitor.

FORMULATIONS, REGIMEN, AND COST:

Forms: Tabs, 250 and 625 mg; oral powder, 50 mg/mL (144 g) at $74.15.

Regimens: 1250 mg bid (tabs); 25 cc bid (oral solution).

AWP: $1169.22/mo.

FOOD: Increases levels 2–3×; take with food, preferably a fatty meal.

RENAL FAILURE: Standard dose.

HEPATIC FAILURE: No recommendation; use with caution.

STORAGE: Room temperature, 15–30°C.

PATIENT ASSISTANCE: 800-777-6637.

ADVANTAGES: Extensive experience; well-tolerated in pregnancy (but not recommended due to low potency).

DISADVANTAGES: Reduced potency compared to most other regimens, need for concurrent fatty meal, diarrhea, inability to effectively boost levels with RTV.

CLINICAL TRIALS: See Table 6.66.

RESISTANCE: The primary resistance mutation is D30N, which is associated with phenotypic resistance to NFV but not to other protease inhibitors (AAC 1998;42:2775). However, the L90M mutation can also occur, and, unlike 30N, it confers cross-resistance to all PIs except TPV/r and DRV/r. Other less important or secondary mutations are 10F/I, 36I, 46I/L, 71V/T, 77I, 82A/F/T/S, 84V, and 88D/S.

PHARMACOLOGY:

Bioavailability: Absorption with meals is 20–80%. Fatty meal increases absorption 2- to 3-fold.

TABLE 6.66 Clinical trials of NFV in treatment-naïve patients

Trial	Regimen	N	Duration (wks)	VL <50	VL <200–400
COMBINE. (Antiviral Ther 2002;7:81)	NFV + AZT/3TC	70	48	50%	60%
	NVP + AZT/3TC	72		65%[a]	75%[a]
SOLO. (AIDS 2004;18:1529)	FPV/r (1400/ 200 qd). + AZT/3TC	322	48	56%	68%
	NFV (1250 bid) + AZT/3TC	327		42%	65%
NEAT. (JAIDS 2004;35:22)	FPV 1400 bid + AZT/3TC	166	48	58%	66%[a]
	NFV 1250 bid + AZT/3TC	83		42%	51%
ACTG 384. (NEJM 2003;349:2293)	EFV + AZT/3TC	155	48	–	88%[a]
	NFV + AZT/3TC	155		–	67%
	NFV + EFV + AZT/ 3TC	178		–	84%
INITIO. (Lancet 2006;368:287)	EFV + ddI + d4T	188	192	74%	–
	NFV + ddI + d4T	162		62%	–
	EFV + NFV + ddI + d4T	155		62%	–
Abbott M98-863. (NEJM 2002;346:2039)	LPV/r + d4T + 3TC	326	48	67%[a]	75%[a]
	NFV + d4T + 3TC	327		52%	63%
BMS 008. (JAIDS 2004;36:684 and. Reyataz pkg insert)	ATV + d4T + 3TC	181	48	33%	67%
	NFV + d4T + 3TC	91		38%	59%

[a] Superior to comparator ($P <0.05$).

$T^{1/2}$: 3.5–5.0 hr (serum).

CNS penetration: No detectable levels in CSF (JAIDS 1999; 20:39).

Excretion: Primarily by cytochrome P450 CYP2C19 (major) and CYP3A4 (minor). Inhibits CYP3A4. Only 1–2% is found in urine; up to 90% is found in stool, primarily as a hydroxylated metabolite designated M8, which is as active as NFV against HIV (AAC 2001;45:1086).

Dose modification in renal or hepatic failure: None. NFV is removed with hemodialysis so that post dialysis dosing is important (AIDS 2000;14:89). The drug is not removed by peritoneal dialysis (JAC 2000;45:709).

Dose modification with hepatic failure: With severe liver disease, consider therapeutic drug monitoring. It appears that autoinduction of NFV metabolism is blunted in severe liver disease, and there is also a reduction in the M8 active metabolite. Standard doses may yield high or low levels.

SIDE EFFECTS:

Diarrhea: About 10–30% of recipients have a secretory diarrhea, characterized by low osmolarity and high sodium, possibly due to chloride secretion (7th CROI, San Francisco, 2000:Abstr. 62). Management strategies include use of several over-the-counter, inexpensive ($4–10/mo) remedies, including oat bran (1500 mg bid), psyllium (1 tsp qd or bid), loperamide (4 mg, then 2 mg every loose stool up to 16/d), or calcium (500 mg bid). Some respond to pancreatic enzymes (1–2 tabs with meals) at a cost of $30–111/mo (CID 2000;30:908).

Class adverse effects: Lipodystrophy, increased levels of triglycerides and/or cholesterol, hyperglycemia with insulin resistance and type 2 diabetes, osteoporosis, and possible increased bleeding with hemophilia (HIV Med 2006;7:85).

DRUG INTERACTIONS:

Drugs that should not be given concurrently: simvastatin, lovastatin, rifampin, rifapentine, alfuzosin, astemizole, fentanyl, terfenadine, eplerenone, ivabradine, flibanserin, lurasidone, dofetilide, lurasidone, cisapride, pimozide, midazolam, triazolam, ranolazine, rivaroxaban, betrixaban, ticagrelor, vorapaxar, silodosin, enzalutamide, mitotane.

high dose sildenafil, ergot derivatives, St. John's wort, amiodarone, quinidine, and proton pump inhibitors.

Drugs that require dose modifications: Anticonvulsants (phenobarbital, carbamazepine, phenytoin) may lower NFV. Edoxaban, apixiban, and dabigatran concentrations may be increased. Anticoagulant dose may need to be decreased based on renal function and indication.

Avoid or use with close monitoring: Oral contraceptives; sildenafil (not to exceed 25 mg/48 hrs); rifabutin (decrease rifabutin dose to 150 mg/d and increase NFV dose to 1,000 mg tid); methadone (no dose change); statins (use pitavastatin, pravastatin, or rosuvastatin); clarithromycin (reduce clarithromycin dose in renal failure; CrCl <30 mL/min); azoles; PIs, and NNRTIs (see Table 6.67);

Colchicine: NFV increases colchicine level.

Buprenorphine: No significant effect. Use standard dose.

PREGNANCY: Category B. Animal teratogenic studies negative; long-term animal carcinogenicity studies show increased tumors in rats given ≥300 mg/kg; minimal to low placental passage. Experience to establish safety in pregnancy is extensive. The pregnancy registry shows birth defects in 47/1212 (3.88%) exposures

---

TABLE 6.67 Nelfinavir combinations with integrase-inhibitors, PIs, and NNRTIs

Drug	Recommendation
RTV, SQV, FPV, IDV, EVG/cobi, RPV, BIC	Inadequate data
NVP, EFV, RAL, DTG	Standard doses
LPV/r, DRV/r, ETR, TPV/r	Avoid combination
MVC	MVC 150 mg bid

(www.apregistry.com, accessed 07/31/2017). The 750 mg tid dose produced variable levels in pregnant women that were generally lower than in nonpregnant women. The 1,250 mg bid regimen produced adequate levels except for variations in the third trimester (CID 2004;39:736). The 2018 DHHS Guidelines on ART in Pregnant Women do not recommend NFV as an alternate PI due to low potency.

Neupogen—see G-CSF

Nevirapine (NVP)

TRADE NAME: Viramune and Viramune XR (Boehringer Ingelheim)
CLASS: Non-nucleoside reverse transcriptase inhibitor (NNRTI).
FORMULATIONS, REGIMEN, AND COST:

- *Forms*: Tabs, 200 mg at $648.19/mo; oral solution, 50 mg/mL (240 mL bottle); at Viramune 400 mg XR tabs at $897.46/mo.
- *Regimens*: 200 mg/d × 2 wks, then 400 mg/d using immediate release tab 200 mg bid or XR tab 400 mg/d. After treatment interruption >7 days should restart with the 200 mg/d regimen. If rash appears during the lead-in period, delay dose escalation until after the rash has resolved, and rule out hepatitis. The lead-in dosing regimen of 200 mg/d should not be continued beyond 28 days. No dose escalation when switching from EFV to NVP; start with NVP 400 mg/d (AIDS 2004;18:572).
- *AWP*: $650.48/mo (200 mg tab); $798.73/mo (XR tab).
- WARNINGS: (1) Avoid initiation of NVP in women with CD4 count >250/mm^3 and men with a CD4 count >400/mm^3 due to high rates of symptomatic hepatitis; (2) see guidelines for discontinuing NVP.

FOOD: No significant effect.

RENAL FAILURE: Patients on dialysis should receive an additional dose of 200 mg following each dialysis treatment.

HEPATIC FAILURE: Contraindicated in patients with moderate or severe liver disease (Child-Pugh B or C).

DISCONTINUATION OF NVP-BASED ART: The concern is NVP monotherapy if all antiretroviral drugs are stopped simultaneously due to the long half-life of NVP. A pharmacokinetic study found that NVP could be detected in 83% if NVP recipients 1 wk after the drug was stopped and 25% at 2 wks (AIDS 2007;21:733). The recommendation is to continue the NRTI "backbone" or other ARVs for an additional 2–4 weeks (2018 DHHS Guidelines). Another option is to substitute a boosted PI for NVP for 2–4 wks before stopping therapy.

PATIENT ASSISTANCE: 800-556-8317 (7:30 AM–5:30 PM CST, Mon.–Fri.).

ADVANTAGES: Extensive experience; 2NN trial suggests antiviral potency nearly comparable to EFV; no food effect; fewer lipid effects than EFV; relatively inexpensive third agent. A safe and effective agent for perinatal transmission prevention in resource-limited setting. but due to rash and hepatoxicity nevirapine-based regimen is no longer recommended for initial therapy in pregnant ARV-naïve women (2018 DHHS Pregnancy and Perinatal Guidelines). A Cochrane Library review (2010) concluded that EFV and NVP are equally effective (with two NRTIs) for initial treatment (Cochrane Database Syst Rev 2010;8:12:CD004246). A retrospective review of the EuroSIDA database also showed long-term durability of NVP was comparable to that of EFV and LPV/r (HIV Med 2010;12:259).

DISADVANTAGES: High rates of serious hepatotoxicity in treatment-naïve women with baseline CD4 counts $>250/mm^3$, high rates of rash, including toxic epidermal necrolysis (TEN) and Stevens-Johnson syndrome; single-resistance mutations often eliminate all therapeutic value; cross-resistance to ETR more likely after failure of NPV than of EFV; single dose for prevention of perinatal transmission may cause resistance. Efficacy data for EFV are more extensive.

CLINICAL TRIALS: See Table 6.68.

2NN: This is the pivotal study comparing EFV and NVP. When combined with NRTIs, ITT analysis at 48 wks showed similar results for NVP bid and EFV, with VL <50 c/mL in 65% and 70%, respectively. The difference was not statistically significant, but the trial failed to show noninferiority according to the FDA definition. The incidence of clinical hepatitis in NVP qd, NVP bid, EFV, and NVP + EFV was 1.4%, 2.1%, 0.3%, and 1.0%, respectively. There was more hepatotoxicity in NVP recipients (9.6% vs. 3.5%), and two deaths were attributed to NVP toxicity (Lancet 2004;363:1253). NVP given once-daily caused more hepatotoxicity (13.6%) and EFV + NVP was inferior virologically compared to EFV + 2 NRTIs.

NEWART Trial: 152 treatment-naïve patients with baseline CD4 counts <250 cells/mm^3 (females) or <400 cells/mm^3 (males) were randomized to NVP (standard dose) or ATV/r, each with TDF/FTC (JAIDS 2010;13:Suppl 4:P4). At 48 wks, VL was <50 c/mL in 61% (NVP) and 65% (ATV/r).

ARTEN: Treatment-naïve patients with appropriate baseline CD4 counts (<250/mm^3 for women or <400/mm^3 for men) were randomized to NVP + TDF/FTC vs. ATV/r + TDF/FTC (Soriano V., Antivir Ther. 2011;16(3):339–48). NVP recipients were in two dose regimens, 400 mg/d or 200 mg bid. The randomization was 1:1:1, but data for the two NVP arms were combined and showed comparable results at 48 wks, with VL <50 c/mL in 67% vs. 65% of NVP vs. ATV/r recipients, respectively (Table 6.68). The rate of failure with twice-daily dosing was 13%, and for once-daily dosing it was 11%. VL decay and time to treatment response were significantly better for NVP recipients. The mean increase in CD4 counts at 1 yr was 193 cells/mm^3 in both groups. The rate of treatment-related discontinuations, including discontinuation due to adverse events and investigator-defined lack of efficacy, was greater with NVP (13.6% vs. 3.6%). The most common NVP-associated side effect was rash, but there were no grade 4 rashes.

TABLE 6.68 NVP trials in treatment-naïve patients

Trial	Regimen	N	Duration (wks)	VL <50	VL <200–500
Atlantic (AIDS 2000;15:2407)	NVP + ddI + d4T	89	48	54%[a]	58%
	IDV + ddI + d4T	100		55%[a]	57%
	3TC + ddI + d4T	109		46%	59%
COMBINE (Antiviral Ther 2002;7:81)	NVP + AZT/3TC	72	48	65%	75%
	NFV + AZT/3TC	70		50%	60%
2NN (Lancet 2004;363:1253)	NVP 400 mg/d + 3TC + d4T	220	48	70%	—
	NVP 200 mg bid + 3TC + d4T	387		65%[b]	
	EFV + 3TC + d4T	400		70%	
	EFV + NVP + 3TC + d4T	209		63%[b]	
ARTEN (49th ICAAC, 2009;Abstr. H924C)	NVP + TDF/FTC	376	48	67%	—
	ATV/r + TDF/FTC	193		65%	
NEWART (JAIDS 2010; 13[S4]:P4)	NVP + TDF/FTC	75	48	61%	—
	ATV/r + TDF/FTC	77		64%	
VERxVE (Gathe. ICAAC 2010:Abstr. H204)	NVP IR + TDF/FTC	506	48	65%	—
	NVP XR + TDF/FTC	505		80%	

[a] Superior to comparators (P<0.05). The P-value in COMBINE was 0.06.
[b] NVP did not meet the noninferiority criteria.

VERxVE: This trial compared 400 mg extended release NVP formulation given once-daily (Viramune XR) to the previously available 200 mg immediate-release formulation given twice-daily to 1013 treatment-naïve patients. Both groups received once-daily TDF/FTC. Criteria for inclusion were absence of baseline resistance and CD4 count <250/mm^3 (women) and <400/mm^3 (men). The median baseline VL was 4.7 log$_{10}$ c/mL, and the mean CD4 count was 228 (Gath J., 18th IAC, 2010, Vienna, THBB 202; Gath J., 50th ICAAC 2010:Abstr. H1808). The 48-wk results showed viral suppression (<50 c/mL) nonsignificant superior results with the XR formulation: 81% vs. 76%, for all participants and 73% vs. 71% for the subset with a baseline VL >100,000 c/mL. Pharmacology studies showed the trough levels for the XR formulation were lower for once-daily XR vs. twice-daily IR but were >13-fold higher than the IC$_{90}$ for wild type HIV.

SWITCH THERAPY: *Switch from EFV- to NVP-based ART due to intolerance to EFV*: In *ACTG 5095*, switching from EFV to NVP was allowed in patients who could not tolerate EFV. The switch was due to EFV-associated CNS toxicity in 47 patients, rash in 18 and "other" in 5. The median CD4 count at the time of switch was 323 cells/mm^3. Resolution of CNS symptoms was noted in 46 of 47 with CNS toxicity and 6 of 15 with rash. Of 70 who switched, 15 (21%) subsequently discontinued NVP due to adverse reactions, including 10 due to grade 3–4 hepatotoxicity and 41 of 67 (67%) achieved viral suppression at 24 wks (CID 2010;50:787).

Switch from PI- to NVP-based ART: A review of data concluded that "a switch from a PI-based regimen to one containing NVP can be accomplished safely while maintaining virologic suppression . . . with no immunologic cost . . . and an overall benefit in the metabolic milieu" (HIV Med 2006;7:537). The switch is associated with good virologic control and rapid improvement in blood lipid changes and insulin resistance with half the patients experiencing positive changes in lipodystrophy (AIDS 1999;13:805; JAIDS 2001;27:229; AIDS 2000;14:807).

The ATHENA study was a review of 125 patients who switched to NVP-based ART compared with 321 who continued PI-based ART. All participants had achieved VL <500 c/mL on PI-based ART. Treatment failure due to toxicity requiring a regimen change (36%) or virologic failure (6%) was greater in the PI continuation group (JID 2002;185:1261).

NVP vs. EFV switch: Retrospective analysis of 162 patients on PI-based ART who had virologic failure or a request for regimen simplification and were given either EFV- or NVP-based ART. Results showed those switched for simplification maintained virologic control at 48 wks, and the two drugs were comparable. For salvage, virologic control was achieved in 13/58 (22%) of NVP recipients and 19/49 (38%) of EFV recipients (HIV Clin Trials 2003;4:244).

NEFA: A trial in which 460 patients receiving PI-based ART were randomized to switch to ABC, NVP, or EFV plus 2 NRTIs. At 48 wks, virologic failure occurred in 13%, 10%, and 6% for these three groups, respectively ($P = 0.1$). Lipodystrophy did not change in any of the groups (NEJM 2003;349:1036).

High baseline viral load: In an analysis of six reports of 416 NVP recipients, viral suppression to <500 c/mL was observed in 83% and 89% of those with baseline viral loads above and below 100,000 c/mL, respectively (HIV Clin Trials 2001;2:317).

TENOR: Single-arm study of 70 patients receiving initial therapy or switching for intolerance of another regimen. Regimen was once-daily NVP (400 mg) + TDF/FTC. At 72 wks, the regimen was continued in 52 (74%), and, of these patients, VL was <400 c/mL in 84% (Eur J Med Res 2009;14:516).

RESISTANCE: Monotherapy is associated with rapid and high-level resistance with primary RT mutations 103N, 100I, 181C/I, 188C/L/H, and 190A resulting in an increase in the IC_{90} of >100-fold (JAIDS 1995;8:141; JID 2000;181:904). Cross-resistance with EFV is universal. NVP is more likely than EFV to select for ETR-resistant virus because of the possibility of the Y181I/C mutations. NVP resistance is challenging in two distinct clinical settings, both related to the relatively long half-life and the low genetic barrier to resistance mutations. The more extensive studies involve resistance associated with single-dose NVP for preventing perinatal transmission, which is a strategy in developing countries. HIVNET 012 found that this was highly effective in perinatal transmission prevention, but resistance mutations were noted using standard assays in 19% of women. In *PACTG 316*, 14/95 women (15%) who received intrapartum NVP developed

NVP resistance mutations 6 wks postpartum (JID 202;186:181). Subsequent studies using real-time PCR to detect minority species, with a detection limit of 0.2%, found that K103N was present in an additional 40% (JID 2005;192:16). The frequency is clade- specific: clade C, 69%; clade D, 36%; clade A, 19% (JAIDS 2006;42:610). *Resistance mutations are also observed in the infants born to exposed mothers and in strains recovered from breast milk* (JID 2005;192:1260). The clinical implications of these observations are unclear, but in one study, women with perinatal NVP exposure who were subsequently treated with NVP-based regimens had a poorer virologic response compared to women who had not been previously exposed to NVP (NEJM 2004;351:217). A report suggests that the NNRTI mutations were no longer detected even in the minority pool after 6-12 mos (NEJM 2007;356:135).

PHARMACOLOGY:

Bioavailability: 93%; not altered by food, fasting, ddI, or antacids. $T^{1/2}$: 25–30 hrs.

CNS penetration: CSF levels are about 45% of peak serum levels (CSF-to-plasma ratio = 0.45). The CNS penetration effectiveness is the highest—class 4 (Neurology 2011;76:693).

Breast milk: Significant concentrations are transferred into breast milk (AZT and 3TC is also transmitted) (AAC 2009;53:1170).

Metabolism: Metabolized by cytochrome P450 (CYP3A4) to hydroxylated metabolites that are excreted primarily in the urine, which accounts for 80% of the oral dose. NVP autoinduces hepatic CYP3A4, reducing its own plasma half–life over 2-4 wks from 45 hrs to 25 hrs (JID 1995;171:537).

Dose modification with renal or hepatic failure: NVP is extensively metabolized by the liver. NVP is contraindicated in moderate and severe liver disease due to hepatotoxicity. NVP metabolites are largely eliminated by the kidney with <5% unchanged in the urine. No dose adjustment is required for patients with renal impairment. Patients on dialysis should receive an additional dose of 200 mg following each dialysis treatment (NVP package insert, 05/2013).

SIDE EFFECTS:

BLACK BOX WARNING: Severe, life-threatening and in some cases fatal hepatoxicity (see below).

Hepatotoxicity: Early hepatotoxicity usually occurs in the first 6 wks and appears to be a hypersensitivity reaction. It may be accompanied by drug rash, eosinophilia, and systemic symptoms (DRESS syndrome). This reaction differs from "transaminitis" noted with PIs and EFV in that it is more likely to progress to liver necrosis and death even with early detection and occurs primarily with high baseline CD4 counts, especially in women. The rate of symptomatic hepatitis in women with a baseline CD4 count $\geq$250 cells/mm^3 is 11% compared to 0.9% in women with lower CD4 counts at baseline. Men also have an increased risk with a CD4 count $\geq$400 cells/mm^3, but the rates are lower, 6.4% vs. 1.2%. Chronic hepatitis B or C do not appear to be risk factors (JID 2005;191:825). The mechanism of this reaction is not known, but the association with high CD4 counts suggests an immune mechanism and a genetic predisposition (CID 2006;43:783). There have been at least 6 deaths in pregnant women given continuous NVP-based ART (JAIDS 2004;36:772). 2018 DHHS Guidelines recommend that NVP not be given to treatment-naïve women with a baseline CD4 count >250 cells/mm^3, or men with a baseline CD4 count of >400 cells/mm^3. Also, the CDC issued a warning against using NVP for PEP based on reports of two healthcare workers (HCW) with severe hepatitis, including one who required a liver transplant (Lancet 2000;57:687; MMWR 2001;49:1153). This concern does not apply to the single dose of NVP given at delivery to prevent perinatal transmission or to persons who have a high CD4 count on other ART regimens who are switching to NVP-based ART. NVP recipients may also develop hepatotoxicity later in the course of treatment, a form of hepatitis that is more benign and similar to hepatitis seen with other anti-HIV drugs. This hepatitis is characterized by an elevation in transaminase levels, it is usually asymptomatic, the frequency is about 10%, and it is more common in those with chronic HBV or HCV co-infection (CID 2004;39:1083). Management guidelines for the severe early form include frequent monitoring of hepatic function in the first 12–18 wks, warning the patient, and prompt discontinuation of NVP if this diagnosis is considered. Guidelines for the later asymptomatic transaminitis are unclear, but many recommend discontinuation of NVP if the ALT is >5 or 10× the ULN (Hepatology 2002;35:182). It should be noted that frequency of hepatotoxicity is highly variable in different geographic areas, but most large series report rates of grade 3 hepatoxicity or hepatic enzyme elevations >3- to 5-fold above ULN at 4–13% and some find no gender difference or CD4 associated risk (JAIDS 2004;35:495; HIV Med 2010;11:650; JID 2005;191:825; Drug Saf 2007;30:1161; HIV Med 2008;9:221; HIV Med 2010;11:334).

Rash: Rash is seen in about 17%. It is usually maculopapular and erythematous with or without pruritus and is located on the trunk, face, and extremities. Some patients with rashes require hospitalization, and 7% of all patients require discontinuation of the drug, compared with 4.3% given DLV, 1.7% given EFV, and 26% given ETR (package insert, PDR). Frequency of severe (grade 3–4) rash in the 2NN trial was 6% in patients with a CD4 count >200/mm^3 and 1–2% in those with a CD4 count <200/mm^3 (AIDS 2005;19:463). Indications for discontinuation of an NNRTI due to rash are rash accompanied by fever, blisters, mucous membrane involvement, conjunctivitis, edema, arthralgias, or malaise. Steroids are not effective (JAIDS 2003;33:41). Stevens-Johnson syndrome and TEN have been reported, and at least three deaths ascribed to rash have been reported with NVP (Lancet 1998;351:567). There is evidence that this NVP-induced rash results from NVP-stimulated CD4 cells that produce IFN-γ (J Pharmacol Exp Ther 2009;331:836). Patients with rash should always be assessed for hepatotoxicity, as the two may occur together. A review of 122 patients with NVP rashes who were switched to EFV showed EFV-associated rashes in 10 (8%), but the rate of EFV rash was 20% among those whose NVP rashes were "severe" (HIV Med 2006;7:378).

Lipid effects: The D:A:D study indicates that NVP increases HDL cholesterol, reduces the total-to-HDL cholesterol index, and does not increase the risk for cardiovascular events (Drugs 2006;66:1971).

DRUG INTERACTIONS: NVP, like rifampin, induces CYP3A4. Maximum induction takes place 2–4 wks after initiating therapy.

Drugs that are contraindicated or not recommended for concurrent use: Rifampin, ketoconazole, St. John's wort, rifapentine, and atazanavir.

Use with antiretroviral agents: See Table 6.69.

NVP may significantly decrease the serum concentrations of amiodarone, carbamazepine, clonazepam, cyclophosphamide, cyclosporin, diltiazem, disopyramide, ergotamine, ethosuximide, fentanyl, itraconazole, lidocaine, midazolam, nifedipine, posaconazole, sirolimus, tacrolimus, verapamil, and voriconazole. Use with close monitoring—warfarin and other oral anticoagulant (rivaroxaban, betrixaban, ticagrelor, vorapaxar, edoxaban, apixiban, and dabigatran)

Drugs that require dose modification with concurrent use:

Oral contraceptives: NVP decreases AUC for ethinyl estradiol by about 30% (JAIDS 2002;29:471); alternative or additional methods of birth control should be used.

Clarithromycin: NVP reduces clarithromycin AUC by 30% but increases levels of the 14-OH metabolite, which is active against *H. influenzae* and *S. pneumonia*, but consider azithromycin for MAC. NVP levels increased 26%. Use standard doses and monitor or use azithromycin.

Fluconazole increases NVP 2-fold. Monitor for toxicity. *Ketoconazole*: AUC and C_{max} levels of ketoconazole are decreased 72% and 44%, respectively. NVP increases by 15–30%: not recommended. *Voriconazole*: No data, but significant potential for decrease of voriconazole and/or increase of NVP serum level.

Rifabutin: AUC increased 17%; no dose alteration.

Rifampin: NVP AUC and C_{max} decreased more than 50%; there is also concern about additive hepatotoxicity (NVP + rifampin in standard doses has been found to be virologically inferior vs. HIV (JAMA 2008;300:530). If co-administration is needed, initiate w/NVP 400 mg/d, but EFV preferred with rifampin (CROI 2010;abstract 602).

Phenobarbital, phenytoin, carbamazepine: No data; monitor anti-convulsant levels; NVP concentrations may be decreased.

Methadone: NVP reduces AUC of methadone by about 50%; opiate withdrawal is a concern and has been reported; methadone dose increases are variable but average 15–25% (CID 2001;33:1595).

Statins: No data; may decrease lovastatin and simvastatin levels; consider pitavastatin, pravastatin, or rosuvastatin.

Buprenorphine: No significant change; use standard dose.

Silodosin: NVP may decrease silodosin concentrations.

Enzalutamide and mitotane: may decrease NVP concentrations. Avoid

PREGNANCY: NVP is used extensively in resource-limited countries for prevention of perinatal HIV transmission and the data addressing multiple issues are also extensive. The two forms of NVP-based treatment are short-term peripartum prophylaxis that usually consists of a single 200 mg dose of NVP to the mother at the onset of labor and a single 2 mg/kg dose to the infant at 48–72 hrs (JID 1998;178:368). This is well-tolerated by the mother regardless of the baseline CD4 count and reduces perinatal transmission by about 50% (Lancet 1999;354:795). The major concern is the long half-life of NVP with a subsequent HIV resistance rate of 19% in HIVNET 012 (AIDS 2001;15:1951) and 15% in PACTG 316 (JID 2002;186:181). Although delay of ART is not recommended, some studies show that NVP can still be used effectively if ART is delayed 6–12 mos (NEJM 2007;356:135; CID 2008;46:611). NVP resistance can also be reduced or avoided with a NRTI "tail" by d/c NVP first with continuation of NRTIs for 2–4 wks (JID 2006;193:482; PloS Med 2009;6:e1000172).

Long-term antenatal NVP-based ART: NVP pharmacokinetics are not notably altered during pregnancy (HIV Med 2008;94:214). The major concern is the risk of NVP hypersensitivity reactions in women with a baseline CD4 count of >250 cells/mm^3. The reactions include potentially life-threatening hepatotoxicity and life-threatening hypersensitivity skin reactions including Stevens-Johnson syndrome

(JAIDS 2004;35:120; Obstet Gynecol 2003;101:1094). These reactions including fatal cases have been described with and without pregnancy, and it appears that pregnancy does not increase the risk (AIDS 2010;24:109). As a consequence of these observations, the 2018 DHHS Guidelines for Use of Antiretroviral Agents in Pregnancy no longer recommend NVP-based ART (EFV and RPV are alternative NNRTI-based regimens). If NVP is the only NNRTI option available, it should be initiated in pregnant women only if the baseline CD4 count is <250 cells/mm³ The Pregnancy Registry reporting of the first-trimester NVP exposures in the United States indicated 32/1135 (2.82%) birth defects (data to July 31, 2017).

Nortriptyline—see also Tricyclic Antidepressants

TRADE NAMES: Aventyl (Eli Lilly), Pamelor (Mallinckrodt), and generic.

CLASS: Tricyclic antidepressant.

FORMULATIONS, REGIMEN, AND COST: Caps: 10 mg, $0.44; 25 mg, $0.88; 50 mg, $1.29; 75 mg, $2.47. Oral suspension: 10 mg/5 mL, 473 mL, $182.95.

INDICATIONS AND DOSE REGIMENS:

Depression: 25 mg hs initially; increase by 25 mg every 3 days until 75 mg, then wait 5 days and obtain level with expectation of 100–150 ng/dL.

Neuropathic pain: 10–25 mg hs; increase dose over 2–3 wks to maximum of 75 mg hs. Draw serum levels if higher doses used.

PHARMACOLOGY:

Bioavailability: >90%.

$T^{1/2}$: 13–79 hrs, mean 31 hrs.

Elimination: Metabolized and excreted renally.

TABLE 6.69 Dose recommendations for NVP + PI combinations

PI	InSTI/PARVI Level	NVP LeNPVel	RegiDosing Recommendation
IDV	↓28%	No change	IDV/r 800/200 mg q12h + NVP standard
RTV	↓11%	No change	RTV as sole PI is not recommended
SQV/r	↓25%	No change	Recommend SQV/r 1,000/100 mg bid
NFV	↑10%	No change	Standard doses
FPV/r	↓25%	may ↓ or ↑	FPV/r 700/100 mg bid + NVP standard dose (Antimicrob Ag Chemother 2006;50:3157).
LPV/r	LPV ↓55%	No change	LPV/r 400/100 mg bid (treatment-naïve) or 600/150 mg bid (treatment-experienced). Consider LPV/r 500/125 mg bid
ATV ATV/c ATV/r	↓	↑	Do not co-administer boosed or unboosted ATV with NVP as NVP ↓; ATV exposure and potential toxicity with ↑ NVP exposure.
TPV/r	may ↓ or↑	may ↓ or ↑	Standard: TPV/r 500/200 mg bid + NVP 200 mg bid. Limited data.
DRV/r DRV/c	No change	↓27%	DRV/r 600/100 mg bid, standard NVP. Limited observational data. Avoid DRV/c with NVP.
RAL	No data. No change likely	No data. No change likely	No data. Usual dose likely

(continued)

TABLE 6.69 Continued

PI	InSTI/PARVI Level	NVP LeNPVel	RegiDosing Recommendation
EVG/r EVG/ cobi	May ↓	May ↑	Avoid
DTG	May ↓	No data. No change likely	Avoid
BIC	May ↓	No data. No change likely	Avoid

SIDE EFFECTS: Anticholinergic effects (dry mouth, dizziness, blurred vision, constipation, urinary hesitancy), orthostatic hypotension (less than with other tricyclics), sedation, sexual dysfunction (decreased libido), and weight gain.

DRUG INTERACTIONS: The following drugs should not be given concurrently: Adrenergic neuronal blocking agents, clonidine, other α-2 agonists, excessive alcohol, fenfluramine, cimetidine, MAO inhibitors, and any drugs that increase nortriptyline levels (cimetidine, quinidine, fluconazole). All PIs, cobicistat, and DLV may increase nortriptyline levels. Avoid in patients with QTc prolongation.

PREGNANCY: Category D. Animal studies are inconclusive, and experience in pregnant women is inadequate. Avoid during first trimester, but decision should be individualized and when possible limit use in the last two trimesters.

Norvir—see Ritonavir

Nystatin

TRADE NAMES: Mycostatin (Bristol-Myers Squibb) and generic.

CLASS: Polyene macrolide similar to amphotericin B.

FORMULATIONS, REGIMEN, AND COST:

Generic:.
- Lozenges: 500,000 units at $0.68/lozenge.
- Cream: 100,000 U/g, 15 g at $17.50.
- Ointment: 100,000 U/g, 15 g at $17.50.
- Powder: 100,000 U/g, 30 g at $53.82.
- Suspension: 100,000 U/mL, (5ml) at $5.05.
- Oral tabs: 500,000 units at $1.42/tab.

PATIENT ASSISTANCE PROGRAM (Bristol-Myers Squibb): 800-272-4878.

ACTIVITY: Active against *C. albicans* at 3 µg/mL and other *Candida* species at higher concentrations.

INDICATIONS AND DOSES:

Thrush: 5 mL suspension to be gargled 4–5×/d × 14 days. Disadvantages: Nystatin has a bitter taste, causes GI side effects, must be given 4×/d, and does not work as well as clotrimazole troches or oral fluconazole (HIV Clin Trials 2000;1:47). Efficacy is dependent on contact time with mucosa.

PHARMACOLOGY:

Bioavailability: Poorly absorbed and undetectable in blood following oral administration. Therapeutic levels persist in saliva for 2 hr after oral dissolution of two lozenges.

SIDE EFFECTS: Infrequent, dose-related GI intolerance (transient nausea, vomiting, diarrhea).

Oxandrolone

TRADE NAME: Oxandrin (BTG).

CLASS: Anabolic steroid.

FORMULATIONS, REGIMEN, AND COST: Tabs, 2.5 and 10 mg.

> *Cost*: Per tab, $5.52 (2.5 mg), $11.25 (10 mg).
>
> PATIENT ASSISTANCE PROGRAM: 866-692-6374.
>
> INDICATION AND DOSES: Wasting. Prior studies showed a modest weight gain after 16 wks with a dose of 15 mg/d (AIDS 1996;10:1657; AIDS 1996;10:745; Br J Nutr 1996;75:129). Another clinical trial with 262 HIV-infected men with 10–20% weight loss showed increases in body weight. Body cell mass gain was noted with only 40 mg/d, but treatment was associated with significant decreases in total and free testosterone levels, increased LDL cholesterol, and elevated transaminase levels (JAIDS 2006;41:304). Natural testosterone esters are preferred for hypogonadal men (CID 2003;36[suppl 2]:S73). A comparison of nutrition counseling, nutrition counseling + oxandrolone, or nutrition counseling + resistance training showed oxandrolone was the least cost-effective at $55,000/QALY (AIDS Care 2007;19:996).

PHARMACOLOGY:

> Bioavailability is 97%.

SIDE EFFECTS: Virilizing complications primarily in women, including deep voice, hirsutism, acne, clitoral enlargement, and menstrual irregularity. Some virilizing changes may be irreversible, even with prompt discontinuation. Men may experience increased acne and increased frequency of erections. Of particular concern is hepatic toxicity with cholestatic hepatitis; discontinue drug if jaundice occurs or abnormal liver function tests are obtained. Drug-induced jaundice is reversible. Peliosis hepatis (blood-filled cysts) has been reported and may result in life-threatening hepatic failure or intraabdominal hemorrhage. *Miscellaneous side effects*: Nausea, vomiting, changes in skin color, ankle swelling, depression, insomnia, and changes in libido. Other potential side effects are increased LDL cholesterol and exacerbation of lipoatrophy.

DRUG INTERACTIONS: Increases activity of oral anticoagulants and oral hypoglycemic agents.

PREGNANCY: Category X. Teratogenic.

Paromomycin

TRADE NAME: Humatin (Monarch Pharmaceuticals and Caraco) and generic.

CLASS: Aminoglycoside (for oral use).

FORMULATIONS, REGIMEN, AND COST: 250 mg cap at $5.67 ($952/21 day course).

> INDICATIONS AND DOSE: Cryptosporidiosis. 1 g po bid or 500 mg po qid.
>
> EFFICACY: The drug is active in vitro and in animal models against *Cryptosporidia* but only at levels far higher than those achieved in humans. There are anecdotal reports of clinical response, but controlled trials show marginal benefit and no cures (CID 1992;15:726; Am J Med 1996;100:370). An uncontrolled trial found good results with paromomycin 1 g bid + azithromycin 600 mg/d × 4 wks, then paromomycin 1 g bid (alone) × 8 wks (JID 1998;178:900), and there are anecdotal case reports supporting this regimen (Parasitol Res 2006;98:593). At present, there is a consensus that there is no effective chemotherapy for cryptosporidiosis except immune reconstitution with ART. Even modest increases in CD4 counts are effective (NEJM 2002;346:1723).

PHARMACOLOGY: Not absorbed; most of the oral dose is excreted unchanged in stool; lesions of the GI tract may facilitate absorption and serum levels may increase in presence of renal failure.

SIDE EFFECTS: GI intolerance (anorexia, nausea, vomiting, epigastric pain), steatorrhea, and malabsorption rare complications include rash, headache; vertigo with absorption and serum levels. There could be ototoxicity and nephrotoxicity with systemic absorption, as with other aminoglycosides.

PREGNANCY: Category C.

Pegylated Interferon

TRADE NAMES: Peginterferon alfa-2a—Pegasys (Roche); peginterferon alfa-2b—Peg-Intron (Schering-Plough).

FORMULATIONS, REGIMEN, AND COST:

- Peginterferon alfa-2a (Pegasys) is supplied as a solution ready for injection, which requires refrigeration and is available at a fixed dose of 180 µg per 1 mL solution at $1,039.83.
- Peginterferon alfa-2b (Peg-Intron) is supplied as lyophilized powder to be reconstituted with 0.7 mL saline; several strengths are available based on body weight (50 µg at $902.60, 80 µg at $947.64, 120 µg at $995.06, 150 µg at $1,044.84).
- PATIENT ASSISTANCE PROGRAM: 877-734-2797 (Pegasys) and 800-521-7157 (Peg-Intron).
- PRODUCT: Recombinant alfa-interferon conjugated with polyethylene glycol (PEG), which decreases the clearance rate of interferon and results in sustained concentrations permitting less frequent dosing.
- CONTRAINDICATIONS: Autoimmune hepatitis and hepatic failure with Child-Pugh score ≥6 before or during treatment. Contraindications to ribavirin: (1) pregnant female, (2) male patient with pregnant partner, and (3) patient with hemoglobinopathies.

TABLE 6.70 Results of four clinical trials of PegIFN + ribavirin for HCV in patients with HIV co-infection

	No. Pts	Regimen × 48 Wks	Rate of SVR	
			Gen 1	Gen 2/3
ACTG A5071 (NEJM 2004;351:451)	66	Peg-IFN 180 mg/wk Ribavirin 600–1,000 mg/d Duration: 48 wks	14%	73%
APRICOT (NEJM 2004;351:451)	289	Peg-IFN 180 mg/wk Ribavirin 800 mg/d Duration: 48 wks	29%	62%
RIBAVIC (JAMA 2004;292:2839)	205	Peg-IFN 180 mg/wk Ribavirin 800 mg/d Duration: 48 wks	15%	—
PRESCO (AIDS Res Hum Retro 2007;23:972)	389	Peg-IFN 180 mg/wk Ribavirin 1,000/d (<75 kg) or 1200/d (75 kg) Duration by Genotype: 1 & 4–72 wks, 2 & 3–48 wks	36%	72%

INDICATIONS: Although FDA indicated in combination with ribavirin, PEG-interferon–based regimens are NOT recommended for in treatment-naïve patients with HCV genotype 1, 2, 3, 4, 5/6 due to better tolerated and more effective directly acting HCV agents.

New agents for HCV with HCV/HIV:

Dose: Pegylated IFN (alfa 2a 180 mg (Pegasys) or alfa 2b 1.5 mg/kg (Peg-Intron) SC/wk.

Dose with renal impairment:

With CrCL 30–50 mL/min: Peg-IFN-alfa-2b 1 μg/kg SQ once weekly or peg-IFN alfa 2a 180 μg SQ once weekly.

With CrCl <30 mL/min +/- HD: Peg-IFN-alfa-2b 1 µg/kg SQ
   once weekly or peg-IFN alfa 2a 135 µg SQ once weekly.
MONITORING.

Toxicity: CBC and comprehensive metabolic panel at baseline,
   2 wks, then every 6 wks. TSH at baseline and then every
   12 wks.

Patients with cardiac disease: EKG at baseline and as needed.

Women of childbearing potential: Urine pregnancy testing every
   4–6 wks.

PHARMACOLOGY:

The differences between the two commercially available peg-IFN
products are that Peg-Intron (alfa–2b) is a linear chain PEG and
Pegasys (alfa–2a) is a branched chain PEG. This structural difference
results in higher serum level and more prolonged $T^{1/2}$ with Pegasys.
Despite the PK difference, the two products appear to be clinically
equivalent. (NEJM 2009;361:580).

Bioavailability: Increases with duration of therapy. Mean trough
   of peg-IFN alfa 2b with 1 µg/kg SQ at week 4 = 94 pg/mL, at
   week 48 = 320 pg/mL. C_{max} mean is 554 pg/mL at 15–44 hrs
   and sustained up to 48–72 hrs. Compared to non-pegylated
   IFN, peg-IFN C_{max} is about 10× greater and AUC is 50×
   greater.

$T^{1/2}$: Peg-IFN alfa 2a = 77 hr; peg-IFN alfa 2b = 40 hr (compared
   with 8 hr for non-pegylated interferon).

Elimination: Renal 30% (7× lower clearance than non-pegylated
   interferon). Eliminated primarily in the bile.

SIDE EFFECTS: Similar to those of IFN; 15–21% in clinical trials
discontinue therapy due to adverse reactions (NEJM 2004;351:438;
NEJM 2004;351:451).

BLACK BOX WARNINGS: Depression, serious bacterial
infections, autoimmune disorder, ischemic disorders.

TABLE 6.71 Criteria for Peg-IFN dose reduction and/or discontinuation

Laboratory Measurement	Criteria for Dose Reduction to 0.5 µg/mL	Criteria for Discontinuation
ANC[a]	<750/mm^3	<500/mm^3
Platelet count	<50,000/mm^3	<25,000/mm^3

[a] Leukopenia generally responds to G-CSF, which may be preferred to avoid dose reduction.

Neuropsychiatric: Depression, suicidal or homicidal ideation, and relapse of substance abuse. Should be used with extreme caution in patients with history of psychiatric disorders. Warn patient and monitor. Depression reported in 21–29%. Suicides reported. Active depression with suicidal ideation is a contraindication. EFV given concurrently has been found to increase mood disorders but did not increase the risk of depression in one report of 53 patients (JAIDS 2008;49:61).

Marrow suppression: ANC decreases in 70%, <500/mm^3 in 1%, platelet counts decrease in 20%, <20,000/mm^3 in 1%. Avoid or discontinue AZT.

Flu-like symptoms: Most common; about 50% will have fever, headache, chills, and myalgias/arthralgias. May decrease with continued treatment. May be treated with NSAIDs or acetaminophen; with liver disease acetaminophen dose should be <2 g/d.

Thyroid: Thyroiditis with hyperthyroidism or hypothyroidism. TSH levels should be measured at baseline and during therapy every 12 wks.

Retinopathy: Obtain baseline retinal evaluation in patients with diabetes, hypertension, or other ocular abnormality.

Injection site reaction: Inflammation, pruritus, pain (mild) in 47%.

GI complaints: Nausea, anorexia, diarrhea, and/or abdominal pain in 15–30%.

Skin/hair: Alopecia (20%), pruritus (10%), and/or rash (6%).

Miscellaneous: Hyperglycemia, cardiac arrhythmias, elevated hepatic transaminase levels 2–5×, colitis, pancreatitis, autoimmune disorders, hypersensitivity reactions.

DRUG INTERACTIONS: Avoid co-administration of marrow suppressive agents including AZT and ganciclovir. Ribavirin should not be given with ddI. ABC should also be avoided with ribavirin.

PREGNANCY: Category C. IFN is not recommended in pregnancy (2018 DHHS Guidelines in Pregnancy). Abortifacient potential in primates and direct antigrowth/antiproliferative effects. Ribavirin is a potent teratogen (Category X) and must be avoided in pregnancy and used with caution in women of childbearing potential and their male sexual partners. Breastfeeding: No data.

Pentam—see Pentamidine

Pentamidine

TRADE NAME: Pentam for IV use; NebuPent for inhalation; APP Pharmaceuticals LLC (American Pharmaceutical Partners).

CLASS: Aromatic diamidine-derivative antiprotozoal agent that is structurally related to stilbamidine.

FORMULATIONS, REGIMEN, AND COST: 300 mg IV vial at $154.06; 300 mg NebuPent inhalation at $154.06.

PATIENT ASSISTANCE PROGRAM: IV and aerosolized pentamidine 888-391-6300.

INDICATIONS AND DOSES:

P. jiroveci pneumonia (PCP) treatment: 4 mg/kg IV given over ≥1 hr × 21 days. The approved dose is 4 mg/kg, but some clinicians prefer 3 mg/kg in patients with ADR. TMP-SMX is preferred (Ann Intern Med 1986;105:37; AIDS 1992;6:301).

PCP prophylaxis: 300 mg/mo delivered by a Respirgard II nebulizer using 300 mg dose diluted in 6 mL sterile water delivered at 6 L/min from a 50 psi compressed air source until the reservoir is dry. TMP-SMX preferred due to superior efficacy in preventing PCP, efficacy in preventing other infections (e.g., CAP, soft tissue infection), reduced cost, and greater convenience (NEJM 1995;332:693). Aerosolized pentamidine should not be used for PCP treatment (Ann Intern Med 1990;113:203).

MONITORING:

Aerosolized pentamidine: This is considered safe for the patient but poses risk of TB to HCWs and other patients. Patient should be evaluated for TB (PPD, X-ray, and sputum examination if indicated). Suspected or confirmed TB should be treated prior to aerosol treatments. Adequate air exchanges with exhaust to outside and appropriate use of particulate air filters are required. Some suggest pregnant HCWs should avoid environmental exposure to pentamidine until risks to fetus are better defined.

Parenteral administration: Adverse effects are common and may be lethal. Due to the risk of hypotension, the drug should be given in supine position, the patient should be hydrated, pentamidine should be delivered over ≥60 minutes, and BP should be monitored during treatment and afterward until stable. Regular laboratory monitoring (daily or every other day) should include creatinine, potassium, calcium, and glucose; other tests for periodic monitoring include CBC, LFTs, and calcium.

PHARMACOLOGY:

Bioavailability: Not absorbed orally. With aerosol, 5% reaches alveolar spaces via Respirgard II nebulizer. Blood levels with monthly aerosol delivery are below detectable limits.

$T^{1/2}$: Parenteral, 6 hr.

Elimination: Primarily nonrenal but may accumulate in renal failure.

Dose modification of parenteral form with renal failure:
CrCl >50 mL/min: 4 mg/kg q24h;
10–50 mL/min: 4 mg/kg q24h–q36h;
<10 mL/min: 4 mg/kg q48h.

SIDE EFFECTS:

Aerosolized pentamidine: Cough and wheezing in 30% (prevented with pretreatment with β2 agonist), sufficiently severe to require discontinuation of treatment in 5% (NEJM 1990;323:769). Other reactions include laryngitis, chest pain, and dyspnea. The role of aerosolized pentamidine in promoting extrapulmonary *P. jiroveci* infection and pneumothorax is unclear. Risk of transmitting TB to patients and HCWs.

Systemic pentamidine: In a review of 106 courses of IV pentamidine, 76 (72%) had adverse reactions; these were sufficiently severe to require drug discontinuation in 31 (18%) (CID 1997;24:854). The most common causes of drug discontinuation were nephrotoxicity and hypoglycemia. A review of PCP treatment efficacy in 3 cohorts with 1,188 episodes of PCP showed 3-mo survival rates of 85% with TMP/SMX treatment, 87% with clindamycin + TMP/SMX treatment, 87% with clindamycin + primaquine, and 70% for pentamidine (JAC 2009;64:1282). The RR of death with pentamidine after adjusting for confounders was 2.0. A review of 29 clinical studies also concluded that pentamidine was inferior to TMP/SMX and clindamycin/primaquine (JAIDS 2008;48:63). *Nephrotoxicity* is noted in 25–50%. It is usually characterized by a gradual increase in creatinine in the second week of treatment but may cause acute renal failure. Risk is increased with dehydration and concurrent use of nephrotoxic drugs.

Hypotension is unusual (6%), but may cause death, most often with rapid infusions; drug should be infused over ≥60 minutes.

Hypoglycemia, with blood glucose 15–59 mg/dL range in 5–10%, can occur after 5–7 days of treatment, sometimes persisting several days after discontinuation. Hypoglycemia may last days or weeks and is treated with IV glucose ± oral diazoxide. Cases of hypoglycemia resulted in discontinuation of pentamidine in 42% of the cases.

Hyperglycemia (2–9%) and insulin-dependent diabetes mellitus may occur with or without prior hypoglycemia.

Leukopenia and thrombocytopenia are noted in 2–13%.

GI intolerance with nausea, vomiting, abdominal pain, anorexia, and/or bad taste is common.

Local reactions include sterile abscesses at IM injection sites (IM no longer advocated) and pain, erythema, tenderness, and induration (chemical phlebitis) at IV infusion sites. *Other reactions* include pancreatitis hepatitis, hypocalcemia (sometimes severe), increased amylase, hypomagnesemia, fever, rash, urticaria, toxic epidermal necrolysis (TEN), confusion, dizziness (without hypotension), anaphylaxis, arrhythmias, including torsade de pointes.

DRUG INTERACTIONS: Avoid concurrent use of parenteral pentamidine with nephrotoxic drugs, including aminoglycosides, amphotericin B, and foscarnet and cidofovir. Amphotericin B: severe hypocalcemia.

PREGNANCY: Category C. Limited experience with pregnant women.

Pravastatin

TRADE NAME: Pravachol (Bristol-Myers Squibb) and generic.

CLASS: Statin (HMG-CoA reductase inhibitor).

FORMULATIONS, REGIMEN, AND COST: Tabs: 10 mg at $3.21, 20 mg at $3.26, 40 mg at $4.79, and 80 mg at $4.79.

INDICATIONS AND DOSES: Elevated total cholesterol, LDL cholesterol, and/or triglycerides and/or low HDL cholesterol.

This is often a favored statin for dyslipidemia associated with PI-based ART due to paucity of drug interactions with PIs with the exception of DRV/r (CID 2003;37:613; CID 2006;43:645), although it may be less effective than other statins. Dose adjusted rosuvastatin, atorvastatin, or standard-dose pitavastatin should be used if a more potent statin is required. For example, a comparative trial vs. rosuvastatin in HIV-infected patients showed better outcome with rosuvastatin (AIDS 2010;24:77), and a review in two large HIV clinics suggested atorvastatin and rosuvastatin are preferred due to greater declines in LDL cholesterol (CID 2011;52:387; CID 2010;51:718). The initial dose for pravastatin is 40 mg/d. If desired cholesterol levels are not achieved with 40 mg/d, 80 mg/d is recommended. A starting dose of 10 mg daily is recommended in patients with a history of significant hepatic or renal dysfunction. Pravastatin can be administered as a single dose at any time of the day. A report of pravastatin use in HIV-infected patients demonstrated improvements in the atherogenic lipid profile within 12 wks without change in inflammatory markers (J Clin Lipidol 2010;4:279). However, another report found pravastatin and rosuvastatin had a highly significant effect on reduction in CRP levels in HIV-infected patients that was independent of any lipid effect (AIDS 2011;25:1123).

MONITORING: Blood lipids at 4-wk intervals until desired results are achieved, then periodically. It is recommended that transaminases be measured prior to the initiation of therapy, prior to the elevation of the dose, and when otherwise clinically indicated. Patients should be warned to report muscle pain, tenderness, or weakness promptly, especially if accompanied by fever or malaise; obtain CPK for suspected myopathy.

PRECAUTIONS: Pravastatin (and other statins) are contraindicated with pregnancy, breastfeeding, concurrent conditions that predispose to renal failure (sepsis, hypotension, etc.), and active hepatic disease. Alcoholism is a relative contraindication.

TABLE 6.72 Pravastatin-ART drug interactions

Antiretroviral Agent	Effect on Pravastatin	Dose Recommendation for Pravastatin
NNRTIs		
EFV	↓ AUC 40%	May need higher dose
ETR	No change	Standard dose
NVP	No data	Interaction unlikely
Integrase Inhibitors		
RAL, DTG, EVG	No data	RAL AUC increased 13%. No data with DTG and EVG. Interaction unlikely. Use standard dose.
PIs		
DRV/r	↑ AUC 81% (single dose); ↑ 23% (at steady-state)	Start with lowest dose or use alternative statin
ATV, ATV/c, DRV/c IDV, NFV, TPV/r,	No data	Standard with low dose, then titrate
LPV/r	↑ AUC 33%	Standard dose
SQV/r	↓ AUC 50%	Standard dose; may need higher dose

Possible interactions with spironolactone, cimetidine, and ketoconazole that reduce cholesterol levels and may effect adrenal and sex hormone production with concurrent use.

Itraconazole increases pravastatin AUC and C_{max} 1.7× and 2.5×, respectively. Cholestyramine and colestipol decrease pravastatin AUC 40%; administer pravastatin 1 hr before or 4 hr after.

Niacin and gemfibrozil: concurrent use with pravastatin increases the risk of myopathy. Rare cases of rhabdomyolysis with acute renal failure secondary to myoglobinuria have been reported with pravastatin and other drugs in this class.

PHARMACOLOGY:

Bioavailability: 14%.

$T^{1/2}$: 1.3–2.7 hr.

Elimination: Fecal (biliary and unabsorbed drug) 70%; renal 20%.

SIDE EFFECTS:

Musculoskeletal: Myopathy with elevated CPK plus muscle tenderness, weakness, or pain + fever or malaise. Rhabdomyolysis with renal failure has been reported.

Hepatic: Elevated transaminase levels in 1–2%; discontinue if otherwise unexplained elevations of ALT and/or AST are >3× ULN.

Miscellaneous: Diarrhea, constipation, nausea, heartburn, stomach pain, dizziness, headache, skin rash (eczematous plaques), insomnia, and impotence (rare).

PREGNANCY: Category X. Contraindicated.

Prezista—see Darunavir

Primaquine

TRADE NAME: Generic primaquine.

CLASS: Aminoquinoline.

FORMULATIONS, REGIMEN, AND COST: 15 mg base tabs (26.3 mg primaquine phosphate) at $1.79.

INDICATIONS AND DOSES: *P. jiroveci* pneumonia: Primaquine 30 mg (base) qd + clindamycin 600–900 mg q8h IV or 450 mg po q6h.

For mild PCP, some prefer primaquine 15 mg (base) qd (+ clindamycin) to decrease the risk of bone marrow suppression.

Note: The published experience and recommendation is for mild to moderately severe PCP (Ann Intern Med 1996;124:792; CID 1994;18:905; CID 1998;27:524). A meta-analysis of published reports of PCP patients who failed initial treatment found that the clindamycin-primaquine regimen was superior to all others with responses in 42 of 48 (87%) (Arch Intern Med 2001;161:1529). A more recent review 1188 cases of PCP showed the 3-mo survival rate with TMP-SMX treatment was 85%, for clindamycin-primaquine 81%, and pentamidine 76% (*p* = 0.009) (JAC 2009;64:1282). The 2018 Guidelines for Prevention and Treatment of Opportunistic Infections in HIV-Infected Adults and Adolescents (www.mmhiv.com/link/2009-OI-NIH-CDC-IDSA) recommend clindamycin-primaquine as an alternative to TMP/SMX for moderate to severe PCP.

PHARMACOLOGY:

Bioavailability: Well absorbed.

$T^{1/2}$: 4–10 hr.

Elimination: Metabolized by liver to an active metabolite (carboxyprimaquine).

SIDE EFFECTS: *Hemolytic anemia* in patients with G6PD deficiency; its severity depends on drug dose and genetics of G6PD deficiency. In African Americans, the reaction is usually mild and self-limited or asymptomatic; in patients of Mediterranean or certain Asian extractions, hemolysis may be severe. Hemolytic anemia may also occur with other forms of hemoglobinopathy. The 2015.

IDSA/NIH/CDC Guidelines recommend screening G6PD deficiency prior to use of primaquine "whenever possible". Note that the prevalence of G6PD deficiency in >63,000 US troops was 2.5%, and it was particularly high for blacks, Asians, and Hispanics (Mil Med 2005;171:905). Warn patient of dark urine as sign and/or measure G6PD level prior to use in susceptible individuals.

Other hematologic side effects: Methemoglobinemia, leukopenia.

GI: Nausea, vomiting, epigastric pain (reduced by administration with meals).

Miscellaneous: Headache, disturbed visual accommodation, pruritus, hypertension, arrhythmias.

PREGNANCY: Category C. Limited experience in pregnant women. There is a theoretical risk of hemolytic anemia if fetus has G6PD deficiency.

Procrit—see Erythropoietin

Pyrazinamide (PZA)

TRADE NAME: Generic pyrazinamide.

CLASS: Derivative of niacinamide.

FORMULATIONS, REGIMEN, AND COST: 500 mg tab at $2.85 (2 g/d at $11.40/d).

INDICATION AND REGIMEN:

Tuberculosis, initial phase of three- to four-drug regimen, usually for 8 wks (MMWR 1998;47[RR-20]; MMWR 2000;49:185). Treatment of latent TB with PZA + rifampin is no longer recommended due to hepatotoxicity (MMWR 2003;52:735).

Usual dose:

    40–55 kg: PZA 1,000 mg/d.

    56–75 kg: PZA 1500 mg/d.

    76 to >90 kg: PZA 2000 mg/d (max dose).

Treatment with Rifater (tabs with 50 mg INH, 120 mg rifampin, and 300 mg PZA):

    <65 kg: 1 tab/10 kg/d.

    >65 kg: 6 tabs/d.

PHARMACOLOGY:

Bioavailability: Well-absorbed, but absorption is reduced by about 25% in patients with advanced HIV infection (Ann Intern Med 1997;127:289).

$T^{1/2}$: 9–10 hr.

CSF levels: Equal to plasma levels.

Elimination: Hydrolyzed in liver; 4–14% of parent compound and 70% of metabolite excreted in urine.

Renal failure: Usual dose unless creatinine clearance <10 mL/min –50% of dose or 12–20 mg/kg/d (increased risk of hyperuricemia).

Hepatic failure: Contraindicated.

SIDE EFFECTS: PZA appears to be the major cause of hepatotoxicity in patients with hepatitis as a complication of TB treatment (Am J Respir Crit Care Med 2003;167:1472; and 2008;177:1391). Hepatotoxicity occurs in up to 15% who receive >3 g/d. The risk is increased with HCV co-infection (Chest 2007;131:803), transient hepatitis with increase in transaminases, jaundice, and a syndrome of fever, anorexia, and hepatomegaly; rarely, acute yellow atrophy. Monitor LFTs monthly if there are abnormal baseline levels, symptoms suggesting hepatitis or elevated levels during therapy that are not high enough to stop treatment (ALT <5× ULN). Hyperuricemia is common, but gout is rare. Nongouty polyarthralgia in up to 40%; hyperuricemia usually responds to uricosuric agents. Use with caution in patients with history of gout. *Rare*: Rash, fever, acne, dysuria, skin discoloration, urticaria, pruritus, GI intolerance, thrombocytopenia, sideroblastic anemia.

PREGNANCY: Category C. Not teratogenic in mice, but limited experience in humans. Risk of teratogenicity is unknown. Currently recommended for treatment of active TB in the United States and by WHO guidelines.

Pyrimethamine

TRADE NAME: Daraprim (Amedra Pharmaceuticals).

CLASS: Aminopyrimidine-derivative antimalarial agent that is structurally related to trimethoprim.

FORMULATIONS, REGIMEN, AND COST: 25 mg tab at $21.15 (~$1,903/mo). *Note*: If pyrimethamine is not covered by insurance due to cost, SMX/TMP is the preferred treatment regimen for toxoplasmosis encephalitis.

Pharmacy wholesalers may not have pyrimethamine. To obtain pyrimethamine for patients: Compounding Pharmacies (e.g., Avella Specialty Pharmacy) can compound patient-specific supply for a fraction of the cost ($1/tab). Walgreens Specialty Pharmacy is the contracted Daraprim supplier: 844-463-2727 ($21.15/tab).

PATIENT ASSISTANCE PROGRAM: daraprimdirect@icsconnect.com.

INDICATIONS AND DOSE REGIMENS: Toxoplasmosis.

Primary prophylaxis: Pyrimethamine 50 mg po/wk + dapsone 50 mg po qd + leucovorin 25 mg/wk or pyrimethamine 75 mg/wk + dapsone 200 mg/wk and leucovorin 25 mg/wk or atovaquone 1500 mg/d ± pyrimethamine 25 mg/d + leucovorin 10 mg/d.

Treatment: Pyrimethamine 200 mg x1, then 50 mg (<60 kg) or 75 mg (>60 kg) po qd + sulfadiazine 1 gm (<60 kg) or 1.5 gm (>60 kg) po qid (plus leucovorin 10-25 mg po qd) x a minimum of 6 weeks, then maintenance with pyrimethamine 25-50 mg/d plus sulfadiazine 2-4 gm/d plus leucovorin 10-25mg/d.

PHARMACOLOGY:

Bioavailability: Well-absorbed.

$T^{1/2}$: 54–148 hr (average 111 hr).

Elimination: Parent compound and metabolites excreted in urine.

Dose modification in renal failure: None.

TABLE 6.73 Toxoplasmosis treatment

Acute (≥ 6 wks)	*Maintenance*
Preferred	*Preferred*
Pyrimethamine 200 mg po × 1, then 50 mg (<60 kg) to 75 mg (>60 kg) po/d + leucovorin 10–25 mg/d + sulfadiazine 1 g (<60 kg) to 1.5 g (>60 kg) po q6h If pyrimethamine not available: TMP-SMX (5 mg TMP/kg) IV or po bid	Pyrimethamine 25–50 mg/d po + leucovorin 10–25 mg/d po + sulfadiazine 2–4 g/d po
Alternatives Pyrimethamine + leucovorin (as above) + 1. Clindamycin 600 mg IV q6h po or IV 2. Atovaquone 1500 mg po bid 3. Azithromycin 900–1200 mg/d	*Alternatives* Pyrimethamine + leucovorin (as above) + 1. Clindamycin 600 mg po q8h 2. Atovaquone 750–1500 mg po12h
Alternative without pyrimethamine 1. Atovaquone 1500 mg po bid + sulfadiazine 1.0–1.5 g po q6h 2. TMP-SMX (5 mg TMP/kg) IV or po bid 3. Atovaquone 1500 mg po bid	*Alternative without pyrimethamine* 1. Atovaquone 750–1500 mg po12h 2. Continue 3. Continue

From 2018 CDC/NIH/IDSA Guidelines for Opportunistic Infections.

SIDE EFFECTS: Reversible marrow suppression due to depletion of folic acid stores with dose-related megaloblastic anemia, leukopenia, thrombocytopenia, and agranulocytosis; prevented or treated with folinic acid (leucovorin).

GI intolerance: Improved by reducing dose or giving drug with meals.

Neurologic: Dose-related ataxia, tremors, or seizures.

Hypersensitivity: Most common with pyrimethamine plus sulfadoxine (Fansidar) and due to sulfonamide component of combination.

Drug interactions: Lorazepam: hepatotoxicity. *AZT, ganciclovir, interferon*: additive bone marrow suppression.

PREGNANCY: Category C. Teratogenic in animals, but limited experience has not shown association with birth defects in humans.

Raltegravir (RAL)

TRADE NAME: Isentress (Merck & Co., Inc).

CLASS: Integrase strand transfer inhibitor (InSTI).

FORMULATIONS, REGIMEN, AND COST: 400 mg tabs and 600 mg HD tabs at $1,667.52/mo; chewable tablets: 25 mg at $1.50/tab and 100 mg at $6.02/tab; orals suspension single-use packet of 100 mg.

PRODUCT INFORMATION: 800-850-3430.

STANDARD REGIMEN: 400 mg po bid OR 1,200 mg (2 HD tabs) po QD with or without food.

Note: RAL HD once-daily only FDA indicated for treatment-naïve patients or virologically suppressed patients on initial RAL bid regimen.

RAL HD once-daily not recommended with ETR, TPV/r, Al, Mg, Ca antacid co-administration.

Renal failure: GFR 50-80 mL/min, standard; GFR <50 mL/min, standard dose likely but no data.

Hepatic failure: Standard dose for mild to moderate hepatic failure; Severe liver disease; standard dose likely, but no data.

STORAGE: Room temperature.

INDICATIONS:

Treatment of HIV infection in combination with other ARV agents in treatment-naïve and ART-experienced patients with evidence of HIV replication despite ongoing ART. Treatment of HIV infection in combination with other ARV agents in ART-naïve patients.

One of the preferred first-line ARV regimen (RAL + TDF/FTC or TAF/FTC) in treatment-naïve patients (2018 DHHS Guidelines).

ADVANTAGES:

Potent antiretroviral agent; transmitted resistance is uncommon; relatively low pill burden (2/d) without food requirements; frequency of adverse reactions is low, there is no significant effect on insulin resistance or blood lipids and no dose-related toxicity has been detected. Clinically important drug interactions are infrequent since RAL does not use, inhibit, or induce the P450 metabolic pathway. More rapid viral load reduction than with PI- and NNRTI-based regimens (not clinically significant).

DISADVANTAGES:

Cross resistance with elvitegravir. Sequential use of EVG and RAL is not recommended. Lower genetic barrier to resistance compared to PI/r.

RESISTANCE: Raltegravir (RAL), elvitegravir (EVG), and dolutegravir (DTG) have lower genetic barriers to resistance compared to PIs and a high level of cross-resistance (JID 2011:203:1204). There are also variations in resistance mutations that are subtype-specific (J Med Virol 2011;83:751). Resistance and failure with RAL in subtype B-infected patients is associated with primary mutations at Q148 or N155. Mutations here confer significant reduction in activity, but the reduction increases when combined with at least one additional mutation, which can emerge rapidly:

155H + (74M/R, 92Q, 97A, 138A/K, 140A/S, 151I, 163R, 183P, 226D/F/H, 230R).

148K/R/H + (140S/A, 138K).

143C/H/R.

Note: In a *BENCHMRK analysis* of 94 failures, 64 (68%) had in vitro resistance (NEJM 2008;359:355). Of these, 48 (75%) had ≥2 or more mutations. The *three most common pathways* in 121 RAL failures were 148 K/R/H (48%), 155 H (31%), and H3 C/R (21%) (JID 2011;203:1204). Strains of HIV resistant to RAL are usually sensitive to dolutegravir and resistant to elvitegravir. Allele-specific sequencing prior to treatment with RAL in BENCHMRK participants found that those who subsequently had virologic failure were twice as likely to have a baseline primary or secondary integrase resistance mutation; secondary mutations were most common (AAC 2011;55:114).

CLINICAL TRIALS:

TREATMENT-NAÏVE: *STARTMRK*: 563 treatment-naïve patients were randomized to RAL + TDF/FTC or EFV/TDF/FTC. Baseline data and 48- and 96-wk results are summarized in Table 6.74 (Lancet 2009;374:796; JAIDS 2010;55:39). The study found (1) rates of viral suppression with VL <50 c/mL were nearly identical (79% vs. 81%), (2) the mean CD4 count increase was significantly greater in the RAL recipients, (3) adverse reactions were significantly more common in EFV recipients, and (4) EFV recipients has significantly higher levels of LDL-cholesterol. Week 96 data from STARTMRK showed viral suppression (<50 c/mL) in 81% and 79% of RAL-recipients and EFV-recipients, respectively. Median CD4 changes were +240 cells/mm^3 (RAL) and 225 cells/mm^3 (EFV). Increases in total cholesterol, LDL cholesterol, and HDL cholesterol were greater in EFV recipients, and side effects were greater in the EFV recipients (78% vs.47%), but the rate of serious side effects was similar (12% and 14%) (JAIDS 2010;55:39). The 156-wk follow-up presented at the 2011 CROI are summarized in Table 6.74. RAL virologic outcome was noninferior (*p* <0.001) (Rockstroh JK, Clin Infect Dis. 2011;53:807).

Protocol 004: This was a phase II multicenter, double-blind, randomized controlled trial with RAL (doses of 100, 200, 400, and 600 mg po bid) vs. EFV 600 mg/d in 198 treatment-naïve patients. Each group received the study drug in combination with TDF/FTC.

TABLE 6.74 STARTMRK: RAL + TDF/FTC vs. EFV/TDF/FTC in treatment-naïve patients: 48-wk

	RAL + TDF/FTC n = 281	EFV/TDF/ FTC n = 282
Baseline		
Mean VL (c/mL)	103,205	106,215
Mean CD4 count (cells/mm^3)	219	217
Results (48 wks)		
VL <50 c/mL	81%[b]	79%
CD4 count increase (cells/mm^3)	189	163
ADRs	16%	32%[a]
• Grade 3 or 4	+ 9	+ 21
• LDL-C mean change (mg/dL)	−4	+ 40
• Triglyceride mean change (mg/dL)	29%	61%
• CNS toxicity	3	11
• Cancer		
Results (96 wks)		
VL <50 c/mL	81%	79%
CD4 count increase (median) (cells/mm^3)	240	225
ADRs requiring discontinuation	4%	6%
Results (156 wks)		
VL <50 c/mL	75%	68%
CD4 count increase (median) (cells/mm^3)	332	295
ADRs requiring discontinuation	5%	7%

From (Lancet 2009;374:796), 96-wk (JAIDS 2010;55:39), and 156-wk results (CID 2011;53:807.

[a] P = <0.05.
[b] Resistance tests showed RAL resistance mutations in 3 of 6 patients tested.

At 48 wks, the pooled outcome data for the 4 RAL dose regimens for 160 patients given RAL were similar to the 38 given EFV-based ART (63% vs. 38%) (JAIDS 2007;6:125; Gotuzzo. 2010CROI;Abstr. 514).

SHIELD: Randomized pilot trial of 35 treatment-naïve patients treated with RAL + ABC/3TC. At 48 wks, 32/35 (91%) had VL <50 c/mL and 35/35 (100%) had VL <400 c/mL, the median CD4 increase was 247/mm^3, and lipid changes were modest (HIV Clin Trials 2010;11:260.

PROGRESS: Treatment-naïve patients randomized to LPV/r + RAL vs. LPV/r + TDF/FTC.

QDMRK: The goal was to determine if RAL could be given once-daily. The study with 770 treatment-naïve patients randomized to RAL 800 mg/d vs. 400 mg bid, each with TDF/FTC (Eron JJ.

Lancet Infect Dis. 2011:907). At 48 wks, the outcome was worse in the once-daily arm compared to the twice-daily arm, with viral suppression to <50 c/mL in 83% vs. 89%, virologic failure in 14% vs. 9%, integrase resistance mutations in 9 vs. 2, and FTC RAMs in 11 vs. 4. The study was stopped prematurely. The differences between arms was most pronounced in those with baseline VL >100,000 c/mL and those with low RAL levels.

TREATMENT-EXPERIENCED: *BENCHMRK*: Trial of safety and efficacy of RAL in 509 treatment experienced subjects with randomized, double-blind, placebo-controlled study design. Entry criteria were age >16 yrs and resistance to ≥1 drug in each class: NRTI, NNRTI, and PI. Participants were randomized 2:1 (RAL:Placebo); each group received optimized background therapy (OBT) or RAL + OBT (see Tables 6.75 and 6.76). The 96-wk data from BENCHMRK-1 and -2 showed sustained viral suppression (<50 c/mL) in 57% of RAL recipients and 26% of placebo recipients. There were no new RAL-related safety concerns (CID 2010;50:605). HIV isolates from 112 RAL failures showed integrase resistance mutations in 73 (65%).

SWITCHMRK: This was a phase III trial designed to determine the safety and efficacy of switching patients with stable viral suppression on LPV/r-based ART to either RAL plus continued NRTIs or to continue the LPV/r-based regimen (Lancet 2010;375:396).

TABLE 6.75 BENCHMRK-1 & -2: 48- and 96-wk results

	RAL + OBT	Placebo + OBT
	n = 462	n = 237
Baseline		
CD4 count (median) (cells/mm^3)	151	158
VL (log$_{10}$ c/mL) (median)	4.6	4.6
Years of prior ART (median)	10	10
No. prior ART (median)	12	12
Results: 48 wks		
VL <50 c/mL[a]	63%	33%
Baseline VL >100,000 c/mL	48%	16%
CD4 count increase (median) (cells/mm^3)	81	11
ADRs requiring discontinuation	2%	3%
Results: 96 wks		
VL <50 c/mL[a]	57%	26%
CD4 count increase (median) (cells/mm^3)	123	49

From NEJM 2008;359:339.

[a] See Table 6.76 for results for VL <50 c/mL by phenotypic and genotypic resistance score of OBT.

TABLE 6.76 BENCHMRK-1 & -2: Correlation of outcome with baseline resistance tests

Genotype Score	OBT	RAL + OBT	Phenotype Score[a]	OBT	RAL + OBT
0	3%	45%	0	2%	51%
1	37%	67%	1	13%	61%
≥2	62%	77%	2	48%	71%

From NEJM 2008;359:355.

[a] Based on the lower/higher cutoff.

Analysis at 24 wks showed persistent viral suppression in 319/352 (91%) on LPV/r vs. 293/347 (84%) on RAL (p <0.05). A post-hoc analysis found that most of the failures in the RAL group had a history of prior virologic failure indicating the importance of combining RAL with two other active drugs (Lancet 2010;375:352).

ACTG 5262: The single-arm trial with DRV/r + RAL showed a virologic failure rate of 27% at 48 wks and was stopped prematurely.

SPIRAL: Open-label trial in which 273 patients with viral suppression (VL <50 c/mL × 6 mos with PI/r-based regimen) were randomized to continue the current regimen or switch to RAL (plus NRTIs). At 48 wks, 89.2% of patients on RAL and 86.6% of those on a PI/r remained free of treatment failure (p = NS and 96.9%) and 95.1% remained free of virologic failure, respectively (p = NS) (AIDS 2010;24:1697). Switching to RAL was associated with improvement in lipid profile.

EASIER-ANRS-138: Multidrug-resistant patients receiving ENF-based ART were randomized to continue the current regimen vs. switch to RAL-based ART (HIV Clin Trials 2010;11:283). Virologic responses were comparable at 48 wks, with significant improvement in quality of life.

TRIO-ANRS-139: This is a noncomparative trial with 100 patients with multidrug-resistant HIV (>3 primary PI mutations, >3 NRTI mutations, <3 DRV mutations, and <3 NNRTI mutations). Baseline VL was 4.2 $\log_{10}$ c/mL and median CD4 count was 258 cells/mm^3. At week 96, there were 5 virologic failures (>50 c/mL), all with low-level viremia.

RAL intensification: 30 patients with VL <50 c/mL for >1 yr on ART were randomized to RAL intensification (400 mg bid) vs. placebo. At 4 and 24 wks, RAL intensification had no significant impact on (1) VL using a single copy assay, (2) measures of T-cell activation, (3) CD4 count, or (4) gut-associated lymphoid tissue (GALT) (Hiroyu-Hatano et al., 2010 CROI;Abstr. 101LB.

NRTI-SPARING: *SPARTAN ATV + RAL*: Pilot study of a NRTI-sparing regimen in treatment-naïve patients using ATV 300 mg + RAL 400 mg bid vs. ATV/r + TDF/FTC once daily. By 24 wks, there were 6 virologic failures in the ATV + RAL arm, including 5 with RAL resistance and 13 (21%) with grade 4 hyperbilirubinemia. Jaundice was also common in this group. The pilot trial was stopped at 24 wks based on these findings (Kozal M., 2010 IAS, Vienna:Abstr. THLBB204).

PROGRESS RAL + LPV/r: LPV/r + RAL vs. LPV/r + TDF/FTC in treatment-naïve patients (Reynes et al.,18th IAS 2010, Vienna; Abstr. MOABO101). At 48 wks, patients in the NRTI sparing arm had virolologic response rates (83% vs. 85% <50 c/mL by TLOVR analysis). Two in each group discontinued due to adverse events, and CD4 count increases were similar. Concerns with this study are low baseline VL (mean VL 18,000 c/mL) and small samples size (NN = 206).

A5262 RAL + DRV/r: The trial was a single arm single-arm open-label study with 112 treatment-naïve patients given DRV/r (800/100 mg/d) + RAL (400 mg bid). At wk 48 there were 28 virologic failures including 11 who rebounded. Of the 28 failures, 13 (46%) had VL 50–200 c/mL. Higher failure rates correlated with low baseline CD4 count and VL >100,000 c/mL. Resistance testing showed 5 five with RAL resistance mutations and no PI resistance mutations (Taiwo B., AIDS. 2011;25:2113.551).

PHARMACOLOGY:

Absorption: Absolute bioavailability not established; median trough 72 ng/mL (range 29–118).

Food Effect: Delays T_{max}, may be taken with or without food.

$T^{1/2}$: 9 hrs; intracellular $T^{1/2}$: 29 hrs.

Elimination: RAL is not a substrate P450 enzyme, and it does not inhibit or induce CYP3A4. RAL is eliminated by hepatic glucuronidation; the glucuronidated metabolite is largely eliminated in stool (51%) and urine (32%) (Drug Metab Dispos 2007;35:1657). Moderate liver impairment and severe renal disease do not alter pharmacokinetics; severe liver disease has not been studied.

CNS Penetration: 7.3%; CSF levels exceed IC_{50} for wild-type HIV by a median of 4.5-fold. The CNS penetration score is 3 in a four-class system (Neurology 2011;76:693).

SIDE EFFECTS: Few dose related side effects. Doses up to 1,600 mg/d were generally well-tolerated (Clin Pharmacol Ther 2008;83:293). There were no adverse events that were significantly more frequent in the RAL recipients than in placebo recipients in BENCHMRK-1 and -2 (NEJM 2008;359:339). The frequency of hepatotoxicity in STARTMRK and BENCHMRK with 743 RAL recipients showed grade 3/4 liver enzyme elevations were infrequent except with HBV and/or HCV coinfection with rates of 2.6–4.0% (Rockstroh. 2010 CROI;Abstr. Q125). The frequency of malignancies in BENCHMRK-1 and -2 was 16/461 (3.5%) in RAL recipients at 48 wks compared to 4/178 (2.6%) in placebo recipients for an OR = 1.5. The difference did not persist with longer follow-up, but post FDA-approval surveillance for malignancies is being carried out. Data from >6000 patients with >3900 patient-years of RAL exposure showed no association (Ann Pharm 2010;44:42). Phase II trials found that 6% of RAL recipients had grade 3–4 elevations of CPK and there have been case reports of rhabdomyolysis (JAIDS 2007;46:125; Ann Pharm 2010;44:42; AIDS 2008;22:1382). The lipid changes at 48 wks in STARTMRK showed significantly greater mean increases in EFV recipients for total cholesterol (+33 vs. +10 mg/dL) and triglyceride levels (+37 vs. –3 mg/dL). Body composition changes were similar (JAIDS 2010;55:39). A case of reversible cerebellar ataxia has been reported (AIDS 2010;24:2757). Hypersensitivity reactions including DRESS syndrome (drug rash with eosinophilia and systemic symptoms).

DRUG INTERACTIONS: RAL is not a substrate, inducer, or inhibitor of the CYP3A4 metabolic pathway. It is consequently not expected to alter pharmacokinetics of PIs, NNRTIs, methadone, statins, azoles, tacrolimus, oral contraceptive, or erectile dysfunction agents. Nevertheless, some possibly important interactions are noted regarding RAL pharmacology. Rifampin decreases RAL levels; avoid or use RAL 800 mg bid (AAC 2009;53:2852). Doubling the RAL dose may not compensate for the low trough levels (JAC 2010;65:2485), although a limited clinical experience suggests the double-dose RAL performs well (JAC 2011;66:951). Rifabutin

TABLE 6.77 RAL drug interactions

Agent	Effect on RAL	Recommendation
Rifampin	RAL AUC ↓40%	RAL 800 mg bid w/co-administration. Limited clinical data.
Rifabutin	RAL AUC ↓19%	Standard dose rifabutin; RAL 400 mg bid
Phenobarbital	May decrease RAL	Avoid; use valproic acid or levetiracetam
Phenytoin	May decrease RAL	Avoid; use valproic acid or levetiracetam
Omeprazole	RAL AUC ↑3×	Standard doses
TDF	RAL AUC ↑49%	Standard doses
TAF	Interaction unlikely	Use standard doses
TPV/r	RAL AUC ↓24% RAL Cmin ↓55%	Case report of hepatic necrosis reported with co-administration; use with caution
EFV	RAL AUC ↓36%	Standard dose RAL; Cmin RAL not affected
ATV/r	RAL AUC ↑40–70%	Standard doses
RTV	RAL unchanged	Standard doses
ETR	RAL unchanged	Standard doses
RPV	Interaction unlikely	Use standard doses
LPV/r	RAL Cmin ↓30%	Standard doses
MVC	RAL AUC ↓40%	Standard doses
DRV/r	DRV Cmin ↓36%	Clinical significance unknown. Standard doses
FPV	RAL AUC ↓37% APV AUC ↓36%	Avoid
FPV/r	RAL AUC ↓55%	Clinical significance unknown. Standard doses

has no clinically significant effect on RAL levels (J Clin Pharmacol 2011;51:943). Omeprazole significantly increases RAL levels presumably due to increased solubility at high pH levels (Drug Metab Dispos 2007;35:1657). With regard to antiretroviral agents, the drugs that decrease RAL levels the most are TPV/r, MVC, and EFV (Ann Pharm 2010;44:42; AAC 2008;52:4338), but the changes are not sufficient to alter dosing. Anecdotal cases of substantial reductions in RAL AUC with concurrent ETR are reported including virologic failure in four cases (AIDS 2009;27:869), but a formal pharmacokinetic study did not support this finding with RAL bid. RAL HD once-daily is not recommended with ETR.

Oral contraceptive: No significant interaction.
Methadone: No significant interaction.

PREGNANCY: Category C. No treatment related effects were observed on embryonic or fetal survival in rodents. There are no studies in pregnant woman to document pharmacokinetics or safety. The 2010 DHHS Guidelines on Antiretroviral Drugs in Pregnant HIV-infected women list RAL as "insufficient data to recommend use.".

Rebetol—see Ribavirin

Retrovir—see Zidovudine (AZT, ZDV)

Ribavirin

TRADE NAME: Rebetol and Rebetron (combined Rebetrol/Intron A) (Schering-Plough); Copegus (Roche), Virazole (Valeant) inhalation.

FORMULATIONS, REGIMEN, AND COST: 200 mg caps at $10.60 (Rebetrol) per cap; 200 mg tab (Copegus) at $23.37 per tab; $13,023.26/6 g vial (Virazole); oral solution 40 mg/mL (100 mL) at $232.80.

Note: Concurrent use with ddI is contraindicated due to increased risk of pancreatitis and/or lactic acidosis. Use with caution when given with AZT (additive anemia) or d4T (potentiation of mitochondrial toxicity). Avoid ABC (potential antagonism).

INDICATION (FDA labeling): Ribavirin in combination with interferon is FDA indicated for treatment of chronic HCV in patients with compensated liver disease who have not previously been treated. However, due to the availability of better tolerated and more effective HCV agents, PEG-IFN plus ribavirin is no longer recommended as initial therapy for HCV.

Ribavirin is recommended as an alternative in combination with paritaprevir/RTV/ombitasvir/dasabuvir for Genotype 1a, treatment-naïve patients without cirrhosis.

In combination with elbasvir/grazoprevir, the addition of ribavirin can be considered as an alternative treatment for the treatment of Genotype 1a in patients with NS5A RASs and compensated cirrhosis.

CONTRAINDICATIONS: Pregnancy in a female patient, pregnancy in the female partner of a male patient, hemoglobinopathies.

Regimen: Dosage range 1,000–1,200 mg/d resulted in improved sustained virologic response (SVR). Recommended weight-based dose.

Standard: <75 kg, 400 mg in AM, 600 mg in PM; >75 kg, 600 mg bid.

CrCl 30–50 mL/min: RBV 200 mg and 400 mg alternating.

CrCL <30 mL/min: RBV 200 mg/d (limited data; monitor for toxicity).

CLINICAL TRIALS: Ribavirin has been used to treat HCV for more than 20 yrs. It appears to be synergistic with interferon-alfa. The mechanism of action is not well established. Several older trials have tested the relative efficacy of HCV treatment using ribavirin + interferon (IFN) vs. IFN alone and show a substantial advantage to including ribavirin. With HIV-HCV co-infection, sustained viral suppression is achieved in only 15–25% with genotype 1 and 70–80% with genotypes 2 and 3 (NEJM 2004;351:451; NEJM 2004;351:438; JAMA 2004;292:2909) before direct-acting HCV treatment became available. Compared to HCV mono-infected patients, these rates of SVR are much lower for genotype 1 and comparable for genotypes 2 and 3 (Lancet 2001;358:958; NEJM 2002;347:975). SVR are much higher (>95%) even with HIV-coinfection with currently approved direct acting HCV antiviral.

PHARMACOLOGY:

> *Oral bioavailability*: 64%; absorption increased with high-fat meal.
>
> *T½*: 30 hr.
>
> *Elimination*: Metabolized by phosphorylation and deribosylation; there are few or no cytochrome P450 enzyme-based drug interactions. Metabolites are excreted in the urine. The drug should not be used with severe renal failure.

SIDE EFFECTS: About 15–20% of patients receiving ribavirin + IFN discontinue therapy due to side effects. The main side effects are anemia, cough, and dyspepsia. Hemolytic anemia is noted in the first 1–2 wks of treatment and usually stabilizes by week 4. In clinical trials without HIV co-infection when combined with IFN, the mean decrease in hemoglobin was 3 g/dL, and 10% of patients had a hemoglobin <10 g/dL. Patients with a hemoglobin <10 g/dL or decrease in hemoglobin ≥2 g/dL and a history of cardiovascular disease should receive a modified regimen of ribavirin 600 mg/d. When combined with dasabuvir, ombitasvir, paritaprevir, and ritonavir, mean Hbg decrease was 2.4 g/dL with <1% of patients with Hbg <8.0 g/dL during treatment. The drugs should be discontinued if the hemoglobulin decreases to ≤8.5 g/dL or if the hemoglobin persists at <12 g/dL in patients with a cardiovascular disease. Erythropoietin (40,000 units SQ every week) is usually effective (Am J Gastro 2001;96:2802). Concurrent use of AZT should be avoided whenever possible. Ribavirin is a nucleoside that may cause mitochondrial toxicity, especially when combined with other NRTIs that cause mitochondrial toxicity, especially ddI and d4T; 2 of 15 patients given this combination developed lactic acidosis (Lancet 2001;357:280). Other side effects ascribed to ribavirin include leukopenia, hyperbilirubinemia, increased uric acid, and dyspnea.

BLACK BOX WARNINGS: Birth defects, fetal death, hemolytic anemia.

DRUG INTERACTIONS: Increased risk of anemia with AZT co-administration; monitor closely (AAC 1997;41:1231; AIDS 1998;14:1661). In combination with ddI, there is potentiation of ddI toxicity due to inhibition of mitochondrial DNA polymerase-γ, resulting in pancreatitis and lactic acidosis (AAC 1987;31:1613; Lancet 2001;72:177). This combination should be avoided. ABC may decrease the efficacy of ribavirin (avoid co-administration).

PREGNANCY: Category X. Potent teratogen. Must be used with caution in women with childbearing potential and in their male sexual partners. Adequate birth control is mandatory.

Rifabutin

TRADE NAME: Mycobutin (Pfizer) and generic.

CLASS: Semisynthetic derivative of rifampin B that is derived from *Streptomyces mediterranei*.

FORMULATIONS, REGIMEN, AND COST: 150 mg cap at $17.49.

INDICATIONS AND DOSES:

M. avium complex (MAC) prophylaxis: 300 mg po qd. Efficacy established (NEJM 1993;329:828); azithromycin or clarithromycin is preferred.

MAC treatment: Rifabutin as the third drug is combined with clarithromycin (or azithromycin) and EMB using 300 mg/d in severe MAC disease in patients with CD4 <50/mm^3. *Note*: dose adjustment needed in patients treated with PIs, COBI, and some NNRTIs co-administration (see below).

Tuberculosis: Preferred over rifampin for use in combination with most PIs or NNRTIs (MMWR 2004;53:37). Usual dose for TB treatment and prophylaxis: 300 mg/d, but dose must be adjusted for concurrent use with PIs. A meta-analysis of cohort studies and meta-analysis to evaluate rifamycin use in combination with antiretroviral agents suggested excessive rates of relapse with 2 mos of rifamycin compared to 8 mos of treatment (OR 3.6; 95% CI, 1.1–11.7) (CID 2010;50:1288).

ACTIVITY: Active against most strains of MAC and rifampin-sensitive *M. tuberculosis*; cross-resistance between rifampin and rifabutin is common with *M. tuberculosis* and MAC.

PATIENT ASSISTANCE PROGRAM: www.PfizerRxPathways. com.

PHARMACOLOGY:

Bioavailability: 12–20%.

$T^{1/2}$: 30–60 hr.

Metabolism: Metabolized via CYP3A4 to 25-0-deacetyl-rifabutin (10% of total antimicrobial activity).

Elimination: Primarily renal and biliary excretion of metabolites.

Dose modification in renal failure: None.

SIDE EFFECTS: *Common*: Brown-orange discoloration of secretions; urine (30%), tears, saliva, sweat, stool, and skin (warn the patient). *Infrequent*: Rash (4%), GI intolerance (3%), neutropenia (2%). *Rare*: Flu-like illness, hepatitis, hemolysis, headache, thrombocytopenia, myositis. Uveitis, which presents as red and painful eye, blurred vision, photophobia, or floaters, is dose-related, usually with doses >450 mg/d, or with standard dose (300 mg/d) plus concurrent use of drugs that increase rifabutin levels including most PIs, clarithromycin, and azoles including fluconazole (NEJM 1994;330:868). These patients should be evaluated by an ophthalmologist and are usually treated with topical corticosteroids and mydriatics.

TABLE 6.78 Rifabutin interactions and dose adjustments with ARVs

ARV	ARV Dose	Rifabutin Dose[aa]
EFV	Standard	450–600 mg/d or 600 mg 2–3×/wk[c]
NVP	Standard	300 mg/d or 3 ×/wk
ETR	Standard	300 mg/d[a]
RPV	50 mg/d	300 mg/d
PI/r (all)	Standard	150 mg/d or 300 mg 3 ×/wk[c]
DRV/r	Standard	150 mg/d or 300 mg 3 ×/wk
FPV/r[b]	Standard	150 mg/d or 300 mg 3 ×/wk
ATV/r	Standard	150 mg/d or 300 mg 3 ×/wk
NFV	Standard	150 mg/d or 300 mg 3 ×/wk
IDV	1,000 mg q8h	150 mg/d or 300 mg 3 ×/wk
MCV	300 mg bid	300 mg/d
RAL	Standard	300 mg/d
DTG	Standard	300 mg/d
EVG/c	Avoid	Avoid
TAF	Avoid	Avoid
BIC/TAF/FTC	Avoid	Avoid
DTG/RPV	Increase RPV to 50 mg/d	Usual dose

From (2018 NIH/CDC/IDSA Recommendations for Opportunistic Infections and DHHS Guidelines for Use of Antiretroviral Agents in Adults and Adolescents and CDC recommendations [last reviewed January, 2018]).

[a] Dose assumes no concurrent PI/r. If combined with ETR and rifabutin, SQV/r or DRV/r not recommended due to potential additive decrease in ETR concentrations.
[b] Avoid unboosted FPV.
[c] Note dose higher than FDA recommendation due to lower concentrations observed in HIV-infected patients.

DRUG INTERACTIONS: Rifabutin induces hepatic microsomal enzymes (cytochrome P450 3A4), although the effect is less pronounced than for rifampin. Dose adjustment for antiretroviral agents when rifabutin is given are summarized in Table 6.78. With EFV, the AUC of rifabutin decreases by a mean of 37%, requiring an increase in rifabutin dose to 450 mg/d (CID 2005;41:1343). Rifabutin reduces the levels of warfarin, barbiturates, benzodiazepines, some β-blockers, chloramphenicol, clofibrate, oral contraceptives, corticosteroids, cyclosporine, some benzodiazepines (midazolam, triazolam, diazepam), dapsone, digitalis, doxycycline, haloperidol, oral hypoglycemics, voriconazole, posaconazole, ketoconazole, phenytoin, quinidine, theophylline, trimethoprim, and verapamil.

Drugs that inhibit cytochrome P450 and prolong the half-life of rifabutin: PIs, erythromycin, clarithromycin (56% increase), and azoles (fluconazole, itraconazole, posaconazole, and ketoconazole). With concurrent rifabutin and fluconazole, the levels of rifabutin are significantly increased, leading to possible rifabutin toxicity (uveitis, nausea, neutropenia) or increased efficacy (CID 1996;23;685).

COMMENTS:

Rifampin and rifabutin are related drugs, but in vitro activity and clinical trials show that rifabutin is preferred for MAC, and rifampin is preferred for *M. tuberculosis*.

Drug interactions are similar for rifabutin and rifampin, although rifabutin is a less potent inducing agent of hepatic microsomal enzymes.

Uveitis requires immediate discontinuation of drug and ophthalmology consult.

All PIs, COBI, and NNRTIs (except for NVP and RPV) require a dose adjustment when given with rifabutin.

PREGNANCY: Category B. Not teratogenic in rats or rabbits. No pharmacologic data or clinical experience in human pregnancy, but no specific concerns in pregnancy. The OI guidelines recommends rifabutin in pregnancy for the treatment of active TB and prophylaxis of MAC (2018 OI Guidelines).

Rifamate—see Isoniazid, or Rifampin

Rifampin

TRADE NAME: Rifadin (Aventis) and generic. Combination with INH: Rifamate. Combination with INH and PZA: Rifater (Aventis).

FORMULATIONS, REGIMEN, AND COST: Caps: 150 mg at $3.24, 300 mg at $2.07. Rifamate: Caps with 150 mg INH + 300 mg rifampin at $6.37 (generic). Rifater: Tabs with 50 mg INH + 120 mg rifampin + 300 mg pyrazinamide at $4.71. IV vials: 600 mg at $135.

INDICATIONS AND DOSE: Tuberculosis (with INH, PZA, and SM or EMB).

Dose: 10 mg/kg/d (600 mg/d max).

DOT: 600 mg 2× to 3×/wk. (HIV-infected patients with CD4 counts <100/mm^3 should receive DOT 3×/wk. The rationale is the observation of acquired rifamycin-resistance in trials of HIV–TB co-infected patients with CD4 counts <100/mm^3 treated with rifapentine once weekly or rifabutin twice weekly, each in combination with INH (Lancet 1999;343:1843; MMWR 2002;51:214).

Prophylaxis (alone or in combination with PZA or EMB): 10 mg/kg/d (600 mg/d max).

Antiretrovirals and TB treatment: Rifamycins should be included in any regimen for active TB. Options with ART include:

Rifampin (standard dose) + EFV: Consider increasing EFV dose to 800 mg/d for patient >60 kg; however, EFV 600 mg/d was effective in clinical trials.

Rifabutin substitution with ETR, RPV, IDV, FPV, NFV, LPV/r, SQV, ATV, DRV/r, and RTV-boosted regimen in which the RTV dose is ≤200 mg bid.

Do not delay antiretroviral therapy in patients with CD4 <50 cells/mm^3. ART must be started within 2 wks of starting TB therapy.

ACTIVE AGAINST: *M. tuberculosis, M. kansasii,* methicillin-sensitive *S. aureus* (use in combination with fluoroquinolones), *H. influenzae, S. pneumoniae, Legionella,* and many anaerobes.

PHARMACOLOGY:

Bioavailability: 90–95%, less with food. Absorption is reduced by 30% in patients with advanced HIV infection; significance is unknown (Ann Intern Med 1997;127:289).

$T^{1/2}$: 1.5–5.0 hr; average 2 hr.

Elimination: Excreted in urine (33%) and metabolized.

Dose modification in renal failure: None.

SIDE EFFECTS:

Common: Orange-brown discoloration of urine, stool, tears (contact lens), sweat, skin (warn patient).

Infrequent: GI intolerance; hepatitis (in 2.7% given INH + RIF), usually cholestatic changes in first month of treatment; jaundice (usually reversible with dose reduction or continued use); hypersensitivity, especially pruritus ± rash (6%); flu-like illness in 0.4–0.7% given rifampin 2×/wk with intermittent use (dyspnea, wheezing, purpura, leukopenia).

Rare: Thrombocytopenia, leukopenia, hemolytic anemia, increased uric acid, and BUN. Frequency of side effects that require discontinuation of drug is 3%.

DRUG INTERACTIONS: Extensive, due to induction of hepatic cytochrome P450 (3A4, 2B6, 2C8, 2C9) enzymes (www.mmhiv.com/link/CDC-NCHHSTP). Rifampin should be avoided with all PIs, NNRTIs (except EFV), EVG/c, BIC, TAF, and COBI. EFV has no significant effect on rifampin levels, but rifampin reduces EFV levels by 20–26%; some recommend EFV 800 mg/d for person >60 kg, but 600 mg/d is effective in clinical trials. Limited experience suggests that NVP may not be appropriate due to increased rates of HIV virologic failure. The 2018 CDC/IDSA/NIH OI Guidelines recommend EFV-based ART when rifampin is used (www.mmhiv.com/link/2009-OI-NIH-CDC- IDSA). The CDC previously recommended dosing NVP at 300 mg bid, but this has subsequently been found to be virologically inferior (JAMA

2008;300:530), and the dose of 300 mg bid is associated with a higher rate of adverse reactions (Antiviral Ther 2008;13:529). With ETR, there is marked decrease in ETR levels; avoid this combination. The MVC AUC decreases 64%; use MVC 600 mg bid (limited clinical data). Rifabutin is preferred. RAL level decreased 40–60%; avoid this combination. If co-administration is needed, increase RAL to 800 mg bid in patients with no RAL-associated mutations (limited clinical data). Consider rifabutin with RAL co-administration (no interaction). DTG concentrations decreased. Increase dose to 50 mg bid (use only in patients without INSTI-associated resistance mutations).

The following drugs inhibit cytochrome P450 enzymes and prolong the half-life of rifampin: Clarithromycin, erythromycin, and azoles (fluconazole, itraconazole, and ketoconazole). Rifampin decreases levels of atovaquone, barbiturates, oral contraceptives, corticosteroids, cyclosporine, dapsone, fluconazole, ketoconazole, methadone, phenytoin, theophylline, trimethoprim, sirolimus, tacrolimus, and many other drugs that are 3A4 substrates. Rifampin should not be used concurrently with atovaquone, clarithromycin, posaconazole, or voriconazole. With fluconazole and itraconazole, it may be necessary to increase the azole dose. The level of dapsone is decreased 7- to 10-fold; consider alternative.

PREGNANCY: Category C. Dose-dependent congenital malformations in animals. Isolated cases of fetal abnormalities noted in patients, but frequency is unknown. Large retrospective studies have shown no risk of congenital abnormalities; case reports of neural tube defects and limb reduction (CID 1995:21[suppl 1]:S24). May cause postnatal hemorrhage in mother and infant if given in last few weeks of pregnancy; give prophylactic vitamin K, 10 mg single dose to the infant.

Rifater—see Isoniazid or Rifampin, or Pyrazinamide
See Ann Intern Med 1995;122:951.

Rilpivirine (RPV)

TRADE NAME: Edurant (Janssen Therapeutics).

CLASS: NNRTI.

FORMULATIONS, REGIMEN, AND COST:

> *Forms:* RPV 25 mg tablet. Price: $ 1,160.10/mo;
> RPV/TDF/FTC 25/300/200 mg tab (Complera) at $3,216.92/mo (1 mo).
>> RPV/TAF/FTC 25/25/200 mg tab (Odefsey) $ 3,009.29/mo.
>> DTG/RPV 50/25 mg tablet (Juluca) at $3,094.80/mo.
> USUAL ADULT DOSE:
>> RPV 25 mg (one tablet) taken once-daily with a meal;
>> RPV/TDF/FTC 1 tab qd with a meal;
>> RPV/TAF/FTC 1 tab qd with a meal;
>> DTG/RPV 50/25mg tab qd with meal. *Note:* FDA indicated for virologically suppressed patients with no known DTG or RPV resistant mutations.
> *Concurrent ART agents:* Standard RPV dose recommended with PI/r, PI/c, MVC, EVG/c, DTG, RAL, and NRTI. Co-administration with ddI is complicated by the need to take ddI on an empty stomach and RPV must be taken with food.
> *Hepatic disease:* No dose adjustment needed for mild to moderate (Child-Pugh A and B) hepatic impairment.
> *Renal insufficiency:* Use standard dose with close monitoring in patient with ESRD. RPV is unlikely to be removed during hemodialysis and peritoneal dialysis.
> *EFV:* RPV should not be given concurrently with EFV; the long EFV T½ and induction properties complicates the EFV→RPV switch. In patients who are virologically suppressed, switching from EFV to RPV is safe (Mills. ICAAC 2011;Abstr. H2-974c).
> ADVANTAGES: Single-tablet co-formulation with DTG, TAF/FTC and TDF/FTC. Well-tolerated; once-daily administration; relatively few drug interactions; minimal effect on

blood lipids; may be used as an alternative NNRTI in pregnancy; low pill burden; active against strains with the K103N mutation.

DISADVANTAGES: Low genetic barrier to resistance; a major resistance mutation (E138K) also confers resistance to ETR; increased rates of failure with baseline VL >100,000 c/mL and CD4 <200 cells/mm^3 compared to EFV; meal requirement; reduction in bioavailability without gastric acid; contraindicated with PPIs; and dose separation is required with H2 blockers and antacids.

CLINICAL TRIALS: The registration trials *ECHO* and *THRIVE* compared RPV to EFV in 1,368 treatment-naïve patients randomized to receive RPV 25 mg or EFV 600 mg/d in combination with TDF/FTC (ECHO) or with investigator's choice of TDF/FTC, AZT/3TC, or ABC/3TC (THRIVE). Criteria for inclusion was a baseline VL ≥5,000 c/mL, susceptibility to NRTIs, and absence of specific NNRTI mutations. The pooled results at 48 and 96 wks are summarized in Table 6.79 and 6.80.

The rate of virologic failure was nearly the same with VL <100,000 c/mL, but there were significantly more failures with a baseline VL>100,000 c/mL.

Caution or use of an alternative agent is recommended with a baseline VL >100,000 c/mL.

RPV was better tolerated, with lower frequency of neurologic psychiatric and rash reactions.

As expected virologic failure was associated with NNRTI and NRTI RAMs. For RPV, the dominant RAM was 138K compared to K103N with EFV. This difference will influence NNRTI resistance sequences, especially with ETR, which is active against 103N but has reduced activity with 138K (see below).

RESISTANCE: High level resistance: 101P and 181LV mutations associated with RPV virologic failure K101E/P, E138K/G. V179l/

TABLE 6.79 Pooled data for ECHO and THRIVE at 48 and 96 wks (package insert)

Variable	RPV n = 686	EFV n = 682
Baseline data		
Age median (yrs)	36	36
Male	76%	76%
Viral load ($\log_{10}$ c/mL) VL >100,000 c/mL	5.0 46%	5.0 52%
CD4 count (median, cells/mm^3)	249	260
NRTI: TDF/FTC	80%	80%
Results		
VL <50 c/mL	83%	80%
Virologic failure	13%	9%
Failure by baseline VL		
<100,000 c/mL	5%	5%
100,000–500,000 c/mL	20%	11%
>500,000 c/mL	29%	17%
CD4 count (mean, cells/mm^3)	+ 192	+ 176
Discontinuation due to adverse events	2%	7%
ADR (Grade 2-4)		
Neurological (H/A, dizziness) Psychiatric (Depression, insomnia,	4%	10%
abnormal dreams)	8%	10%
Rash	3%	11%

From Drugs Today 2011;47:5.

L, Y181C, V189l, H221Y, F227C/L, and M230L. The most common mutation associated with failure is E138K, which increases resistance by 2.8-fold without M184I and 6.7-fold with M184I. With RPV resistance, there is cross-resistance to ETR in 89% and cross-resistance to NVP in 63%.

TABLE 6.80 Resistance-associated mutations (RAMs) in patients with virologic failure: pooled 96-wk results for ECHO and THRIVE Trials

	RPV	EFV
Number Tested	86	42
Number NNRTI RAMs	46 (53%)	20 (48%) K103N 14
Predominant RAM	E138K 31 (36%)	(33%)
Number NNRTI RAMs	48 (56%)	11 (26%) M184V 6
Predominant RAM	M184I 32 (37%)[a]	(14%)

From Cohen CJ, IAS 2011, Rome;Abstr. TULBPE032.

[a] The M184I substitution was more frequent than M184V due to a replication advantage when combined with M138K (Hu. 2011 CROI:Abstr. 594). The M184I substitution confers resistance to 3TC and FTC and, combined with E138K, increases resistance to RPV compared to E138K alone.

PHARMACOLOGY:

Food (normal or high fat meal) improves RPV absorption. Fasted condition or high-protein drink decreases RPV absorption by 40–50%.

Protein binding: High; 99.7%.

Excretion: RPV undergoes oxidative metabolism via CYP3A4. Parent drug and metabolite are primarily excreted in feces (85%) and urine (6.1%).

$T^{1/2}$: 50 hrs.

SIDE EFFECTS:

Depressive disorders including depressed mood, major depression and suicidal ideation. During phase III trials, the rate of depression, regardless of causality, was 8%; most were mild or moderate in severity. The rate of grade 3 or 4 depression was 1%.

Fat redistribution including increased visceral fat with central obesity, dorsocervical fat enlargement, breast enlargement, and peripheral fat wasting has been observed. The mechanism and causal role of RPV is unclear.

Dose dependent QTc prolongation: (QTc increased 4.8, 10.7, 23.3 msec with 25 mg, 75 mg, 300 mg dose, respectively.

Lipids: There is virtually no impact on serum lipids.

ECHO and THRIVE trials: Pooled at 96 wks (Cohen CJ, et al., IAS 2011;Abstr. TULBPE032). RPV was better tolerated than EFV. The relative frequencies of grades 2–4 toxicities for RPV and EFV, each with TDF/FTC, are summarized in Table 6.81.

TABLE 6.81 Side effects[a] noted in ECHO and THRIVE for RPV and EFV

Results Based on wk 48 Results (Complera Package Insert)	RPV n = 550	EFV n = 546
Symptomatic		
Nausea	1%	2%
Headache	2%	2%
Dizziness	1%	7%
Insomnia	2%	2%
Abnormal dreams	1%	3%
Depressive disorders	1%	2%
Rash	1%	5%
Laboratory changes		
Creatinine elevation >1.3 ULN	<1%	1%
AST elevation >2.5 × ULN	5–6%	10%
LDL-C >160 mg/dL	6%	13%
Total cholesterol >240 mg/dL	4–5%	17%
Triglyceride >500 mg/dL	1–2%	2%

[a] Grade 2–4 toxicity (DAIDS toxicity range).

DRUG INTERACTIONS:
RPV should not be co-administered with several anticonvulsants (phenytoin, phenobarbital, oxcarbazepine), proton pump inhibitors (omeprazole, pantoprazole, rabeprazole, lansoprazole, esomeprazole), more than a single dose of systemic dexamethasone (at steady-state), St. John's wort, enzalutamide, mitotane, rifampin, or rifapentine.

Avoid co-administration with any other NNRTI (e.g., EFV, ETR, NVP).

TDF AUC increased 23%; RPV concentrations not affected.

ddI: No significant interaction if ddI taken 2 hrs before RPV; RPV concentrations not affected.

DRV/r and LPV/r increase RPV AUC 130% and 52%, respectively; use standard dose. Use with caution in patients with QTc prolongation. SQV/r may increase RPV concentrations. Avoid in patients with QTc >450 msec.

Rifampin, rifabutin, and rifapentine decrease RPV AUC by 80% and 46%, respectively. Avoid rifampin and rifapentine. Increase RPV dose to 50 mg/d with rifabutin co-administration. Other CYP 3A4 inducers may also significantly decrease RPV serum concentrations.

Omeprazole decreases RPV AUC 40%. *Proton pump inhibitors* (PPIs) may also significantly decrease RPV absorption and are contraindicated. If acid suppression is needed, H2 blockers can be considered; these must be given 12 hrs before or 4 hrs after RPV. Antacid should also be administered >2 hrs before or 4 hrs after RPV.

Ketoconazole increases RPV AUC 49%; ketoconazole AUC decreased by 24%.

Other azole antifungals (e.g., fluconazole, itraconazole, posaconazole, voriconazole) may also increase RPV concentrations. Monitor for QTc prolongation and antifungal efficacy.

Macrolide antibiotics (e.g., clarithromycin, troleandomycin, erythromycin) may increase RPV concentrations. Monitor for QTc prolongation. Consider azithromycin with co-administration.

Avoid RPV co-administration with drugs that can significantly prolong QTc (e.g., tricyclic antidepressants, haloperidol, terfenadine, astemizole, sotalol, procainamide, amiodarone, pimozide, disopyramide and high-dose methadone).

Methadone: No change in rilpivirine concentrations; (active R-isomer) AUC decreased by 16%; use standard dose and monitor for withdrawal symptoms. Dose adjustment may be needed in some patients.

Ethinyl estradiol AUC increased 14%; and norethindrone decreased 11%. Clinical significance unknown. No change in RPV.

Sildenafil: No significant interaction.

Atorvastatin hydroxy metabolites increased by 23–39%. Clinical significance unknown. Use standard-dose atorvastatin.

PREGNANCY: Category B. No human data. Not teratogenic and no embryonic toxicity observed in animal studies. RPV recommended as an alternative NNRTI in pregnancy (2018 Pregnancy and Perinatal Guidelines)

Ritonavir (RTV)

TRADE NAME: Norvir (Abbott Laboratories).

CLASS: Protease inhibitor.

FORMULATIONS, REGIMEN, AND COST: 100 mg soft-gel capsules and tablets at $10.28; 100 mg/d booster at $308.60/mo Liquid formulation 80 mg/mL at $1,728/240 mL.

STORAGE: Caps can be left at room temperature (up to 25°C or 77°F) for up to 30 days. Oral solution should not be refrigerated; store tablet at room temperature.

PATIENT ASSISTANCE PROGRAM: 800-659-9050 (8 AM–5 PM CST, Mon.– Fri.).

Dose: Almost always used to boost other PIs. When dose is ≤400 mg/d it is subtherapeutic and should not be considered an antiretroviral agent, hence the designation "/r." The dose is 600 mg bid when used as a single PI, but this is poorly tolerated, not recommended, and never used. Administration with food improves tolerability but is not required for absorption.

Recommended regimens for PI-boosting: See Table 6.82.

TABLE 6.82 RTV boosting of PIs and EVG

PI/r	Dose PI/r		AUC PI. (-Fold Increase)[a]
	Treatment-Naïve	Treatment-Experienced	
ATV/r	300/100 mg/d	300/100 mg/d	2.4
DRV/r	800/100 mg/d	600/100 mg bid or 800/100 mg/d if no DRV mutations	14
FPV/r	1400/100–200 mg/d. 700/100 mg bid	700/100 mg bid	4
IDV/r	800/100 mg bid		2–5
LPV/r	400/100 mg bid. 800/200 mg/d	400/100 mg bid.	15–20
SQV/r	1,000/100 mg bid	1,000/100 mg/d	20
TPV/r		500/200 mg bid	11
EVG	EVG/r 85 mg/d + ATV/r 300/100 mg/d. EVG/r 85 mg/d + LPV 400/100 mg bid. EVG/r 150 mg/d + DRV/r 600/100 mg bid. EVG/r 150 mg/d + FPV/r 700/100 mg bid. EVG 150 mg/d + TPV/r 500/200 mg bid		

[a] Based on data from Ogden RC and Flexner CW, eds, Protease Inhibitors in AIDS Therapy at 166–171, 173 (New York: M Dekker, 2001) and 2018 DHHS Guidelines.

PHARMACOLOGY:

Bioavailability: Not well-determined. Levels increased from about 4% to ≥15% when taken with meals. CNS penetration: No detectable levels in CSF.

$T^{1/2}$: 3–5 hr.

Elimination: Metabolized by cytochrome P450 CYP3A4 >2D6. RTV is a potent inhibitor of cytochrome P450 CYP3A4>2D6, and an inducer of CYP3A4 and CYP1A2 at steady state.

Dose modification in renal or hepatic failure: Use standard doses for renal failure. With hemodialysis, a small amount is dialyzed: dose post-hemodialysis (Nephron 2001;87:186). There are no data for peritoneal dialysis, but it is probably not removed and should be dosed post-dialysis. Consider empiric dose reduction in severe hepatic disease.

SIDE EFFECTS: The most frequently reported adverse events with full-dose therapy are GI intolerance (nausea, diarrhea, vomiting, anorexia, abdominal pain, taste perversion), circumoral and peripheral paresthesias, and asthenia. GI intolerance is dose-related and may be severe (JAIDS 2000;23:236) and can improve with continued administration for ≥1 mo. Hepatotoxicity with elevated transaminase levels is dose-related and there appears to be a modestly increased risk with hepatitis B or C co-infection (JAMA 2000;238:74; JAIDS 2000;23:236; CID 2000;31:1234). Laboratory changes include elevated triglycerides, cholesterol, transaminases, CPK, and uric acid, as well as a prolonged QTc and PR interval w/RTV 400 mg bid.

Class adverse reactions: Insulin-resistant hyperglycemia, fat accumulation, elevated triglycerides and cholesterol, and possible increased bleeding with hemophilia. Hypercholesterolemia and triglyceridemia may be more frequent and severe with full-dose RTV compared with other PIs (JAIDS 2000;23:236; JAIDS 2000;23:261). Much of the effect on lipids is attributed to the higher levels of the concurrent PI caused by RTV, rather than by RTV per se; the effect may be due to both.

DRUG INTERACTIONS: RTV is a potent inhibitor of cytochrome P450 enzymes, including CYP3A4 and 2D6, and can produce large increases in the plasma concentrations of drugs that are metabolized by those mechanisms. The extensive drug interactions summarized below is largely based on data generated for FDA approval when the standard dose is 600 mg bid (CID 1996;23:685). Current doses of 100–400 mg/d also result in significant drug–drug interactions that require avoidance or change of the co-administered medication.

Use with the following agents should be avoided: Alfuzosin, amiodarone, astemizole, bepridil, eplerenone, lurasidone, ivabradine, flibanserin, dofetilide, ranolazine, dexameth-asone (at steady-state), cisapride, flecainide, lovastatin, midazolam, ergot alkaloids, pimozide, propafenone, quin-idine, dronedarone, simvastatin, terfenadine, trazodone, triazolam, St. John's wort, rifapentine, voriconazole (with ≥400 mg/d RTV), high-dose sildenafil, fentanyl, lurasidone, ranolazine, rivaroxaban, betrixaban, ticagrelor, vorapaxar, silodosin, enzalutamide, mitotane.

Dose adjustment needed with edoxaban, apixiban, and dabigatran based on renal function and indication.

Should not be used in patients with prolonged QTc at baseline and with drugs that can prolong QTc (salmeterol, type I and II antiarrhythmics, erythromycin).

Fluticasone: RTV increased fluticasone AUC 350-fold, resulting in an 86% decrease in plasma cortisol AUC. Cushing syndrome and adrenal suppression reported. *FDA warning*: Avoid use concurrently only if benefit outweighs risk (consider alterna-tive such as beclomethasone).

Drugs that require dose modification: Clarithromycin AUC increased 77% (CID 1996;23:685); reduce clarithromycin dose for renal failure. *Methadone* levels are decreased by 36% with high dose RTV; monitor for withdrawal. *Desipramine* levels are increased by 145%; decrease desipramine dose. *ddI*, buffered form, reduces absorption of RTV and should be taken ≥2 hrs apart or use ddI EC. *Ketoconazole* levels are increased 3-fold; do not exceed 200 mg ketoconazole/d.

Itraconazole: No data, but concern with itraconazole doses >400 mg/d; monitor itraconazole levels.

Rifampin reduces RTV levels 35%; limited data on combination use and concern for hepatotoxicity. Avoid.

Rifabutin levels increased 4-fold; rifabutin dose of 150 mg q24h. Consider rifabutin TDM with standard RTV dose for all PI/r regimens.

Ethinyl estradiol levels decreased by 40%; use alternative or additional method of birth control.

Theophylline levels decreased by 47%; monitor theophylline levels.

Phenobarbital, phenytoin, and carbamazepine: Interaction anticipated; carbamazepine toxicity reported. May decrease RTV levels; avoid. Monitor anticonvulsant levels.

Sildenafil: AUC increased 11-fold; do not use >25 mg/48 hrs;

Vardenafil levels increased 49×; do not exceed 2.5 mg q72h.

Tadalafil increased 129%; do not exceed 10 mg/72 hr.

Trazodone: RTV increase trazodone AUC 2.4-fold causing nausea, dizziness, hypotension, and syncope; avoid.

MDMA: A potentially fatal reaction has been reported with MDMA (Ecstasy) (Arch Intern Med 1999;159:2221).

Voriconazole: AUC decreased 82% with RTV 400 mg bid; RTV AUC unchanged. Avoid combination with RTV ≥400 mg bid. Low-dose RTV (100 mg bid) decreases voriconazole AUC by 39%. Use with close monitoring and consider voriconazole TDM; alternative antifungal preferred.

Atorvastatin levels increased 450% with RTV; use lowest atorvastatin dose or use pravastatin, pitavastatin, or rosuvastatin.

Pravastatin levels decreased 50% with concomitant RTV; may need increased pravastatin dose based on lipid response.

Lovastatin and simvastatin are contraindicated. Calcium channel and β-blockers concentration may increase. Use with close monitoring.

Colchicine: RTV can significantly increases colchicine level. Use only after RTV has reached steady-state (10–14 days). Administer a lower colchicine dose (0.6 mg, then 0.3 mg 1 hr later).

PREGNANCY: Category B. Negative rodent teratogenic assays; placental passage studies in rodents show newborn: maternal drug ratio of 1.15 at midterm and 0.15–0.64 at late term. LPV/r is the preferred PI-based regimen. Data from the Pregnancy Registry indicate birth defects in 63/2720 (2.3%) first-trimester exposures. This is below the expected rate (accessed July 31, 2015).

Saquinavir (SQV)

TRADE NAME: Invirase (hard-gel capsule) (Genetech/Roche). The Fortovase formulation was discontinued in February 2006.

CLASS: Protease inhibitor.

FORMULATIONS, REGIMEN, AND COST:.

Forms: Invirase: 200 mg hard gel caps and 500 mg film-coated tabs.
Regimens: Give only with RTV, SQV/r 1,000/100 mg bid.
AWP: $1,260.01/mo (price does not include RTV boosting).
FOOD: Take within 2 hr of a meal.
RENAL FAILURE: Standard regimen.
HEPATIC FAILURE: With mild hepatic disease, use standard regimen. No data for moderately severe or severe liver disease; use with caution.
STORAGE: Room temperature, 15–30°C.
PATIENT ASSISTANCE PROGRAM: 866-422-2377.
Note: Most studies were performed with the Fortovase formulation, which is no longer available.

CLINICAL STUDIES: *Invirase vs. Fortovase formulations of SQV:* The first PI approved by the FDA was Invirase, the hard-gel formulation of SQV. Later, Fortovase soft-gel formulation was introduced (but no longer available), which showed equivalence to IDV/r in treatment-naïve patients in MaxCMin-1 (JID 2003;188:635). MaxCMin-2 compared SQV/r (Fortovase) 1,000/100 mg bid to LPV/r in a mixed population of treatment-experienced and -naïve patients (Antiviral Ther 2005;10:735; HIV Med 2007;8:529). At 48 wks, there was no significant difference in virologic outcome and a better lipid profile in SQV recipients. However, a significantly greater number in the SQV/r group discontinued treatment due to GI intolerance.

A comparison of the Invirase and Fortovase formulations indicated that Invirase was better tolerated and, with RTV boosting, had a better pharmacokinetic profile (HIV Med 2003;4:94). Fortovase was discontinued and a new 500-mg hard-gel cap of Invirase became available to reduce the pill burden.

GEMINI: This was a 48-wk phase III trial in 337 treatment-naïve patients with CD4 counts <350/mm^3 and VL >10,000 c/mL randomized to either SQV/r (Invirase) 1,000/100 mg bid or LPV/r 400/100 mg bid, each in combination with TDF/FTC. The ITT analysis at 48 wks for 337 participants is summarized in Table 6.83 (JAIDS 2009;50:367).

TABLE 6.83 SQV/r (Invirase) vs. LPV/r in treatment-naïve patients (GEMINI trial)

	LPV/r n = 170	SQV/r n = 167
VL <400 c/mL	75%	73%
VL <50 c/mL	64%	65%
CD4 increase (mean) (cells/mm^3)	178	204
Discontinuation for ADR	12	5
Virologic failure	3%	7%
New PI mutations	0	1
Elevated LDL-C	24%	34%
Lipid elevation: Statin Rx	7	6

This interim analysis supports the conclusion that this SQV/r regimen appears virologically equivalent to LPV/r, possibly with less GI intolerance and hyperlipidemia.

STACCATO (Lancet 2006;368:459): In this trial of SQV/r (1500–1600/100 qd) plus 2 NRTIs, participants were randomized to treatment interruption (TI) or continuous therapy (CT) at a ratio of 2:1 (TI:CT). Criteria for entry were a CD4 count >350/mm^3 and a VL <50 c/mL. Those in the TI group discontinued ART when the CD4 count was >350/mm^3. Mean duration of treatment was 21.9 mos; the TI group received 12 wks of continuous ART at the end of treatment. Median CD4 increase was 459/mm^3 for the TI group (n = 284) vs. 655/mm^3 for the CT group (n = 148; P <0.05) and rates of 7% and 8%, respectively, for achieving VL <50 c/mL. A major difference between this study and the SMART study is the CD4 count threshold for treatment interruption: 350 cells/mm^3 in STACCATO and 250 cells/mm^3 in SMART.

RESISTANCE: Major resistance mutations selected with in vitro passage are L90M (most common; 3-fold in IC$_{50}$) and G48V (less common and 8-fold increase IC$_{50}$). Mutations noted in isolates with reduced susceptibility that emerged during treatment with Invirase include 48V and 90M and the following secondary mutations: 10I/R/V, 24I, 54V/L, 62V, 71V/T, 73S, 77I, 82A/F/T/S, and 84V. Similar to other boosted PI, treatment-naïve patients with virologic failure with SQV/r usually have no PI resistance mutations (Antiviral Ther 2006;11:631).

PHARMACOLOGY:

EC$_{50}$: 50 ng/mL. C$_{min}$ with SQV/r 1,000/100 mg bid is usually >500 ng/mL (JAC 2005;56:908).

Bioavailability: Absorption of SQV is not influenced by food when taken with RTV. There is essentially no CNS penetration (CSF-to-serum ratio = 0.02). SQV is category 1 (poor) in the four-class CNS penetration scoring (Neurology 2011;76:693). AUC and trough levels are significantly higher in women compared to men (JID 2004;189:1176).

Pharmacokinetics: Current dosing recommendations are based on pharmacokinetic studies in volunteers using the Invirase formulation. SQV/r regimens of 1,000/100 mg bid and 2,000/100 mg/d give desirable C_{min} and AUC values (JAC 2004;54:785). The 2,000/100 mg/d regimen resulted in a higher AUC (82 vs. 55 mg·hr/L) but lower C_{min} (0.28 vs. 1.02 mg/L) than the bid regimen (JAC 2004;54:785).

$T^{1/2}$: 1–2 hr.

Elimination: Metabolism is by cytochrome P450 isoenzymes CYP3A4 and CYP3A5 in the liver and gut (Clin Pharmacol Ther 2005;78:65); 96% biliary excretion; 1% urinary excretion.

Storage: Room temperature.

Dose modification in renal or hepatic failure: Use standard dose for renal failure. The drug is not removed by hemodialysis (Nephron 2001;87:186) and is unlikely to be removed by peritoneal dialysis.

SIDE EFFECTS: Gastrointestinal intolerance with nausea, abdominal pain, diarrhea in 5–15%; headache, and hepatic toxicity; case reports of hypoglycemia in patients with type 2 diabetes (Ann Intern Med 1999;131:980). Class adverse effects include fat accumulation, insulin resistance, and type 2 diabetes. SQV appears to have a similar effect on blood lipids compared to most other PIs other than ATV and DRV (JID 2004;189:1056). In the GEMINI trial, the change in total cholesterol was slightly worse with LPV/r and slightly worse with SQV/r for LDL cholesterol (JAIDS 2009;50:367). Dose-dependent prolongation of QT and PR intervals: the FDA issued a "safety communication" on February 23, 2011, stating concern for data showing that SQV/r (1,000 mg/100) given to healthy adults caused a dose-dependent prolongation of the QT and PR intervals. This risk is increased in persons taking other drugs that cause QT prolongation, primarily Class IA (such as quinidine or Class III antiarrhythmics (such as amiodarone) or patients who have a history QT prolongation.

The background data are from a placebo-controlled cross-over study in 59 healthy volunteers who were given SQV/r in doses of 1,000/100 mg and 1500/100 mg. The corrected QTc for these two dose regimens were 19 and 30 msec, respectively. The PR interval prolongation was >200 msec in 40% and 47% of the subjects, respectively. The specific FDA recommendations:

An EKG should be obtained before SQV is prescribed.

Not recommended if: (1) pre-treatment QT >450 msec, (2) refractory decreases with serum hypocalcemia or hypomagnesemia, (3) SQV co- administration with other meds that increase QTc (TCAs, RPV, antiarrhythmics), and (4) patients at increased risk of AV block.

Discontinue SQV if an on-therapy EKC at day 3–4 shows a QT interval >450 msec or >20 msec over pretreatment levels.

A cardiology consultation is recommended if drug discontinuation is considered.

Patients should be advised to contact a HCW immediately if they develop symptoms of heart block.

Report adverse events to FDA Med Watch.

DRUG INTERACTIONS:

Drugs should be avoided with SQV/r: Alfuzosin, terfenadine, astemizole, cisapride, triazolam, midazolam, rifampin, pimozide, ergot alkaloids, simvastatin, lovastatin, St. John's wort, alfuzosin, amiodarone, bepridil, flecainide, propafenone, quinidine, rifapentine, dofetilide, salmeterol, eplerenone, ivabradine, flibanserin, lurasidone, ranolazine, and trazodone.

Drugs that should be avoided: Salmeterol and fluticasone, fentanyl. Rivaroxaban, betrixaban, ticagrelor, vorapaxar, silodosin, enzalutamide, mitotane,

Drugs that may require regimen modification:

TABLE 6.84 SQV/r (Invirase) + second PI or NNRTI

Drug	AUC[a]	Regimen[a]
RTV	SQV ↑ 20×, RTV no change	SQV/r 1,000/100 bid
Dual PI combinations	SQV concentrations increased (except with TPV)	Dual boosted PIs are generally no longer recommended. In vitro antagonism with IDV, DRV and FPV levels are decreased, SQV levels decreased with TPV; Avoid.
EFV	EFV ↓ 12%, SQV no change	SQV/r 1,000/100 bid
NVP	NVP no change, SQV ↓ 25%	Consider NVP standard dose plus SQV/r 1,000/100 bid
ETR	ETR ↓ 33% SQV no change	SQV/r 1,000/100 mg bid. ETR standard dose
RPV	May significantly increase RPV	May increase risk of QTc prolongation; avoid
MVC	MVC ↑ 10×	MVC 150 mg bid

Anticoagulant: Dose adjustment needed with edoxaban, apixiban, and dabigatran based on renal function and indication.

Dexamethasone may decrease SQV levels.

Phenobarbital, phenytoin, and carbamazepine may decrease SQV levels substantially; monitor anticonvulsant levels or, preferably, use alternative agent (e.g., levetiracetam).

Ketoconazole increases SQV levels 3×; use standard dose. Monitor for SQV GI toxicity if ketoconazole dose is >200 mg/d. *Itraconazole* has bidirectional interaction with SQV; monitor itraconazole levels and monitor for SQV toxicity.

Clarithromycin increases SQV levels 177% and SQV increases clarithromycin levels 45%; reduce clarithromycin with renal failure.

Oral contraceptives: May decrease ethinyl estradiol. Recommend alternative form of contraception.

Sildenafil AUC increased 2×; use 25 mg starting dose; tadalafil: start with 5 mg dose and do not exceed 10 mg/72 hr; *vardenafil*: start with 2.5 mg dose and do not exceed 2.5 mg/72 hr.

Rifampin reduces SQV levels by 80%; contraindicated. A volunteer study showed marked elevations in transaminase. Rifampin + SQV/r should not be used (AIDS 2006;20:302; Roche letter to care providers, February 2005). *Rifabutin* reduces SQV levels 40%. With any combination of SQV/r use rifabutin 150 mg/d or 300 mg 3x/wk. For the treatment of TB, most experts recommend rifabutin TDM.

Voriconazole levels may decrease with SQV/r 1,000/100 mg bid. Monitor for efficacy of and toxicity to both drugs. Voriconazole TDM recommended.

Atorvastatin levels increase 450% with SQV/r; use lowest starting dose of atorvastatin, or use pitavastatin or pravastatin. *Pravastatin* levels are reduced 50% by SQV/r; may need to increase pravastatin dose.

Methadone: With FTV there is a 10–20% reduction in methadone levels; may increase QTc; avoid co-administration.

Colchicine: SQV/r significantly increases colchicine level; use reduced dose colchicine only after SQV/r is at steady-state.

Garlic supplements decrease SQV AUC, C_{max} and C_{min} levels by about 50% (CID 2002;34:234).

Grapefruit juice increases SQV levels.

Other drugs that induce CYP3A4 (phenobarbital, phenytoin, dexamethasone, carbamazepine, and NVP) may decrease SQV levels; these combinations should be avoided if possible.

Fluticasone: Avoid long-term co-administration. Use beclomethasone.

Tricyclic antidepressants: May increase QTc; avoid.

Interaction with other antiretroviral drugs: See Table 6.84.

PREGNANCY: Category B. Studies in rats showed no teratogenicity or embryotoxicity. The PK data suggests SQV/r at 1,000/100 mg bid provides good levels in pregnancy (Antivir Ther 2009;14:443–50). The 2018 DHHS Guidelines do not recommend SQV/r 1,000/100 mg bid as an alternate to ATV/r or DRV/r in patients with QTc and/or PR prolongation.

Sporanox—see Itraconazole

Stavudine (d4T)

TRADE NAME: Zerit (Bristol-Myers Squibb) and generics.

CLASS: NRTI.

FORMULATIONS, REGIMEN, AND COST:

Forms: Caps: 15, 20, 30, and 40 mg; oral solution: 1 mg/mL (200 mL bottle).

Regimens: For patients weighing >60 kg, 30–40 mg bid; <60 kg, 30 mg bid. *Note*: The WHO has endorsed 30 mg as the standard dose for all patients based on concerns for high rates of peripheral neuropathy and lactic acidosis in low-resource countries. Review of available data supported use of the lower dose (Expert Opin Pharacother 2007;8:679), although the FDA has not endorsed this change.

COST: $403.25/mo (d4T 30 mg bid).

FOOD: No effect.

RENAL FAILURE: See Table 6.85.

HEPATIC FAILURE: No dose recommendation.

PATIENT ASSISTANCE: 800-272-4878.

CLINICAL TRIALS: There is extensive experience with d4T combined with 3TC or ddI. ACTG 384 showed that EFV + AZT/3TC had greater activity and less toxicity compared with EFV + ddI + d4T (see Table 6.86) (NEJM 2003;349:2293). GS-903 compared d4T and TDF in 600 treatment-naïve patients who were randomized to

TABLE 6.85 d4T dosing in renal failure

Wt.	CrCl (mL/min)			
	>50	26–50	10–25	Dialysis
>60kg	40 mg bid [a]	20 mg bid	20 mg/d	20 mg/d
<60kg	30 mg bid	15 mg bid	15 mg/d	15 mg/d

[a] May consider 30 mg bid.

receive TDF or d4T, each with 3TC and EFV. Both regimens were highly effective at 3 yrs, but d4T was associated with more neuropathy, hyperlipidemia, and lipodystrophy than TDF. The CLASS trial examined 3 regimens given over 96 wks. All regimens included ABC/3TC with d4T, EFV or FPV/r. At 48 wks, outcome was superior for EFV + 3TC/ABC vs. d4T + ABC/3TC (JAIDS 2006;43:284). The 301A trial showed once-daily FTC was superior to d4T when combined with ddI + EFV. ACTG 384 showed AZT/3TC + EFV was superior to other combinations including d4T + ddI. AI 454-152 found that d4T + ddI + NFV was equivalent to AZT/3TC + NFV. See Table 6.86.

RESISTANCE: In vivo d4T resistance is mediated primarily by thymidine analog mutations (TAMs) (e.g., 41L, 67N, 70R, 210W, 215Y/F, 219Q/E), and d4T also selects for these mutations. Mutations at 44D and 118I increase resistance to AZT and d4T in the presence of TAMs (JID 2002;185:8998). As with AZT, the M184V mutation increases susceptibility to d4T although the clinical significance is unknown. The multinucleoside resistance mutations (Q151M complex and the T69-insertion mutation) result in resistance to d4T. This agent sometimes selects for the K65R mutation, especially in patients with non-subtype B virus, although it appears to have minimal effect on d4T susceptibility.

PHARMACOLOGY:

Bioavailability: 86% and not influenced by food or fasting.
$T^{1/2}$: Serum, 1 hr; intracellular $T^{1/2}$, 3.5 hr.

TABLE 6.86 Trials in treatment-naïve patients comparing d4T with other antiretrovirals

Study	Regimen	N	Dur (wks)	VL <50	VL <200–500
START-1. (AIDS 2000;14:1591)	d4T + 3TC + IDV	101	48	49%	52%
	AZT/3TC + IDV	103		47%	52%
CLASS. (JAIDS 2006;43:284)	d4T + ABC/3TC	98	48	81%	81%
	FPV/r + ABC/3TC	96		80%	80%
	EFV + ABC/3TC	97		90%[a]	90%[a]
ACTG 384 (NEJM 003;349:2293)	d4T + ddI + EFV	155	48		62%
	d4T + ddI + NFV	155			63%
	AZT/3TC + EFV	155			89%[a]
	AZT/3TC + NFV	155			66%
FTC 301A. (JAMA 2004;292:180)	FTC + ddI + EFV	286	48	78%[a]	81%[a]
	d4T + ddI + EFV	285		59%	68%
GS-903. (JAMA 2004;292:191)	TDF + 3TC + EFV	299	144	68%[b]	71%[a]
	d4T + 3TC + EFV	301		63%	68%
AI 454-152. (JAIDS 2002;31:399)	d4T + ddI + NFV	258	48	33%	55%
	AZT/3TC + NFV	253		33%	56%

[a] Superior to comparator (p <0.05).
[b] TDF + 3TC significantly less toxic.

CNS penetration: 30–40% (JAIDS 1998;17:235) (CSF-to-plasma ratio = 0.16–0.97). Ranks 2 in the four-class CNS penetration score (Neurology 2011;76:693).

Elimination: Renal, 40%.

Dose modification in severe liver disease: No guidelines; use standard dose with caution.

SIDE EFFECTS:

Mitochondrial toxicity: d4T is an important cause of side effects attributed to mitochondrial toxicity, including lactic acidosis with hepatic steatosis, peripheral neuropathy, and lipoatrophy. In most studies of lactic acidosis, d4T is the most frequent NRTI accounting for 33 of 34 reported cases for 2000–2001 (CID 2002;31:838), and d4T was implicated in the majority of reported cases in resource limited countries in more recent reports (AIDS 2007;21:2455; CID 2007;45:254; S Afr Med J 2006;96;722). Frequency is 5–15% but as high as 24% in some early trials. This side effect is dose- and duration-related, and it appears to be caused by depletion of mitochondrial DNA (NEJM 2002;346:811). The relative binding of mammalian mitochondrial DNA is 13–36 times greater for ddI and d4T compared to other NRTIs (TDF, ABC, 3TC, FTC) (J Biol Chem 2001;276:40847). As expected the risk of mitochondrial toxicity is substantially increased when d4T is combined with ddI (AIDS 2000;14:273). Onset is usually noted at 2–6 mos of treatment and usually resolves if d4T is promptly stopped, although the recovery is generally slow. Peripheral neuropathy due to HIV infection or another drug (INH, long-term metronidazole, B6, vincristine, dapsone, thalidomide) or ddI represents a contraindication to d4T.

With regard to d4T doses, a systemic review of 9 trials and 6 cohort reports supported 30 mg bid as the standard dose (Expert Opin Pharmacother 2007;8:679). This lower dose appears to be comparable in antiviral efficacy based on 5 studies, and there was strong evidence of reduced peripheral neuropathy with the lower dose. There was a trend lower lipid effect and less lipoatrophy, but these findings were less conclusive. The WHO has now adopted the 30 mg dose as standard for all patients, and this has been endorsed by PEPFAR (www.pepfar.gov). The FDA has not revised its labeling to reflect the WHO recommended dose of 30 mg bid.

HIV-associated neuromuscular weakness syndrome: A syndrome of ascending motor weakness characterized by variable changes, including progressive sensorimotor polyneuropathy with areflexia and ascending neuromuscular weakness. EMG and pathology show changes in nerves, muscles, or both. Of 69 cases reviewed, 61 were thought to be due to d4T, and many (36%) had onset of symptoms after d4T was stopped. Lactate levels are usually elevated (AIDS 2004;18:1403). The weakness was accompanied by lactic acidosis and is presumed to be a result of mitochondrial toxicity.

Lipoatrophy and hyperlipidemia: d4T is associated with lipoatrophy and hyperlipidemia (CID 2006;43:645) The lipoatrophy is a cosmetic effect that is most obvious in the malar (cheek) area, extremities, and buttocks. These effects persist for prolonged periods after d4T is discontinued, although some studies show slow but significant increase in malar and extremity fat after several months (AIDS 2006;20:243; AIDS 2004;18:1029). Serum lipid changes ascribed to d4T are most significant for triglyceride elevations but also for increased LDL cholesterol (JAMA 2004;292:191). Reversal of lipid effects is noted with switch to alternative NRTIs such as TDF or ABC (JAIDS 2005;38:263; AIDS 2005;19:15; AIDS 2006;20:2043).

> *Other clinical side effects*: Complaints are infrequent and include headache, GI intolerance with diarrhea, or esophageal ulcers.
> *Macrocytosis* with MVC >100, which is inconsequential (JID 2000;40:160).

DRUG INTERACTIONS:

> *NRTIs: AZT*, pharmacologic antagonism; avoid. ddI, increased risk of pancreatitis, lactic acidosis, and peripheral neuropathy; avoid.
> *Drugs that cause peripheral neuropathy should be used with caution or avoided*: ddI, ethionamide, EMB, INH, phenytoin, vincristine, glutethimide, gold, hydralazine, thalidomide, and long-term metronidazole.
> *Methadone* reduces the AUC of d4T by 24%, but this is not thought to be sufficiently severe to require d4T dose adjustment; d4T has no effect on methadone levels (JAIDS 2000;24:241).
> Use with caution when combined with ribavirin.

PREGNANCY: Category C. The pregnancy registry shows birth defects in 21/811 (2.59%) of first-trimester d4T exposures compared to overall prevalence of birth defects of 2.7% (www.apregistry. com, accessed July 31, 2017). d4T is no longer recommended as an alternative to ABC/3TCor TDF/FTC in the 2018 Guidelines for Antiretroviral Drugs for Pregnant Women. Although early studies in pregnancy indicate good short-term tolerability and pharmacokinetics (JID 2004;190:2167), but due to risk of mitochondrial toxicity, lactic acidosis, and hepatic steatosis d4t +/– ddI is not recommended (Sex Trans Infect 2002;78:58) and should not be given with AZT due to pharmacologic antagonism (FDA black box warning).

Stocrin—see Efavirenz

Sulfadiazine

TRADE NAME: Generic.

CLASS: Synthetic derivatives of sulfanilamide that inhibit folic acid synthesis.

FORMULATIONS, REGIMEN, AND COST: 500 mg tab at $4.59.

INDICATIONS AND DOSES:

Toxoplasmosis: Initial treatment 1.0 g po qid (<65 kg) or 1.5 g po qid (>65 kg); maintenance dose: half of prior dose (in combination w/pyrimethamine and leucovorin).

Nocardia: 1 g po qid × ≥6 mos.

UTIs: 500 mg, 1 g po bid × 3–14 days.

PHARMACOLOGY:

Bioavailability: >70%.

$T^{1/2}$: 7–17 hr.

Elimination: Hepatic acetylation and renal excretion of parent compound and metabolites.

CNS penetration: 40–80% of serum levels.

Serum levels for systemic infections: goal is 100–150 μg/mL.

Dose modifications in renal failure: CrCl >50 mL/min, 1.0–1.5 g q6h; CrCl 10–50 mL/min, 1.0– 1.5 g q12h (half dose); CrCl <10 mL/min, 1–1.5 g 24h.

SIDE EFFECTS: Hypersensitivity with rash, drug fever, serum-sickness, urticaria; crystalluria reduced with adequate urine volume (≥1,500 mL/d) and alkaline urine (use with care in renal failure); marrow suppression (anemia, thrombocytopenia, leukopenia, hemolytic anemia due to G6PD deficiency).

DRUG INTERACTIONS: Decreased effect of cyclosporine, digoxin; increased effect of Coumadin, oral hypoglycemics, methotrexate, and phenytoin. Use with caution with ribavirin (anemia).

PREGNANCY: Category C. Competes with bilirubin for albumin to cause kernicterus; avoid in near-term or nursing mothers.

Sulfamethoxazole-Trimethoprim—see
Trimethoprim-Sulfamethoxazole

Sustiva—see Efavirenz

Telzir—see Fosamprenavir

Tenofovir Disoproxil Fumarate (TDF)/ Tenofovir Alafenamide (TAF)

TRADE NAME: TDF: Viread (Gilead Sciences).

Combination with FTC: Truvada (Gilead Sciences).
Combination with 3TC: Cimduo (Mylan)

Combination with FTC + EFV: Atripla (Gilead Sciences and Bristol-Myers Squibb).

Combination with 3TC + EFV: Symfi and Symfi Lo (Mylan)

Combination with FTC + RPV: Complera (Gilead Sciences).

TAF co-formulated with FTC: Descovy (Gilead).

TAF co-formulated with EVG/COBI/FTC: Genvoya (Gilead).

TAF co-formulated with RPV/FTC: Odefsey (Gilead).

TAF co-formulated with DRV/c/FTC: Symtuza (Janssen)

TAF co-formulated with BIC/FTC: Biktarvy (Gilead)

CLASS: Nucleotide analog reverse transcriptase inhibitor (NtRTI, NRTI).

FORMULATIONS, REGIMEN, AND COST: TDF: 300 mg tab (1 po qd) and oral powder (40 mg/g) 60 g;

Truvada (TDF/FTC): 300/200 mg (1 po qd).

Atripla (EFV/TDF/FTC): 600/300/200 mg (1 po qd).

Complera (RPV/TDF/FTC): 25/300/200 mg (1 po qd with a meal).

Stribild (EVG/COBI/TDF/FTC): 150/150/300/200 mg 1 tablet once-daily with food.

Descovy (TAF/FTC): 25/200 mg tab 1 po qd with or without food (in combination with InSTI, PI/r, or NNRTI.

Genvoya (EVG/COBI/TAF/FTC): 150/150/10/200 mg tab 1 po qd with food.

Odefsey (RPV/TAF/FTC): 25/25/200 mg tab 1 po qd with food.

Symtuza (DRV/COBI/TAF/FTC): 800/150/10/200 mg tab 1 po qd with our without food.

Biktarvy (BIC/TAF/FTC): 50m/25m/200 mg tablet with or without food.

Cost: Viread $ 1,279.94/mo; Truvada $ 1,881.14/mo; Atripla $3,057.89/mo.

Complera $ 3,216.92/mo; Descovy: $1,881.14; Genvoya: $ 3,306.92/mo; Odefsey $ 3,009.29.; Biktarvy $3,534.78/mo. Symtuza $4178/mo.

PATIENT ASSISTANCE PROGRAM: 800-226-2056 (9 AM–8 PM EST).

TABLE 6.87 TDF dose adjustments for renal impairment

CrCl. (mL/min/1.73m²)	TDF	TDF/FTC (Truvada)
≥ 50	300 mg/d	1 tab qd
30–49[a]	300 mg q48h (consider TAF)	1 tab q 48 hr
10–29[a]	300 mg q72–96h (consider TAF)	Not recommended
<10	Consider 300 mg/wk	Not recommended
Hemodialysis	300 mg/wk or after 12 hrs of hemodialysis	Not recommended

[a] Note: Most authorities avoid TDF with a creatinine clearance <50 mL/min due to confusion about the contribution of TDF with progression of disease; the exception is with end-stage renal disease.

TAF dose adjustment for renal impairment:
   CrCL >15 mL/min: 25mg po q24h.
   CrCL <15 mL/min: Avoid, but clinical significance unknown.
TAF coformulations dose adjustment in renal impairment:
   CrCL ≥30 mL/min: Usual dose of BIC/TAF/FTC; EVG/ COBI/TAF/FTC; RPV/TAF/FTC, and TAF/FTC co- formulations: 1 tab po once-daily.
   CrCL <30mL/min: No data; avoid TAF co-formulations.
FOOD: No clinically significant effect on TDF, but fatty meals increase EFV absorption by 40% with co-formulated EFV/TDF/FTC. High fat meals increase TAF absorption by 75%.
RENAL FAILURE: See Table 6.87.
HEPATIC FAILURE: No dose change recommended.

CLINICAL TRIALS:
GS-97-901: Median decrease in VL at 28 days with monotherapy in treatment-naïve patients using 300 mg dose was 1.2 $\log_{10}$ c/mL (AAC 2001;45:2733).

GS-98-902: Dose-finding/toxicity study using 75, 150, and 300 mg added to antiretroviral regimen in 189 treatment-experienced patients with VL 400–100,000 c/mL. At 48 wks, the mean VL decrease was 0.62 $\log_{10}$ c/mL among 54 patients receiving 300 mg/d (JAIDS 2003;33:15).

GS-907: Placebo-controlled trial in treated patients with VL 400–10,000 c/mL given 300 mg tenofovir. At 24 wks (n = 550), the mean decrease in VL was 0.61 $\log_{10}$ c/mL among tenofovir recipients compared with 0.03 $\log_{10}$ c/mL in placebo recipients.

GS-903: Randomized, placebo-controlled trial comparing TDF vs. d4T, each in combination with 3TC + EFV for treatment of ART-naïve patients (JAMA 2004;292:191). By ITT (missing = failure) analysis at 144 wks, 73% of TDF recipients and 69% of d4T recipients had a VL <50 c/mL (p = NS) (JAMA 2004;292:191). The drop-out rate was low, but d4T recipients had higher rates of peripheral neuropathy, and higher rates of 184V resistance mutations, lipoatrophy, and elevated fasting/levels of total and LDL cholesterol and triglycerides.

ESS 30009: A trial comparing the triple NRTI regimen of TDF + ABC/3TC with EFV + ABC/3TC in 194 treatment-naïve patients. The trial was stopped at 12 wks due to high rates of virologic failure in the triple NRTI arm (49% vs. 5%); resistance testing showed a high frequency of M184V (100%) and K65R (64%) in 36 with virologic failure (JID 2005;192:1821).

ACTG 5202: 1,858 treatment-naïve patients were randomized to ABC/3TC vs. TDF/FTC, plus either EFV or LPV/r (NEJM 2009;361:2230). The DSMB unblinded the study for the subset of patients with a baseline VL >100,000 c/mL after a medium follow-up at 60 wks because of a higher rate of virologic failure with ABC/3TC compared to TDF/FTC. The respective failure rates were 14% and 7%; OR 2.33, 95% CI, 1.46–3.72; P = <0.001.

GS-934: 517 treatment-naïve patients were randomized to receive co-formulated AZT/3TC + EFV or TDF/FTC + EFV. Results at 48 wks in 487 participants by modified ITT showed TDF/FTC was superior to AZT/3TC in these categories: virologic suppression to <400 c/mL (77% vs. 68%), mean increase in CD4 count (190 cells/

mm^3 vs. 171 cells/mm^3), lower increase in LDL cholesterol (13 mg/dL vs. 20 mg/dL), less limb fat loss, less 184V resistance mutation (2 vs. 9), and fewer drug discontinuations for ADRs (4% vs. 9%) (NEJM 2006;354:251; JAIDS 2006;43:535). The difference was explained primarily by the higher proportion of discontinuations due to adverse events in the AZT/3TC arm (9% vs. 4%), most of which were due to anemia. At 96 wks, there was significantly greater limb fat (8.9 vs. 6.9 kg) and a significantly lower number of M184V mutations (2 vs. 7) among patients on TDF/FTC (JAIDS 2006;43:535). Results at 144 wks show TDF/FTC superior to AZT/3TC in viral suppression (71% vs. 58%) and in median total limb fat (7.9 vs. 5.4 kg) (JAIDS 2008;47:74). A subsequent report found TDF and AZT to have divergent effects on proinflammatory effects, including a strong reduction in interleukin (IL)-10 by TDF (JAIDS 2011;57:265).

ASSERT Trial (TDF/FTC vs. ABC/3TC): Comparisons of these two combinations agents in terms of viral response and toxicity are summarized in Table 6.88.

TDF + ddI: This NRTI combination should be avoided due to (1) increased ddI toxicity reflecting increased intracellular ddI concentrations (J Clin Pharm 205;45:1360; CID 2003;36:1082); (2) blunted CD4 response (AIDS 2004;18:459; AIDS 2005;19:569; CID 2005;41:901); (3) high rates of virologic failure (AIDS 2004;13:180; AIDS 2005;19:1183; AIDS 2005;19:1695); and (4) rapid selection of the K65R resistance mutation (AIDS 2005;19:1695; Antivir Ther 2005;10:171; AIDS 2005;19:213).

HBV: TDF is active against HBV has been FDA approved for that indication and, along with FTC, is considered a preferred agent based on potency and durability (CID 2010;51:1201). In patients with HIV and a positive HBeAg, the inclusion of TDF in the HIV regimen results in a decrease of 4–5 log$_{10}$ in HBV DNA levels, including those with 3TC-resistant strains (AIDS 2003;17:F7; JID 2003;186:1844; CID 2004;38[suppl2]:S98; CID 2003;37:1678; JID 2004;189:1185). In a review of literature comparing the 6 FDA-approved drugs for HBV, TDF was the most active and durable in reducing HBV DNA and promoting histologic improvement (CID

TABLE 6.88 TDF/FTC vs ABC/3TC

	ACTG 5202 (pg 100) NEJM 2009;361:2230	HEAT (pg 181) AIDS 2009;23:1547	ASSERT (pg 182) JAIDS 2010;55:49 CID 2010;51:963
Sponsor	NIH	GSK	GSK
Number	1858	688	385
Trial Design	Double-blind	Double-blind	Randomized
Primary Result	Time to virologic failure (60 wks)	VL<50 c/mL (48 wks)	Toxicity and VL (48 wks)
Result (Duration)	Superior virologic response with TDF with baseline VL >100,000 c/mL (14% vs 7%)	Viral suppression equal (67% vs 68%)	• TDF superior in VL <50 c/mL (71% vs 59%) • No difference in eGFR but TDF showed more tubular dysfunction • Greater ↓ in BMD with TDF/FTC than ABC/3TC

eGFR, estimated glomerular filtration rate; BMD, bone mineral density.

2010;51:1201). A report of 426 patients with HBV monoinfection treated with TDF 144 wks showed no HBV resistance and 13 (3%) failures attributed to nonadherence (Hepatology 2010;51:73). One report found that prolonged exposure to TDF in patients with HBV–HIV co-infection was associated with increased rates of HBeAg clearance (HIV Clin Trials 2009;10:3). The addition of 3TC does not augment TDF activity against HBV, but the addition of TDF to 3TC protects against HBV resistance to 3TC (JID 2004;189:1185). FTC is also active against HBV. Practical application of these data is to use coformulated TDF/FTC in patients with HBV-HIV co-infection.

RESISTANCE: Susceptibility of HIV is decreased in patients with 3 or more thymidine analog mutations (TAMs) that include the 41L and 210W mutations. Susceptibility is maintained with other TAM mutations and increased with 184V. TDF, ddI, and ABC select for the 65R mutation, which confers resistance to all three drugs, as well as to 3TC and FTC (AAC 2004;48:1413). Resistance testing in 14 patients with virologic failure in GS-903 showed no K65R mutations at 96 wks. There is substantial loss of susceptibility with T69 insertion mutation (AAC 2004;48:992); susceptibility is maintained with Q151M complex. Partial phenotypic susceptibility may be maintained despite presence at K65R when M184V is also present. Mutants with K65R and 184V on the same genome were detected in 50% of samples from failures with ddI + TDF + 3TC in patients (Antiviral Ther 2010;15:437).

PHARMACOLOGY:

> *Bioavailability:* TDF: 25% (fasting) to 40% (with food); improvement with food, especially high-fat meal, but levels are adequate when taken in a fasting state.
>
> *CNS penetration:* Poor; score 1 (lowest) in the CNS penetration score (Neurology 2011;76:693).
>
> High-fat meals increase TAF absorption by 75%. May be taken with or without food.
>
> $T^{1/2}$:
>
> > TDF: Serum $T^{1/2}$ 17 hr; intracellular $T^{1/2}$ >60 hr.
> >
> > TAF: Serum $T^{1/2}$ 0.51h; intracellular $T^{1/2}$ of active metabolite 150–180 hr.
>
> *Elimination:*
>
> > TDF: Renal, glomerular filtration, and active tubular secretion.
> >
> > TAF: 80% of oral dose metabolized with 31.7% excreted in feces and <1% excreted in urine. Mild to moderate renal

insufficiency does not affect TAF pharmacokinetics. No data with CrCL <30 mL/min.

No dose adjustment needed with mild to moderate (CP A and B). No data in ESLD.

Drug interaction with TDF:

ATV: ATV AUC is decreased 25%; use standard dose TDF + ATV/ r (300/100 mg) qd.

ddI EC: TDF and ddI co-administration is not generally recommended.

Miscellaneous: Ganciclovir, valganciclovir, probenecid, and *cidofovir* compete for active tubular secretion with increased levels of either tenofovir or the companion drug; monitor for toxicities. LPV/r increases levels of TDF 30% with co-administration. This appears to be due to decreased tenofovir clearance, but the mechanism and significance is unclear (Clin Pharm Ther 2008;83:265).

DRV: tenofovir levels and AUC increase by a mean of 20–25% (2011 DHHS Guidelines). Use standard doses but watch for renal toxicity. Several studies suggest that PI-based ART with TDF is associated with a greater decline in renal function than TDF combined with NNRTIs (JID 2008;197:7; AIDS 2009;23:1971-5).

Drug interaction with TAF: TAF is a substrate of P-gp, BCRP, OATP1B1, and OATP1B3. Inducers of P-gp may significantly decrease TAF concentrations. Avoid TPV/r, inducing anticonvulsants (e.g., carbamazepine, oxcarbazepine, phenobarbital, phenytoin), rifamycins (rifabutin, rifampin, rifapentine) high tenofovir intracellular concentrations observed with rifamycin co-administration (CROI 20918 abstract 282B), St. John's wort.

No significant interactions observed between TAF and DRV/r, BIC, DTG, EFV, or RPV co-administration.

ATV/r increase TAF by 91%; Cobicistat increase TAF by 165%; LPV/r increase TAF by 47%. Co-administered ARV not affected by TAF.

SIDE EFFECTS: *GI intolerance* reported, but it is infrequent. *TDF*: Flatulence occurred more often in TDF-treated patients than placebo-treated patients. *TAF*: Generally well tolerated with only 0.9% discontinuation rate. When co-administered with EVG/COBI/FTC, nausea (10%) was most commonly reported.

Nephrotoxicity: TDF and related drugs (adefovir and cidofovir) may cause renal injury, including the Fanconi syndrome, which is characterized by hypophosphatemia, hypouricemia, proteinuria, normoglycemic glycosuria, and, in some cases, acute renal failure (JAIDS 2004;35:269; AIDS 2004;18:960; CID 2003;37:e174). The mechanism is unclear, but one report suggests mitochondrial toxicity (Kidney Int 2010;78:1060). In the early stages, this may be asymptomatic or cause myalgias; most resolve when the drug is discontinued (JAIDS 2004;35:269). Risk factors are low body weight, preexisting renal disease (AAC 2001;45:2733), and concurrent use of nephrotoxic agents. With TDF there is a dose or TDF exposure relationship, but there were no cases among patients given double dose of TDF (J Med VIrol 2007;79:105). Combination with ddI may contribute through mitochondrial toxicity and competition for uptake by proximal renal tubular cells (Mayo Clin Proc 2007;82:1103). Numerous studies have examined the rate of TDF-associated nephrotoxicity. A large cohort study showed a minimal but statistically significant reduction in creatinine clearance and increase in anion gap with a mean follow-up of 1.7 yrs; treatment duration was not a significant association (HIV Med 2006;7:105). A EuroSIDA review of 6,842 patients showed the risk of chronic renal disease defined as a 25% decrease in CrCl was 2.4/100 person-years compared to 0.7/100 p-y in ART recipients not given TDF. Risks with TDF-associated CRD were increasing age, HBP, HCV, and low CD4 count (AIDS 2010;24:1667). Others have found lower rates. Analysis of 600 participants in GS-903 with calculated CrCl >60 mL/min and serum phosphorus ≥2.2 mg/dL at baseline showed no change in mean serum creatinine or phosphorus levels at week 144 (Nephrol Dial Transplant 2005;20:743). A longer follow-up of GS-903 found that the difference in median GFR at 7 yrs in mL/min/1.73 M^2 was 112 in TDF recipients vs. 120 in controls (17th IAC;Abstr. TUPE0057). In another study of 1,058 TDF recipients, 9 (0.9%) developed an otherwise unexplained increase in serum creatinine (JAIDS 2004;37:1489). Other studies have shown modest declines in creatinine clearance in clinical cohorts (CID 2005;40:1194). A review from Johns Hopkins comparing GFR for 201 TDF recipients and 231 given alternative NRTIs (AIDS 2009;23:197) showed a slight decline in eGFR in the first 180 days that stabilized from day 180 to 720. The change in eGFR was more common with TDF combined with PIs rather than NNRTIs (decrease of 8 mL/min vs. 4 mL/min (CID 2005;40:1194). The conclusion is that TDF may cause nephrotoxicity, but it is infrequent and usually modest in severity and reversible, especially in patients with normal baseline renal function and relatively high baseline CD4 counts (AIDS 2010;24:223:2239). Nevertheless, there are anecdotal reports of severe kidney disease, including acute renal failure.

TAF: When combined with EVG/COBI/FTC in patients with normal renal function, the mean Scr increase from baseline was 0.1 mg/dL at 48 wks. However, no change in urine protein-to-creatinine ratio observed. Urine protein-to-creatinine ratio decrease from 61 mg/g to 46 mg/g at 48 wks after switching from TDF to TAF. In patients with mild to moderate renal impairment (eGFR 30–69 mL/min), EVG/COBI/TAF/FTC did not result in progression of renal impairment at 24 wks.

Monitoring renal function with TDF treatment according to the 2018 DHHS Guidelines should include:

Baseline urinalysis and chemistry profile.

Patients with a CrCl <50 mL/min should not receive TDF since progressive deterioration would make it difficult to distinguish the effect of TDF and the primary renal disease; an exception might be the patient with total renal failure.

Renal function monitoring during TDF treatment should include a baseline chemistry profile (for creatinine and creatinine clearance) and a urinalysis. The chemistry profile should be repeated at 2–8 wks then every 3–6 mos. The urinalysis should be repeated every 6 mos during TDF treatment. More frequent monitoring is recommended with other risks for renal disease such as diabetes or hypertension.

Evaluation for TDF nephrotoxicity should include serum phosphate levels, and urine dipstick for glucose and protein. Glycosuria in a non-diabetic with a normal serum glucose is diagnostic of tubular dysfunction, whereas proteinuria may be due to other causes. Hypophosphatemia is nonspecific unless persistent; the fractional excretion of phosphate is a more useful measure of tubular phosphate wasting and should be calculated in patients with evidence of glomerular or tubular dysfunction.

Bone toxicity: Initiation of many antiretroviral regimens results in a modest non-progressive decline in bone density. Bone density declines observed in TDF-treated patients are generally of greater magnitude than those seen in patients treated with other NRTI. The most comprehensive study with long term follow-up is ACTG A5224, a substudy of ACTG A5202, in which DXA scans were done sequentially in 269 patients randomized to ABC/3TC or TDF/FTC (JID 2011;203:1791). Analysis at 196 wks showed the rate of fractures was 5.4% and was equal by treatment categories. DXA scans showed a decrease in BMD that was 1.4–2.0% greater at 96 wks for TDF/FTC recipients, especially when this was combined with ATV/r. Most of the changes occurred in the first 6 mos; the BMD then stabilized and increased at 1–2 yrs (JID 2011;203:1705). *TAF*: Mean BMD decrease 1.3% at the lumbar spine and 0.66% observed at 48 wks in patients treated with EVG/COBI/TAF/FTC. Fractures reported in 0.8% in these patients. Improvement in BMD observed in 799 patients who were switched from TDF to TAF at week

48 with a mean increase of 1.86% at the lumbar spine and 1.95% at the total hip.

Other: The incidence of laboratory and clinical adverse events has been similar to placebo in controlled clinical trials.

PREGNANCY: Category B. Studies of high-dose TDF exposure in fetal monkeys (doses that produced TDF levels 25-fold higher than in humans) produced a slight reduction in bone porosity and lower levels of insulin-like growth factor (IGF)-1, which regulates linear growth (JAIDS 2002;29:207). Continued administration of TDF to the previously exposed infant primates resulted in a significant reduction in growth and reduced bone porosity. Studies in children (and adults) show bone demineralization with chronic use, which is of uncertain significance (Pediatrics 2006;118:e711; AIDS 2002;16:1257). Pharmacokinetic studies demonstrated a lower AUC in pregnancy but normal trough levels (Mirochnick M. JAIDS 2011;Epub Ahead:PMCID PMC 3125419). However, due to the demonstrated safety in pregnancy, the 2018 DHHS Guidelines on Use of Antiretroviral Agents in Pregnancy recommend TDF/FTC as one of the preferred NRTIs when used in combination with RAL, ATV/r, or DRV/r. The Pregnancy Registry through July 31, 2017, showed birth defects in 76/3342 (2.27%) first-trimester TDF exposures; this is comparable to CDC population-based surveillance data (2.7%). No data with TAF.

Telzir—see Fosamprenavir

Testosterone

FORMULATIONS, REGIME, AND COST:.
Testosterone cypionate (various generic manufacturers).
Testosterone enanthate (various generic manufacturers).

Testosterone patch (Androderm, Watson).

Testosterone gel (AndroGel, Unimed, Testim, Auxilium) Testosterone Cream (First-Testosterone MC Transdermal) 2%.

Testim 1% gel.

Testosterone buccal (Striant, Columbia Laboratories).

Cost: Vials of 100 mg/mL and 200 mg/mL at $28.63/200 mg.

Androderm 24-hr patch at $8.08/2 mg or $16.16/4 mg.

AndroGel 5 g packet at $19.56.

Striant 30 mg at $9.91.

INDICATIONS (for men only, except where noted):

Hypogonadism: Normal testosterone levels in adult men are 300–1,000 ng/dL at 8 AM, representing peak levels with circadian rhythm. Reports from the pre-HAART era showed subnormal testosterone levels in 45% of patients with AIDS and in 20–30% of HIV-infected patients without AIDS (Am J Med 1988;84:611; AIDS 1994;7:46; J Clin Endocrinol 1996;81:4108). At that time, the frequency of hypogonadism correlated with low CD4 counts and symptomatic HIV (Am J Med 1988;84:611). Patients are now living longer, so age-related decline in testosterone levels becomes a complicating factor that generally supersedes the impact of immunosuppression. The CHAMPS study (Cohort of HIV At-risk Aging: Men's Prospective Study) with men age >49 yrs with and without HIV infection found that hypogonadism (<300 ng/mL) was unrelated to HIV serostatus or CD4 count, but was correlated with a VL >10,000 c/mL (CID 2005;41:1794). Indications for testing testosterone levels in men with HIV infection are symptoms of low libido, low bone mineral density, and low BMI despite response to ART. Recommendations for testosterone therapy from the Endocrine Society (J Clin Endoc Rinol Metab 2010;95:2536) are "for symptomatic men with classical androgen deficiency syndromes aimed at inducing and maintaining secondary sex characteristics and at improving sexual function, sense of well being and bone mineral density." Contraindications and precautions are (1) breast or prostate cancer, (2) exclude prostate cancer with prostate digital exam or PSA <4 ng/mL (<3 ng/mL in high-risk men), (3) hematocrit >50%, (4) severe lower urinary tract symptoms, (5) untreated severe sleep apnea, (6) poorly controlled heart failure, or (7) desire for fertility. The goal of therapy is normal free testosterone level, measured in the morning. In men ≥40 yrs, there should be a baseline PSA and a digital exam at 3–6 mos and then according to standard guidelines. In a small placebo-controlled trial of testosterone gel vs. placebo in men >65 yrs with total serum testosterone levels 100–350 ng/dL; testosterone recipients had increased cardiovascular, respiratory and dermatologic events compared to placebo recipients (NEJM 2010;363:109). (Benefits included increased strength.) A review of 51 reports (2003–2008) concluded that the only statistically significant adverse effects were an increase in hemoglobin and a small decrease in HDL cholesterol (J Clin Endocrinol Metab (2010;95:2560). There was no significant effect on mortality, cardiovascular events, or prostate cancer.

Therapeutic trials with testosterone treatment of HIV-infected hypogonadal men show substantial improvements in quality of life with increased libido, reduced fatigue, and reduced depression (Arch Gen Psych 2000;57:141; HIV Clin Trials 2007;8:412). Benefit has also been shown in eugonadal HIV-infected men receiving twice the physiological dose (200 mg/wk), but long-term toxicity should be considered (Ann Intern Med 2000;133:348).

Wasting: Testosterone is an anabolic steroid that may restore nitrogen balance and lean body mass in patients with wasting (JAIDS 1996;11:510; JAIDS 1997;16:254; Ann Intern Med 1998;129:18). A placebo-controlled trial of 51 hypogonadal men with AIDS-associated wasting found that replacement dosing (testosterone enanthate 300 mg IM q3wk) was associated with an average gain of 2.6 kg lean body mass over 6 mos (Ann Intern Med 1998;129:18); these results were sustained over 12 mos in an open-label extension (CID 1999;31:1240).

Lipodystrophy: Testosterone may reduce visceral fat and reduce cholesterol; however, studies show minimal effect on body weight or muscle mass (J Clin Eudocrinol Metals 2005;90:1531), and risks include reduced HDL cholesterol, hepatotoxicity, and risk of prostatic cancer (CID 2002;34:248).

Testosterone for wasting in women: A placebo-controlled trial of women with HIV infection and androgen deficiency defined as free testosterone ≤3 pg/mL demonstrated substantial benefit from testosterone patches of 300 μg 2 ×/wk for ≥18 mos (AIDS 2009;23:951). Testosterone was well-tolerated. Benefits included increases in BMI, lean mass, bone mineral density, and sexual function and a decrease in depression.

Indication: Free testosterone <3 pg/mL; weight <90% of ideal body weight or weight loss >10%.

Treatment: Androderm patch (2.5–5.0 mg patch) 2×/wk regimen (men).

Intramuscular: 200–400 mg IM every 2 wks. The dose and dosing interval may need adjustment; many use 100–200 mg IM every week given by self-administration to avoid low levels in the second week; many initiate therapy for wasting with 300–400 mg every 2 wks, with taper to 200 mg when weight is restored, or combine with other anabolic steroids. Replacement doses are 100 mg/wk (CID 2003;36:S73).

Transdermal systems: Advantages are rapid absorption, controlled rate of delivery with less day-to-day variation in testosterone levels, avoidance of first-pass hepatic metabolism, avoidance of IM injections, and possibly less testicular shrinkage. Two delivery systems are available: Skin patches and a topical gel (Androderm) are available in 2–4 mg sizes. Serum testosterone levels peak at 3–8 hrs. After 1 mo, a morning testosterone level should be obtained. The usual dose is a system that delivers 4 mg/d. AndroGel and Testim are rubbed on the skin starting with 5 mg/d. Gel formulations have the advantage of permitting dose titration based on serum testosterone levels.

Controlled substance: Schedule C-lll.

PHARMACOLOGY:

Bioavailability: Poor absorption and rapid metabolism with oral administration. The cypionate and enanthate esters are absorbed slowly from IM injection sites.

Elimination: Hepatic metabolism to 17 ketosteroids that are excreted in urine.

SIDE EFFECTS: Androgenic effects include acne, flushing, gynecomastia, increased libido, priapism, and edema. Other side effects include aggravation of sleep apnea, sodium retention, increased hematocrit, possible promotion of KS, and promotion of breast or prostate cancer. In women, there may be virilization with voice change, hirsutism, and clitoral enlargement. Androgens may cause cholestatic hepatitis. Patches are associated with local reactions, especially pruritus and occasionally blistering, erythema, and pain.

DRUG INTERACTIONS: May potentiate action of oral anticoagulants.

PREGNANCY: Category X. Contraindicated.

Thalidomide

TRADE NAME: Thalomid (Celgene).

FORMULATIONS, REGIMEN, AND COST: 50, 100, and 200 mg capsules; 100 mg cap at $332.88.

AVAILABILITY: Thalidomide is FDA-approved for marketing through a restricted distribution program, System for Thalidomide Education and Prescribing Safety (STEPS). The STEPS Program is designed to eliminate the risk of birth defects by requiring registration of prescribing physicians, patients, and pharmacists, combined with informed consent, rigorous counseling, accountability, and a patient survey. Only physicians registered with STEPS may prescribe thalidomide. Call 888-423-5436 (option 1) to register and receive necessary forms.

Requirements for prescribing: (1) Agreement to patient counseling as indicated in the consent form, (2) patient consent form with one copy sent to Boston University, and (3) completion of the physician monitoring survey. Patients are registered if they (1) agree to use two reliable methods of contraception, (2) have pregnancy tests performed regularly (females), (3) use latex condoms when having sex with women (males), and (4) agree to participate in mandatory and confidential patient survey. Pharmacies must register to dispense thalidomide by agreeing to (1) collect and file informed consent forms, (2) register patients by phone or fax, (3) prescribe no more than a 28-day supply within 7 days of the prescription date, and (4) verify patient registry with refills.

PATIENT ASSISTANCE: 888-423-5436 (press 2).

FDA LABELING: Approved for moderate to severe erythema nodosum leprosum and multiple myeloma.

Regimen: Usual dose is 50–200 mg/d, most commonly 100 mg hs to reduce sedative side effect. Often start at 100–200 mg/d and titrate down to 50 mg/d or give intermittent dosing (JID 2001;183:343). Doses >200–300 mg/d are poorly tolerated (NEJM 1997;336:1487; CID 1997;24:1223).

MECHANISM: Presumed mechanism for HIV-associated wasting is the reduction in TNF-α production (J Exp Med 1991;173:699). Thalidomide also has numerous other antiinflammatory and immunomodulatory properties (Int J Dermatol 1974;13:20; PNAS USA 1993;90:5974; Mol Med 1995;1:384; J Exp Med 1993;177:1675; JAIDS 1997;13:1047).

CLINICAL TRIALS:

Aphthous ulcers: In a placebo-controlled trial using thalidomide (200 mg/d) in patients with oral aphthous ulcers, 16/29 (53%) in the thalidomide arm responded compared with 2/28 (7%) in the placebo group (NEJM 1997;336:1489). ACTG 251 was a placebo-controlled trial involving 45 patients given thalidomide (200 mg/d × 4 wks followed by 100 mg/d for responders and 400 mg/d for nonresponders for oral or esophageal ulcers). Among 23 recipients of thalidomide, 14 (61%) had a complete remission in 4 wks, and 21 (91%) had a complete remission or partial response. In another ACTG trial for patients with aphthous ulcers of the esophagus, thalidomide (200 mg/d) was associated with a complete response at 4 wks in 8 of 11 (73%) (JID 1999;180:61). Ulcers usually heal in 7–28 days. The usual dose for aphthous ulcers is 100–200 mg/d, with increases up to 400–600 mg/d if unresponsive; after healing, discontinue or use maintenance dose of 50 mg/d (J Am Acad Dermatol 1993;28:271; Gen Dent 2007;55:537).

Wasting: Two placebo-controlled trials and three open-label studies demonstrated that thalidomide (daily doses of 50–300 mg/d) for 2–12 wks was associated with significant weight gains. The largest trial showed a dose of 100 mg/d × 8 wks was associated with a mean weight gain of 1.7 kg compared to placebo; half was lean body mass (AIDS Res Hum Retro 2000;16:1345). The recommended dose is 100 mg/d because larger doses do not increase weight gain but cause more side effects (CID 2003;36[suppl 2]:S74).

Miscellaneous conditions: HIV-associated complications with a limited but favorable reported experience include refractory colitis (CID 2008;47:133), Castleman's disease (AIDS 2008;22:1232; Am J Hematol 2006;81:303; Clin Nephrol 2004;61:352), and IRIS (generally not recommended) (Curr HIV/AIDS Rep 2009;6:162).

PHARMACOLOGY:
See AAC 1997;41:2797.

Bioavailability: Well-absorbed.

$T^{1/2}$: 6–8 hr. Peak levels with 200 mg dose are 1.7 µg/mL; levels >4 µg/mL are required to inhibit TNF-α (PNAS USA 1993;90:5974; J Exp Med 1993;177:1675; J Am Acad Dermatol 1996;35:969). It is not known whether thalidomide is present in semen.

Elimination: Nonrenal mechanisms, primarily nonenzymatic hydrolysis in plasma to multiple metabolites. There are no recommendations for dose changes in renal or hepatic failure.

SIDE EFFECTS:

Teratogenic effects: Major concern is use in pregnant women due to high potential for birth defects, including absent or abnormal limbs; cleft lip; absent ears; heart, renal, or genital abnormalities; and other severe defects (Nat Med 1997;3:8). Maximum vulnerability is 35–50 days after the last menstrual period, when a single dose is sufficient to cause severe limb abnormalities in most patients (J Am Acad Dermatol 1996;35:969). It is critical that any woman of childbearing potential not receive thalidomide unless great precautions are taken to prevent pregnancy (pills and barrier protection). Because thalidomide may be present in semen, condom use is recommended for men. Company records indicate that, through January 2001, there were 26,968 patients treated, and there were no documented exposures during pregnancy. Several male exposures followed by conception were noted, but none resulted in birth defects.

Dose effect: Teratogenic effects occur even with single dose. Neuropathy, rash, constipation, neutropenia, and sedation are common dose-related side effects found in up to 50% of AIDS patients and are more frequent with low CD4 cell counts (CID 1997;24:1223; JID 2002;185:1359).

Drowsiness: Most common side effect is the sedation for which the drug was initially marketed. Administer at bedtime and reduce dose to minimize this side effect. There may be morning somnolence or "hangover.".

Rash: Usually pruritic, erythematous, and macular over trunk, back, and proximal extremities. TEN and Stevens-Johnson syndrome have been reported. Rechallenge following erythematous rash has resulted in severe reactions and should only be done with caution.

Neuropathy: Dose-related paresthesias and/or pain of extremities, especially with high doses or prolonged use. This complication may or may not be reversible; it is not known whether the risk is increased by diabetes, alcoholism, or use of neurotoxic drugs including ddI and d4T. Symptoms may start after the drug is discontinued. Neuropathy is a contra-indication to the drug, and neurologic monitoring should be performed for all patients.

HIV: Thalidomide may cause modest increase in plasma levels of HIV RNA ($0.4 \log_{10}$/mL) (NEJM 1997:336:1487).

Neutropenia: Discontinue thalidomide if ANC is <750/mm^3 without an alternative cause.

Constipation: Common; use stool softener, hydration, milk of magnesia, etc.

Less common side effects include dizziness, mood changes, brady-cardia, tachycardia, bitter taste, headache, nausea, pruritus, dry mouth, dry skin, or hypotension.

DRUG INTERACTIONS: The greatest concern is in women of childbearing potential who take concurrent medications, such as rifamycin and possibly PIs, EVG/c, and NNRTIs, that interfere with the effectiveness of contraceptive. Barrier of contraception must be used. Concurrent use of drugs that cause sedation or peripheral neu-ropathy (e.g., ddI, d4T) may increase the frequency and severity of these side effects.

PREGNANCY: Category X (contraindicated).

Tipranavir (TPV)

TRADE NAME: Aptivus (Boehringer-Ingelheim).

CLASS: Protease inhibitor.

FORMULATIONS, REGIMEN, AND COST: Caps, 250 mg at $13.25/cap, $1,590.18/mo; solution 100 mg/mL as 95 mL bottle at $530.04 (price does not include price of required RTV booster).

PATIENT ASSISTANCE: 800-556-8317.

STANDARD DOSE: TPV/r 500/200 mg bid with food.

AVOID: With severe liver disease (Child Pugh Score Class B or C) and avoid use in combination with other PIs, TAF, ETR, EVG/COBI.

STORAGE: TPV must be used within 60 days if stored at room temperature (up to 25°C [77°F]). Refrigerated TPV caps are stable until date on label.

ADVANTAGES: Active against most PI-resistant HIV (Curr HIV Res 2010;8:347); established efficacy in salvage therapy (JAIDS 2007;45:401).

DISADVANTAGES:

Elevated transaminase levels and hyperlipidemia; reduced efficacy with extensive PI resistance (see "Resistance"); multiple drug interactions and inability to combine with other PIs, TAF, EVG/COBI, and ETR; RTV 400 mg/d boosting requirement; higher incidence of hepatitis and hyperlipidemia than other PIs; black box warning of potential for intracranial hemorrhage and hepatic failure; bid dosing; and DRV/r is better tolerated and typically active against most PI-resistant virus.

INDICATION: Highly pretreated adults with resistance to multiple PIs and susceptibility to TPV (preferably those with virus more susceptible to TPV than to DRV). It requires RTV boosting and initially was most effective when combined with ENF in ENF-naïve patients.

CLINICAL TRIALS:

RESIST-1 and -2: Phase III trials of patients who failed at least 2 PI-based regimens, had VL >1,000 c/mL and had at least one primary PI mutation and no more than two at codons 33, 82, 84, and 90. RESIST-1 was conducted with 620 subjects in the United States, Canada, and Australia; RESIST-2 was conducted with 539 evaluable patients in Europe and South America. Participants were randomized to receive TPV/r or one of four alternative boosted PI regimens: LPV/r, IDV/r, SQV/r, or APV/r (Lancet 2006;368:466).

The 1,159 participants had a median baseline VL of 4.8 $\log_{10}$ c/mL, a median CD4 count of 155 cells/mm^3, and an average of 10 PI resistance mutations. Participants with no virologic response in control arm were allowed to roll over to trial 1182.17, which included TPV/r. The NRTI backbone was individualized. Results are summarized in Table 6.89. Response rates correlated with use of enfuvirtide, higher TPV trough level, baseline phenotype resistance test, and by the "TPV score" (0–2 vs. 5–6), determined by the number of the following PI mutations: 10V, 13V, 20M/R, 33F, 35G, 36I, 43T, 46L, 47V, 54A/M/V, 58E, 69K, 74P, 82L/T, 83D, 84V. Virologic results with these variables are summarized in Table 6.90.

BI 1182.52: This dose-finding study in 216 patients who failed ≥2 PI-based regimens (CROI 2003:Abstr. 596) showed that patients with ≥3 of 4 PRAMs (PI resistance-associated mutations at codons 33, 82, 84, and 90) had a reduced response. This was the reason for the limitation of ≤2 PRAMs as an entry criterion for RESIST.

BI 1182.51: This study enrolled simultaneously with RESIST but was restricted to the patients with 3 or 4 PRAMs (JAIDS 2008;47:429). Patients were randomized to TPV/r (n = 61) or to LPV/r (n = 79), APV/r (n = 76), or SQV/r (n = 75). After 14 days TPV/r was added to the regimens of patients in the other three arms. Patients on TPV/r had a median VL decrease of 1.2 $\log_{10}$ c/mL compared to <0.4 $\log_{10}$ c/mL in each of the other arms; the addition of TPV/r to the other regimens resulted in a substantial boost to viral suppression to a median total decrease of 1.2 $\log_{10}$ c/mL at 4 wks. The suppression noted above was not sustained, indicating the need for additional active agents. Pharmacokinetic studies of the dual PI-boosted regimens showed that TPV reduced C_{min} of the concurrent PIs by 55–81%, presumably due to P450 and P-gp induction. For this reason, dual-boosted PI therapy with these TPV combinations is not recommended.

TPV/r vs. LPV/r: A subset analysis of RESIST-1 compared 24-wk results for patients randomized to either TPV/r or LPV/r. Response was significantly better in the TPV/r recipients in terms of VL reduction ≥1 $\log_{10}$ c/mL (40% vs. 21%), proportion with VL <400 c/mL (34% vs. 25%) and mean CD4 response (+31/mm^3 vs. +6/mm^3)

TABLE 6.89 RESIST-1 and -2: Results at 48 wks

	TPV/r n = 749	CPI/r[a] n = 737
Baseline[b]		
VL ($\log_{10}$ c/mL) (mean)	4.7	4.7
CD4 count (mean;/mm³)	196	195
PI mutations (median)	10	10
Prior antiretroviral agents (median)	12	12
Results at 48 wks		
Completed 48 wks	541 (73%)	230 (31%)[c]
VL <400 c/mL with ENF without ENF	30.4%.	13.8%[c].
	43%.	19%[c].
	27%	13%[c]
VL <50 c/mL	23%	10%[c]
Reduction in VL ($\log_{10}$ c/mL) with ENF	–1.14	0.5
CD4 count increase	48/mm³	21/mm³[c]
Withdrawals for adverse event/ 100 pt-yr exposure	12.4	10.6
Grade 3/4 events/100 pt-yr exposure[d]	64	64
Results at 96 wks[e]		
VL <400 c/mL	26.9%	10.9%
VL <50 c/mL.	20.4%.	9.1%.
with ENF	35%	14%

From Lancet 2006;368:466.

[a] Comparator PI: LPV/r, IDV/r, SQV/r or APV/r.

[b] All results are mean values unless otherwise indicated.

[c] P ≤0.0001.

[d] TPV was associated with significantly more grade 3/4 elevations of triglycerides (31% vs. 23%) and ALT (10% vs. 3%).

[e] 8th Int Congress on Drug Therapy in HIV Infection, Glasgow, 2006, Abstr. P23.

TABLE 6.90 Response correlates in RESIST-1 and -2

		VL Decrease $\log_{10}$ c/mL
TPV score (6 mo)	0–1 mutations	–2.10
	2–3 mutations	–0.89
	4–7 mutations	–0.46
	8–9 mutations	–0.08
Baseline phenotype (48 wks)	IC_{90} fold change 0–3	–1.02
	IC90 fold change >3–10	–0.27
ENF (48 wks)	ENF	–1.67
	No ENF	–0.98

From Lancet 2006;368:466 and package insert (11/15/06).

(AIDS 2007;21:2734). Virologic response was greater in both groups when ENF was used concurrently; VL decreased >1 $\log_{10}$ c/mL at 24 wks in 58% of 293 TPV/r recipients and 26% of 290 LPV/r recipients.

Utilize: Observational study at 40 US sites in which 236 patients failing a PI-based regimen had resistance tests showing 139 (59%) had a PI resistance mutation, and >50% were sensitive to DRV or TPV; other PIs showed that <22% were sensitive (Curr HIV Res 2010;8:347). These data suggest that the most predictably active PIs in patients with multiple PI failures are DRV and TPV.

RESISTANCE: Mutations that contribute to resistance are 10V, 13V, 20M/R/V, 33F, 35G, 36I, 43T, 46L, 47V, 54A/M/V, 56E, 69K, 74P, 82L/T, 83D, and 84V (Topics HIV Med 2008;16:62; J Virol 2006;80:10794). Accumulation of these mutations reduces response. The best response is seen with ≤1 TPV mutation. Intermediate response is seen with 2–7 mutations; with ≥8 mutations, response is minimal. Nevertheless, some of these are more important. The mutations with the greatest impact on resistance are 74P, 47V, 58E, and 82L/T (AIDS Rev 2008;10:125). Clinical cutoffs for TPV susceptibility using the PhenoSense or PhenoSense GT assays are changes of 2- and 8-fold. Corresponding cutoffs using the VircoTYPE assay are 1.2 and 5.4. Mutations at 30N, 50V, and 88D are associated with TPV hypersusceptibility (HIV Clin Trials 2004;5:371; Expert Rev Anti Infect Ther 2005;3:9; Antivir Ther 2010;15:959).

An alternative TPV-weighted mutation score has been proposed based on week 8 of treatment (Antiviral Ther 2010;15:1011). Mutations are assigned the following score:

4 + : 74P, 82 L/T, 83D and 47V.
3 + : 58E and 84V.
2 + : 36I, 43T and 54A/M/V.
1 + : 10V, 33F and 46L.
−2: 76V.
−4: 50L/V.
−6: 54L.

(Score interpretation: sensitive, ≤3; partially sensitive, 4–9; resistant, ≥10.).

The most common TPV-associated resistance mutations that occur during failed TPV therapy are 10I, 13V, 33V/F, 36V/I/L, 82/T/L, and 84V (AIDS 2007;21:179). Note that DRV failures are often associated with the 54L mutation, which confers with TPV hypersusceptibility (AAC 2010;54:3018). Other reports indicate that resistance to both DRV and TPV is rare (AAC 2010;54:2479).

PHARMACOLOGY:

Bioavailability: Oral absorption is substantially improved with a concurrent high-fat meal. RTV given concurrently increases TPV 29-fold and should always be used in combination with TPV. CNS penetration is poor (Neurology 2011;76:693).

$T^{1/2}$: 6 hr.

Excretion: Most of TPV is eliminated in stool; 5% is found in urine.

Dose adjustment for renal failure: None.

Dose adjustment for hepatic failure: Not established. TPV/r is contraindicated with moderate or severe hepatic disease (Child-Pugh class B or C).

TPV is a substrate of CYP3A4 and Pgp. TPV/r has a net inhibitory effect on CYP3A4 and is a potent inducer of Pgp.

DRUG INTERACTIONS:

RTV: RTV 200 mg bid increases TPV levels 29-fold and is required for TPV to achieve therapeutic levels.

NRTIs: Must be dosed ≥2 hr before or after ddI EC; ddI AUC decreased by 40%; clinical significance not known. AZT and ABC concentrations decreased by 40–50%; dose adjustment is not established (package insert). No clinically significant interactions with 3TC, d4T, or TDF (2018 DHHS Guidelines). TAF may be decreased; avoid.

MVC: No dose adjustment necessary; use standard dose.

RAL: RAL C_{min} ↓55%, but no change in AUC; use standard dose.

DTG: Cmin decreased 76%. DTG 50 mg bid can be used with TPV/r only in patients with no INSTI resistant mutations.

EVG/COBI: No data; avoid; May be co-administered with EVG 150 mg/d + TPV/r 500/200 mg bid.

BIC: No data. Avoid.

NNRTIs: No interaction with EFV or NVP. ETR AUC decreased by 76%; avoid.

PIs: Studies combining PIs with TPV/r showed that the drug induced P450 and Pgp, resulting in a 50–80% reduction in the C_{min} levels of LPV, FPV, ATV, and SQV. Therefore, these PIs should not be co-administered with TPV. There are no data for concurrent administration of NFV, IDV, or DRV, but the assumption is that these drugs will be affected in a similar way.

Drugs to avoid: Antiarrhythmics (amiodarone, bepridil, flecainide, propafenone, quinidine, dronedarone), ergot derivatives, lovastatin, simvastatin, pimozide, rifampin, rifapentine, triazolam, midazolam, St. John's wort, astemizole, terfenadine, cisapride, ranolazine, lurasidone, dronedarone, alfuzosin, dofetilide, eplerenone, lurasidone, ivabradine, flibanserin, dexamethasone (at steady-state) salmeterol, fluticasone, fentanyl, rivaroxaban, betrixaban, vorapaxar, silodosin, enzalutamide, mitotane.

Dose adjustment needed with edoxaban, apixiban, and dabigatran based on renal function and indication.

Other drugs use with caution: Alprazolam: increase alprazolam levels; consider lorazepam, temazepam, oxazepam.

Antacids: decrease TPV AUC 25–30%; take ≥2 hr apart.

Antiplatelet drugs (ASA, NSAIDs, clopidogrel, ticlopidine, ticagrelor): May increase risk of bleeding. Avoid co-administration. *Atorvastatin*: atorvastatin AUC increased 9×; use with caution starting with lowest dose (10 mg) and avoiding high doses (e.g., >40 mg/d) or use rosuvastatin (AUC increased 37%; start with 5 mg) or pitavastin, pravastatin.

Buprenorphine: Norbuprenorphine AUC decreased by 80%. TPV trough decreased by 19–40%. Consider TPV TDM.

Benzodiazepines: Avoid clorazepate, estazolam, flurazepam; consider lorazepam, oxazepam, or temazepam.

Calcium channel blockers: May increase levels of calcium channel blockers; monitor closely.

Carbamazepine: AUC increased 26%; may decrease TPV levels; consider valproic acid, lamotrigine, levetiracetam, or topiramate.

Clarithromycin: Increases TPV and clarithromycin levels; no dose adjustment necessary with normal renal function; decrease clarithromycin dose by 75% with CrCl <30 mL/min and by 50% with CrCl 30–60 mL/min.

Colchicine: TPV/r increases colchicine level; co-administer dose adjusted colchicine only after TPV/r has reached steady-state (7 days).

Corticosteroids (dexamethasone with multiple dose): May decrease TPV levels, use with caution.

Cyclosporine: May increase cyclosporine levels; monitor levels.

ddI EC: Separate doses of TPV and ddI EC by 2 hrs.

Desipramine: May increase desipramine, reduce desipramine dose and monitor.

Disulfiram/metronidazole: TPV caps contain 76% alcohol per 100-mg cap and may cause disulfiram-like reactions; avoid.

Ethinyl estradiol: EE AUC reduced 50%; use alternative birth control.

Fluticasone: Risk of increased steroid levels; avoid combination; consider beclomethasone.

Flecainide: Flecainide levels increased; contraindicated.

Fluconazole: TPV AUC increased 56%; limit fluconazole dose to ≤200 mg/d; monitor LFTs. Consider alternative PI if fluconazole >250 mg is needed.

Halofantrine (not available in the United States), *lumefantrine*: Not recommended; risk of inducing torsades de pointes.

Itraconazole and ketonazole: Azole and TPV levels may be increased; consider fluconazole.

Meperidine: May decrease meperidine levels and increase metabolite normeperidine, which may cause seizures.

Methadone: Decrease R-methadone AUC levels 50%. May need to increase methadone dose.

Nifedipine: May increase nifedipine levels; avoid.

Paclitaxel: Possible increase in paclitaxel levels; monitor closely.

Phenobarbital/Phenytoin: May decrease TPV levels and increase or decrease phenobarbital levels; consider valproic acid, lamotrigine, levetiracetam, or topiramate.

Rifampin: Decrease TPV levels; contraindicated.

Rifabutin: RBT levels increased 2.9×; use RBT 150 mg q24h. Consider rifabutin TDM.

Sildenafil: Increased sildenafil levels; limit to ≤25 mg in 48 hr.
Tacrolimus: increased levels of tacrolimus; use reduced doses.
Tadalafil: ≤10 mg q72h. For the treatment of pulmonary hypertension; start with tadalafil 20 mg/d only after TPV/r has reached steady state (>7 days).

Theophylline: may increase levels of theophylline; consider therapeutic monitoring.

Vardenafil: increased levels of vardenafil; do not exceed 2.5 mg q72h (with RTV).

Voriconazole: may decrease voriconazole levels and increase TPV levels; avoid (use amphotericin or caspofungin) or monitor voriconazole levels carefully.

SIDE EFFECTS: With the exceptions of hepatitis and hyperlipidemia, and GI intolerance, the side effects profile is similar to that of other PIs. The most common side effects are GI intolerance, headache, hypertriglyceridemia, rash, fatigue, and increases in transaminase levels (grade 3/4 increases in 8%).

Hepatotoxicity with clinical hepatitis, sometimes with hepatic failure and death, has been reported. Hepatotoxicity is more common in patients with HBV or HBC co-infection. Indications to discontinue TPV/r based on grade 3/4 transaminase increases are unclear.

GI intolerance includes nausea (5%) and diarrhea (4–10%). Less frequent side effects are fatigue, headache, and abdominal pain.

Rash: More common in women (13% vs. 8%).

Hyperlipidemia: Increases in total cholesterol, LDL-C, and triglycerides (grade 3/4 increases in triglyceride elevations in 31% of RESIST participants who received TPV/r vs. 23% of controls) are common; serum lipid levels should be monitored.

Intracranial bleeding: Includes fatal and nonfatal cases, but did not correlate with abnormal coagulation parameters. Most had recent head surgery, head trauma, or similar risk factors. Review of Boehringer-Ingelheim records found 13 cases, including 8 fatal intracranial hemorrhages in 6,840 HIV-infected patients in clinical trials (J Infect 2008;57:85). The cause may be related to inhibition of platelet aggregation.

BLACK BOX WARNING: Fatal and nonfatal intracranial hemorrhage and clinical hepatitis including fatal cases.

PREGNANCY: Category C. The 2018 DHHS Guidelines on Antiretroviral Agents in Pregnancy list TPV as "not recommended in treatment-naïve patients.".

Trazodone

TRADE NAME: Desyrel (Bristol-Myers Squibb) and generic.

CLASS: Nontricyclic antidepressant.

FORMULATIONS, REGIMEN, AND COST: Tabs: 50 mg at $0.56, 100 mg at $0.73, 150 mg at $1.46, 300 mg at $5.43. Extended release tablet-24 h 150 mg and 300 mg tablet at $3.84.

INDICATIONS AND DOSE REGIMENS:

Depression: Especially when associated with anxiety or insomnia: 400–600 mg hs. Increase dose 50 mg every 3–4 days up to maximum dose of 400 mg/d for outpatients and 600 mg/d for hospitalized patients.

Insomnia: 50–150 mg qhs.

PHARMACOLOGY:

Bioavailability: >90%, improved if taken with meals.

$T^{1/2}$: 6 hr.

Elimination: Hepatic metabolism, then renal excretion.

SIDE EFFECTS: Adverse effects are dose- and duration-related and are usually seen with doses >300 mg/d; may decrease with continued use, dose reduction, or schedule change.

Major side effects: Sedation in 15–20%; orthostatic hypotension (5%); nervousness; fatigue; dizziness; nausea; vomiting; and anticholinergic effects (dry mouth, blurred vision, constipation, urinary retention). *Rare:* Priapism (1/6,000); agitation; cardiovascular; and anticholinergic side effects are less frequent and less severe than with tricyclics.

DRUG INTERACTIONS: LPV/r, COBI and RTV increase trazodone levels; avoid or use low dose trazodone. Trazodone may increase levels of phenytoin and digoxin; alcohol and other CNS depressants potentiate sedative side effects. Contraindicated with SQV/r due to potential for additive QTc prolongation.

PREGNANCY: Category C.

Tricyclic Antidepressants—see also Nortriptyline

Tricyclic antidepressants elevate mood, increase physical activity, improve appetite, improve sleep patterns, and reduce morbid preoccupations in most patients with major depression. The following principles apply:

FORMULATIONS, REGIMEN, AND COST:

INDICATIONS:

Psychiatric indications: Major depression: Response rates are 60–70%. Low doses are commonly used for adjustment disorders including depression and anxiety. Usual therapeutic dose for depression is 50–150 mg hs for nortriptyline and 100–300 mg hs for amitriptyline.

Peripheral neuropathy: Controlled trials have not shown benefit in AIDS-associated peripheral neuropathy, but clinical experience is extensive and results in diabetic neuropathy are good. If used, choice of agents depends on time of symptoms (JAMA 1998;280:1590).

Night pain: Amitriptyline (most sedating) start with 25 mg hs. *Day pain*: Nortriptyline (less sedating and less of an anticholinergic effect) start with 25 mg hs. Some recommend therapeutic drug monitoring for depression, but generally not for peripheral neuropathy.

Dose: Initial treatment of depression is 4–8 wks, required for therapeutic response. Initial dose is usually given at bedtime, especially with insomnia or if sedation is a side effect.

Common mistakes are use of an initial dose that is too high, resulting in excessive anticholinergic side effects or oversedation. The dose is increased every 3–4 days depending on tolerance and response. Treatment of major depression usually requires continuation for 4–5 mos after response. Multiple recurrences may require long-term treatment.

SERUM LEVELS: Efficacy correlates with serum levels of nortriptyline when used as an antidepressant. Therapeutic monitoring of drug levels allows dose titration. Target level for nortriptyline is 70–125 ng/dL.

PHARMACOLOGY: Well-absorbed, extensively metabolized, long half-life, variable use of serum levels (see below).

SIDE EFFECTS: Anticholinergic effects (dry mouth, dizziness, blurred vision, constipation, tachycardia, urinary hesitancy, sedation), sexual dysfunction, orthostatic hypotension, weight gain, QTc prolongation (with PIs use with caution).

RELATIVE CONTRAINDICATIONS: Cardiac conduction block (avoid with RTV >400 bid). With PI/r, PI/c, EVG/c co-administration, decrease TCA dose and titrate slowly. Prostatism and narrow angle glaucoma reported. *Less common side effects*: Mania, hypomania, allergic skin reactions, marrow suppression, seizures, tardive dyskinesia, tremor, speech blockage, anxiety, insomnia, parkinsonism, hyponatremia; cardiac conduction disturbances and arrhythmias (most common serious side effects are with overdosage).

Trimethoprim (TMP)

TRADE NAME: Generic.

FORMULATIONS, REGIMEN, AND COST: Tabs: 100 mg at $0.68; oral solution 50 mg/5 mL (473 mL) at $480.00.

INDICATIONS AND DOSE REGIMENS:

PCP (with sulfamethoxazole as TMP-SMX or with dapsone): 5 mg/kg po tid (usually 300 mg tid or qid) × 21 days.

UTIs (uncomplicated): 100 mg po bid or 200 mg/d × 3–14 days.

PHARMACOLOGY:

Bioavailability: >90%.

$T^{1/2}$: 9–11 hrs.

Excretion: Renal.

Dose modification with renal failure: CrCl >50 mL/min, full dose; 10–50 mL/min, one-half to two-thirds dose; <30 mL/min, one-third to one-half dose.

SIDE EFFECTS: Usually well-tolerated; most common are pruritus and skin rash; GI intolerance; marrow suppression (anemia, neutropenia, thrombocytopenia); antifolate effects (prevent with leucovorin; reversible hyperkalemia in 20–50% of AIDS patients given high doses) (Ann Intern Med 1993;119:291,296; NEJM 1993;238:703).

DRUG INTERACTIONS: Increased activity of phenytoin (monitor levels) and procainamide; levels of both dapsone and trimethoprim are increased when given concurrently.

PREGNANCY: Category C. Teratogenic in rats with high doses; limited experience in patients shows no association with congenital abnormalities.

Trimethoprim-Sulfamethoxazole (TMP-SMX, cotrimoxazole)

TRADE NAME: Bactrim (Roche), Septra (Monarch), and generic.

FORMULATIONS, REGIMEN, AND COST: TMP/SMX 80/400 mg (SS) tabs at $0.66; 160/800 mg (DS) tabs at $1.72. oral suspension 200/40 mg per 5 mL (473 mL) at $112.94. For IV use: 10 mL vials with 16/80 mg/mL at $5.35/10 mL.

INDICATIONS AND DOSE REGIMENS.

PCP prophylaxis: 1 DS qd or 1 SS qd; alternative is 1 DS 3×/wk. Discontinuation of PCP prophylaxis after ART-associated immune reconstitution (CD4 >200/mm^3 for >3 mos) is safe and avoids significant toxicity (CID 2001;33:1901; MMWR 2002;51[RR-8]:4). PCP prophylaxis with TMP-SMX reduces the frequency of bacterial pneumonia and other bacterial infections (CID 2006;43:90).

Graduated initiation to reduce adverse effects (ACTG 268) (JAIDS 2000;24:337): Oral preparation (40 mg trimethoprim and 200 mg sulfamethoxazole/5 mL), 1 mL qd × 3 d, then 2 mL qd × 3 d, then 5 mL qd × 3 d, then 10 mL qd × 3 d, then 20 mL qd × 3 d, then 1 TMP- SMX DS tab qd.

PCP treatment: 5 mg/kg (trimethoprim component) po or IV q8h × 21 days, usually 2 DS po q8h (70 kg). A review of 1,188 episodes of HIV-associated PCP in Europe showed TMP-SMX was the most frequent first line agent (81%), had the lowest rate of drug change for failure or toxicity (21%) and the best survival rate (85%) (JAC 2009;64:1282).

Toxoplasmosis prophylaxis: 1 DS qd.

Toxoplasmosis treatment: Alternative to pyrimethamine/sulfadiazine: acute therapy (>6 wks) TMP-SMX 5 mg/kg (TMP) PO or IV bid × ≥6 wks, then maintenance at half dose (Eur J Clin Microbiol Infect Dis 1992;11:125; AAC 1998;42:1346; Cochrane Database Syst Rev 2006;19:CD005420).

Isospora: 1 DS po qid × 10 days; may need maintenance with 1–2 DS/d. *IDSA recommendation*: TMP-SMX 1 DS bid × 7–10 days, then 1 DS 3×/wk or 1 Fansidar/wk indefinitely.

Salmonella: 1 DS po bid × 5–7 days; treat >14 days if relapsing.

Nocardia: 4–6 DS/d × ≥6 mos.

Urinary tract infections: 1 DS bid × 3–14 days.

Prophylaxis for cystitis: Half SS tab daily.

Malaria prophylaxis: TMP-SMX is effective prophylaxis for PCP and has proved highly effective for preventing malaria (Lancet 2006;367:1256). Initial results in malaria-endemic areas shows TMP-SMX prophylaxis for PCP does not select for TMP-SMX–resistant malaria (Ann J Trop Med Hyg 2006;75:375).

ACTIVITY: TMP-SMX is effective in the treatment or prophylaxis of infections involving *P. jiroveci*, most methicillin-sensitive *S. aureus* (MSSA), >80% of community-associated MRSA (USA

300 strains), *Legionella, Listeria,* and common urinary tract pathogens. TMP/SMX is used preferentially in low-resource countries for CNS toxoplasmosis with good results (Am J Trop Med Hyg 2009;80:583) and is the preferred agent if pyrimethamine/sulfadiazine is not available (2017 OI guidelines). Some studies show increasing rates of mutations in the dihydropteroate synthase gene of *P. jiroveci* that are associated with increased resistance to sulfonamides and dapsone (JID 1999;180:1969); a meta-analysis found that this mutation is associated with prolonged exposure to sulfonamides, but the clinical significance of these mutations in terms of reduced response is unclear (Emerg Infect Dis 2004;10:1760). In clinical trials, clinical outcome has not been worse with DHS mutation when these patients were treated with TMP-SMX (Lancet 2001;358:545; Emerg Infect Dis 2004;10:1721; Proc Am Therac Soc 2006;3:655). Current rates of resistance of *S. pneumoniae* to TMP-SMX are about 15–30% (AAC 2002;46:2651; NEJM 2000;343:1917), but their significance is questioned (Proc Am Thoracic Soc 2006;3:655). A systematic review of the literature suggested that TMP-SMX prophylaxis does not promote resistance to other antibiotics (CID 2011;52:1184).

PHARMACOLOGY:

Bioavailability: >90% absorbed with oral administration (both drugs).

$T^{1/2}$: Trimethoprim, 8–15 hr; sulfamethoxazole 7–12 hr.

Elimination: Renal; $T^{1/2}$ in renal failure increases to 24 hrs for trimethoprim and 22–50 hrs for sulfamethoxazole.

Renal failure: CrCl >30 mL/min, usual dose; 10–30 mL/min, one-half to two-thirds dose; <10 mL/min, manufacturer recommends avoidance, but one-third to one-half dose may be used for PCP.

SIDE EFFECTS: Noted in 10% of patients without HIV infection and about 50% of patients with HIV. The gradual initiation of TMP-SMX noted above results in a 50% reduction in adverse reactions (JAIDS 2000;24:337), suggesting that it is not a true hypersensitivity reaction. The prevailing opinion is that these side effects are usually due to toxic metabolites ascribed to altered metabolism of TMP-SMX with HIV infection. The presumed benefit from gradual initiation is to permit time for enzyme induction. A Cochrane Library review examined three strategies with TMP-SMX reaction: treat through, rechallenge, or desensitize (Cochrane Database Syst Rev 2007;CD005646). Best results were achieved with desensitization (see Tables 6.91 and 6.92).

> *Most common*: Nausea, vomiting, pruritus, rash, fever, neutropenia, and increased transaminases. Many HIV-infected patients may be treated despite side effects (GI intolerance and rash) if symptoms are not disabling; alternative with PCP prophylaxis is dose reduction usually after drug holiday (1–2 wks) and/or "desensitization" (see below).
>
> *Rash*: Most common is erythematous, maculopapular, morbilliform, and/or pruritic rash, usually 7–14 days after treatment is started. Less common are erythema multiforme, epidermal necrolysis, exfoliative dermatitis, Stevens-Johnson syndrome, urticaria, and Henoch-Schönlein purpura.

TABLE 6.91 Rapid TMP-SMX desensitization schedule

Time (hr)	Dose (TMP/SMX)	Dilution
0	0.004/0.02 mg	1:10,000 (5 mL)
1	0.04/0.2 mg	1:1,000 (5 mL)
2	0.4/2.0 mg	1:100 (5 mL)
3	4/20 mg	1:10 (5 mL)
4	40/200 mg	(5 mL)
5	160/800 mg	Tablet

TABLE 6.92 Eight-Day TMP-SMX desensitization schedule

Day	Dilution
1	1:1,000,000
2	1:100,000
3	1:10,000
4	1:1,000
5	1:100
6	1:10
7	1:1
8	Standard suspension – 1 mL 40 mg SMX – 8 mg TMP
9	1 DS tab/d

GI intolerance is common with nausea, vomiting, anorexia, and abdominal pain; rare side effects include *C. difficile* diarrhea/colitis and pancreatitis.

Hematologic side effects include neutropenia, anemia, and/or thrombocytopenia. The rate of anemia is increased in patients with HIV infection and with folate depletion. Some respond to leucovorin (5–15 mg/d), but this is not routinely recommended.

Neurologic toxicity may include tremor, ataxia, apathy, aseptic meningitis, and ankle clonus (Am J Med Sci 1996;312:27).

Hepatitis with cholestatic jaundice and hepatic necrosis has been described.

Hyperkalemia in 20–50% of patients given trimethoprim in doses >15 mg/kg/d (NEJM 1993;328:703). The risk is particularly great with co-administration of ACE inhibitors, Arbs, β-blockers, and potassium-sparing diuretics.

Interstitial nephritis with or without urine eosinophils: Pseudo-elevation of serum creatinine of ≥17.6% without affecting GFR (Chemotherapy 1981;27:229).

Altered flora: Chronic administration of TMP-SMX may increase rates of resistance to this and other antibiotics for bacteria in the normal flora including *E. coli* and *S. pneumoniae* (JAIDS 2008;47:585; J Infect 2008;56:171).

PROTOCOL FOR ORAL DESENSITIZATION OR "DETOXIFICATION":

Rapid desensitization (CID 1995;20:849): Serial 10-fold dilutions of oral suspension (40 mg TMP, 200 mg SMX/5 mL) given hourly over 4 hrs.

Note: A prospective trial showed no difference in outcome with desensitization compared with rechallenge (Biomed Pharmacother 2000;54:45).

8-day protocol: Serial dilutions prepared by pharmacists using oral suspension (40 mg TMP, 200 mg SMX/5 mL). Medication is given 4 times daily for 7 days in doses of 1 cc, 2 cc, 4 cc, and 8 cc using the following dilutions: Table 6.92

DRUG INTERACTIONS: Increased levels of oral anticoagulants, phenytoin, and procainamide. Risk of megaloblastic anemia with methotrexate.

PREGNANCY: Category C. The two issues are birth defects with first-trimester exposures and hyperbilirubinemia and kernicterus with exposure near delivery. A systematic review of data through July 2005 showed minimal risk of kernicterus with late pregnancy exposures; with first-trimester exposures there was "mixed evidence linking first-trimester exposures to cleft lips, neural tube defects, cardiovascular defects, and urinary tract defects" (AIDS Rev 2006;8:24). The conclusion is that the risk is small, and TMP-SMX is considered safe for pregnant women in developing countries as currently recommended by the WHO. In the US, recommendation is to use TMP-SMX with caution due to possible kernicterus, although no cases of kernicterus have been reported (CID 1995;21[suppl 1]:S24). The 2018 DHHS Opportunistic Infection Guidelines recommend TMP-SMX in pregnancy when indicated, while acknowledging a small increased risk of birth defects associated with first-trimester exposure. This should be accompanied by the standard folic acid supplement of 0.4 mg/d; it is unclear if higher doses would provide additional protection. Ultrasound at weeks 18–20 is recommended due to possible kernicterus, although no cases of kernicterus have been reported (CID 1995;21[suppl 1]:S24).

Trizivir—see Zidovudine, Lamivudine, and Abacavir

Truvada—see Tenofovir and Emtricitabine

Valacyclovir—see Acyclovir

Valganciclovir—see Ganciclovir

Valcyte—see Ganciclovir

Vibramycin—see Doxycycline

Videx—see Didanosine

Viracept—see Nelfinavir

Viramune—see Nevirapine

Vitrasert—see Ganciclovir

Voriconazole

TRADE NAME: Vfend (Pfizer) and generic.
CLASS: Triazole antifungal.

FORMULATIONS, REGIMEN, AND COST: Tabs: 50 mg at $11.71, 200 mg at $46.91; Vial for IV use: 200 mg at $152.58. Oral suspension (200 mg/5 mL) at $1055.30 per 75-mL bottle.

Regimens:

Oral: 300 mg (6 mg/kg) po bid × 1 day (loading dose), then 4 mg/kg (200–300) mg po bid on an empty stomach. Avoid high-fat meal. Usual dose for aspergillosis or severe infections is 300 mg bid; 100–150 mg bid for patients <40 kg. Monitor voriconazole concentrations due to high degree of variability in voriconazole levels attributed to variable metabolism due to age, hepatic disease, genetic polymorphisms and drug interactions, especially omeprazole (CID 2008;46:201).

IV: 6 mg/kg IV q12h × 2 doses (loading dose), then 3–4 mg/kg IV q12h.

Hepatic failure: 6 mg/kg q12h ×2 doses, then use half-dose 2 mg/kg q12h.

Renal failure: Use standard oral dose.

In vitro activity: Active against most *Candida* species, including many fluconazole-resistant strains. Voriconazole is 16- to 32-fold more active than fluconazole against *Candida* (JCL 2007;45:70). Active against >98% of *C. albicans, C. krusei, C. tropicalis,* and *C. parapsilosis* (AAC 2002;46:1032; J Med Microbiol 2002;51:479; J Clin Microbiol 2002;40:852). Very active against most *Aspergillus*; more active in vitro than itraconazole (J Infect Chemotherapy 2000;6:101; CID 2002;34:563; JCL 2002;40:2648; AAC 2002;46:1032). More recent reviews indicate persistence of good activity (Med Mycol 2008;12:1).

Zygomycetes (mucor) are less susceptible; posaconazole preferred (AAC 2002;46:2708; AAC 2002;46:1581; AAC 2002;46:1032). Activity against *Scedosporium apiospermum* (*Pseudoallescheria boydii*) is variable (AAC 2002;46:62). Most dermatophytes are sensitive (AAC 2001;45:2524). *C. neoformans* is usually highly susceptible with in vitro activity superior to both fluconazole and itraconazole but minimal experience clinically (Eur J Clin Microbiol 2000;19:317; AAC 1999;43:1463; AAC 1999;43:169). Also active in vitro against *H. capsulatum, B. dermatitidis,* and *Penicillium marneffei.*

FDA APPROVAL: Voriconazole is approved for treatment of (1) invasive aspergillosis, (2) serious infections caused by *Scedosporium apiospermum* and *Fusarium* spp., (3) esophageal candidiasis, and (4) candidemia in the non-neutropenic host.

CLINICAL TRIALS: Major clinical trial compared voriconazole (6 mg/kg IV q12h × 2 doses, then 4 mg/kg IV q12h × ≥7 days, then oral voriconazole 200 mg bid) with amphotericin B (1.0–1.5 mg/kg/ d IV) in 277 patients with invasive *Aspergillus*. Voriconazole had a significantly better response rate (53% vs. 32%), better 12-wk survival (71% vs. 58%), and less toxicity (NEJM 2002;347:408).

PHARMACOLOGY:

Oral bioavailability: 96%; AUC reduced by 24% when taken with high-fat meal.

Tissue penetration: Autopsy studies show good penetration into lung, brain, liver, kidneys, spleen, and myocardium (AAC 2010;2011;55:925). Preliminary data suggest that effective levels are achieved in CSF (Br J Harmalol 1997:97:663).

Loading dose: Day 1; without loading dose, the maintenance dose requires 6 days to reach steady state.

Metabolism: Metabolized primarily by P450 CYP2C19 >> 2C9 > 3A4 enzymes. >94% of metabolite is excreted in urine; metabolites have little or no antifungal activity; <2% parenteral formulation is excreted in urine. Review of 181 level measurements showed great variation ranging from <1 mg/L in 25% to >5.5 mg/L in 31% (CID 2008;46:201). The high levels were associated with omeprazole co- therapy and IV therapy; there was CNS toxicity with high levels that cleared when the drug was stopped.

Hepatic failure: AUC increases 2.3-fold; use 100 mg bid.

$T^{1/2}$: 6–24 hr.

Levels: Target C_{min} >2.05 µg/mL (Antimicrob Ag Chem 2006;50:1570) and C_{trough} <5.5 µg/mL (CID 2008;46:212).

SIDE EFFECTS:

Visual effects are most common; 30% in clinical trials; these include altered visual perception, color change, blurred vision, and/or photophobia. Changes are dose related, reversible, and infrequently require discontinuing therapy, but patients should be warned.

Rash in 6%, including rare cases of Stevens-Johnson syndrome, erythema multiforme, and toxic epidermal necrolysis.

Hepatotoxicity: Elevated transaminases in 13%, usually resolves with continued drug administration. Serious hepatic toxicity is rare, but manufacturer recommends monitoring liver enzymes.

Toxic encephalopathy attributed to high levels has been reported (AAC 2007;51:137; CID 2008;46:212). Response has been rapid and complete with stopping the drug.

DRUG INTERACTIONS: Inhibition of P450 enzymes primarily CYP2C19 and to a lesser extent 2C9 and 3A4 (AAC 2002;46:3091). Drug interactions with boosted PIs, NNRTIs, and MVC are extensive (Ann Pharm 2008/42:698).

Contraindicated for concurrent use: Decreased voriconazole levels: Rifampin, rifabutin, rifabutin, carbamazepine, ritonavir (≥400 mg bid), St. John's Wort, and phenobarbital. *Increased concurrent drug levels*: Sirolimus, terfenadine, astemizole, cisapride, pimozide, quinidine, ergot derivatives.

Alter dose:

May significantly increase silodosin, dospirenone, rivaroxaban, betrixaban, ticagrelor, vorapaxar, edoxaban, apixiban, and dabigatran. Consult FDA labeling for dose modification.

Cyclosporine: Increased cyclosporine; use half dose cyclosporine and monitor levels.

Tacrolimus: increased tacrolimus levels 3-fold; use one-third dose tacrolimus; monitor levels.

Warfarin: May increase prothrombin time; monitor.

Statins: Increased simvastatin lovastatin levels; consider pravastatin, pitavastatin, rosuvastatin, or atorvastatin.

Benzodiazepines: Midazolam, triazolam, and alprazolam increased levels expected; reduce benzodiazepine dose or consider lorazepam.

Calcium channel blockers: Nifedipine and felodipine level increases expected; may need dose decrease.

Methadone: Increases methadone's pharmacologically active R-enantiomer by a mean of 47%. There were no cases of withdrawal or detectable overdose among 16 methadone recipients given voriconazole 200 mg/d (AAC 2007;51:110). Caution is advised, since reduced dose of methadone may be indicated.

Sulfonylureas: Tolbutamide, glipizide and glyburide level increases expected; monitor blood glucose.

Vinca alkaloids: Increased vincristine and vinblastine levels expected; dose may be reduced to avoid neurotoxicity.

Phenytoin: Decreased voriconazole 70% and increase phenytoin levels 80%; use voriconazole 400 mg po q12h or 5 mg/kg q12h; monitor phenytoin levels.

Omeprazole: AUC increased 4-fold; voriconazole C_{max} and AUC increased 15% and 40%, respectively; reduce omeprazole to half dose (Br J Clin Pharm 2003;56 Suppl 1:56).

Oral contraceptives: Ethinyl estradiol AUC increased 61%, norethindrone AUC increased 53%; monitor for ADRs related to these oral contraceptives.

Clopidogrel: May decrease efficacy of clopidogrel; avoid.

Colchicine: voriconazole may increase colchicine level; consider decreasing colchicine dose.

PREGNANCY: Category D. Avoid; teratogenic in rodents and congenital anomalies in rabbits.

Xanax—see Alprazolam

Zerit—see Stavudine

Ziagen—see Abacavir

Zidovudine (AZT, ZDV)

TRADE NAME: Retrovir, Combivir (AZT/3TC), Trizivir (AZT/3TC/ABC) (ViiV Healthcare/GlaxoSmithKline), and generic.

CLASS: Nucleoside analog reverse transcriptase inhibitor (NRTI).

FORMULATIONS, REGIMEN, AND COST:

Forms:
   AZT: 100 and 300 mg tabs (Retrovir and generic); 10 mg/mL IV solution; 10 mg/mL oral solution.
   AZT/3TC: 300/150 mg tabs (Combivir and generic).
   AZT/3TC/ABC: 300/150/300 mg tabs (Trizivir and generic).
Regimens: AZT: 300 mg bid or 200 mg tid; AZT/3TC or AZT/3TC/ABC: 1 tab bid.
AWP: AZT, $361.8/mo; AZT/3TC, $931.61/mo; AZT/3TC/ABC, $1,738.46/mo. Generic AZT is now available at $6.02/300 mg tab; AZT/3TC at $15.53/tab; and AZT/ABC/3TC at $28.97.
Food: No effect.
Renal failure: CrCl < 15 mL/min, 100 mg tid or 300 mg/d. AZT/3TC (Combivir) and AZT/3TC/ABC (Trizivir) co-formation: not recommended with CrCl < 50 mL/min.
Hepatic failure: Trizivir contraindicated with severe liver disease. AZT, Combivir: standard dose.
Combination to avoid: AZT/d4T (antagonism).
Combination to use with caution:
   AZT plus ganciclovir or valganciclovir: marrow suppression.

AZT plus ribavirin: Additive anemia; may need EPO.

AZT plus EPO: Hold EPO when Hgb >13 g/dL (see EPO).

AZT plus cancer chemotherapy: marrow suppression.

ACTG 076 protocol: Intrapartum regimen is 2 mg/kg IV over 1 hr, then 1 mg/kg/hr until delivery.

PATIENT ASSISTANCE PROGRAM: 866-518-4357.

CLINICAL TRIALS: FDA-approved in 1987 based on a controlled clinical trial showing significant short-term benefit in preventing AIDS-defining opportunistic infections and death (NEJM 1987;317:185). Early studies (ACTG 019, 076, 175, Concord, etc.) became sentinel reports. Despite 15 yrs of use, resistance in recently transmitted strains is only about 2–10% (NEJM 2002;347:385). AZT is commonly paired with 3TC (Combivir) or ABC/3TC (Trizivir) as the nucleoside components of ART regimens. Potency of these regimens is well-established.

ACTG 384 showed that AZT/3TC/EFV was superior to ddI/d4T/EFV (NEJM 2003;349:2293), but in *GS-934* TDF/FTC/EFV was superior to AZT/3TC + EFV in terms of viral suppression to <50 c/mL (80% vs. 70%), rates of toxicity, CD4 response at 48 wks (+ 90/mm^3 vs. + 58/mm^3), and adverse reactions requiring discontinuation (4% vs. 9%; NEJM 2006;354:251). Follow-up at 96 wks demonstrated greater loss of limb fat and more M184V mutations in patients in the AZT/3TC arm (JAIDS 2006;43:535). A Cochrane Review comparing AZT and TDF containing ART regimens concluded that TDF was superior in terms of CD4 response, tolerance, adherence, and less resistance (Cochrane Database Syst Rev 2010;6:CD008740).

RESISTANCE: The thymidine analog mutations (TAMs) are 41L, 67N, 70R, 210W, 215Y/F, and 219Q/E. A total of 3–6 mutations result in a 100-fold decrease in sensitivity. About 5–10% of recipients of AZT + ddI as dual NRTI therapy develop the Q151M complex, and a larger number develop the T69S insertion mutation, both of which confer high-level resistance to AZT, ddI, ddC, d4T, 3TC, and ABC. The M184V mutation that confers high-level 3TC resistance delays resistance or improves susceptibility to AZT unless there are multiple TAMs. It may also prevent the emergence of multinucleoside mutations, which are now very uncommon. Analysis of patients with early HIV infection indicates that 2–10% have genotypic mutations associated with reduced susceptibility to AZT (NEJM 2002;347:385).

PHARMACOLOGY:

Bioavailability: 60%; high-fat meals may decrease absorption. CSF levels: 60% serum levels (CSF-to-plasma ratio = 0.3–1.35) (Lancet 1998;351:1547). Another report showed a median CSF concentration of 6% of plasma levels which was 4.3-fold above the IC_{50} for wild-type virus (Arch Neurol 2008;65:65: AIDS 2009;23:1359). CNS penetration score is highest: rank 4 (Neurology 2011;76:693).

$T^{1/2}$: 1.1 hr; Renal failure: 1.4 hr; intracellular: 3 hr.

Elimination: Metabolized by liver to glucuronide (GAZT) that is renally excreted.

Dose modification in renal failure or hepatic failure: Excreted in urine as active drug (14–18%) and GAZT metabolite (60–74%). In severe renal failure (CrCl <18 mL/min), AZT half-life is increased from 1.1 to 1.4 hrs and GAZT half-life increased from 0.9 to 8.0 hrs. *Dosing recommendation*: GFR >15 mL/min, 300 mg bid; GFR <15 mL/mm, 300 mg/d; hemodialysis and peritoneal dialysis, 300 mg/d. No dose modification with liver disease.

SIDE EFFECTS:

GI intolerance, altered taste (dysgeusia), insomnia, myalgias, asthenia, malaise, and/or headaches are common and are dose related (Ann Intern Med 1993;118:913). Most patients can be managed with symptomatic treatment.

Marrow suppression: Related to marrow reserve, dose and duration of treatment, and stage of disease (J Viral Hepatol 2006;13:683; HIV Med 2007;8:483). Anemia may occur within 4–6 wks, and neutropenia is usually seen after 12–24 wks. Marrow examination in patients with AZT-induced anemia may be normal or show reduced RBC precursors. Severe anemia should be managed by discontinuing AZT or giving erythropoietin concurrently. Neutropenia and ANC <750/mm^3 should be managed by discontinuing AZT or giving G-CSF concurrently. Most patients with preexisting HIV-associated anemia have increased Hb with ART that includes AZT, but this response is slower than with other NRTIs (JAIDS 2008;48:163).

Myopathy: Rare dose-related complication possibly due to mitochondrial toxicity. Clinical features are leg and gluteal muscle weakness and/or pain, elevated LDH and CPK, muscle biopsy showing ragged red fibers, and abnormal mitochondria (NEJM 1990;322:1098); response to discontinuation of AZT occurs within 2–4 wks. The mechanism is unclear (Pharmacology 2008;82:83).

Macrocytosis: Noted within 4 wks of starting AZT in virtually all patients and serves as crude indicator of adherence.

Class adverse reaction: Lactic acidosis, often with steatosis, is a complication ascribed to all NRTIs but primarily to d4T, and, to a lesser degree, ddI and AZT. This complication should be considered in patients with fatigue, abdominal pain, nausea, vomiting, and dyspnea. Laboratory tests show elevated serum lactate, CPK, ALT, and/or LDH, and reduced serum bicarbonate ± increased anion gap. Abdominal CT scan or liver biopsy may show steatosis. This is a life-threatening complication. Pregnant women and obese women appear to be at increased risk. NRTIs should be stopped or there should be a change to another ARV class or to NRTIs that are unlikely to cause mitochondrial toxicity such as TDF and ABC. Lipoatrophy, also most commonly associated with d4T or d4T + ddI, also occurs with AZT therapy. In ACTG 384, lipoatrophy was observed in both the ddI + d4T and AZT/3TC arms, but its onset was slower in the AZT/3TC-treated patients. There is also evidence that AZT-induced lipoatrophy may be less reversible than lipoatrophy caused by d4T.

Fingernail discoloration with dark bluish discoloration at base of nail noted at 2–6 wks.

Carcinogenicity: Long-term treatment with high doses in mice caused vaginal neoplasms; relevance to humans is not known.

DRUG INTERACTIONS: Use with caution with ribavirin (anemia). Additive or synergistic against HIV with ddI, ABC, IFN-alfa, and foscarnet in vitro; antagonism with ganciclovir and d4T. AZT and d4T should not be given concurrently due to in vitro and in vivo evidence of antagonism resulting from competition for phosphorylation (JID 2000;182:321). Clinical significance of interaction with ganciclovir (in vitro) is unknown, but combination should be avoided due to additive bone marrow suppression. Methadone increases levels of AZT 30–40%; AZT has no effect on methadone levels (JAIDS 1998;18:435).

Other marrow-suppressing drugs should be used with caution: TMP-SMX, dapsone, pyrimethamine, flucytosine, interferon, Adriamycin, vinblastine, sulfadiazine, vincristine, amphotericin B, and hydroxyurea. Probenecid increases levels of AZT and concurrent use is complicated by a high incidence of rash reactions to probenecid.

Fluconazole, atovaquone, valproic acid may increase AZT levels.

PREGNANCY: Category C. AZT is an alternative NRTI (preferred TDF and ABC) (with 3TC and a third agent) for all pregnant women to prevent perinatal transmission and for maternal health. The data on efficacy of AZT for preventing prenatal HIV transmission were well-established with ACTG 076 (NEJM 1994;331:1173). This effect is presumably due to reduction in maternal VL, but also by other mechanisms that are poorly understood (NEJM 1996;335:484). Studies show that the rates of HIV transmission are far lower with HAART than with AZT monotherapy (0–2% vs. 8.8%) (JAIDS 2002;29:484). Extensive pharmacokinetic studies show that AZT levels are not significantly altered by pregnancy so standard doses are advocated (NEJM 1994;331:1173).

With regard to infant safety, concerns have been raised regarding hypospadias, vaginal and other tumors, and mitochondrial toxicity. One report showed an increased rate of hypospadias (7/752 vs. 2/895 [p = 0.007]) (JAIDS 2007;44:299), but this risk has not been observed in other studies or in the HIV Pregnancy Registry with more than 1,500 cases. Two transplacental carcinogenicity studies in mice showed increases in rates of tumors, especially vaginal cancer (J Natl Cancer Inst 1997;89:1602; Fundam Appl Toxicol 1997;38:195). The relevance of these studies is not established since doses used produced far higher AZT exposures than are seen clinically, the relevance of such animal models of carcinogenesis is not established, and the HIV Pregnancy Registry has not confirmed the association, with reports on more than 1,500 AZT exposures. The rate of birth defects associated with AZT first-trimester exposures in the Registry reported through July 31, 2017, was 134/4,160 (3.22%).

An earlier report from France found evidence of mitochondrial toxicity with neurologic consequences in 12 infants exposed to AZT in utero (Lancet 1999;354:1084). Subsequent reviews with data on 20,000 infants exposed to AZT failed to show any neurologic, immunologic, oncologic, or cardiac complications (NEJM 2000;343:759; NEJM 2000;343:805; AIDS 1998;12:1805; JAMA 1999;281:151; JAIDS 1999;20:464). An expert NIH panel concluded that the benefit of decreasing risk of perinatal transmission exceeded the hypothetical concerns of transplacental carcinogenesis, and these complications have not been supported in the Pregnancy Registry as just summarized.

Zithromax—see Azithromycin

Zovirax—see Acyclovir

7

Infection Management

Aspergillosis

SOURCE DOCUMENT: Aspergillosis last reviewed by Patterson et al., Clin Infect Dis 2016;63:112. US DHHS Guidelines: Aspergillosis is no longer addressed because of the low incidence among people living with HIV (PLWH) without other underlying risk factors and management is similar to that in persons with other immunodeficiencies.

EPIDEMIOLOGY: Aspergillus spp. are ubiquitous fungi in the environment and are inhaled into the lungs, making it almost impossible to avoid exposure. Aspergillus infections manifest in three main forms: invasive aspergillosis (IA), chronic (saprophytic), and allergic. IA is associated with more disease severity and may present as invasive pulmonary aspergillosis (IPA), *Aspergillus* sinusitis, disseminated aspergillosis, or single-organ IA. IA was a modestly common opportunistic infection (OI) in the era preceding highly active antiretroviral therapy (HAART) in patients with advanced HIV infection, particularly those with additional risk factors of corticosteroid use, neutropenia, broad-spectrum antibiotic treatment, and underlying lung disease. It is far less frequent in the HAART era. The most frequent pathogen is *Aspergillus fumigatus*, although other species are occasionally implicated.

CLINICAL FEATURES: The most common site of infection is the lung with pneumonia or tracheobronchitis. The pulmonary form shows an infiltrate that might be diffuse, focal, or cavitary; the "halo sign" or "air crescent sign" on computed tomography (CT) scan specifically suggests this diagnosis. Clinical symptoms include fever, cough, dyspnea, pleurisy, hemoptysis, and/or hypoxemia. With tracheobronchitis, there is an ulcerative or an exudative pseudo-membrane that is adherent to the trachea and can be detected with bronchoscopy. Symptoms include cough, fever, dyspnea, stridor, and/or wheezing. Extrapulmonary forms of aspergillosis include meningoencephalitis, osteomyelitis, sinusitis, brain abscess, and skin/soft tissue infections.

DIAGNOSIS: Diagnosis is made through histopathologic/cytologic and culture of tissue and fluid specimens. Where there are concerns for resistance or atypical growth of the organisms, molecular methods should be employed in diagnosis. Polymerase chain reaction (PCR) testing, though sensitive, is not currently approved as a primary identification method due to variability in reporting by commercial laboratories. Bronchoscopy with bronchoalveolar lavage (BAL) is recommended in all patients with suspicion for IPA. BAL galactomannan (GM) is recommended as an accurate marker for diagnosis in IPA. Serum GM is not recommended in routine blood screening; $(1\rightarrow3)$-β-D-glucan is recommend for diagnosing IA in high-risk patients, but it is not specific for *Aspergillus*.

PREVENTION: As noted, exposure to the organism is uniform, al-though avoidance of dusty areas such as construction sites may re-duce the extent of exposure.

TREATMENT: Per current guidelines, voriconazole is the drug of choice for the treatment of all forms of IA. Initiation of antifungal therapy is recommended while evaluating patients with suspi-cion of IA. Alternative regimens include liposomal amphotericin B. Echinocandins may be employed in salvage therapy and should not be used as first-line agents. Combination of triazoles or amphotericin B with echinocandins have been suggested to have synergistic effects in some studies and might be employed in sal-vage therapy. In refractory disease, switching antifungal class is recommended.

Surgery is sometimes employed in cases of IA such as in localized skin infections, osteomyelitis, and sinusitis. CNS infections are managed medically, and surgery employed where rational. Azoles therapeutic drug monitoring (TDM) should be employed especially when there are concerns of treatment failure or interactions between triazoles and other drugs.

Preferred: Voriconazole 6 mg/kg IV q12h on day 1 (2 doses), then 4 mg/kg IV q12h until clinical improvement, then

> For patients >40 kg: Voriconazole 200 mg po q12h (consider 300 mg for severe infections).
> For patients <40 kg: Voriconazole 100 mg po q12h (consider 150 mg for severe infections). Dose adjusts based on serum concentrations (Target trough >2.05 µg/mL)

Treatment duration: until resolution or stabilization.

Alternatives:

> Lipid amphotericin B IV 3–5 mg/kg/d
> Amphotericin B deoxycholate IV 1 mg/kg/d
> Isavuconazole 372 mg IV tid for 6 doses, then 372 mg IV or po qd
> Caspofungin 70 mg IV × 1, then 50 mg IV qd
> Micafungin 100–150 mg IV qd
> Anidulafungin 200 mg IV × 1, then 100 mg IV qd

Posaconazole IV or ER tablet 300 mg bid po for first 2 doses, then 300 mg IV qd until stable, then transition to 300 mg po qd. Target trough levels >1.25 µg/mL.

Duration of above regimens: Until CD4 count is >200 cells/mL and disease resolution/stabilization.

Immune reconstitution inflammatory syndrome (IRIS): Rare with aspergillosis; recurrent symptoms more strongly suggest relapse.

STARTING ART: This should be started soon after initiating antifungal treatment, since IRIS is not an issue. Drug–drug interactions between azoles and cobicistat, non-nucleoside reverse transcriptase inhibitors (NNRTIs), protease inhibitors (PIs), and other CYP450 inducers/inhibitors are problematic.

Treatment failure: The prognosis with untreated IA is poor, so emphasis should be placed on adequate antifungal treatment and initiation of antiretroviral therapy (ART).

Prevention of recurrence: There is no experience with long-term suppression.

Bartonellosis

SOURCE DOCUMENT: Bartonellosis: NIH & DHHS guidance last reviewed March 13, 2017 (http://aidsinfo.nih.gov.guidelines).

EPIDEMIOLOGY: Bartonella includes 24 species and causes retinitis, trench fever, relapsing bacteremia, endocarditis, bacillary angiomatosis (BA), and bacillary peliosis hepatis. However, BA in PLWH is caused by either *B. henselae* or *B. quintana*. BA is seen when the CD4 count decreases to <50/mL. BA can be complicated by chronic illness and intermittent bacteremia which can last for months to years.

CLINICAL FEATURES: The most common form in AIDS patients is BA which represents disseminated disease with characteristic red papular lesions that resemble Kaposi sarcoma. Most patients have evidence of systemic disease with fever, night sweats, hepatosplenomegaly, weight loss, and intermittent bacteremia. This infection should also be considered in patients with advanced HIV infection who present with an FUO since it is a major cause in AIDS. Although infection is typically seen with CD4 of <50 mL, it should also be considered in the differential diagnosis with CD4 of <100/ mL. Important clues are systemic features of a chronic infection, cat exposure ("cat scratch fever"), the characteristic skin lesions, and a chronic febrile condition often lasting months.

DIAGNOSIS: The diagnosis is usually obtained by appropriate cultures, biopsies, and tissue stains using Warthin-Starry stain to demonstrate characteristic bacilli. Gram stain and acid fast stains are not useful. A serologic test from the Centers for Disease Control (CDC) is available in some state health labs and some private laboratories, although quality control may be an issue because sensitivity and specificity have not been evaluated. Seroconversion is sometimes delayed for up to 6 weeks with acute infection, but this is not usually problematic since many patients have been infected for several months. Up to 25% of patients failed to seroconvert; those who do will often sero-revert indicating response to treatment which can be used to correlate for resolution and recurrence. Blood cultures using EDTA tubes have occasionally proven useful, but the yield is low. PCR tests are in development, but not readily available.

PREVENTION: Primary chemoprophylaxis for *Bartonella* is not recommended.

TREATMENT:
Duration: At least 3 months. Bacillary angiomatosis, bacteremia, osteomyelitis, and peliosis hepatis.
  Preferred:

Doxycycline 100 mg po/IV q12h or
Erythromycin 500 mg po/IV q6h (generally not recommended with cobicistat, PIs, and NNRTIs)

CNS infection:

Doxycycline 100 mg po/IV q12h +/- rifampin 300 mg po/IV q12h (see page 624 for drug–drug interactions)

Confirmed Bartonella endocarditis:

Doxycycline100 mg IV q12h + Gentamicin 1 mg/kg IV q8 h × 2 weeks, then continue Doxycycline 100 mg IV/po q12h
For renal insufficiency: Doxycycline 100 mg IV q12h + rifampin 300 mg IV/po q12h) × 2 weeks, then continue with doxycycline 100 mg IV/po q12h

Other severe infections:

Doxycycline 100 mg po or IV q12h or erythromycin 500 mg po or IV q12h *plus* rifampin 300 mg po or IV q12h.

Alternatives for Bartonella infections excluding endocarditis and CNS infections:

Azithromycin 500 mg po/d *or*
Clarithromycin 500 mg po bid

If a relapse occurs after a ≥3 month course of primary treatment:

Macrolide or doxycycline until CD4 count is >200/mL

Indications to discontinue long-term treatment:

Treatment at least 3–4 months and CD4 count >200/mL for at least 6 months

Note regarding in vitro susceptibility tests: These tests often fail to predict response and lesions have reportedly developed in the presence of TMP/SMX, fluoroquinolones, and β-lactams. These drugs should not be used even if active in vitro.

Response: Bartonella serology with IgG titers should be determined at diagnosis. If positive, this test should be used to monitor response to therapy with titers at 6–8 week intervals until a 4-fold decrease is observed. This test is available from the CDC and several commercial labs.

STARTING ART: If ART-naïve with central nervous system (CNS) or ophthalmic lesions, patient should probably be treated with doxycycline and rifampin 2–4 weeks prior to starting ARV therapy.

IRIS: This is not reported with *Bartonella* infections complicating HIV infection.

Management of treatment failure: Defined as patient who fails treatment one or more times; use an alternative regimen for at least 3 months. If antibody titers are increasing while on treatment, continue until 4-fold decrease in titers is documented.

Prevention of recurrence: If there is a relapse after at least 3 months of primary treatment, the recommendation is long-term suppression with doxycycline or a macrolide until the CD4 count is >200/mL for 6 months. Some experts prefer to continue treatment until the *Bartonella* titers decrease at least 4-fold.

Pregnancy: Erythromycin should be used instead of tetracyclines due to teratogenicity. Second-line can be a third-generation cephalosporin (e.g., ceftriaxone can be considered). Do not use first- or second-generation cephalosporins because they are ineffective.

Mucocutaneous Candidiasis

SOURCE DOCUMENT: Mucocutaneous Candidiasis; NIH & DHHS guidance last updated October 18, 2017 (http://aidsinfo.nih.gov. guidelines).

EPIDEMIOLOGY: Oropharyngeal and esophageal candidiasis are common complications of late-stage HIV infection (CD4 <200/mL). The majority of infections are due to *Candida albicans*, but non-albicans species have been reported worldwide and are becoming more prevalent. Vulvovaginal candidiasis is common in the general population and does *not* reflect immune deficiency or HIV infection. Nevertheless, these lesions may be more common and severe in women with advanced HIV infection. In women with advanced HIV, oropharyngeal candidiasis is far more common than vulvovaginal candidiasis, which is rarely refractory to treatment with azoles.

PRESENTATION: The oral lesions ("thrush") are characterized as painless, white plaque-like lesions on oral mucosa. In contrast to oral hairy leukoplakia (OHL), candidiasis plaques can easily be scraped away, and the typical OHL lesions are more often located on the lateral surface of the tongue. Less commonly, red erythematous plaques in the posterior oropharynx can be noted as well. Esophageal candidiasis generally reflects lower CD4 counts and is accompanied by substernal chest pain and odynophagia. However, the patient can present without any symptoms as well. Endoscopic exam shows these the same white plaques lining of the esophagus.

DIAGNOSIS: Thrush is generally diagnosed by visual appearance of typical lesions in the oral mucosa, but it can be confirmed with

KOH prep or culture of scraped lesions. Esophageal candidiasis is diagnosed clinically with odynophagia in the presence of oropharyngeal thrush but can be confirmed by endoscopic exam with typical histopathology on mucosal biopsies. The same principles apply to vulvovaginal candidiasis. Most cases are caused by *C. albicans*, and culture is infrequently needed, but may be useful to detect non-albicans species such as *C. glabrata* and *C. krusei*.

PREVENTION: Although clinical trials have shown that fluconazole can prevent most forms of mucosal candidiasis in patients with HIV infection, there has been occasional resistance noted in *C. albicans*. In patients exposed to azoles or with long-term treatment, emergence of non-albicans *Candida* spp. (especially *C. glabrata*) can occur. Prospective randomized trial data showed there may be improved outcomes with primary prophylaxis. However, mucocutaneous candidiasis is treated very efficiently with acute therapy and has very low associated morbidity/mortality. Prolonged use has a higher risk to benefit ratio attributable to cost, increased resistance, and drug interactions. Therefore, routine primary prophylaxis is not recommended.

TREATMENT:
Oropharyngeal candidiasis:

> *Preferred oral treatment*: Fluconazole 100 mg po/d × 7–14 days
> *Alternative oral therapy*:
> Itraconazole oral solution 200 mg po/d × 7–14 days
> Posaconazole 400 mg po suspension po bid ×1 day, then 400 mg daily

> *Preferred topical treatment*:

> Clotrimazole troches 10 po 5×/d × 7–14 days
> Miconazole buccal tablet 50 mg qd applied to cover the canine fossa × 7–14 days

Alternative topical treatment:

Nystatin suspension 4–6 mL or 1–2 flavored pastilles 4–5
times daily

Esophageal candidiasis: Treatment is empiric. Failure of symptom
resolution requires further evaluation (i.e., EGD) to assess for resistant organisms vs. other causes (e.g., HSV, CMV, etc.).

Preferred therapy:

Fluconazole 200 mg to 400 mg (3–6 mg/kg) po × 14–21 days
or IV/d
Itraconazole oral solution 200 mg po/d × 14–21 days

Alternatives: All 14–21 days of therapy

Voriconazole 200 mg po/IV bid
Isavuconazole 200 mg po loading dose then 50 mg po/d
Isavuconazole 400 mg po loading dose then 100 mg po/d
Isavuconazole 400 mg po once-weekly
Caspofungin 50 mg IV/d
Micafungin 150 mg IV/d
Anidulafungin 100 mg IV × 1 dose then 50 mg IV/d
Amphotericin B deoxycholate 0.6 mg/kg IV/d or liposomal
Ampho 3–4 mg/kg IV/d

Uncomplicated vulvovaginal candidiasis:

Preferred therapy:
Fluconazole 150 mg × 1 dose po
Topical azoles:
Clotrimazole: Apply 1% applicator PV qhs × 1–2 weeks
Butoconazole: Apply 5 g once PV ×1

Miconazole: Apply 2% applicator PV qhs × 1 week

Terconazole: Apply 0.8% applicator PV qhs or 80 mg supp PV qhs × 3 days

Topical treatment duration: ≥ 7 days for severe/recurrent vulvovaginal candidiasis.

Alternative therapy:

Itraconazole solution 200 mg po/d for 3–7 days

Severe/recurrent esophageal candidiasis:

Consider fluconazole 100–200 mg qd

Note: Increase risk of azole resistance with chronic suppression. Check for potential ARV drug–drug interactions with azoles.

Cytomegalovirus

SOURCE DOCUMENT: Cytomegalovirus disease (NIH, DHHS guidelines http://aidsinfo.nih.gov/guidelines- Last Updated: November 4, 2015; Last Reviewed: January 27, 2017).

EPIDEMIOLOGY: Cytomegalovirus (CMV) plays an important role in end-organ disease in patients with advanced HIV infection with CD4 counts <50/mL. In the pre-HAART era, this was a common late-stage complication. During the HAART era, the frequency of these infections decreased >90% (JID 2015;211:169) and are now seen primarily in patients with undetected late-stage HIV infection or those with failed ART.

CLINICAL FEATURES: CMV complicating HIV infection occurs primarily in the eye (retinitis), 80–90%; gastrointestinal tract (esophagitis and colitis), 5–15%; neurologic system (ventriculoencephalitis, encephalitis, and radiculomyelopathy), <2%; and rarely the lung (pneumonitis). Most CMV complications occur in patients with latent CMV infections, so disease represents reactivation of a dormant potential pathogen due to failed immune control.

CMV retinitis: Clinical presentation is a patient with late stage HIV infection (CD4<50) complaining of variable visual problems depending which part of the retina is affected; complaints include scotomas, decreasing visual acuity, peripheral and central visual field loss, floaters, and flashing lights. Of these, floaters and flashing lights are the most likely predictors of CMV retinitis (Ophthalmology 2004;111:1326). Funduscopic exam typically shows perivascular yellow-white retinal infiltrates +/– intra-retinal hemorrhage, sometimes referred to as "scrambled eggs and ketchup." Little to no inflammation is noted in the vitreous body. If left untreated, the disease progresses in 2–3 weeks to blindness. The diagnosis is usually established on the basis of the combination of typical funduscopic changes in the patient with advanced HIV infection. CMV can be detected by PCR in vitreous and aqueous humor and is highly specific, but usually unnecessary. *Differential diagnosis*: Toxoplasmosis, HSV, VZV, syphilis, TB.

IRU: Immune reconstitution uveitis is an ocular form of IRIS which typically occurs between 2 and 84 weeks (median 20 weeks) after initiation of ART though it can happen at any time (months–year). It manifests as floaters, blurry vision, photophobia or even vision loss. Any patient with new visual symptoms with history of CMV retinitis and immune recovery should be immediately evaluated for IRU given high chance of ocular morbidity including blindness. Ophthalmological findings reveal inflammation of anterior chamber and vitreous cavity.

CMV colitis: The usual presentation is subacute with fever, weight loss, abdominal pain, diarrhea, and/or gastrointestinal (GI) bleeding, or rarely perforation in the patient with advanced HIV infection (CD4<50). Diagnosis is made by endoscopy which can vary from small superficial punctate erosions to large deep ulcers surrounded by healthy tissue to near full-thickness necrotizing colitis. Histopathology ranges from nonspecific inflammation to neutrophilic infiltration with vascular endothelial damage with the presence of characteristic inclusion bodies by immunostaining.

CMV esophagitis: Clinical presentation is a patient with advanced HIV infection complaining of fever and odynophagia, with or without retrosternal pain that is usually well-localized by the patient. The diagnosis is established by endoscopic evidence of large, shallow, mucosal ulcers plus microscopic evidence of intranuclear and intracytoplasmic inclusions with an inflammatory response at the ulcer edge. The pathologic diagnosis is based on detection of inclusion bodies and typical histopathologic findings. *Differential diagnosis*: HSV, Candida

CMV pneumonitis: Extremely uncommon cause of pneumonitis in AIDS patients. Frequently isolated in BAL with PCR or cytology, and significance as a true pathogen in this patient population remains unclear. Workup should continue for a more likely causative agent. *Clinical presentation*: Fever, dyspnea with CXR, or CT showing diffuse pulmonary infiltrates. *Diagnosis*: Positive PCR CMV from BAL, typical cytopathological induced by CMV noted on cytology *without* any other pathogens isolated or lung biopsy showing pneumonitis with CMV inclusions.

CMV neurologic disease: Clinical features: encephalitis versus myelitis versus polyradiculopathy. Encephalitis is usually subacute with confusion, headache, fevers, and lethargy making it hard to distinguish between HIV encephalopathy. Rapid progression with cognitive decline, delirium, cranial nerve deficits, ataxia, and nystagmus are also seen, which is less common in HIV encephalopathy. *Diagnosis*: Lumbar puncture (LP) findings are mononuclear pleocytosis and increased protein with PCR positive for CMV; magnetic resonance imaging (MRI) showing periventricular enhancement and/or meningeal enhancement also support this diagnosis.

Polyradiculopathy presents with an ascending paralysis with initial symptoms of leg pain and sacral paresthesia followed by progressive leg paresis, then bladder and bowel dysfunction. *Diagnosis*: Cerebrospinal fluid (CSF) shows a polymorphonuclear pleocytosis with low glucose in one-third of patients, and increased protein similar to bacterial meningitis (J Gen Intern Med 1996;11:47). CMV PCR is also typically positive (JID 1997;176:348).

Myelitis manifests with lower extremity weakness with hyperactive reflexes. MRI of spine shows no masses and hyperintensity in the anterior horns on T2-weighted imaging, which distinguishes it from HIV myelitis (no enhancement and is subacute). *Diagnosis*: CSF shows moderate pleocytosis with elevated protein. CMV PCR positivity is variable and so diagnosis is based on clinical context in the setting of PLWH with CD4 <50, with exclusion of other viral and neoplastic illness.

DIAGNOSIS: CMV viremia can be tested by PCR, culture, or CMV antigen assay. However, this testing is not adequately sensitive or specific. Diagnosis varies depending on the organ involved.

PREVENTION: CMV disease in patients with HIV infection generally represents activation of latent CMV infection, so avoidance of CMV exposure is sometimes recommended in persons who are CMV seronegative. Risks for CMV infection include MSM sex exposure, injection drug use, and extensive exposure to children, such as at daycare centers. More realistic recommendations for prevention with low CD4 counts is good hygienic practices and, especially important, adequate management of HIV infection to prevent advanced immunosuppression. Oral primary prophylaxis is no longer recommended and was supported by a study that showed overall high all-cause mortality in this vulnerable patient population (HIV Clin Trials 2009;10:143).

TREATMENT:

CMV retinitis:
Sight-threatening retinitis (within 1,500 μm from fovea): Intravitreal ganciclovir (2 mg/injection), or foscarnet (2.4 mg/injection) either for 1–4 doses over a period of 7–10 days to rapidly achieve high intraocular levels, *plus* systemic therapy (NB: systemic therapy required to prevent disease in the other eye):

> *Preferred*: Valganciclovir 900 mg po bid for 14–21 days; then qd
> *Alternatives*:
> Ganciclovir 5 mg/kg IV q12h × 14–21 days, then 5 mg/kg IV/d
> Ganciclovir 5 mg/kg IV q12h × 14–21 days, then valganciclovir 900 mg po/d
> Foscarnet 90 mg/kg IV q12h × 14–21 d, then 90–120 mg/kg IV q24hr

Cidofovir 5 mg/kg/week IV × 2 wks, then 5 mg/kg every other week with saline hydration before and after therapy and probenecid 2 g po 3 hrs before dosing, plus 1 g po 2 hr post dose & 1 g 8 hr later (total of 4 g). *Note*: Avoid this option in patients with sulfa allergy.

Peripheral lesions: Give one of the systemic antiviral therapy regimens listed above for 3–6 months: this decision should be made in consultation with an ophthalmologist and should include consideration of the anatomic location of the retinal lesion, condition of the contralateral eye, the patient's immunologic and virologic status, and his or her response to ART.

Relapsed disease: If non–vision-threatening and recently started ART, repeat induction with ganciclovir or foscarnet therapy.

For patients with no response to single-drug CMV therapy, and patients with multiple relapses, combination therapy is superior and recommended (Arch Ophthalmol 1996; 114(1):23–33).

Ganciclovir reinduction:

Ganciclovir 5 mg/kg IV q12H or valganciclovir 900 mg po bid *plus* continue Foscarnet 90 mg/kg IV q24 × 2 wks

or

Foscarnet reinduction:

Foscarnet 90 mg/kg IV q12H × 2 wks *plus* continue Ganciclovir 5 mg/kg IV q24H or valganciclovir 900 mg po qd

Maintenance:

Ganciclovir 5 mg/kg IV q24H or valganciclovir 900 mg po qd *plus* Foscarnet 90 mg/kg IV q 24H as long as possible based on tolerability

Ophthalmological exam should be performed 2 weeks after induction therapy, monthly until immune recovery occurs, and then every 3 months.

STARTING ART: In resource-rich countries, consider initiation of therapy 14 days after initiation of CMV treatment, as CMV levels are usually minimal and thus have a lower incidence of IRU.

Immune reconstitution uveitis: (1) Minimize by treating CMV retinal lesions until there is immune recovery and (2) treat immune reconstitution uveitis with periocular corticosteroids or a short course of systemic steroids.

Discontinuation of retinitis treatment:

1. CMV treatment for at least 3–6 months of ART and no active lesions, and CD4 >100 for 3–6 months;
2. Decision should be made in consultation with the ophthalmologist; considerations should include CD4 response, anatomic location of the lesion, vision in the contralateral eye, and availability of regular ophthalmologic follow-up, which is desired at 3-month intervals to detect relapse or immune reconstitution uveitis.

Reinstitution of maintenance therapy: CD4 count<100/mL
CMV esophagitis and colitis:
Preferred: Ganciclovir 5 mg/kg IV q12h; may switch to valganciclovir 900 mg/kg po q12h when the patient can absorb and tolerate po therapy
Alternative treatments:

For treatment limiting toxicity or ganciclovir resistance: foscarnet: 60 mg/kg IV q8h or 90 mg/kg IV q12h
Mild cases: a consider withholding further CMV treatment if ART is given with response

Duration of CMV therapy: 3–6 weeks or until symptoms have resolved

Maintenance treatment: Not necessary but should be considered with relapsing disease, or with concurrent CMV retinitis

CMV pneumonitis: Similar to CMV retinitis; duration and role of valganciclovir is not established in this setting.

CMV neurologic disease:
Dual therapy at high doses until neurological symptoms improve:

Ganciclovir 5 mg/kg IV q12h *plus* foscarnet 90 mg/kg IV q12h
until neurological symptoms improve
ART should be not delayed.
If patient cannot tolerate high doses, either or both drug doses
can be halved. If patient cannot tolerate dual therapy,
monotherapy at high dose is recommended.

Maintenance:

Similar to CMV retinitis
Valganciclovir 900 mg po qd until VL suppressed, and CD4 >100
for 6 months.

Cryptococcus Neoformans

SOURCE DOCUMENTS: (1) NIH/DHHS guidance (last updated
August 17, 2016; last reviewed June 14, 2017 (http://aidsinfo.
nih.gov/guidelines 2017), and (2) IDSA Guidelines: Clin Infect Dis
2010;50:291.

EPIDEMIOLOGY: C. neoformans is found worldwide. The frequency
of cryptococcosis in the pre-HAART era was 5–8% in PLWH. This OI
has now become relatively rare in the United States and seen almost
exclusively in those with a CD4 count of <100/mL.

PRESENTATION: The usual port of entry is the lung, and many have
pneumonitis, although it may be subclinical. The most common
clinical presentation is subacute meningitis with fever, headache,
malaise, and altered mental status in a patient with a CD4 count of
<100 cells/mm^3. Any organ of the body can be involved, and it is usu-
ally disseminated when diagnosed in a PLWH. Other less common
clinical presentations include vesicular or papular skin lesions
that may resemble molluscum. Alternatively the presentation

may be pneumonitis with a consolidated pneumonia on imaging accompanied by cough, fever, and dyspnea.

DIAGNOSIS: The diagnosis of cryptococcal meningitis is usually easy with positive blood cultures in 55%, positive serum crypto-coccal antigen (CrAg test) in >95%, positive CSF CrAg in >95%, and positive India ink test in 60–80% (many labs in the United States no longer perform the test). LP usually shows elevated pressure (>250 mm H_2O) in 60–80% of patients, and CSF shows mildly elevated levels of serum protein (50–150 mg/dl), low-to-normal glucose concentrations, and pleocytosis (5–100 cells/LPF) made up of mostly lymphocytes; some may have low inflammatory cells on CSF (indicative of poor prognosis). *Note* that a positive serum CrAg test may indicate cryptococcal meningitis or cryptococcal infection at an extrameningeal site. An unexplained positive test should prompt an LP for CSF analysis. Methods of CrAg testing include latex agglutination, immunoassay, and the more recently developed lateral flow assay.

Caution: Focal neurologic signs or obtundation may indicate a mass lesion that would contraindicate the LP, necessitating CNS imaging first.

TREATMENT: There are three phases of treatment: induction for ≥2 weeks with combination antifungals with amphotericin B and flucytosine. Liposomal amphotericin B has proven to have a safer side-effect profile in terms of renal toxicity and tolerability compared to amphotericin B deoxycholate in recent noncomparative studies and is preferred. Flucytosine is preferred to fluconazole as an initial combination antifungal because it has lower relapse rates and more rapid CSF Cryptococcus clearance. Higher doses of fluconazole (800 mg qd) might have a better efficacy compared to 400 mg qd. Induction is followed by consolidation with fluconazole 400 mg qd for another 8 weeks and then maintenance with fluconazole 200 mg qd to complete at least 1 yr of antifungal treatment.

Cryptococcal meningitis, extrapulmonary, and diffuse pulmonary disease:

Induction therapy: ≥2 weeks until clinical improvement and negative CSF crypto culture, then consolidation therapy.

Preferred regimens:

Liposomal ampho B 3–4 mg/kg IV daily plus flucytosine 25 mg/kg po qid

or

If cost is an issue: Ampho B deoxycholate 0.7–1.0 mg/kg IV daily plus flucytosine 25 mg/kg po qid

Alternative induction regimens:

Ampho B lipid complex 5 mg/kg IV daily *plus* flucytosine 25 mg/kg po qid

Liposomal ampho B 3–4 mg/kg *or* Ampho B lipid complex 5 mg/kg IV daily *or*

Ampho B deoxycholate 0.7–1.0 mg/kg IV daily *plus* fluconazole 800 mg po or IV daily

Liposomal amphotericin B 3–4 mg/kg IV daily alone *or*

Amphotericin B deoxycholate 0.7–1.0 mg/kg IV daily alone

Fluconazole (400 mg or 800 mg) po or IV daily plus flucytosine 25 mg/kg po qid

Fluconazole 1200 mg po or IV daily alone

Consolidation therapy: ≥8 Weeks, followed by maintenance therapy

Preferred regimen:

Fluconazole 400 mg po or IV once daily

Alternative regimen:

Itraconazole 200 mg po bid

Maintenance therapy:
Preferred regimen:

Fluconazole 200 mg po for ≥ 1 yr

Focal cryptococcal pulmonary disease and cryptococcal antigenemia:

Fluconazole 400 mg po qd × 12 months.

Management of increased intracranial pressure: This is critical since it accounts for more than 90% of deaths in the first 2 weeks and 40% of deaths in weeks 3–10. Recommendations are (1) determine baseline CSF pressure unless focal neurologic signs or impaired mentation requires CT or MRI imaging; (2) if CSF opening pressure is >25 mm H_2O with symptoms of increased pressure, reduce pressure with LP drainage to 50% (usually 20–30 mL of CSF); if ICP is very high, reduce to <20 mm; if persistent elevation >25 mm and symptoms, repeat LP daily until pressure and symptoms stabilized >2 days; (3) consider temporary percutaneous drains or ventriculostomy if daily LP is repeatedly required; and (4) consider permanent VP shunt only if antifungal therapy and conservative methods to control intracranial pressure have failed.

Cryptococcus gattii: This yeast differs from *C. neoformans* as it more frequently occurs in immunocompetent hosts, is infrequently found in PLWH, appears to be less sensitive to standard antifungal agents, and is geographically unique. Historically, this agent was most common in tropical and subtropical areas, but more recently has been found in Canada and the northwest United States. Most strains are susceptible to amphotericin B (MIC 90 <1 µg/mL) and relative resistance to flucytosine (MIC-50 of 2–4 µg/mL)

Comments on therapy:

Repeat LP: This is indicated to control elevated intracranial pressure and sometimes recommended at the end of induction therapy (i.e., at 2 weeks) since positive cultures at this time predict poor outcome suggesting continuation of the induction (e.g., 2 additional weeks of induction therapy).

Amphotericin B is associated with more rapid clearance of *C. neoformans* than fluconazole (10% vs. 31% at 2 weeks); *flucytosine + amphotericin B* is associated with more rapid clearance of *C. neoformans* compared to amphotericin B alone and also may reduce the rate of relapse and decrease mortality.

Fluconazole alone: Response appears to be dose-related with doses of 1,200 mg/d superior to 800 mg/d. If fluconazole is used alone in patients unable to tolerate Amphotericin + flucytosine, use fluconazole 1,200 mg/d; *fluconazole 400 mg + flucytosine* is less effective than Amphotericin B + flucytosine.

Flucytosine: Blood levels should be measured at 2 hours post dose, and it is recommended to keep the dose between 25 mg/L and 100 mg/L. Dose should be reduced with creatinine clearance <40 mL/min.

Resistance: Amphotericin B resistance is rare; resistance to flucytosine develops rapidly with flucytosine monotherapy; fluconazole resistance is rare.

Lipid amphotericin B: Best data are for Ambisome at 4–6 mg/kg/d; a dose of 6 mg/kg is recommended for severe disease.

Primary prophylactic fluconazole or itraconazole: Significantly reduces the frequency of cryptococcal meningitis in patients with CD4 counts <50 cells/mL. Nevertheless, primary prophylaxis is not recommended due to concern for resistance and drug interactions.

Cryptococcal clearance from CSF: This is most rapid with amphotericin B + flucytosine, then amphotericin B plus fluconazole, then fluconazole alone.

Drug toxicity: Fluconazole, monitor for hepatotoxicity (but this is rare); *amphotericin B*, monitor for nephrotoxicity and electrolyte abnormalities (Mg^{+2} and K^+); reduce risk with preinfusion 500–1,000 mL normal saline and reduce symptomatic reactions with pretreatment acetaminophen and diphenhydramine +/– corticosteroid 30 minutes before amphotericin B (note that corticosteroids are rarely needed). *Flucytosine*, monitor for neutropenia and GI toxicity; 2 hr post dose blood levels should be 25–100 µg/mL.

Response: Mortality with the recommended three-phase regimen is about 5% and CSF cultures are sterile at 2 weeks in 60–70%. Factors associated with a poor response are altered mental status at presentation, high fungal load, low CSF WBC, high intracranial pressure, and slow fungal clearance. The major early concern is elevated intracranial pressure, which can lead to cranial nerve deficits, or herniation and death. *Management of elevated intracranial pressure with repeated LPs is critical since this is the major cause of mortality.* The relapse rate with fluconazole therapy in phase 3 is 2%. It is recommended to obtain CSF culture at 2 weeks. Serum CrAg titer is not useful for following response to therapy, but CSF CrAg may be. Monitoring CrAg titers in CSF or blood to evaluate response to therapy is not recommended. Treatment failure is defined by lack of clinical response and positive cultures after 2 weeks of appropriate treatment; relapse is defined as initial clinical response followed by recurrence of symptoms with a positive CSF culture after ≥4 weeks of treatment. Patients who fail fluconazole monotherapy should be treated with amphotericin B +/– flucytosine. Failure with Amphotericin should be treated by continuing Amphotericin B, or switch to liposomal amphotericin (4–6 mg/kg/d) or lipid complex amphotericin (5 mg/kg/d). An alternative strategy is high dose (800 mg) fluconazole plus flucytosine. Newer azoles such as voriconazole and posaconazole are active vs. *C. neoformans* but not thought to have any advantage over fluconazole. *Echinocandins* have no activity against *Cryptococcus* spp. and are not recommended for management

IRIS: The frequency of IRIS is about 30%. The usual presentation is worsening clinical symptoms despite negative CSF fungal culture. The recommended management is to continue ART, continue antifungal treatment, and consider a short course of corticosteroids. To minimize the risk of crypto IRIS, delay 2–10 weeks before initiating ART.

STARTING ART: Optimal timing of ART is not known. ART should generally be started at the time of starting chronic suppressive therapy (after the induction and consolidation phases of treatment), and concurrent with fluconazole (200 mg/d) for chronic suppressive therapy. Starting ART early (i.e., within 1–2 weeks) has been associated with increased mortality (NEJM 2014;370:2487); therefore, it is considered prudent to delay initiation of ART until at least 2 weeks of antifungal induction therapy. Delay in ART is especially important in patients with low (<5 cells/µgL) CSF cell count and increased intracranial pressure.

Chronic suppressive therapy: Fluconazole suppressive therapy is continued until CD4 >100, no detectable HIV for >3 months, and chronic suppressive therapy for at least 1 yr.

Cryptosporidiosis

SOURCE DOCUMENT: Cryptosporidiosis NIH DHHS Guidance, last updated June 14, 2013; last reviewed June 2017 (http://aidsinfo.nih.gov/guidelines).

EPIDEMIOLOGY: Cryptosporidiosis was a common cause of chronic diarrhea in patients with advanced HIV infection in the pre-HAART era and continues to be an important opportunistic pathogen in AIDS patients in developing countries and in patients with advanced HIV infection due to delayed diagnosis or inadequate ART. The most common species is *C. parvum*; less common are *C. hominis* and *C. meleagridis*. Diarrhea is usually caused by one species although it may be caused mixed species. Cryptosporidiosis has become an infrequent enteric pathogen in patients with early-stage disease or those receiving ART with immune response. The major risk is advanced HIV infection with a CD4 count <100/mm³. The usual source is ingestion of food or fluids contaminated with stool or water sources including pools, lakes, and water supplies, despite chlorination. Person-to-person transmission is infrequent and is most common in sexually active MSM.

CLINICAL FEATURES: Most common is acute watery diarrhea that is often accompanied by cramps, nausea, and vomiting. About one-third have fever. Involvement of the biliary tract is common leading to sclerosing cholangitis and pancreatitis. Disease patterns described in patients with AIDS include asymptomatic carriage (5%), self-limited diarrhea of <2 months duration (29%), chronic diarrhea lasting >2 months (60%) and fulminant, severe cholera-like diarrhea with >10 L/d. Pulmonary disease has been reported, but is not often diagnosed.

DIAGNOSIS: The standard test is microscopic exam of stool or tissue using acid-fast stain. Immunofluorescence staining appears to be 10× more sensitive compared and is now the gold standard test. Additional staining tests include enzyme immunoassay (EIA) and immunochromatographic tests which detect stool antigens. PCR testing is the most sensitive and can detect as few as five oocytes. A single specimen is usually adequate for a patient with severe diarrhea, but repeat testing is advised for those with less severe symptoms. Microscopic exam of small bowel pathology sections is useful in patients with enteritis.

PREVENTION: Patients at risk should be counseled to avoid potentially contaminated food and water; practice careful hygiene with handwashing after handling pets, soil contact, or diapering babies; avoid eating raw oysters, drinking water during travel to developing countries, and having oral-anal contact; and use condoms with penile-anal contact. This risk is magnified by CD4 counts <100 cells/mm^3 and notably reduced with immune response to ART. Rifabutin and possibly clarithromycin/azithromycin when taken for M. avium prophylaxis might confer some protection against cryptosporidiosis.

TREATMENT: Most important is ART with immune reconstitution to a CD4 count >100 cells/mm^3. Symptomatic disease may be severe and require aggressive oral and IV rehydration plus electrolyte replacement. Total parenteral nutrition may be used in patients with severe diarrhea with nutritional deficiencies. Treatment of severe diarrhea should include tincture of opium (more effective) or loperamide. Antimicrobials recommended include nitazoxanide (500–1,000 mg po bid × 14 days with food) or paromomycin 500 mg po qid × 14–21 days. However, there is limited efficacy of these drugs in immunocompromised patients, and immune reconstitution remains paramount.

Special considerations: In pregnant women, initiation of ART is important both in restoring immunity and in preventing maternal-to-child transmission. Loperamide use may be associated with birth defects and should be avoided during the first trimester unless benefits outweigh potential risk. Paromycin and nitazoxanide can be considered after the first trimester in severe symptoms.

Herpes Simplex Virus

SOURCE DOCUMENT: Herpes Simplex Virus Disease NIH, DHHS; last reviewed January 27, 2017 (http://aidsinfo.nih.gov/guidelines).

EPIDEMIOLOGY: Seroprevalence rates of HSV-1 and HSV-2 in US adults are approximately ~50% and 12%, respectively (https://www.cdc.gov/nchs/data/databriefs/db304.pdf). Among PLWH, 95% are HSV-1 seropositive and 70% HSV-2 seropositive (JAIDS 2004;35:435). Most infections are asymptomatic and chronic; however, there is risk of viral shedding and transmission.

CLINICAL FEATURES: Orolabial herpes: Most commonly caused by HSV-1. The usual presentation is a sensory prodrome followed by rapid evolution of papule, then vesicle, ulcer and crusting. The usual course is 5–10 days if left untreated, and it can be precipitated by stress or sunlight.

Genital herpes: Most commonly caused by HSV-2, and similar to HSV-1, it can cause genital mucosal or skin lesions through various stages as above. It can be accompanied by pain, pruritus, vaginal or urethral discharge, and inguinal lymphadenopathy.

HSV-1 and HSV-2 lesions are indistinguishable.

HSV can cause proctitis in HIV-infected MSM without causing external anal ulcers (Sex Transm Dis 2013;40:768). In patients with CD4<100 cells/mL, deep, extensive nonhealing ulcers can occur, which may be associated with acyclovir resistance (Antimicrob Agents Chemother 1994;38:1246).

Rare manifestation of pseudotumor-like, hypertrophic HSV genital lesions that mimic neoplasia and require immunomodulators for treatment have been reported (CID 2013;57:1648).

Nonmucocutaneous HSV infections include keratitis, encephalitis, hepatitis, and retinitis.

DIAGNOSIS: Frequently, the diagnosis can be made clinically. Ideally, lesions suspicious for herpes should be confirmed by lab diagnosis. The preferred diagnostic tests are PCR and viral culture. PCR testing is most sensitive method. The diagnostic yield of viral culture is highest in early stage of lesion (J Clin Microbiol 1981;13:913). HSV typing should be done with genital lesions since HSV-2 is more likely to cause recurrent infections.

PREVENTION: Condom use (Ann Intern Med 2005;143:707) and partner disclosure (JID 2006;194:42) reduces HSV-2 acquisition/transmission. Use of suppressive acyclovir in PLWH did not prevent transmission of HSV-2 (JID 2013;208:1366); hence, suppressive therapy is not recommended. TDF and TDF/FTC has been shown to reduce risk of HSV-2 transmission in HIV-1/HSV-2 negative persons with HIV positive partners; however, this has not been studied in PLWH so it cannot be recommended (Ann Intern Med 2014;161:11). Also, there are no studies of postexposure prophylaxis to guide this potential method of prevention.

TREATMENT:
Orolabial/initial or recurrent genital HSV: (1) Valacyclovir: 1 g po bid, or (2) famciclovir 500 mg po bid, or (3) acyclovir 400 mg po tid for 5–10 days.

Severe mucocutaneous HSV: Acyclovir 5 mg/kg IV q8h; change to po when lesions begin to regress and continue until lesions are healed.

Suppressive therapy: Indications: (1) Severe and frequent recurrences (JID 2003;188:1009), (2) in patients with a CD4 count of <250 cells/mL who are starting ART and are at risk of genital ulcer disease. Suppressive therapy decreases HIV RNA levels in blood and genital secretions in PLWH not on ART, but has not been shown to decrease transmission or impact progression of HIV disease (Lancet 2010; 375:824); (NEJM 2010;362:427).

Options: (1) Valacyclovir: 500 mg po bid, (2) famciclovir 500 mg po bid, (3) acyclovir 400 mg po bid.

The need to continue therapy should be reassessed periodically.

Treatment failure: Resistance to antivirals should be suspected in patients whose lesions do not respond to therapy after 7–10 days. Viral culture and phenotype testing for susceptibility should be performed.

Preferred therapy: IV foscarnet 80–120 mg/kg/d IV in 2–3 doses until lesions resolve.

Alternative: (1) Cidofovir 5 mg/kg IV weekly (× 2 weeks, then every other week); (2) topical trifluridine, cidofovir 1% gel (compounding by pharmacy), or imiquimod 5% cream 3× week.

Monitoring for response and adverse effects of therapy: HSV infections should not influence the decision to start ART. Immune reconstitution after starting ART reduces recurrence and severity of episodes, but not viral shedding.

Renal function should be monitored in patients on high-dose acyclovir therapy.

Pregnancy: Acyclovir is treatment of choice during pregnancy due to its extensive use and safety. (Birth Defects Res A Clin Mol Teratol 2004;70:201). Valacyclovir and famciclovir are also well-tolerated. The maximum risk of transmission to fetus is during delivery due to viral shedding. Caesarian delivery should be done in women with active genital lesions. Suppressive therapy with acyclovir or valacyclovir is recommended at 36 weeks in women with recurrent genital herpes during pregnancy (Obstet Gynecol 2010;116:1492).

Impact of HSV infection on HIV: HIV acquisition: In a meta-analysis of 18 studies, HSV-2 infection was associated with 2- to 3-fold increase in HIV acquisition (AIDS 2006;20:73). Studies have shown an increased number of genital dendritic cells in HSV-2 positive, HIV-uninfected individuals, which may increase the risk of HIV acquisition (AIDS 2007;21:589; JID 2011;203:602).

HIV transmission: Increased HIV viral shedding has been observed in HSV genital lesions (JAMA 1998;280:61). A randomized placebo controlled trial in Africa to assess if HSV suppression with acyclovir decreased transmission of HIV in discordant couples showed reduced occurrence of genital ulcers and lower HIV RNA levels but did not decrease transmission of HIV when compared to placebo (NEJM 2010;362:427).

HIV progression: Some studies have shown increased HIV RNA levels in patients with HSV infection, but no significant impact on CD4 count (JID 1997;176:766). In another study of 84 HIV- and HSV-2–positive individuals, HSV was not associated with any inflammatory or immune markers (AIDS Res Hum Retroviruses 2015;31:276).

Microsporidiosis

SOURCE DOCUMENT: Microsporidiosis; NIH; DHHS guidance (http://aidsinfo.nih.gov/guidelines); last updated May 7, 2013, last reviewed: June 14, 2017.

EPIDEMIOLOGY: Microsporidia are ubiquitous fungus-like organisms (classified as protists) defined by the presence of a unique invasive organelle consisting of a single polar tube that coils around the interior of the spore.

In the pre-HAART era, microsporidia were relatively common causes of diarrhea in late stage HIV infection with a CD4 of <100/mL, but the reported frequency was highly variable depending largely on the diagnostic studies performed. One large series with 733 PLWH with diarrhea found 11 (1.5%) had microsporidiosis (Hum Pathol 1990;21:475).

CLINICAL FEATURES: There are multiple species but only two are commonly implicated in PLWH: *Enterocytozoon bieneusi* causing diarrhea, malabsorption, and cholangitis; and *E. intestinalis* causing diarrhea, disseminated infection, and keratoconjunctivitis.

Multiple additional species in this class have been implicated in HIV-related infectious complications, but these two appear to be most important. A brief list of microsporidial diseases can be found at https://www.cdc.gov/dpdx/microsporidiosis/index.html.

DIAGNOSIS: Microscopic detection of microsporidia is limited by small size (spores 1–5 μm) in stool samples and other body fluids. Effective morphologic demonstration of microsporidia by light microscopy can be accomplished with staining methods that produce differential contrast between the spores of the microsporidia and the cells and debris. Magnification up to 1,000-fold is often required, combined with special stains such as Chromotrope 2Rand "fluorescent brighteners" such as calcofluor white and Uvitex 2B. In biopsy specimens, microsporidia can be detected with Giemsa, tissue Gram stains (Brown-Hopps Gram stain), calcofluor white, Warthin-Starry Silver, or Chromotrope 2A. For diarrhea, a three-stool exam using chromotrope and chemofluorescent stains is often sufficient. If stool exam is negative despite suspected microsporidiosis, consider small bowel biopsy.

Species identification can be made by PCR with species-specific primers, electron microscopy, or staining with species-specific antibodies.

PREVENTION: PLWH with a CD4 count of <200/mL should avoid contaminated water, undercooked meat, or seafood and practice good hygiene. ART is critically important. There are no recommended antimicrobials for prevention of this category of pathogens in susceptible hosts.

TREATMENT: Treatment of diarrheal disease is usually ART combined with nonspecific agents. Administration of ART with immune restoration (an increase in CD4 to >100 cells/μL) is associated with resolution of symptoms of enteric microsporidiosis. Patients should be given fluid support, nutritional supplementation, and antimotility agents. No specific antimicrobial agent can be recommended for microsporidiosis in general, nor specifically for

E. bieneuzi-associated diarrhea. Fumagillin 60 mg po daily and TNP-470 are two agents that have some effectiveness (not available in the US).

Agents that do not appear effective include albendazole, metronidazole, atovaquone, and furazolidone. There is weak evidence supporting use of nitazoxanide in patients with higher CD4 count.

Albendazole 400 mg bid until CD4 count is >200 cells/mm^3 × 6 months + ART appears effective for treating microsporidia other than *E. bieneusi* or *V. corneae*.

Microsporidial keratoconjunctivitis: Topical fumagillin bicylohexylammonium 3 mg/mL in saline (fumagillin 70 µg/mL), 2 gtt every 2 hours × 4 days, then 2 drops qid (investigational use only in US) + albendazole 400 mg po bid (for systemic infection) plus ART.

STARTING ART: This is indicated promptly, as noted earlier. IRIS has been reported with *E. bieneusi* infection, but it is rare and should not dissuade initiating ART.

Progressive Multifocal Leukoencephalopathy (PML)/JC Virus Infection

SOURCE DOCUMENT: Progressive multifocal leukoencephalopathy; NIH, DHHS guidance, last updated May 6, 2017, http://aidsinfo.nih.gov/guidelines.

EPIDEMIOLOGY: JC virus is worldwide in distribution, with up to 70% of healthy adults demonstrating exposure based on serologic studies, while 20–30% of healthy immunocompetent adults have detectable JC virus DNA in urine. Progressive multifocal leukoencephalopathy (PML) is rare except in patients with advanced HIV infection and patients treated with immunosuppressants or immunomodulatory humanized antibodies, such as natalizumab or rituximab. Most patients have advanced immunosuppression with CD4 counts <50/mL; however, rare cases occur in patients with CD4 counts >200/mL, and some develop as an expression of IRIS.

In the pre-HAART era, 3–7% of HIV-infected patients developed PML, which was usually fatal. In the HAART era, the frequency of PML complicating HIV infection is rare, but mortality continues to be high.

CLINICAL FEATURES: PML is a focal demyelination neurologic syndrome with insidious onset over several weeks with neurologic deficits based on the site of cerebral involvement. Variable presentations include ataxia and dysmetria reflecting cerebellar involvement; aphasia, hemiparesis, and sensory deficits reflecting involvement of frontal and parietal lobes; and hemianopsia reflecting involvement of occipital lobes. Seizures occur in up to 18% of patients. Involvement of the spinal cord and the optic nerves is rare. There is a lack of inflammation, and headaches and fever are uncommon.

DIAGNOSIS: MRI is the preferred imaging method and typically shows hyperintense white matter lesions on T2-weighted images in areas which correlate with neurologic deficits. CSF analysis typically shows little evidence of an inflammatory response with most cases exhibiting no pleocytosis, minimally decreased glucose, and normal or mildly elevated protein. PCR for JC virus DNA is 70–90% sensitive but reduced to less than 60% for patients receiving ART. Some cases may require a brain biopsy to confirm the diagnosis. In such cases, there are highly characteristic cytologic findings.

PREVENTION: ART with immune reconstitution is the most effective and possibly the only effective method to prevent PML.

TREATMENT: No effective therapy currently exists other than the use of ART to achieve immune reconstitution. In previously untreated patients, ART should be initiated immediately, while patients currently receiving ART should have therapy adjusted if they are not fully virologically suppressed.

Response to ART: Quantitation of CSF JCV DNA is possibly useful to monitor response. *Note* that PML may also occur as a complication of ART (PML IRIS) (Nat Clin Pract Neurol 2006;2:557). Corticosteroids are sometimes recommended based on case reports of clinical and virologic benefit. Contrast-enhanced MRI may be helpful in documenting response. Treatment failure has been defined by continued positive CSF JCV at 3 months. Despite therapy, neurologic deficits are often irreversible. In patients who continue to deteriorate, MRI should be repeated. IRIS has been reported to complicate PML, usually within the first few months of ART, with more rapid deterioration and MRI findings of edema, contrast enhancement, and mass effect. Some authors have reported benefit from corticosteroids; however, this should be balanced against the potential further immunosuppressive effects.

Failed response to ART therapy: There are no clear recommendations for management of failed therapy based on clinical trials. Therapies including mefloquine, cidofovir, maraviroc, and cytarabine have not shown consistent benefit. Evidence for other treatments, including maraviroc and mirtazapine, are limited to anecdotal reports.

Mycobacterium avium Complex Infection

SOURCE DOCUMENTS: Guidelines for the Prevention and Treatment of Opportunistic Infections in HIV-infected Adults and Adolescents: Disseminated *Mycobacterium avium* Complex disease, last reviewed June 14, 2017, at http://aidsinfo.nih.gov/guidelines.

EPIDEMIOLOGY: Mycobacterium avium complex (MAC) is ubiquitous and is thought to be acquired via inhalation or ingestion. Person-to-person transmission is less likely. No specific environmental exposure or activity has been defined as a risk. The incidence of disseminated MAC in patients with a CD4 cell count of < 100 cells/mL in the absence of ART and MAC prophylaxis is 20–40%. The incidence of disseminated MAC in the HAART era has decreased by more than 10-fold to 2.5 cases per 1,000 person years. Risk factors include a CD4 of < 50 cells/mL, HIV viral load > 100,000 copies/mL, and previous OI (AIDS 2010;24:1549).

PRESENTATION: The usual symptoms of MAC infection include fever, night sweats, weight loss, fatigue, diarrhea, and abdominal pain. Lab tests at presentation frequently include anemia and an elevated alkaline phosphatase. Physical exam often shows hepatosplenomegaly and/or diffuse generalized lymphadenopathy. Localized infections such as pneumonitis, osteomyelitis, pericarditis, lymphadenitis, soft tissue abscesses, genital ulcers, or CNS involvement are seen commonly in patients who have received ART with improved immune function or as a manifestation of IRIS.

DIAGNOSIS: Isolation of MAC from blood cultures, lymph nodes, bone marrow, or other sterile body sites helps in diagnosis. In addition to microscopic exam and staining for acid fast bacilli, clinical specimens are inoculated in solid media like Middlebrook 7H11 and in liquid media such as BACTEC 12B broth. Growth of MAC can take 2–4 weeks in solid media and 7–14 days using BACTEC system. Identification of species is done by DNA probes or high-performance liquid chromatography (HPLC). Blood cultures have >90% sensitivity in disseminated disease. Respiratory and stool specimens have poor sensitivities, 22% and 20%, respectively, but good positive predictive value (60%) for bacteremia (JID 1994;169:289).

Prophylaxis: DHHS guidelines recommend starting prophylaxis to prevent MAC disease if CD4 is <50 cells/mL. Primary MAC prophylaxis is no longer recommended by the IAS guidelines (JAMA 2018;320:379). No specific measures are recommended to prevent environmental exposure.

Preferred: Azithromycin 1,200 mg weekly or clarithromycin 500 mg bid.

Prior to starting prophylaxis, disseminated MAC should be ruled out by clinical assessment and AFB blood cultures should be ordered if necessary. Routine screening with respiratory and stool cultures is not recommended to rule out MAC infection.

Alternative: Rifabutin 300 mg qd for those who cannot tolerate macrolides, but TB should be excluded before using rifabutin.

Discontinuation: Discontinue treatment when CD4 count is >100 cells/mL for >3 months. Two randomized placebo-controlled studies have shown that the risk of acquiring MAC after discontinuing prophylaxis is minimal. This helps reduce pill burden and potential drug–drug interactions.

The IAS-USA panel (JAMA 2018;320:379) recommends against primary prophylaxis for MAC if effective ART is initiated immediately and viral suppression is achieved, since studies have shown no significant mortality difference once MAC disease develops irrespective of whether patients have received MAC prophylaxis or not (JID 2015;212:1366).

TREATMENT: Initial treatment should be with two or more drugs to prevent and delay the development of drug resistance. Susceptibility testing for macrolides is recommended.

Preferred:.(1) Clarithromycin 500 mg po bid plus ethambutol 15 mg/kg po qd is the preferred regimen. (2) Azithromycin 500–600 mg/d plus ethambutol 15 mg/kg po qd may be substituted due to intolerance or drug interactions with clarithromycin.

Additional third agent: The addition of rifabutin 300 mg po qd is suggested when there is a high MAC load (>200 CFU/mL), advanced immunosuppression (CD4 <50 cells/mL), or absence of effective ART.

Randomized clinical trials have shown that addition of rifabutin improved survival and delayed emergence of resistance (CID 1999;28:1080).

Alternative additional agents include (1) amikacin 10–15 mg/kg IV qd; (2) streptomycin 1g IV or IM qd; (3) moxifloxacin 400 mg po qd; and (4) levofloxacin 500 mg po qd. However, there are no controlled trials that have tested their efficacy.

STARTING ART: ART should be started as soon as possible after 2 weeks of MAC treatment to reduce pill burden, drug interactions, and risk of IRIS initially.

ACTG 5164 was a randomized trial showing that early ART (within 14 days) in patients with acute OIs had less progression to death and no increase in adverse events as compared to deferred ART (within 45 days) (PLoS ONE 4:e5575).

Response to therapy: Clinical improvement with decline in fever and symptoms should be noted within 2–4 weeks. Blood cultures should be obtained at 4–8 weeks in patients who fail to show clinical response. Therapeutic response may be expected to be delayed in patients who have more extensive disease and/or very advanced immunosuppression at baseline.

Drug side effects and interactions:

Clarithromycin/azithromycin: Can cause nausea, vomiting, abdominal pain, and transaminitis. Clarithromycin in doses >1 g has been associated with increased mortality and is not recommended. A comparative trial for treatment of MAC bacteremia showed clarithromycin superior in time to clearance of cultures, but another trial indicated these drugs were comparable when used with ethambutol (CID1998;27:1278).
PIs can increase clarithromycin levels, and efavirenz can decrease levels. Azithromycin does not have significant interactions with them.

Rifabutin: Can cause uveitis, arthralgias. It also a substrate and inducer of cytochrome P450 3A4 and can cause complex drug interactions with cobicistat, PIs, and NNRTIs, thus requiring dose adjustments.

Discontinuation of secondary prophylaxis: Criteria include at least 12 months of complete treatment along with improvement in clinical symptoms and a CD4 count of >100 cells/mL for ≥6 months.

Secondary prophylaxis should be reinstituted if CD4 count is <100 cells/mL. Primary prophylaxis should be reinstituted if the CD4 count decreases to <50 cells/mL.

Treatment failure: This is defined by lack of clinical response and persistence of positive blood cultures after 4–8 weeks of recommended treatment. Repeat drug susceptibility testing must be done in patients with relapsed disease. Based on sensitivity testing, a new regimen that includes at least two new, previously unused agents should be started (e.g., a fluoroquinolone, amikacin, rifabutin, or ethambutol). The benefit of using macrolides despite development of resistance is unknown. Clofazimine is not recommended as trials have shown no efficacy and increased mortality with its use. Also important is use of appropriate ART regimen.

Treatment in pregnancy: Clarithromycin has been associated with increased birth defects in certain animal studies; its use in the first trimester in humans showed increased risk of spontaneous abortion in one study, so its use is not recommended in pregnant women. Azithromycin is recommended for primary prophylaxis and ethambutol plus azithromycin for secondary prophylaxis.

IRIS: IRIS is a relatively common feature of MAC treatment and occurs most frequently in the first 8 months post treatment, especially in months 1–3 after initiating ART. Most common signs are fever and a focal inflammatory reaction such as lymphadenitis, pneumonitis, pericarditis, osteomyelitis, thoracic spine abscess, keratitis, peritonitis, and skin abscesses. The incidence of MAC IRIS is reported as 3%, with three main clinical presentations: peripheral lymphadenitis, thoracic disease, and intraabdominal disease. Blood cultures are usually negative, but it is important to rule out therapeutic failure. Management of MAC IRIS includes continuation of ART and MAC therapy. Mild symptoms can be treated with nonsteroidal antiinflammatory drugs (NSAIDs); for severe disease, prednisone (20–60 mg/d) with slow taper can be used.

Mycobacterium Tuberculosis

SOURCE DOCUMENT: Mycobacterium tuberculosis infection and disease; NIH and DHHS Guidance, last updated September 22, 2017 (http://aidsinfo.nih.gov.guidelines).

EPIDEMIOLOGY: The major source of active TB in PLWH in the US is reactivation of latent TB infection (LTBI). The prevalence of LTBI in the US is about 4–5%. Risk of reactivation increases soon after HIV infection, and, if HIV is untreated, the annual risk is 3–16%, which applies to all CD4 strata but increases with progressive decline of CD4. ART substantially reduces this risk so that current rates of active TB in the US have decreased to about 500 new cases/yr in the population of PLWH. In the US, risk is highest in foreign-born PLWH.

PREVENTION: As noted, the major predisposing factor for TB in persons with HIV infection is birth or residence outside the US. This observation supports the high priority to test for LTBI in PLWH returning from extensive stays at international sites of high TB prevalence.

Latent TB infection: TB is acquired by inhalation of droplet nuclei containing bacilli of *M. tuberculosis* group, followed by the immune response that usually controls and sequesters viable bacilli, usually for years, as "latent TB," as indicated by positive tuberculin skin test (TST) and/or interferon gamma release assay (IGRA) tests. The annual risk of active TB with HIV infection plus LTBI is magnified 3- to 12-fold, and the probability of reactivation in the absence of anti-TB therapy depends largely on immune competence based on CD4 counts. Active TB has been shown to increase HIV viral loads, potentially leading to more rapid HIV disease progression. Treatment of LTBI decreases the risk of active TB by about 60% and the risk of death by about 25%. This observation supports the recommendation for testing all patients with HIV infection for LTBI with the TST or IGRA. A positive result with either test should prompt a review of symptoms for active TB (e.g., cough, fever, sweats, weight loss, or lymphadenopathy). Screening should also include chest x-ray. Prior US practice favored the TST (skin) test, but the IGRA test has higher specificity and requires only a single patient visit. Both tests are less sensitive in advanced immunosuppression. At present, either test is recommended; using a combination of both TST with IGRA is not recommended in the US. Criteria for a positive TST is >5 mm induration at 48–72 hrs in a PLWH.

DIAGNOSIS: The sensitivity of classic TB symptoms (cough, fever, night sweats, weight loss) is decreased among patients taking ART. In addition, pulmonary cavitation becomes less common and extrapulmonary disease more common as CD4 counts fall below 200 cells/µL, while chest radiography becomes less sensitive. Sputum is commonly smear-negative in PLWH; however, culture and nucleic acid amplification (NAA) testing remains reliable. Pleural, pericardial, and CSF fluid; urine; and lymph node aspirates should be obtained as clinically indicated, and NAA testing may also be useful although of lower yield from these specimens. Next-generation NAA testing is now also able to detect rifampin resistance (Xpert MTB/RIF assay).

Lipoarabinomannan (LAM), a component of the *Mycobacterium* TB cell wall, is detectable in urine and has high specificity but variable sensitivity which increases with disease burden.

TREATMENT:

Latent tuberculosis prophylaxis-screening: PLWH who have a positive screening test for LTBI and no evidence of active TB by clinical review, including a negative chest x-ray, are considered to have LTBI. PLWH who are anergic and have no recent TB contact should not receive LTBI treatment.

Treatment of latent TB:

Preferred:

Isoniazid (INH) 300 mg po qd + plus pyridoxine 25 mg/d × 9 mo *or* INH 900 mg po twice weekly with directly observed therapy (DOT) + pyridoxine 25 mg/d × 9 mo

Alternative:

Rifampin 600 mg po daily × 4 mo *or* rifabutin (dose adjusted based on ART regimen) × 4 months *or* rifapentine 900 mg (or 750 mg if 32–49.9 kg) po weekly + INH 15 mg/kg weekly (up to 900 mg) + pyridoxine 50 mg weekly × 12 weeks in patients receiving EFV or RAL based ART.

If drug-resistant TB is suspected, select drugs based on consultation with a TB expert.

Treatment of active TB: DOT is recommended for all HIV-related TB. Intensive phase (2 months) INH + (RIF or RFB) + PZA + EMB. Treatment for 5–7 days/week or twice weekly and preferably DOT in the intensive phase. If drug sensitivity testing shows INH and RIF are active, EMB and PZA can be discontinued. Continue INH + (RIF or RBT) dosing at 5–7 days/wk for duration depending on site of infection and sensitivity:

Pulmonary, drug-sensitive: 6 mos
Pulmonary TB + positive culture at 2 mos of therapy: 9 mos
Extrapulmonary; CNS: 9–12 mos
Bone or joint: 6–9 mos
Other sites: 6 mos

Note: Duration of therapy should be based on doses received; not time span given.

Drug-resistant TB:

Empiric treatment for suspected RIF +/- additional drug resistance: INH + (RIF or RFB) + PZA + EMB + (moxifloxacin or levofloxacin) + (aminoglycoside or capreomycin)

INH resistance: (RIF or RFB) + EMB + PZA + (moxifloxacin or levofloxacin) × 2 mo, then (RIF or RFB) + EMB + (moxifloxacin or levofloxacin) × 7 mo

Resistance to rifamycin or other agents: consult with TB expert.

Note that treatment should be modified by results of sensitivity testing, and a TB expert should be consulted for resistant TB.

Adjunctive steroids: Recommended for HIV-related TB involving CNS or pericardium.

Dexamethasone 0.3–0.4 mg/kg/d × 2–4 wks then taper by 0.1 mg/kg/d weekly until 0.1 mg/kg/d, then 4 mg/d, tapered by 1 mg/d weekly for total of 12 weeks of therapy.

Alternative: Prednisone or prednisolone for pericardial disease, 60 mg/d, tapered by 10 mg weekly for total of 6 weeks

STARTING ART: Co-treatment of HIV and TB is complicated because of large pill burden, high adherence demands, potential drug–drug interactions (especially between the rifamycins and most ART), overlapping side effects, and risk of development of IRIS. Current evidence supports the initiation of ART before completion of TB therapy. For ART-naive patients with CD4 of <50, ART should be started within 2 weeks after TB treatment initiation; for those with higher CD4 counts (≥50 cells/mL), ART should be started within 8 weeks of starting anti-TB treatment, but most experts recommend starting within 2–4 weeks with advanced HIV disease. Due to interactions with rifampin, a regimen including 2 NRTIs with efavirenz is usually favored, although increased doses of raltegravir

(800 mg bid) or dolutegravir (50 mg bid) are also acceptable options. Bictegravir is contraindicated with rifampin.

Pneumocystis jirovecii (Formerly Pneumocystis carinii) Pneumonia

CLASSIFICATION AND NOMENCLATURE: Prior to 2002, the ubiquitous fungus *Pneumocystis jirovecii* was classified as a protozoan with the official name of *P. carinii*. Further investigation led to the discovery of two distinct species: *P. carinii* now refers strictly to a species which is specific to rats, while *P. jirovecii* is the opportunistic human pathogen. However, the abbreviation PCP continues to be used to refer to pneumocystis pneumonia.

EPIDEMIOLOGY: The majority of children develop serologic evidence of exposure by the age of 4 yrs. Disease can represent reactivation of latent disease or reinfection, as suggested by occasional outbreaks.

  PCP was the leading OI in patients with AIDS in the pre-HAART era, but rates of this infection have decreased substantially since the beginning of the HAART era in 1996 with the combination of ART and PCP prophylaxis. Most cases now occur in patients with undiagnosed HIV infection and those with known HIV infection who are not receiving adequate ART and PCP prophylaxis. The major risk is a CD4 count of <200 cells/mL, previous PCP, or other factors that correlate with advanced HIV such as thrush, weight loss, and high HIV viral loads.

CLINICAL FEATURES: PCP should be suspected in any patient with known or suspected HIV infection, a CD4 count of <200/mL, and typical clinical findings. The usual presentation is subacute onset and gradual progression of exertional dyspnea, nonproductive cough, fever, and chest pain. These symptoms evolve over several days or weeks. Physical exam is often negative except for fever, tachypnea, and tachycardia, with or without diffuse bilateral fine rales. Rarely, extrapulmonary disease is seen and is associated with use of pentamidine for prophylaxis. Many patients show other signs of advanced HIV infection including thrush and wasting. Patients with suspected PCP should have blood gases and HIV serology if HIV infection has not been confirmed.

Radiographic findings: Chest imaging usually shows diffuse bilateral, symmetrical interstitial infiltrates but can be normal during early stages. Less common findings include unilateral or apical infiltrates (especially in those receiving aerosolized pentamidine prophylaxis), cysts, pneumatoceles, adenopathy, effusion, or pneumothorax. Up to 18% of patients with PCP have a second process, including bacterial pneumonia or TB. CT scan is helpful if chest radiography is equivocal or normal.

Laboratory findings: Hypoxemia is the cardinal finding of PCP. Blood gas testing typically shows reduced arterial O_2 and an increased alveolar-arterial (A-a) gradient that may be mild (A-a gradient <35 mm Hg), moderate (A-a gradient 35–45 mm Hg), or severe (A-a gradient >45 mm Hg). Post-exercise oxygen desaturation may facilitate the diagnosis in mild cases. Elevations of lactate dehydrogenase (>500 mg/dL), and 1,3 β-D-glucan are both sensitive but nonspecific.

Definitive diagnosis is usually established by demonstrating typical organisms in BAL fluid or the less sensitive induced-sputum specimens. Biopsies are also highly sensitive (whether bronchoscopic, transbronchial, or via open biopsy), while spontaneously expectorated sputum is not recommended due to very low yield. Several stains are useful for detecting the characteristic cystic and trophic forms or cell walls of *P. jirovecii*. Sensitivity depends on the organism load, specimen quality, specimen source, and microbiologist's skill. Organisms remain detectable for several days after initiation of therapy; therefore, treatment should not be delayed in order to make the diagnosis.

PCR is highly sensitive and is increasingly utilized for diagnosis, although specificity can be as low as 85%. Although usually performed on BAL specimens, it has the advantage of being able to detect organisms in upper respiratory samples, including induced sputum and oral washes. A newer quantitative PCR may be a better at distinguishing between colonization and infection.

PREVENTION:

Indications for primary PCP prophylaxis: (1) CD4 count of <200 cells/mL or CD4% <14%, (2) history of thrush, or (3) history of an AIDS-defining infection.

Prophylaxis regimens: TMP/SMX is the preferred agent due to efficacy and additional protection against toxoplasmosis and several bacterial infections when given at the recommended dose of 1 DS tab po daily. Lower dose of 1 SS tab daily or 1 DS tablet 3 times/week is also effective and may be better tolerated.

Alternative PCP prophylaxis regimens: (1) Dapsone 100 mg/d; (2) dapsone 50 mg/d + pyrimethamine 50 mg/week + leucovorin 25 mg/week, (3) atovaquone 1,500 mg po daily with meals, or (4) aerosolized pentamidine 300 mg by nebulization with a Respigard II nebulizer given monthly (the efficacy of other devices is unproven; also does not protect against toxoplasmosis).

Stopping PCP prophylaxis: Prophylaxis can be stopped when the CD4 count has been >200 cells/mL for >3 months. Patients on ART with suppressed viral load and CD4 100–200 cells/mL remain at low risk for PCP.

TREATMENT: All courses are for 21 days. Trimethoprim-sulfamethoxazole (TMP/SMX) remains the first-line agent and must be adjusted for renal function. Deterioration or lack of improvement within the first several days is common, and regimen should not be changed due to failure for at least 4–8 days.

Mild to moderate disease:

Preferred: TMP/SMX 2 tabs tid (or total 5 mg/kg/dose tid based on TMP component).

Alternatives: (1) Dapsone 100 mg po daily + TMP 15 mg/kg/d divided q8h, (2) primaquine 30 mg base po daily + clindamycin 450 mg po q6h, (3) atovaquone 750 mg po bid with food (less effective compared to TMP/SMX).

Moderate to severe disease:

Preferred: TMP-SMX 5 mg/kg/dose (TMP component) IV q8h × 21 days.

Alternatives: (1) Primaquine 30 mg base po daily + clindamycin
600 mg iv q6h, (2) pentamidine 4 mg/kg IV daily (reduce to 3
mg/kg/d for side effects).

Treatment with corticosteroids is associated with decreased mortality in severe disease. Patients with a PaO_2 of <70 on room
air or A-a gradient of ≥35 mm HG should receive prednisone 40 mg po bid × 5 days, then 40 mg daily × 5 days, then
20 mg daily for 11 days (or methylprednisolone at 75% of
prednisone dose).

Secondary prophylaxis should begin as soon as the 21-day regimen is completed and is identical to primary prophylaxis in
dosing and discontinuation.

Comments on management: Relative efficacy of treatments: ACTG
108 showed TMP/SMX, TMP/dapsone, and clindamycin to be equally
effective for mild to moderate PCP (Ann Intern Med 1996;124:792).
A review of 1,122 HIV infected patients in Denmark showed comparable 3-month survival rates for HIV-associated PCP with TMP/
SMX (85%), primaquine/clindamycin (81%), and IV pentamidine
(76%) (JAC 2009;64:1282). Aerosolized pentamidine should not be
used for PCP therapy.

Resistance of *P jirovecii* to sulfonamides is suggested by
mutations on the dihydropteroate synthase gene, but there does
not appear to be an association with therapeutic failure. Patients
who develop PCP despite TMP/SMX prophylaxis do not require alternate therapy.

Adverse drug reactions (ADRs): Adverse reactions to TMP/SMX
for PCP have been reported in up to 80% of patients, primarily
rash (30–50%), leukopenia (30–40%), azotemia ((1–5%), hepatitis (20%), and thrombocytopenia (15%). Most can be treated
through use of antihistamines for rashes, antipyretics for fever, and
antiemetics for nausea. The side effects of dapsone and primaquine
include methemoglobinemia and hemolysis; pentamidine when
administered systemically can cause hypoglycemia, hypotension,
cardiac dysrhythmia, azotemia, and electrolyte abnormalities.

Pregnancy: Therapy is identical to standard dosing, although primaquine should be avoided due to risk of maternal hemolysis. Folic acid 0.4 mg/d can be given to reduce risk of neural tube defect from TMP/SMX; however, addition of folinic acid has led to increased treatment failure and mortality. Therefore, folate supplementation should only be given within the first trimester.

Toxoplasmosis

SOURCE DOCUMENT: Toxoplasma gondii Encephalitis (NIH/DHHS Guidelines), last updated July 25, 2017, http://aidsinfo.nih.gov/guidelines.

EPIDEMIOLOGY: T. gondii is a protozoan that causes toxoplasma encephalitis (TE). Disease results from reactivation of latent cysts primarily in patients with advanced HIV infection with CD4<200/mL.

The geographic prevalence of positive anti-*Toxoplasma* antibody (IgG), indicating latent infection, varies greatly, averaging about 11% in the US, and 50–80% in most of Europe, Latin America, and African countries. The greatest risk for TE is latent infection and a CD4 count of <50 cells/mL, but a CD4 count of <200 cells/mL is also considered a risk. PLWH who are seronegative have a very low incidence of toxoplasmosis. If disease does occur, it represents (a) primary infection (b) erroneous serological testing, or (c) reactivation of latent disease in patients who cannot produce antibodies.

Sources of *T. gondii* infection in the US include consumption of undercooked meat, eating raw shellfish, or exposure to cat stool. Note that these exposures may be remote and long forgotten. There is no person-to-person transmission.

CLINICAL FEATURES: The usual clinical presentation is fever, headache, and confusion with or without focal neurologic deficits in a patient with advanced HIV infection. Early disease may present with headache and fever. Some patients may have nonfocal manifestations and psychiatric disturbances. However, more commonly, the disease presents with focal neurologic findings that may progress to seizures, stupor, and then coma. Extracranial involvement, such as retinochoroiditis or pneumonia, may be present but is less common.

DIAGNOSIS: Positive serology (anti-*Toxoplasma* immunoglobulin G or Toxo IgG) is the screening test that indicates prior infection. In the absence of Toxo IgG, a diagnosis of toxoplasmosis is highly unlikely, but not impossible. Anti-toxoplasma IgM antibodies usually are absent and therefore not helpful.

Definitive diagnosis requires a compatible clinical syndrome, typical imaging findings, and detection of the organism in a clinical sample.

The second critical test is head imaging by CT or MRI. CT or MRI of the brain typically shows multiple contrast-enhancing lesions in the gray matter of the cortex or basal ganglia with associated edema. Less commonly, it manifests as a single brain lesion or diffuse encephalitis. MRI is more sensitive than CT and should be obtained when CT is negative or equivocal, and there is enough suspicion. Positron emission tomography (PET) scans may be helpful in distinguishing TE and CNS lymphoma.

When feasible, an LP should be performed for CSF PCR. *Note* that the CSF PCR for *T. gondii* has low sensitivity of about 50%, but good specificity of 96–100%.

Many clinicians rely on response to empiric anti-toxoplasma therapy if the imaging, serology, and/or CSF PCR support this diagnosis and alternative diagnoses are considered unlikely. In this case, brain biopsy is reserved for therapeutic failures. A definitive diagnosis can be made with brain biopsy, most commonly by stereotactic CT-guided needle biopsy. Hematoxylin and eosin stains can be used for the detection of *T. gondii*, but sensitivity is significantly by immunoperoxidase staining.

The differential diagnosis of focal neurological disease in patients with AIDS includes primary CNS lymphoma and progressive multifocal leukoencephalopathy (PML). Less common causes of focal neurologic disease in patients with AIDS include mycobacterial infection (especially TB); fungal infection, such as cryptococcosis; Chagas disease; pyogenic brain abscess (particularly in IV drug users); and primary and metastatic brain tumors.

PREVENTION: PLWH should be tested for IgG antibody to *Toxoplasma* soon after diagnosis to detect latent infection.

To reduce risk of acquisition, PLWH should be advised not to eat raw or undercooked meat or raw shellfish. They should wash their hands after contact with raw meat and after contact with soil; they should also wash fruits and vegetables well before eating them raw. PLWH who are seronegative and own cats should be advised to have someone who is HIV-negative and not pregnant change the litter box daily.

TREATMENT: PLWH with positive *Toxoplasma* serology and a CD4 of <100/mL should receive prophylaxis with 1DS TMP/SMX qd (as indicated for PCP prophylaxis). The alternative is dapsone/pyrimethamine/leucovorin, which is also active against PCP.

Prophylaxis may be discontinued when the CD4 has increased to >200/mL for ≥3 months (can also consider discontinuing if CD4 is 100–200/mL and HIV RNA levels remain below limits of detection for at least 3–6 mos).

Preferred regimen:

TMP-SMX 1 DS po daily

Alternative regimens:

TMP-SMX 1 DS po three times weekly, *or*
TMP-SMX SS po daily, *or*
Dapsone 50 mg po daily + (pyrimethamine 50 mg + leucovorin 25 mg) po weekly, *or*
Dapsone 200 mg + pyrimethamine 75 mg + leucovorin 25 mg po weekly, *or*
Atovaquone 1,500 mg po daily, *or*
Atovaquone 1,500 mg + pyrimethamine 25 mg + leucovorin 10 mg po daily

Toxoplasmosis encephalitis:
Initial treatment:

Pyrimethamine 200 mg po once, followed by dose based on body
weight:
  Body weight ≤60 kg: Pyrimethamine 50 mg po daily + sulfadiazine 1,000 mg po q6h + leucovorin 10–25 mg po
  daily (can increase to 50 mg daily or bid if bone marrow
  suppression)
  Body weight >60 kg: Pyrimethamine 75 mg po daily + sulfadiazine 1,500 mg po q6h + leucovorin 10–25 mg po daily (can
  increase to 50 mg daily or bid if bone marrow suppression).

Alternative regimens:

Pyrimethamine/leucovorin (doses above) + clindamycin 600 mg
  po or IV q6h
TMP (5 mg/kg) + SMX (25 mg/kg) po or IV bid
Atovaquone 1,500 mg po bid + pyrimethamine/leucovorin, *or*
Atovaquone 1,500 mg po bid + sulfadiazine, *or*
Atovaquone 1,500 mg po bid
Pyrimethamine/leucovorin + azithromycin 900–1,200 mg po qd
  (based on a small cohort study)

Duration of above regimens: Treatment should continue for
at least 6 weeks for acute infection, longer if clinical or imaging
studies indicate extensive disease or response is incomplete at
6 weeks.
Maintenance therapy:
Preferred regimen:

Pyrimethamine 25–50 mg po daily + sulfadiazine 2,000–4,000
  mg po daily (in 2 to 4 divided doses) + leucovorin 10–25 mg
  po daily

Alternative regimen:

Clindamycin 600 mg po q8h + (pyrimethamine 25–50 mg + leucovorin 10–25 mg) po daily; must add additional agent to prevent PCP *or*

TMP-SMX DS 1 tablet bid, *or*

TMP-SMX DS 1 tablet daily (if low pill burden is important), *or*

Atovaquone 750–1,500 mg po bid + (pyrimethamine 25 mg + leucovorin 10 mg) po daily, *or*

Atovaquone 750–1500 mg po bid + sulfadiazine 2000–4000 mg po daily (in 2 to 4 divided doses), *or*

Atovaquone 750–1500 mg po bid

Stopping therapy: Therapy can be halted after completion of the course and the patient is asymptomatic from TE infection and has a CD4 count of >200/mL for >6 months.

Indications to restart TE prophylaxis or maintenance: CD4 <200/mL

Adjunctive steroids: Use only to treat mass effect and discontinue as soon as possible.

Antiepileptics: Use for history of seizure and continue through acute treatment; avoid use for seizure prophylaxis.

Zoster

SOURCE DOCUMENT: Varicella-Zoster Disease (NIH & DHHS Guidance) hppt://aidsinfo.nih.gov/guidelines, last updated July 8, 2013; last reviewed July 25, 2017.

EPIDEMIOLOGY: More than 95% of adults born in the US have immunity to varicella-zoster virus (VZV), most frequently from primary VZV infection (chickenpox). Reactivation of latent VZV results in herpes zoster infection (shingles). A person's lifetime risk for shingles is 15–20%, with increased rates in the elderly and immunocompromised. The incidence rate for adult PLWH is 15-fold higher versus age-matched controls. Although all adults with HIV infection are at increased risk, the risk is highest in those with a CD4 count of <200/mL. Rates also appear to be higher immediately after ART initiation.

CLINICAL FEATURES: The usual presentation is a prodrome with pain in the region of the involved dermatome that evolves within days to a characteristic dermatomal vesicular rash that evolves over 3–5 days. A review of 282 cases of zoster in PLWH showed 67% had a single dermatome involved, 41% were thoracic (JAIDS 2005;40:169). The frequency of postherpetic neuralgia was 18%, and about 10% have a recurrence within 1 yr of the initial event.

Most VZV-related complications in HIV, including disseminated zoster, occur in patients with a CD4 of <200/mL. The CNS is the main target organ. Major VZV-related neurologic complications include CNS vasculitis, multifocal leukoencephalitis, ventriculitis, myelitis, myeloradiculitis, optic neuritis, cranial nerve palsies, aseptic meningitis, acute retinal necrosis (ARN), progressive outer retinal necrosis (PORN), disseminated zoster, and brainstem lesions.

ARN and PORN are variants of necrotizing retinal disease seen in PLWH. PORN occurs almost exclusively in patients with a CD4 of <100/mL, while ARN can occur in immunocompetent as well as immunosuppressed patients. Both of these ocular infections have high rates of vision loss.

DIAGNOSIS: VZV infections are usually easy to diagnose based on clinical presentation with vesicular lesions. Varicella (chickenpox) infection is associated with seroconversion; zoster has the typical dermatomal distribution. When there is confusion, the etiologic virus may be detected by PCR, direct fluorescent antigen, or culture using fresh swabs from typical lesions or by tissue biopsy. PCR is most sensitive and specific. Serology is not generally recommended.

PREVENTION: (1) PLWH who are susceptible to VZV (i.e., persons who have no history of varicella or shingles, who are seronegative for VZV, and who have no history of vaccination against VZV) should avoid exposure to individuals with active varicella or herpes zoster. (2) Household contacts of PLWH without immunity should be vaccinated if they themselves are also without immunity. (3) Long-term prophylaxis is not recommended

TREATMENT:

Herpes zoster (shingles): Prompt antiviral therapy should be instituted in all PLWH whose herpes zoster is diagnosed within 1 week of rash onset (or any time before full crusting of lesions).

Localized dermatomal:
Preferred:

Valacyclovir 1 g po tid × 7–10 d *or*
Famciclovir 500 mg po tid × 7–10 d

Alternative:

Acyclovir 800 mg po 5×/d × 7–10 d
Longer duration should be considered, if lesions resolve slowly

Extensive cutaneous lesions or visceral involvement:

Acyclovir 10–15 mg/kg IV q8h until clinical improvement, then
  oral valacyclovir 1g tid, famciclovir 500 mg tid, or acyclovir
  800 mg po 5×/d × 10–14 d

ARN/PORN:
Recommended:

Involvement of an experienced ophthalmologist
plus
Optimized ART
plus
VZV antiviral:
  PORN: Ganciclovir 5 mg/kg q12h and/or foscarnet 90 mg/
    kg IV q12h
  plus Intravitreal ganciclovir 2 mg/0.05 mL and/or foscarnet
    1.2 mg/0.05 mL twice weekly

ARN: Acyclovir 10–15 mg/kg IV q8h for 10–14 days, followed by valacyclovir 1 g po tid for 6 weeks *plus* Intravitreal ganciclovir 2 mg/0.05 mL twice weekly × 1–2 doses

Duration should be determined based on clinical, virologic, and immunologic response in consultation with an ophthalmologist.

8

Systems Review

Cardiovascular Disease

Cardiovascular disease (CVD) is the major cause of death in the United States and a major cause of death with HIV infection in the HAART era (AIDS 2010;24:1537). There are substantial data indicating that HIV infection increases the risk of an acute myocardial infarction (MI) by approximately 60% compared to age-matched controls (J Clin Endocrin Metab 2007;92:2506). This risk is multifactorial, including some factors that are reversible and many that are HIV-related. The relative risks for an acute MI by the D:A:D analysis are summarized in Table 8.1.

SPECIFIC FACTORS:

- *HIV viral load (VL)*: An analysis of 6,517 patients in a Boston healthcare system from 1998 to 2008 found a significant risk associated with a VL of >100,000 c/mL (odds ratio [OR] 2.2; $p = 0.01$) and a decreased risk with a VL of <400 c/mL (OR 0.6; $p = 0.6$). Similarly, a CD4 count of <200/mL appeared to be a significant risk (OR 1.5; $p = 0.02$), and increasing the CD4 by 50/mL correlated with a decreased risk (OR 0.95; $p = 0.001$) (JAIDS 2010;55:615).
- There are also substantial data suggesting HIV treatment may be an important risk factor (see later discussion). The possible central role of immune activation, as indicated by elevated inflammatory markers, is consistently shown, but causally enigmatic (PLoS Med 2008;5:e203; JID 2010;201:1788; Curr Infect Dis Rep 2011;13:94). Large population-based

TABLE 8.1 Risk factors for an acute myocardial infarction (MI) in D:A:D[a]

Risk Category	RR[b]
PI exposure (/yr)	1.1
Age (/5)	1.2
Male sex	2.1
BMI 30	1.3
Smoking	2.9
Current	1.6
Former	
Prior CVD event	4.6
Diabetes	1.7
Hypertension	1.3
Total cholesterol (mmol/L)	1.3
Family history	1.4

[a] D:A:D data (NEJM 2007;356:1723).
[b] RR, Adjusted relative risk.

trials, including SMART, have shown that ART reduces markers of inflammation but does not normalize them (AIDS 2010;24:1657). Nevertheless, discontinuation of ART in the SMART trial was associated with a substantially increased risk of major cardiovascular events (OR 1.6; $p = 0.05$) (NEJM 2006;355:2283).

- *Agents*: D:A:D is a large, observational cohort of PLWH designed to evaluate CVD. It is robust in numbers and methods that includes review of all CVD events by blinded cardiologists. Early studies based on the analysis of 23,000 PLWH showed that the highest risk was in patients with RTV-boosted PIs (JID 2004;189:1056). The presumed mechanism was drug-induced lipid elevation. RTV at a dose of 100 mg bid in seronegative patients increased TG levels 27%, LDL-C 16%, and total cholesterol 17% (HIV Med 2005;6:421; NEJM 1995;333:1528). LPV/r did not increase TG or LDL-C levels more, but did increase the total cholesterol. FPV, DRV, and TPV all show this effect, with increases in TG and LDL-C with RTV boosting; the magnitude of the change is dependent on the dose of RTV (Lancet 2006;368;476; Lancet 2007;369:1169), and there is an independent effect of the protease inhibitor (PI) on cholesterol. The exception is ATV, which has no apparent independent effect on lipids, but a very modest effect with RTV boosting at 100 mg/d (AIDS 2006;20:711). d4T and AZT are also associated with elevated triglyceride levels (JAIDS 2006;43:535; JAMA 2004;292:191). A D:A:D analysis based on 178,835 person-years of follow-up and 580 MIs found a significant risk with only four ART agents: recent exposure to ABC or ddI and cumulative exposure to IDV/r or LPV/r (JID 2010;201:318). The data for ABC are particularly controversial due to conflicting results in both prospective and retrospective studies. With regard to lipids and other ART agents, effects are less or nil with NVP and RPV compared to EFV (AIDS 2003;17:1195; Curr Infect Dis Rep 2011;13:1). MVC caused less dyslipidemia than EFV in the MERIT trial (Clin Trials 2008;30:1228). RAL does not appear to alter blood lipids (NEJM 2008;359:339; Lancet 2010;375:396). DTG has a similar impact on blood lipids as RAL. Mild increases in TC, LDL, and TG can be seen (Clin Drug Investig 2015;35;211). ART-associated changes are usually apparent within 2–3 mos of initiating therapy.

- *ATV* is the exception to PI-associated CVD risk. ATV is associated with an unconjugated hyperbilirubinemia, and bilirubin is a natural antioxidant that prevents oxidative stress associated with the atherosclerotic cascade. Recent studies have begun to demonstrate how this translates to CVD risk reduction. A Veterans Administration (VA) study of 9,500 patients showed lower risk for MI and stroke in patients who received ATV containing regimens versus those who received other PIs, non-nucleoside reverse transcriptase inhibitors (NNRTIs), or integrase strand transfer inhibitors (INSTIs) (AIDS 2017;31:2095).

- *Risk*: An increased risk of cardiovascular disease associated with ART was initially assumed based on serum lipid changes. The D:A:D data (just summarized) showed 126 MIs among 23,468 patients with a relative risk (RR) of 1.25; for smoking it was 2.2 (NEJM 2003;349:1993). With long-term follow-up (>4 yrs), the rate of MIs in patients receiving ART was about 26% above predicted rates (HIV Med 2006;7:218). A review of nine studies indicated a significant risk of CVD in seven reports (Circulation 2008;118:e29); other reports also show a modest increased OR for coronary events with use of ART (JAMA 2003;289:2978; AIDS 2003;17:1179). These data collectively indicate that HIV infection is associated with an increased risk of CVD and MIs, and contributing factors include HIV infection per se, selected ART regimens, and traditional risks such as smoking.

- *Hyperlipidemia*: Changes in blood lipids are an important concern in patients with HIV infection, with and without ART. Studies in the pre-HAART era indicated that HIV infection was associated with elevated TG levels and decreased levels of LDL-C and HDL-C (Am J Med 1991;90:154; JAMA 2003;289:2978). The decrease in HDL-C and increase in TG levels increased the risk of CVD; studies comparing people living with HIV (PLWH) and HIV-negative individuals demonstrate a 1.5- to 2.0-fold increase in CVD associated with HIV infection (Circulation 2008;118:198). Although the rate of CVD is significantly higher, the absolute rate is low.

- *Biomarkers*: The markers most commonly used to measure immune activation in research studies have been hsCRP and interleukin (IL)-6 (and D-dimer) (PLoS Med 2008;5:e203). Studies in patients without HIV have found the best outcomes in those with a hsCRP <2 mg/L and LDL <70 mg/dL (J Am Coll Cardiol 2005;45:1644). IL-6 is another favored marker used in the SMART trial. These markers also predicted death in participants in SMART when adjusted for CD4 count and VL (JAIDS 2003;32:2010; JID 2010;201:1796). D-Dimer, a marker of thrombotic activity, has also been predictive of death in persons with and without HIV infection (AIDS 2009;23:929). The data show that these biomarkers predict CVD and death and that levels are increased with HIV infection and that they decrease, but do not return to normal, with ART (Curr Opin AIDS 2010;5:511; JID 2010;201:1788). For more information, see the section on immune activation biomarkers.

SPECIFIC RECOMMENDATIONS:

- Risk assessment should include a review of other CV risk factors as defined below based on updated 2013 American College of Cardiology/American Heart Association (ACC/AHA) guidelines, ASCVD risk calculator, and AIDS Clinical Trials Group (ACTG)/Infectious Diseases Society of America (IDSA).
  - CVD risk assessment recommendations:
    - Obtain fasting lipid panel prior to starting ART, and at 4–8 wks with new regimen.
    - Assess for traditional CVD risk factors and repeat every 4–6 yrs in patients who are low risk (ASCVD risk <7.5%).
    - Identify these three high-risk groups for primary prevention: Diabetes and age 40–75, LDL >190 mg/dL, clinical ASCVD (history of MI, ACS, stable or unstable angina, coronary or other arterial revascularization, stroke/TIA, peripheral arterial disease).
    - If not included in one of the above risk groups, and age 40–75, calculate ASCVD 10-yr risk.
    - Refer to ACC/AHA guidelines for primary prevention for high-risk groups (Circulation 2014;129:S2).
    - For 10-yr risk <5%, LDL <190 mg/dL, non-diabetics age 40–75 with CVD risk factors consider lifestyle changes.
    - Address non–lipid modifiable risk factors including smoking, obesity, and diet.

- ASCVD calculator is an estimate of 10-yr risk for cardio-vascular disease and stroke. Components include (1) age 40–79; (2) sex; (3) race, including non-Hispanic white and African American; (4) total cholesterol, HDL, and LDL; (5) systolic blood pressure; (6) tobacco use; (7) treatment for hypertension; (8) diabetes; (9) current aspirin use; (10) current statin use.
- The calculation is readily available from multiple sources including: http://my.americanheart.org/cvriskcalculator
- The ACC/AHA guidelines and ASCVD calculator are estimates of CVD risk based on a non-HIV population. Predictive models for CVD in PLWH are under investigation but have yet to be incorporated into clinical practice. One such predictive model is the D:A:D CVD prediction model (Eur J Prev Cardiol 2015:23;214). The predictive model includes traditional CVD risk factors (age, gender, CVD family history, smoking history, systolic blood pressure, HDL, total cholesterol, diabetes) in addition to cumulative NNRTI and PI exposure, current ABC use, and CD4 count. In comparison to the Framingham predictive model, the D:A:D predictive model estimated CVD risk more accurately (Eur J Prev Cardiol 2015:23;214).
- *Management*: Recommendations are from the ACC/AHA (Circulation 2014:129:S2), ACTG, and IDSA (CID 2003;37:613), the Academic Consortium (CID 2006;43:645), IAS-USA Guidelines, and the European AIDS Clinical Society Guidelines 2008.

GUIDELINES FOR PREVENTION:

- Hyperlipidemia: (see Table 8.3)
  - The updated 2013 ACC/AHA guidelines reflect that no randomized controlled trials (RCTs) demonstrated clear benefit for target HDL and LDL goals. Instead, recommendations are to use maximum tolerated statin intensity in benefited groups (Circulation 2014;129).

- There is also a shift in conclusions about HDL-cholesterol, "the good cholesterol." HDL is atheroprotective by promoting efflux of cholesterol from macrophages. HDL cholesterol can be converted to a dysfunctional form, so levels may be deceptive. Thus, it is the HDL efflux capacity that is most relevant (NEJM 2011;264:127).
- *Baseline assessment*: Lipid panel, including cholesterol, LDL and HDL cholesterol, and triglycerides after fasting at least 8 hrs (preferably 12 hrs). Nonfasting lipid panels can also provide useful information about cholesterol subsets. Fasting is necessary for accurate measurement of triglycerides and the calculation of LDL but has minimal effect on total cholesterol. LDL-C is calculated by the Friedewald equation: LDL-C = TC − (HDL-C) − TG/5 (JAIDS 2002;31:257). LDL cholesterol measurements are unreliable with triglyceride levels >400 mg/dL. In this situation, clinicians can subtract HDL levels from total cholesterol to obtain a non-HDL cholesterol level (JAMA 2001;285:2486) or can use direct LDL measurements. Interpretation must take into account secondary causes of dyslipidemia including nephrosis, alcoholism, thiazides, testosterone treatment, estrogen treatment, hypogonadism, uncontrolled diabetes, and cocaine abuse.
- *Hypertension*: See J Am Coll Cardiol November 7, 2017.
  - Treat for blood pressure >130/80 in patients with clinical ASCVD and 10-yr risk >10%.
  - Treat for blood pressure >140/90 in patients with no clinical ASCVD and 10-yr risk <10%.
  - Therapy should include nonpharmacologic therapy: physical activity, DASH diet, sodium reduction, weight loss, reduction in alcohol consumption.
- *Acetylsalicylic acid (ASA)/aspirin*:
  - Recommendations are from US Preventive Services Task Force (USPTF) and AHA guidelines on primary prevention of stroke and cardiovascular disease (Circulation 2002;106:388–391).

- Men age 45–79 and women age 55–79 with high risk of CVD, for whom benefits outweigh risks (GI bleed and hemorrhagic stroke):
  - *Aspirin* 81–325 mg, no benefit with use of higher doses. *Lifestyle modifications* for patients with elevated blood pressure and hyperlipidemia (Circulation 2014;129:S76–S99).
  - *Diet*: Rich in fruits and vegetables, whole grain, high fiber, fish (especially oily fish >2 ×/wk); reduce intake of saturated fat, cholesterol, alcohol, sodium, and glucose.
  - *Physical activity*: 3–4 sessions per week, 40 minutes each
  - *Tobacco cessation*
  - *Consider marijuana cessation* in high-risk patients. Components in marijuana have been implicated in endovascular injury. An increased risk for CVD is suggested in patients without HIV, but studies showing this association have been inconclusive (Ann Intern Med January 23, 2018).
- *Chronic kidney disease (CKD)*:
  - Patients with high risk for CVD in addition to CKD are at especially high risk for CVD and CKD events and should be monitored accordingly (PLoS Med. 2017;14:e1002424). See section on renal complications.
- *Antiviral substitution*:
  - *NRTIs*: A review of the CNICS cohort with 2,267 treated patients found that tenofovir disoproxil (TDF), 3TC, and ABC had minimal impact compared to the thymidine analogs, ddI was associated with the highest LDL-C increases, and d4T recipients had the highest triglyceride increases (AIDS 2011;25:185).
  - PI/r regimens often have the poorest atherogenic lipid profile—most marked with LPV/r (ATAZIP: JAIDS 2009;23:16) and RTV (CASTLE: JAIDS 2010;53:323 and a meta-analysis, JAC 2010;65:1878). ATV appears to be essentially "lipid neutral" without boosting (JAIDS 2009;57:153). RTV promotes an atherogenic lipid pattern

in a dose-dependent fashion, as shown in the LESS trial (HIV Clin Trials 2010;11:239).

- Substituting an NNRTI, ATV, or ATV/r for another boosted PI has improved lipid profiles (JAIDS 2005;39:174; AIDS 2005;19:917).
- *NNRTIs*: EFV has a modest impact on LDL-C and TG levels, as shown in the MERIT trial, with comparison to MVC (HIV Clin Trials 2011;12:24), and compared to RAL in STARTMRK (JAIDS 2010;55:39). According to the SPIRIT study, switch from boosted PI regimens to RPV-FTC-TDF resulted in improved TC, TG, LDL, and TC:HDL ratio (AIDS 2014:28:335). A similar decrease in TC, LDL, and TG was shown with RPV in comparison to EFV (BMC Infect Dis 2017: 17;511).
- *INSTI*: RAL appears to be lipid-neutral according to the SWITCHMRK (Lancet 2010;375:396) and SPIRAL (AIDS 2010;24:1697) studies. DTG appears to be lipid-neutral as well. Smaller increases in TC, LDL, and TG are seen with DTG, in comparison to EFV and ritonavir-boosted darunavir (Clin Drug Invest 2015; 35:211).
- *Switch versus statin therapy*: One report found that statin therapy was more effective than changing antiretroviral agents (AIDS 2005;19:1051). In another study comparing statin introduction to switch therapy, rosuvastatin added to boosted PI regimens resulted in greater decreases in TC and LDL compared to switch therapy to a non-PI regimen (HIV Med 2016;17:605).

TREATMENT OF HYPERLIPIDEMIA:
See Circulation 2014;129:S2.

- Updated ACC/AHA 2013 guidelines removed specific LDL targets and have identified four major high-risk groups that would benefit from statin therapy for primary and secondary prevention of CVD.
- The maximum tolerated statin therapy is recommended based on the risk group (see Table 8.2).

TABLE 8.2 Statins

Agent[a]	Intensity	Form	Dose (FDA)		Decrease LDL
			Initial mg/day	Max mg/day	
Atorvastatin (Lipitor)	Moderate: 10–20 mg High: 40–80 mg	Tabs – 10, 20, 40, 80 mg	10	80	35–60%
Pravastatin (Pravachol)	Low: 10–20 mg Moderate: 40–80 mg	Tabs – 10, 20, 40, 80 mg	20–40	80	30–40%
Rosuvastatin (Crestor)	Moderate: 5–10 mg High: 20–40 mg	Tabs – 5, 10, 20, 40 mg	10	40	45–60%
Pitavastatin (Livalo)	Low: 1 mg Moderate 2–4 mg	Tabs- 1, 2, 4 mg	2	4	30–50%

[a] Lovastatin (Mevacor) and simvastatin (Zocor) are not included due to major drug interactions with all PIs and cobicistat. Fluvastatin not included due to low potency, lack of safety data, and interactions with PIs and NNRTIs.

- Lifestyle modifications are recommended in addition to statin therapy.
- Lipid panels should be obtained 4–12 wks after start of therapy to monitor for compliance with medications and lifestyle modifications.
- LDL reductions are used for monitoring compliance and not for goal targeted therapy.
- Repeat every 3–12 mos.

TREATMENT OF HYPERTRIGLYCERIDEMIA:
See *Circulation* 2001;123:243.

- Drug therapy (Table 8.4):
  - *Statins*: These are the most effective drugs for reducing LDL-C; they also decrease TG. The clinical benefit correlates with the LDL-C decrease. An analysis of 700 PLWH showed that lipid goals were achieved more frequently with atorvastatin or rosuvastatin compared to pravastatin (CID 2011; 52:387) A meta-analysis of 58 placebo-controlled trials found that all-cause mortality was reduced by 10% for every 1.0 mmol/L decrease in LDL cholesterol with no threshold (Lancet 2010; 376:1670). Once started, statins are usually continued for a lifetime. If stopped, lipid levels return to baseline within 2–3 wks.
  - Statins have beneficial antiinflammatory effects that are not completely explained by lipid reduction. The JUPITER study with rosuvastatin showed that the cardiac event rate and the hsCRP results were significantly reduced even after adjusting for the change in LDL-cholesterol (Am J Cardiovasc Drugs 2010;10:383). Statin therapy has been noted to reduce hsCRP levels (Arch Med Res 2010;41:464). This has been noted in PLWH as well (AIDS 2011;25:1128). The latter report showed a median decrease of hsCRP of 3.0–2.4/L (p <0.001) that did not correlate with changes in lipids.
  - *PI interactions*: Most statins are metabolized using cytochrome P3A4; all PIs inhibit CYP3A4. The greatest effect is with lovastatin and simvastatin; atorvastatin is only partially metabolized by CYP3A4; pravastatin and rosuvastatin are not metabolized by this mechanism, except for the interaction of DRV/r and pravastatin (see Table 8.4). Inhibition of CYP3A4 causes significant toxicity potential when used with PIs but not NNRTIs.

TABLE 8.3 Treatment of hyperlipidemia

Risk Group	Therapy
Clinical ASCVD	High intensity statin
LDL >190 mg/dL	High intensity statin
Diabetes and age 40–75	Moderate intensity statin
10 yr risk >7.5%	Moderate intensity statin

From Circulation 2014;129:S2.

- *Adverse effects*: In a review of 700 PLWH given statins, 6.4% discontinued treatment due to toxicity, and rates were nearly equal for pravastatin, atorvastatin, and rosuvastatin (CID 2011;52:387). The most common was CPK elevation,

TABLE 8.4 Drug interactions: Effect of ARV agents on AUC of statins

Statin[a]	ATV[a]	DRV/r[b]	EFV	ETR	FPV/r	LPV/r	SQV/r	TPV
Atorvastatin	ND	↑4.0	ND	ND	1.5	↑4.9	↑0.8	↑8.0
Pravastatin	ND	↑1.8	↓0.4	↔	ND	↑1.33	↓0.5	ND
Rosuvastatin	↑2.1	↑–	ND	↔	–	↑2.0	↑–	↑1.2
Pitavastatin	↑0.31	↔	↔	ND	ND	↔	ND	ND

Adapted from the 2017 DHHS Guidelines.

ND, No data; ↔, no significant effect.

[a] For atorvastatin—concurrent ATV/cobi increases atorvastatin conc. 9.2-fold (Avoid). DRV/cobi increases atorvastatin concentrations 3.9-fold (do not exceed 20mg/d).

[b] For rosuvastatin-concurrent ATV/cobi increases rosuvastatin concentrations 3.4-fold (use rosuvastatin 20 mg/d). DRV/cobi increases rosuvastatin dose 1.9-fold (use rosuvastatin 10 mg/d).

Lovastatin and simvastatin are not included—both are contraindicated for concurrent use with PIs and cobicistat. Both may be used with EFV and ETR with doses based on lipid response without exceeding the recommended dose.

TABLE 8.5 Triglycerides: Preferred fibrates

Agent	Form	Regimen
Gemfibrozil (Lopid and generic)	Tabs – 600 mg	600 mg bid before meals
Fenofibrate (TriCor and generic)	Tabs: 48, 145 mg Caps: 67, 100, 200 mg	48–145 mg/d 200 mg/d

and the most severe was rhabdomyolysis with renal failure. Obtain baseline CPK levels and repeat the test if myalgias develop; some recommend discontinuing statins or lowering the dose if the level is 3–5× ULN (Treatment Guidelines, Med Letter 2003;3:15). Other adverse drug reactions (ADRs) include gastrointestinal symptoms and increased transaminase levels in 1–2%, which are often corrected by use of an alternative statin. A rare polyneuropathy has been reported (Neurology 2002;58:1333).

- *Fibrates*: These agents (fenofibrate and gemfibrozil) are used to treat triglyceride levels >400–500 mg/dL (Table 8.5). Levels <150 mg/dL are considered normal, and levels >400 mg/dL represent an independent risk for cardiovascular disease. These drugs can be used concurrently with statins as shown in ACTG5087, which found good results with the combination (J Clin Lipidol 2010;4:279).

  - *Triglyceride levels >400 mg/dL*: Preferred treatment is with fibrates, either micronized fenofibrate 48–145 mg/d, or gemfibrozil 100 mg bid. If triglyceride levels remain >500 mg/dL, consider fish oil 3–6 g/d (CID 2005;41:1498).

- *Niacin*: Reduces LDL-C and triglycerides. Concerns are flushing, minimal published experience in PLWH with dyslipidemia, and possible insulin resistance (Antivir Ther 2006;11:1081). One report showed favorable results with a mean decrease of 34% in TG with ER niacin, combined with ASA pretreatment to avoid flushing. Recently, the AIM-HIGH study, a large clinical trial in which niacin was used to increase HDL-C in patients with coronary heart disease, was halted when it became clear that elevations in HDL-C did not decrease cardiovascular risk.

- *Fish oil*: Active components are omega-3 fatty acids, which are used to treat high TG. The usual dose in 3–6 g/d, it is generally well tolerated, and data supporting efficacy in PLWH are modest but good (CID 2005;41:1498; Antiviral Ther 2006;11:1081). Use is generally reserved for patients who fail fibrates.
- *Ezetimibe*: This agent in a dose of 10 mg/d reduces absorption of cholesterol. Ezetimibe lowers LDL in patients intolerant to statin therapies and in patients who need additional LDL lowering in combination with statins. Benefits in cardiovascular endpoints are seen in combination with statin therapy (J Am Coll Cardiol 2016;67:353). A report with 44 PLWH given ezetimibe and a statin showed good tolerance and good LDL response (AIDS 2009;23:2133).

Dilated Cardiomyopathy

Note that the prior classic study (NEJM 1998;339:1092) has been withdrawn for reasons that are not clear.

CAUSE: Unknown, but likely multifactorial. Current hypotheses include:

1. Mitochondrial toxicity from zidovudine (Cardiovasc Res 2003;60:147; CID 2003;37:109; JAIDS 2004;37:S30; Chem Res Toxicol 2008;21:990).
2. Direct HIV myocardial damage (Cardiovasc Toxicol 2004;4:97; Am J Physiol 2000;279:H3138; Am J Physiol 2004;286:C1).
3. Nutritional deficiencies from L-carnitine and selenium deficiency (Curr HIV Res 2007;5:129; NEJM 1999;340:732).
4. Proinflammatory cytokines: Tumor necrosis (TNF)-α, IL-1β and IL-6 (Int J Cardiol 2007;120:150; Cytokine2007;39:157; AIDS 2008;22:585).

5. Autoimmune mechanisms (AIDS 2003;17(suppl 1):S21; Heart 1998;79:599).
6. Opportunistic infections (Wien Klin Wochenschr 2008; 120:77).

FREQUENCY: With the advent of HAART, HIV cardiomyopathy has changed from severe, dilated cardiomyopathy to a minimally symptomatic, mildly reduced EF with various degrees of impaired diastolic function (Circulation 2014;129:1781). Longitudinal studies in the pre-HAART era described rates of 6–8% for symptomatic cardiomyopathy (Eur Heart J 1992;13:1452; Clin Immunol Immunopathol 1993;68:234). Rates of left ventricular diastolic dysfunction with routine echocardiography are much higher and correlate with stage of immunosuppression (Heart 1998;80:184). Rates are thought to have decreased during the HAART era by as much as 7-fold (Wein Klin Wocheuschr 2008;120:77; Am Heart J 2006;151:1147). Nevertheless, the SUN study, with echocardiographs in 656 unselected PLWH with average age of 41 yrs and median CD4 count of 462 cells/mm^3, found that 18% had left ventricular dysfunction, 40% had left atrial enlargement, and 57% had pulmonary hypertension (CID 2011;52:378). These changes correlated with elevated hsCRP.

SYMPTOMS: Congestive heart failure (CHF)-associated symptoms include progressive dyspnea with exertion, impaired exercise capacity, orthopnea, paroxysmal nocturnal dyspnea, peripheral edema, arrhythmias, and/or syncope.

DIAGNOSIS: Echocardiogram showing ejection fraction (EF) <50% normal ± arrhythmias on electrocardiogram (EKG), not otherwise explained. Criterion for dilated cardiomyopathy in the major study was an EF <45% and end diastolic volume index >80 mL/M^2 (NEJM 1998;339:1093). Myocardial biopsies in 76 patients in this study showed myocarditis with inflammatory cells in 63; biopsy cultures yielded coxsackie B in 15 and cytomegalovirus (CMV) in 4.

TREATMENT:
See Circulation 2014;129:1781.

Optimal therapy for HIV cardiomyopathy is poorly understood. No randomized trials of heart failure medications have been performed in this patient population. Therapy is therefore guideline-driven from HIV negative cardiomyopathy patients.

- *ART*: Use non–AZT-containing regimen. Several studies have found that HAART has reduced rates of HIV cardiomyopathy (AIDS 2012;26:2027; J Infect 2000;40;282). A few case reports showed regression and normalization of heart function with ART (South Med J 2006;99:274;Cardiol Young2003;13:373). However, concrete evidence showing ART reversal of HIV-associated cardiomyopathy is not currently available.
- *Angiotensin converting enzyme (ACE) inhibitor/angiotensin receptor blocker (ARB)*: Lisinopril 10 mg/d titrated up to 40 mg/d as tolerated.
  - *Alternatives*: Enalapril 2.5 mg bid and titrate up to 20 mg bid; captopril 6.25 mg tid up to 50 mg tid. Can use ARB if patient is ACE inhibitor intolerant.
  - *Allergy or contraindication to both ACE inhibitor and ARB*: consider combination with hydralazine and isosorbide dinitrate.
- *β-Blocker*: Metoprolol succinate (metoprolol-XL) 25 mg/d titrated up to 200 qd, or carvedilol 3.125 mg bid titrated up to 25 mg bid, or bisoprolol 2.5 mg/d titrated up to 20 mg/d.
- *Persistent symptoms*: add diuretic-furosemide 10–40 mg/d (up to 240 mg bid) or bumetanide. Also, consider spironolactone 25 mg/d (up to 50 mg bid), hydrochlorothiazide, or metolazone.
- *Refractory*: consider digoxin 0.125–0.25 mg/d.
- *Automatic implantable cardioverter-defibrillator (AICD) devices*: Little is known about the effect of device therapy in PLWH with cardiomyopathy as the rate and effectiveness of implantable devices have not been reported in patients with HIV cardiomyopathy (J Am Coll Cardiol 2012;59:1891).
- *Other options*: Treat hypertension, treat hyperlipidemia, discontinue alcohol, limit salt intake, avoid cocaine use, and smoking cessation. Some recommend supplemental

antioxidants, such as carnitine and/or selenium (200 μg/d), if deficient (NEJM 1999;340:732).

- *Immunotherapy*: Intravenous immunoglobulin (IVIG) and etanercept. Very limited data show benefits from these agents and further studies are needed (Circulation 1995;92:2220; Circulation. 2001;103:1044).

Myocarditis

The prevalence of HIV myocarditis has decreased since the widespread use of HAART. HIV myocardial disease ranges from incidental asymptomatic myocarditis seen on echocardiogram to symptomatic cardiomyopathy (AIDS Res Hum Retroviruses 1998;14:1071). Treatment of symptomatic heart failure is as described in the preceding section.

CAUSE: Myocarditis is thought to be multifactorial with several proposed mechanisms of cardiovascular injury.

1. *HIV direct invasion* (Mod Pathol 1990;3:625; Curr Opin HIV AIDS 2017;12:561).
2. *Co-infection with other viruses*: EBV facilitating HIV entry into cells (Dev Biol Stand 1990;72:309).
3. *Opportunistic infections*: CMV, HSV, toxoplasmosis, NTM (Curr Opin HIV AIDS 2017;12:561).
4. *Immune dysregulation*: Proinflammatory state and subsequent vascular injury and myopathy (Int J Cardiol 2007;120:150; Cardiovasc Toxicol 2004;4:97).
5. *Drug-induced*: Dolutegravir (Medicine [Baltimore] 2016; 95:e5465).

Pericarditis/Pericardial Effusion

In the pre-ART era, pericardial disease was the most common clinical manifestation of HIV cardiac disease.

CAUSE: In asymptomatic patients, the etiology of pericardial effusion is often unknown (Eur Heart J 2013;34:3538). In the symptomatic patient, infectious etiologies and neoplastic processes are the most common etiologies. Mycobacterial infections are the most common infectious causes (Angiology 2003;54:469). In sub-Saharan Africa, >90% of pericardial effusions are due to *M. tuberculosis* (Heart 2013;99:1146). Other infectious etiologies include *S. aureus, Cryptococcus, Nocardia, Streptococcus pneumoniae, Listeria monocytogenes*, and *Chlamydia trachomatis*. Lymphoma and Kaposi sarcoma are the most common neoplastic causes (Angiology 2003;54:469).

FREQUENCY: In a German prospective cohort of 800 subjects (85% on ART), only 2 patients had pericardial disease (Eur J Med Res 2011;16:480). However, in resource-limited settings, the prevalence of pericardial disease in PLWH is similar to that reported from pre-ART studies (Eur Heart J 2013;34:3538). In a South African study of 518 subjects, pericardial disease was diagnosed in 25% (Eur Heart J 2012;33:866).

SYMPTOMS: Patients are usually asymptomatic with small pericardial effusion on imaging. Symptomatic disease manifests with dyspnea, fever, pleuritic chest pain, and pericardial friction rub. In severe cases, cardiac tamponade can occur which presents with tachycardia, decreased blood pressure, and elevated jugular venous pressure.

DIAGNOSIS: Echocardiogram is the study of choice. For symptomatic patients, pericardiocentesis should be performed to obtain fluid and/or tissue for microbiological and cytological analysis.

TREATMENT: The management of pericardial effusion in PLWH depends on the severity and etiology of the pericardial disease. The majority of patients with a pericardial effusion have small effusions causing no symptoms. Asymptomatic disease requires no further testing except for follow-up (Am J Cardiol 1994;74:94). If symptomatic, pericardiocentesis is recommended for diagnostic and therapeutic evaluation. If tamponade occurs, immediate pericardiocentesis is required. Additional management is warranted depending on the identified or suspected etiology. If the patient is not already taking ART, initiation of ART should be strongly considered.

Dermatologic Complications

Skin manifestations may be the first indication of HIV infection, especially certain mucocutaneous conditions which serve as proxy indicators of advanced HIV infection. (Int J Dermatol 2007;46 Suppl 2:14). A 2016 review noted that there is a paucity of up-to-date and comprehensive evidence-based guidelines for treatment of HIV-related skin conditions at an international level (AIDS Res Treat 2016;2016: 3272483).

An older review of 897 patients with HIV infection referred for a dermatology consult in Baltimore from 1996 to 2002 found that the most frequent diagnoses were folliculitis (18%), condyloma acuminatum (12%), seborrhea (11%), xerosis cutis (10%), dermatophytic infection (7%), warts (7%), hyperpigmentation (6%), and prurigo nodularis (6%) (J Am Acad Dermatol 2006;54:581). Most of these conditions were associated with low CD4 counts (folliculitis, idiopathic pruritus, prurigo nodularis, molluscum, and seborrhea). Pruritus was especially common and often unexplained ("idiopathic pruritus"); this is thought to result from immune dysregulation and is sometimes accompanied by eosinophilia (JID 1996;54:266).

Papular Pruritic Eruption (PPE)

Typical presentation is pruritic darkened papules 0.2–1.0 cm diameter most common on extremities. A hypersensitivity to insect bites is often the cause (JAMA 2004;292:2614). Insect bite reaction occurs on the exposed surfaces of the body and can be a reaction to the bite of any insect. PPE in patients receiving ART is associated with a greater HIV viral load at initiation. The differential diagnosis

TABLE 8.6 Common skin conditions in PLWH

Condition	Cause	Presentation	Diagnosis	Treatment
Folliculitis	Usually *S. aureus*, can be caused by intrafollicular yeast or intrafollicular mites.	Pustules, with pruritus	Microbiological: Culture	*S. aureus*: topical erythromycin or clindamycin, or systemic antistaphylococcal antibiotic *Pityrosporum ovale*: topical or systemic antifungal agents *Demodex folliculorum*: permethrin cream or topical metronidazole
Eosinophilic folliculitis	A noninfectious, inflammatory dermatosis of unknown etiology that principally affects the hair follicles (J Dermatol 2016;43:919)	Very pruritic lesions that resemble acne or PPE but preferentially located on the upper body including the neck, head, and upper chest. More pruritic than acne. Less skin discoloration than PPE.	Clinical: Follicular inflammation ± follicular destruction and abscess formation. Histological: PAS and B+B Multiple eosinophils destroying the hair follicle wall and eosinophilic abscesses are seen in eosinophilic folliculitis	Topical steroids (47% efficacy), phototherapy with UVB and/or PUVA. Regimen trends between 1965 and 2013 were characterized by frequent use of antifungals and UV (16% and 14% of 133 regimens), efficacies of 70% and 94%, respectively. Tacrolimus, retinoids, and diaminodiphenyl sulfone also effective (90%, 89%, and 100%, respectively). (J Dermatol 2016;43:847)

Psoriasis	Possibly related to expanded CD8+ memory T cells and imbalanced CD4/CD8 ratio	Frequently severe generalized erythema, pruritus, pain, and fine scaling +/- pustular form.	May be presenting sign of HIV infection or develop after diagnosis.	ART is important. Phototherapy is considered first-line and may be effective. Acitretin (Soriatane) 25–50 mg/day can be considered as second-line. Data are limited on biologic agents in PLWH. (J Am Acad Dermatol 2010;62:291).
Scabies	Sarcoptes scabiei	Small red papules that are intensely pruritic, especially at night. "Burrow": a 3–15 mm line which is the superficial tunnel the female mite digs at 2 mm/d. Found in interdigital webs of the fingers, volar aspect of the wrist, periumbilical area, axilla, thighs, buttocks, genitalia, feet, and breasts.	Detection of mite: 0.4 × 0.3 mm, 8-legged, and shaped like a turtle. Scrape infected area, place on a slide with a coverslip, and examine under 10× magnification to demonstrate mites or eggs.	Treatment should include family members and close contacts treated at the same time. Permethrin cream (5%) applied to total body. Retreat at 1–2 wks. Lindane (1%): rare resistance occurs. Ivermectin 200 µg/kg po repeated at 2 wks (NEJM 1995;333:26). Rash and pruritus may persist up to 2 wks post-treatment. Bedding and clothing must be decontaminated.

(continued)

TABLE 8.6 Continued

Condition	Cause	Presentation	Diagnosis	Treatment
		Scabies crustosus (Norwegian scabies): severe form seen in immunocompromised hosts with uncontrolled spread; involves large areas, sometimes the total skin surface with scales and crusts that show thousands of mites		Scabies crustosus: isolate immediately and use strict barrier precautions. Treat with ivermectin 200 μg/kg po followed by a second dose in 1–2 wks
Seborrheic dermatitis	Yeast. Prevalence ~ 35% among patients with early HIV infection and up to 85% among patients with AIDS.	Erythematous plaques with greasy scales and indistinct margins, located on the scalp, central face, post-auricular area, presternal, axillary, and occasionally pubic area	Clinical, based on presentation	ART Short-term (≤4 wks) treatment with mild potency steroid ± ketoconazole 2% cream for the duration of the flare only, and tar-based shampoos, selenium sulfide, or zinc pyrithione applied qd, or ketoconazole shampoo.

May be a
manifestation
of IRIS (Clin
Exp Dermatol
2010;35:477)

In studies comparing topical
ketoconazole with topical
corticosteroids, both agents
had similar efficacy, although
topical corticosteroids
showed a 2-fold greater risk
of side effects compared with
ketoconazole.

Itraconazole 200 mg/d for
7 days followed by varying
intermittent therapy for 2–11
mos.

includes eosinophilic folliculitis and prurigo nodularis. The diagnosis can usually be established by a skin biopsy. The best treatment is ART, but this usually requires >16 wks for a good response. Other treatments include topical steroids or topical capsaicin (Top HIV Med 2010;18:16).

Bacillary Angiomatosis

See Arch Intern Med 1994;154:524; Dermatology 2000;21:326; CID 2005;40:S154.

Uncommon in ART era but still may be seen in people with CD4 counts of <100/mL. *Bartonella henselae* and *B. quintana* can both cause cutaneous manifestations. The usual presentation is papular, nodular, pedunculated, and/or verrucous lesions that start as red or purple papules and gradually expand to nodules or pedunculated masses. They appear vascular and may bleed extensively with trauma. There are usually one or several lesions, but there may be hundreds. Subcutaneous lesions may develop as deep-seated, tender nodules with erythematous or normal-appearing overlying skin (CID 1993;17:612). Infrequently, these lesions can develop as an enlarging deep suppurative ulcer (Arch Dermatol 1995;131:963). Cat and flea exposure have been associated with *B. henselae* infections and body louse exposure with *B. quintana*. The differential diagnosis includes Kaposi sarcoma, cherry angioma, hemangioma, pyogenic granuloma, and dermatofibroma. Diagnosis is based on skin biopsy showing lobular vascular proliferation with inflammation, and Warthin-Starry silver stain showing typical organisms as small black clusters. Serology is available (immunofluorescence assay [IFA] and enzyme immunoassay [EIA]); IFA titers >1:256 usually indicates active infection. In resource-limited settings where diagnostic pathology is not available, it may be misdiagnosed as Kaposi sarcoma (J Int Assoc Provid AIDS Care 2015;14:21). See section on *Bartonella*.

Cryptococcosis

See CID 2000;30:652 and section on Cryptococcus.

Typical presentation is nodular, papular, follicular, or ulcerative skin lesions; often resembling molluscum (i.e. centrally umbilicated papular lesions). Usual locations are face, neck, and scalp. Diagnosis is made with serum cryptococcal antigen assay and biopsy with Gomori methenamine silver stain to show typical encapsulated, budding yeast and positive culture. Perform LP in any patient with a positive serum cryptococcal antigen or blood culture with *C. neoformans* (if positive, see *Cryptococcus* section). Treatment, if negative LP, fluconazole 400 mg/d po × 8 wks, then 200 mg/d. If positive LP, see pg. Cryptococcus section.

Drug Eruptions

See J Allergy Clin Immunol 2008;121:826.

CAUSE: Most common are antibiotics, especially sulfonamides (TMP/SMX), β-lactams, anticonvulsants, NNRTIs, and TPV, FPV, and DRV, all of which include sulfa moieties. Some data show cross-reactivity between DRV and TMP/SMX (AIDS 2015;29:785). However, these reactions are rarely severe (AIDS 2015;29:2213). An increase in the CD8:CD4 ratio in the dermis of PLWH with toxic epidermal necrolysis (TEN) versus HIV-negative patients with TEN may contribute to the greater incidence of TEN in HIV (J Am Acad Dermatol 2014;70:1096).

PRESENTATION: The usual presentation is a morbilliform, erythematous, usually pruritic ± low grade fever, usually within 2 wks of new drug, or days after reexposure. Most common is a maculopapular rash that starts on the chest, face, and arms. Less common and more severe forms include urticaria (intensely pruritic, edematous, and circumscribed), anaphylaxis (laryngeal edema, nausea, vomiting ± shock), or hypersensitivity syndrome (severe reaction with rash and fever ± hepatitis, arthralgias, lymphadenopathy, and hematologic changes with eosinophilia and atypical lymphocytes, usually at 2–6 wks after drug is started; NEJM 1994;331:1272; see also later sections on abacavir and nevirapine), Stevens-Johnson syndrome (SJS) (fever, erosive stomatitis, disseminated erosions ± blisters dark red macules, ocular involvement; mortality 5%), and TEN.

TREATMENT: In severe symptomatic reactions, discontinue implicated agent (for TMP-SMX, see pg. 409) and treat. Use antihistamines and topical corticosteroids for uncomplicated drug rashes. SJS and TEN are managed as burns with supportive care. There is no role for corticosteroids in these cases (Cutis 1996;57:223). Complete avoidance required for ABC, NVP hepatotoxicity, and any other drug implicated in SJS or TEN. Desensitization protocol is available for TMP-SMX (see pg. 411).

Folliculitis

A review of 897 PLWH referred for a dermatology consultation found that folliculitis was the most common diagnosis, accounting for 18% (J Am Acad Derm 2006;54:581; NEJM 1988;318:1183; Arch Dermatol 1995;131:360). See Table.

Furunculosis

See Staphylococcus aureus section.

Herpes Simplex

See CID 2005;40:S167 and HSV Section.

Herpes Zoster

See VZV Section.

Prurigo Nodularis

See Int J Dermatol 1999;37:401.

Most common with CD4 count of <200/mL. The cause is unknown. The presentation is intense pruritus with excoriated nodules >1 cm diameter that are hyperpigmented. The lesions are generally symmetric, start on the arms, and then spread to the upper trunk. Unreachable areas such as the mid-back are usually spared. This may be a variant of PPE or other primary dermatologic condition. The major treatment modality is symptomatic to prevent vicious cycle pruritus: pruritus → scratch trauma → lichenification → increased pruritus.

Treatment includes occlusive dressings, high-potency steroids, hydroxyzine 10–25 mg hs or doxepin 10–25 mg hs, or mirtazipine 15–30 mg hs. Phototherapy may help. Thalidomide and lenalidomide have reported benefit in refractory cases (Dermatol Ther [Heidelb] 2016;6:397).

Pruritus

Pruritus is a very common problem in PLWH (Curr Infect Dis Rep 2015;17:464; Semin Cutan Med Surg 2011;30:101; Int J STD AIDS 2012;23:255). One cross-sectional study found a prevalence of 45% in general PLWH (J Am Acad Dermatol 2014;70:659); half reported that itching significantly impacted their quality of life. In addition to primary skin conditions, hepatitis, lymphoma, and psychiatric disorders can all lead to itching. After evaluating for a primary skin disease and infestation by scabies, pruritus can usually be treated by topical steroids. Sometimes treating HIV itself will improve itching. Other treatment options include antihistamines, anticonvulsants (e.g., gabapentin and pregabalin), serotonin and norepinephrine reuptake inhibitors (SNRIs), and selective serotonin reuptake inhibitors (SSRIs).

Psoriasis

Psoriasis may be a presenting sign of HIV infection, often occurring with advanced HIV disease. Skin rash has been noted to be more severe and persistent than in HIV-negative psoriasis (Best Pract

Res Clin Rheumatol 2015;29:244). It may also manifest as an immune reconstitution inflammatory syndrome (IRIS) process (J Am Acad Dermatol 2015;72:e35). Expansion of the CD8+ memory T-cell subset and imbalanced CD4:CD8 ratio may contribute to development of psoriasis in HIV (Dermatol Online J 2007;13:4). ART should be started promptly, and some cases may respond to ART alone. Phototherapy is considered first-line by the National Psoriasis Foundation for HIV-associated psoriasis; acitretin is considered second-line therapy (J Am Acad Dermatol 2010;62:291). Topical therapies are supplemental.

Scabies

See MMWR 2002;51[RR-6]:68) and Table 8.6.

Seborrheic Dermatitis

See J Am Acad Dermatol 1992;27:37 and Table 8.6.

Gastrointestinal Complications

Oral Lesions

Aphthous Ulcers

CAUSE: Unknown. Lesions appear as single or multiple white, or yellow circumscribed ulcers with a red halo. The differential includes HSV, CMV, drug-induced ulcers; biopsy is recommended for nonhealing ulcers. Aphthous ulcers often recur. Presentation may be associated with aphthous ulcers in the esophagus.

CLASSIFICATION:

- *Minor*: <0.5 cm diameter, usually self-limiting with healing in 7–10 days.

- *Major*: >0.5 cm, deep, prolonged (may last for months), heal slowly, cause pain especially with eating, and may prevent oral intake. High potential for scarring (AIDS 1992;6:963; Oral Surg Oral Med Oral Pathol 1996;81:141; Am J Clin Dermatol 2003;4:669).

TREATMENT:

- *ART*: Response may be dramatic (days to weeks) (Int J Infect Dis 2006;11:278).
- Topical treatment with applications 2× to 4×/d; achieve pain relief and may reduce duration of ulcers.
  - *Lidocaine* solution before meals.
  - *Triamcinolone hexacetonide* in Orabase—preferred (J Am Dent Assoc 2003;134:200).
  - *Fluocinonide gel* (Lidex) 0.05% ointment mixed 1:1 with Orabase or covered with Orabase.
  - *Amlexanox* (Aphthasol) 5% oral paste (J Oral Maxillofac Surg 1993;51:243).
- Oral and intralesional therapy (refractory cases):
  - *Prednisone* 40 mg/d po × 1–2 wks then taper (Am J Clin Dermatol 2003;4:669)
  - *Colchicine* 1.5 mg/d (J Am Acad Dermatol 1994;31:459). *Note*: dose reduction required with PI/r or cobicistat co-administration.
  - *Dapsone* 100 mg/d
  - *Pentoxifylline* (Trental) 400 mg po tid with meals
  - *Thalidomide* 200 mg/d po × 4–6 wks ± maintenance with 200 mg 2×/wk. *Note*: Thalidomide is "experimental" for aphthous ulcers. Thalidomide has strict requirements for use, but is very effective; data support use in treatment of persistent lesions, but less data to support utility in prevention of aphthous ulcers (CID 1995;20:250; NEJM 1997;337:1086; JID 2001;183:343; Am J Clin Dermatol. 2003;4:669).

Gingivitis

CAUSE: Caused initially by plaque formation, leading to hardening of the gumline (tartar), ultimately leading to irritation of the gingiva and infection. Gingival infection is mainly provoked by anaerobic bacteria, such as *Prevotella* and *Fusobacterium* spp.

PHASES: Linear gingival erythema → necrotizing gingivitis → necrotizing periodontitis → necrotizing stomatitis.

TREATMENT:

- *Routine dental care:* Brush and floss ± topical antiseptics.
  - *Listerine* swish × 30–60 seconds bid, Peridex, etc.
- Dental consultation for curettage and debridement.
- *Antibiotics (necrotizing stomatitis):* Metronidazole; alternatives—clindamycin or amoxicillin-clavulanate.

Herpes Simplex

See HSV section.

Oral Hairy Leukoplakia (OHL)

CAUSE: Intense replication of EBV (CID 1997;25:1392).

PRESENTATION: Unilateral or bilateral adherent white/gray patches on lingual lateral margins ± dorsal, or ventral surface of tongue. Patches are irregular folds and projections.

DIFFERENTIAL:

- *Candidiasis:* OHL does not respond to azoles and cannot be scraped off (unlike candidiasis).
- *Others:* Squamous cell carcinoma or traumatic leukoplakia.

DIAGNOSIS: Diagnosis is usually clinical; biopsy is sometimes advocated for lesions that require therapy and do not respond, but is rarely necessary.

IMPLICATIONS: Found almost exclusively with HIV, indicates low CD4 count, predicts AIDS, and responds to ART.

TREATMENT: See CID 1997;25:1392. Rarely symptomatic and rarely treated, but occasional patients have pain or have concern about appearance. The options include:

- *ART* (preferred)
- *Topical therapy*:
  - *Podophyllin* 25% topical cream +/− acyclovir topical cream 5%, applied once weekly (World J Clin Cases 2014;2:253).
  - Combination topical therapy has been shown to be effective with low recurrence rate of leukoplakia.
- *Systemic anti-EBV treatment*:
  - *Acyclovir* 800 mg po 5×/d × 2–3 wks
  - Other effective antivirals include famciclovir, valacyclovir (JID 2003;188:883). Foscarnet, ganciclovir, and valganciclovir are also effective, but generally not recommended for OHL due to side-effect profiles. Lesions frequently recur when treatment is discontinued.

Salivary Gland Enlargement

CAUSE: The most common cause is diffuse infiltrative lymphocytosis syndrome (DILS), a condition associated with HIV and Sjögren's syndrome (Ann Intern Med 1996;125:494; Arthritis Rheum 2006;55:466). May also be seen with IRIS (Int J STD AIDS 2008;19:305). More prevalent among children. PIs have been associated with salivary gland enlargement and decreased salivary flow rates (Oral Dis 2009;15:52).

PRESENTATION: Parotid enlargement, cystic, unilateral or bilateral, nontender, usually asymptomatic; may be painful, cosmetically disfiguring, or cause xerostomia (Ear Nose Throat J 1990;69:475; Arthritis Rheum 2006;55:466; Rheumatology 2008;47:952).

DIFFERENTIAL: Differential diagnosis includes reactive lymphadenopathy, lymphoepithelial cysts, abscess, malignancy (Diagn

Cytopathol 2012;40:684). Must differentiate cystic from solid lesion with computed tomography (CT) scan (Laryngoscope 1998;98:772) and/or fine needle aspiration (FNA). FNA is useful for microbiology, cytology, and decompression. May require biopsy to exclude tumor, especially lymphoma. Biopsy usually shows histology resembling Sjögren's syndrome; characteristic features are severe salivary duct atypia and foci of lymphocytes, predominantly CD8+ lymphocytes (Arch Pathol Lab Med 2000;124:1773; J Oral Pathol Med 2003;32:544); alternatively, there may be "nonspecific chronic sialadenitis" (Oral Dis 2003;9:55). If infection is present, the most common pathogens are mycobacteria and CMV. The frequency of this complication has decreased substantially during the HAART era (Arthritis Rheum 2006;55:466).

TREATMENT:

- *FNA* for decompression of fluid-filled parotid cysts; may require large-bore needle for aspiration.
- *Xerostomia*: Sugarless chewing gum, artificial saliva, muscarinic agonists such as pilocarpine.

Candidiasis, Oropharyngeal (Thrush)

See Candidiasis section.

Esophagitis

DIFFERENTIAL: Potential causes vary significantly by CD4 count. Consider non–HIV-related causes, especially if CD4 is >200/mL. Most common etiologies are medication-related or food-related esophagitis and gastroesophageal reflux disease (GERD). Presenting symptoms include odynophagia and dysphagia. With CD4 of <200/mL, the most common cause of esophagitis is candidiasis. *Candida* esophagitis mainly causes plaques (rather than ulcers), and odynophagia may be severe. *C. albicans* is the most frequent cause of *Candida* esophagitis; other *Candida* spp. are marginally involved.

TABLE 8.7 Differential diagnosis and characteristics of oral lesions

Lesion	Character	Location	Pain	Biopsy Required?
Candidiasis	White or yellow plaques	Palate, tongue, buccal mucosa	None or mild	No
Oral hairy leukoplakia	White, corrugated	Lateral tongue	None	No
Herpes simplex	Vesicular ulcers	Vermillion border (gingiva), palate	Mild-moderate	No
Aphthous ulcers	White, yellow ulcers	Soft palate mucosa	Severe	No
Necrotizing gingivitis	Yellow ulcers necrotic	Anywhere	Severe	Yes
Bacterial gingivitis	Necrotic, putrid	Local or generalized	Severe	No
Kaposi sarcoma	Red, purple nodule	Anywhere, especially palate	None-moderate	Yes
Squamous cell cancer	Red, white indurated	Anywhere, especially tongue	None-severe	Yes

From Classification of the ACTG Subcommittee Oral HIV/AIDS Research Alliance) (J Oral Pathol Med 2009;38:481.

Esophageal ulcers are usually due to CMV (45%), or they are idiopathic aphthous ulcers (40%); HSV accounts for only 5% (Ann Intern Med 1995;122:143). Other causes to consider include drug-induced dysphagia (Am J Med 1988;88:512), including from AZT (Ann Intern Med 1990;162:65), as well as infections with M. avium, tuberculosis (TB), cryptosporidium, P. jirovecii, primary HIV infection, histoplasmosis, KS, or lymphoma (Gastrointest Endosc 1986;32:96; BMJ 1988;296:92).

DIAGNOSIS: Endoscopy assists in establishing the diagnosis in about 70–95% of cases (Arch Intern Med 1991;151:1567); yield with barium swallow is low (20–30%).

TREATMENT: Response to empiric treatment often precludes need for endoscopic diagnosis of candida esophagitis. Typically, treat with antifungal for 1–2 wks and plan endoscopy if no clinical response. Fluconazole is the preferred treatment for candidiasis because of established efficacy, more predictable absorption, and fewer drug interactions compared with alternative azoles. Other antifungals (voriconazole, posaconazole, anidulafungin, caspofungin, micafungin) are also approved by the US Food and Drug Administration (FDA) for esophageal candidiasis but are infrequently required and generally reserved for fluconazole-resistant candida.

Anorexia, Nausea, Vomiting

MAJOR CAUSES: Medications (especially ARVs, antibiotics, opiates, and nonsteroidal antiinflammatory drugs [NSAIDs]), depression or anxiety, intracranial pathology, infectious and noninfectious GI disease, hypogonadism, pregnancy, lactic acidosis, acute gastroenteritis, small bowel overgrowth, idiopathic AIDS enteropathy, renal dysfunction.

ART: Nausea ± vomiting and/or abdominal pain are reported in 2–17% of patients given PIs (JAIDS 2004;37:1111). The most common agents, in rank order, are RTV, IDV, LPV/r, TPV/r, FPV, SQV, DRV, and ATV. The effect is dose-related and most common with boosted PIs with >200 mg RTV/d. Symptoms can occur at any time but are most frequently seen early in the treatment course (J Med Toxicol 2014;10:26). Similar symptoms are frequent with AZT and ddI (buffered). While seen less frequently, the integrase inhibitors most common adverse effects are nausea and diarrhea (Expert Opin Drug Saf 2014;13:431).

TABLE 8.8 Esophageal disease in patients with HIV infection

	Candida	CMV	HSV	Aphthous Ulcers
Frequency	50–70%	10–20%	2–5%	10–20%
Clinical features				
Dysphagia	+++	+	+	+
Odynophagia	++	+++	+++	+++
Thrush	50–70%	<25%	<5%	<10%
Oral ulcers	Rare	Uncommon	Often	Uncommon
Pain	Diffuse	Focal	Focal	Focal
Fever	Infrequent	Often	Infrequent	Infrequent
Diagnosis				
Endoscopy	Usually treated empirically. Pseudo-membranous plaques; may involve entire esophagus.	Biopsy required for diagnosis. Erythema and erosions/ulcers, single or multiple discrete lesions, often distal.	Biopsy required for diagnosis. Erythema and erosions/ulcers, usually small, coalescing, and shallow	Similar in appearance and location to CMV ulcers. Biopsy required to rule out CMV and HSV.

(continued)

TABLE 8.8 Continued

	Candida	CMV	HSV	Aphthous Ulcers
Micro-biology	Brush: Yeast and pseudo-mycelium on KOH prep or PAS Culture with sensitivities may be useful with suspected resistance	Biopsy: Intracellular inclusions and/or positive culture. Highest yield with histopath of biopsy and culture. Culture not recommended false positives.	Brush/biopsy: Intracytoplasmic inclusions + multinucleate giant cells, FA stain, and/or positive culture.	Negative studies for candida, HSV, CMV, and other diagnoses.

EVALUATION: If relationship to medication is unclear, consider medication change, morning testosterone level, GI evaluation (endoscopy, CT scan), intracranial evaluation (head CT scan or magnetic resonance imaging [MRI]), or empiric treatment. A thorough evaluation for opportunistic infections (OI) and malignancy should be undertaken for any patient with wasting syndrome, and reversible causes of weight loss should be excluded prior to any consideration for nutritional supplementation.

TREATMENT: Treat underlying condition first.

- *Anorexia*:
  - *Megestrol* 400–800 mg/d. Weight gain is mostly fat. May decrease testosterone level or increase blood sugar. Consider megestrol (pg. 324) + testosterone (pg. 394).
  - *Dronabinol* 2.5 mg po bid; active ingredient of marijuana. Weight gain is mostly fat.
- *Nausea and vomiting*:
  - *Prochlorperazine* 5–10 mg po q6–8h
  - *Trimethobenzamide* 250 mg po q6–8h
  - *Metoclopramide* 5–10 mg po q6–8h
  - *Dimenhydrinate* 50 mg po q6h–q8h
  - *Lorazepam* 0.025–0.05 mg/kg IV or IM
  - *Haloperidol* 1–5 mg bid po or IM
  - *Dronabinol* 2.5–5 mg po bid; ondansetron 0.2 mg/kg IV or IM.
  - Note: Phenothiazines (haloperidol, metoclopramide, prochlorperazine, trimethobenzamide) may cause dystonia. Metoclopramide is preferable to dimenhydrinate, oxazepam, and ondansetron.
  - *PEG*: Percutaneous endoscopic gastrostomy (PEG) may be required to deliver nutrition and medications, including ART regimen. The European Society for Clinical Nutrition and Metabolism (ESPEN) guidelines provide considerations for when such therapy may be indicated (Clin Nutr 2006;25:319).

Diarrhea

Note that most studies of acute and chronic diarrhea were done in the pre-HAART era when this complication was often associated with advanced immunosuppression and high rates of "AIDS enteropathy" and OI complications (MAC, CMV, and cryptosporidiosis), which are now far less common (AIDS 2005;18:107).

- *Acute diarrhea* is defined as >3 loose or watery stools/d for 3–10 days.
- *Chronic diarrhea* is defined as diarrhea lasting more than 4 wks.

EPIDEMIOLOGY: A review in 44,778 PLWH followed at >100 medical facilities in the United States from 1992 to 2002, found an annual incidence of 7.2 cases of bacterial diarrhea per 1,000 patient-yrs and yielded bacterial pathogens in 1,115 (CID 2005;41:1621). The most common bacterial pathogens, in rank order, were *C. difficile* (598 cases; 54%), *Shigella* (156, 14%), *C. jejuni* (154; 14%), *Salmonella* (82; 7%), *S. aureus* (43, 4%), and MAC (22; 2%). With introduction of HAART, incidence of noninfectious causes of diarrhea has significantly increased, with the majority of cases now attributed to medication (Am J Gastroenterol 2000;95:3142; CID 2012;55:860). Up to 19% of patients on HAART experience moderate to severe diarrhea that is suspected to be secondary to ART (AIDS Rev 2009;11:30).

DIAGNOSTIC EVALUATION:

- *Medication-related*: Main antiretroviral agents: all PIs (especially NFV, LPV/r, SQV, fosamprenavir/r). PIs have been demonstrated in in vitro models to negatively impact epithelial cell barrier function and increase chloride secretion (Antivir Ther 2005;10:645; BMC Gastroenterol 2010;10:90). Newer PIs (ATV, DRV) are much less frequently associated with diarrhea (Dig Dis Sci 2015;60:2236). ddI and other NRTIs can also provoke diarrhea, while NNRTIs are less commonly associated with diarrhea. While diarrhea is not commonly seen with integrase inhibitors, diarrhea is one of the most common adverse effects of this class of medication (Infect Dis Ther 2014;3:103).

MANAGEMENT:
See CID 2000;30:908.

- *Loperamide* 4 mg, then 2 mg every loose stool, up to 16 mg/d
  - Calcium 500 mg bid
  - Psyllium 1 tsp qd–bid or 2 bars qd–bid
  - Oat bran 1,500 mg bid
  - Pancreatic enzymes 1–2 tabs with meals
  Pathogen detection: See CID 2001;32:331; Arch Pathol Lab Med 2001;125:1042):
- *Blood culture*: MAC, *Salmonella Campylobacter, E. coli, Shigella.*
- *Stool culture: Salmonella, Shigella, C. jejuni, Vibrio, Yersinia, E. coli* 0157.
- Stool assay for *C. difficile* toxin A and B by EIA, polymerase chain reaction (PCR), or a combination test for toxin.
- *O&P examination* + modified acid-fast stain (*Cryptosporidia, Cyclospora, Isospora, Entamoeba histolytica*), trichrome or other stain for microsporidia, and antigen detection (*Giardia*).
- Consider diagnostic testing for CMV, histoplasmosis, and *Cryptococcus* which may present as diarrhea with systemic symptoms in the context of low CD4 counts OFF

RADIOLOGY:

- CT scan with contrast—*C. difficile* colitis, CMV colitis, and lymphoma.

ENDOSCOPY:

- Most useful for CMV, Kaposi sarcoma, and lymphoma

CAMPYLOBACTER JEJUNI: Approximately 4–8% of PLWH with acute diarrhea; rates are increased up to 39-fold in men who have sex with men (MSM) (CID 1997;24:1107; CID 1998;26:91; CID 2005;40:S152). PLWH with low CD4 counts are at increased risk for enteric infection and for bacteremia with non-*jejuni* species of Campylobacter including *Campylobacter coli, cineadi, fennelliae, laridis, fetus,* and *upsaliensis.* Most labs cannot recover these agents in stool cultures but can usually detect them in blood cultures. Clinical features of *C. jejuni* enteric infection are watery diarrhea or bloody flux, and fever; fecal leukocytes are variable; any CD4 count. Warn the lab if any other Campylobacter species in stool are suspected. Blood cultures give the highest yield with these non-*C. jejuni* species.

TREATMENT: See CID 2001;32:331,

Ciprofloxacin 500 mg po bid or azithromycin 500 mg po qd. Modify according to in vitro activity. Ciprofloxacin resistance is increasing (Emerg Infect Dis 2002;8:237; Microb Drug Resist 2013;19:110).

With bacteremia: ADD an aminoglycoside to ciprofloxacin to limit the emergence of resistance.

Azithromycin not recommended with bacteremia. Duration for mild or moderate disease is 7 days; for bacteremia, it is ≥2 wks.

CLOSTRIDIUM DIFFICILE: The most frequent single cause of infectious diarrhea in PLWH. HIV infection is a risk factor for the development of *C. difficile* infection and risk was associated with low immunoglobulin and low albumin levels (BMC ID 2015;15:194). In addition, a CD4 count of <50 increases risk of *C. difficile* infection (AIDS 2013;27(17):2799).

ENTERIC VIRUSES:

Account for >30% of acute diarrhea in PLWH.

Clinical features: Watery diarrhea, acute, but one-third can become chronic; seen at any CD4 cell count.

Major agents: Norovirus, adenovirus (serotypes 40 and 41), astrovirus, picornavirus, calicivirus (NEJM 1993;329:14). Etiologic diagnosis is rarely indicated and is usually performed if concern for disease outbreak; however, diagnosis of norovirus and adenovirus 40 and 41 is occurring more frequently in clinical labs.

NOROVIRUS: This virus is the major cause of infectious diarrhea in the world and is also the leading cause of outbreaks of diarrhea associated with foodborne disease, residents of healthcare facilities, passengers on cruise ships, travelers, and immunocompromised patients (CID 2009;49:1061; Discov Med 2010;10:61). Major symptoms are vomiting and diarrhea, often in the winter ("winter vomiting disease"), though outbreaks can occur at any time. The diagnosis can be established with reverse transcription (RT)-PCR of stools or emesis. The classic diagnostic criteria are "Kaplan's Criteria": (1) duration of 12–60 hrs, (2) incubation period of 24–48 hrs, (3) >50% of affected persons have vomiting, and (4) there is no bacterial pathogen found. Management is infection control and symptomatic treatment of patients.

IDIOPATHIC: 25–40% of PLWH with acute diarrhea have noninfectious causes; rule out medication, diet, irritable bowel syndrome, malabsorption, and the like. Infectious causes should be excluded if symptoms are severe or chronic, including culture, O&P examination, and *C. difficile* test. Obtain stool elastase to evaluate for pancreatic dysfunction (Curr Opin Infect Dis 2016;29:486).

CRYPTOSPORIDIA: Varying with geographical location, between 15–40% of cases of diarrhea in AIDS is estimated to be attributable to cryptosporidium infection (CID 1998;27:536; Interdiscip Perspect ID 2010:2010; Eur J Clin Microbiol ID 2011;30:1461). Infection causes a secretory diarrhea and, in the setting of AIDS infection, is often chronic and may cause severe wasting.

CYTOMEGALOVIRUS: Disease is noted in the context of CD4 counts of <50/µL. Diarrhea is frequently bloody, occurring in the context of fever, anorexia, and abdominal pain.

ISOSPORA BELLI: Also known as *Cystoisospora belli*. The parasite is found globally, but infections are more common in tropical areas. Infection results in watery, nonbloody, malabsorptive, secretory diarrhea.

MICROSPORIDIA: ENTEROCYTOZOON BIENEUSI OR ENTERO-CYTOZOON (SEPTATA) INTESTINALIS: Routine examination for ova and parasites does not usually detect microsporidial spores. Rather, modified trichrome stain, calcofluor white, or microsporidia indirect immunofluorescent stains should be requested if this pathogen is suspected. Occurs mainly in the context of very low CD4 count (<50/μL). Diarrhea is secretory and usually nonbloody.

MYCOBACTERIUM AVIUM COMPLEX (MAC): See *M. avium* section. Diarrhea is seen as part of a systemic infection with symptoms of high fever, night sweats, weight loss, cough; manifesting only in patients with very low CD4 count. Plaques and nodules are frequently seen at sites of infection without mucosal exudation; the duodenum is most frequently affected, followed by the rectum (J Clin Gastroenterol 1995;21:323; Gastrointest Endosc 2005;61:775).

EMPIRIC TREATMENT, SEVERE ACUTE IDIOPATHIC DIARRHEA

- *Empiric Lomotil or loperamide*: Note that some consider *C. difficile* infection to be a contraindication to these antiperistaltic agents, but supporting evidence is slim (CID 2009;48:598).

    Crofelemer (Fulyzaq) is a newly approved medication for treatment of noninfectious chronic secretory diarrhea in AIDS; it inhibits water loss in diarrhea by inhibiting epithelial cell chloride secretion into the lumen (Am J Gastroenterol 1999; 94:3267; HIV AIDS [Auckl] 2013;5:153; Dig Dis Sci 2015;60:2236; Expert Rev Clin Pharmacol 2015;8:683). Patients with noninfectious diarrhea for >1 mo on ART (majority of patients were on PIs) treated with crofelemer were more likely to have <2 watery bowel movement per week compared to placebo (17.6% vs. 8%). At a cost of ~$600/mo, its role in the management of noninfectious chronic secretory diarrhea in patients on non–PIs-based regimens remains to be determined.

HIV Enteropathy

Described in the pre-HAART era as a diarrheal syndrome associated with advanced immunosuppression (CD4 <100/mL) with no identified pathogen and characterized by nonspecific pathologic changes in the small bowel (AIDS 2005;19:107; ID Clin Pract 2010;5:293). HIV enteropathy is always a diagnosis of exclusion made after all other causes are ruled out (Gastroenterology 2009;136:1952). Postulated mechanisms included defective transport (AIDS 1998;12:43), changes in intestinal microtubule cytoskeleton (AIDS 2001;15:123), or HIV infection of the GI epithelial cells (J Biomed Sci 2003;10:156).

Hematologic Complications

Hematologic abnormalities, including anemia, thrombocytopenia, and neutropenia, were major issues in HIV care in all areas of the world in the pre-HAART era but are now major concerns primarily in resource-limited settings. The ACTG PEARLS (Prospective Evaluation of Antiretrovirals in Resource-Limited Settings) study reviewed prevalence data for these complications among 1,571 ART-naïve patients in Brazil, Haiti, India, Malawi, South Africa, Thailand, Zimbabwe, and the United States from 2005 to 2007. Participants had CD4 counts of <300/mL and no acute illness (Int J Infect Dis 2010;14:e1088). The main findings:

- *Anemia* (Hgb ≤10 g/dL): Prevalence 11.9%; 50% macrocytic; highest rates in Africa and Haiti.
- *Thrombocytopenia* (platelet count <120,000/mL): Prevalence 7.2% with highest rates in India, Brazil, Malawi, and the United States.

- *Neutropenia* (ANC <1,300/mL): Prevalence 4.3%; greatest in Africa, Haiti, and the United States.

Anemia

SYMPTOMS: Oxygen delivery is impaired with activity when Hgb levels are <8–9 g/dL and becomes impaired at rest with hemoglobin levels <5 g/dL (JAMA 1998;279:217). Chronic anemia is frequently asymptomatic but can manifest with nonspecific symptoms, such as exertional dyspnea, fatigue, weakness, and difficulty concentrating. Late complications include confusion, CHF, angina, and restless leg syndrome (NEJM 2015; 372:1832).

CAUSES: Multiple potential causes:

- *HIV and immune activation*: HIV infection of marrow progenitor cells (CID 2000;30:504). Incidence correlates with immune state: 12% with CD4 <200/mL, 37% with AIDS-defining OI (Blood 1998;91:301). Anemia predicts death independent of CD4 count and VL (Semin Hematol Suppl 4;6:18; AIDS 1999;13:943; AIDS Rev 2002;4:13; JAIDS 2004;37:1245; Antivir Ther 2008;13:959; HIV Med 2010;11:143). More recent studies suggest anemia, like hsCRP and IL-6, is an expression of immune activation.
  - *Findings*: Normocytic, normochromic, low reticulocyte count, low erythropoietin (EPO) level (NEJM 2005; 352:1011).
  - Factors that correlate with anemia are CD4 <200/mL, high VL (>50,000 copies/mL), female sex, use of AZT, reduced body mass index (BMI), and black race (CID 2004; 38:1454; JAIDS 2004;37:1245) and biomarkers of immune activation.
  - *Treatment*: ART. With immune reconstitution, prior reports show increases in Hgb of 1.0–2.0 g/dL at 6 mos (AIDS 1999;13:943; JAIDS 2001;28:221; AIDS Res Ther 2015;12:26), but results are inconsistent (CID 2000;30:504).

Consider EPO (starting at 100 units/kg TIW) with symptomatic and refractory cases. It should also be noted that this would not address the issue of immune activation.

- *Marrow-infiltrating infection or tumor* (lymphoma or Kaposi sarcoma, rare), or infection (MAC, TB, CMV, histoplasmosis): Findings include normocytic, normochromic, low platelet count, evidence of etiologic mechanism. Bone marrow biopsy is critical for diagnosis.
- *Parvovirus B19*: Infects erythroid precursors; symptoms reflect marginal reserve (sickle cell disease, etc.) and inability to eradicate infection due to immune deficiency. More recent studies suggest parvovirus B19 is a very rare cause of anemia in patients with HIV (CID 2010;50:115).
  - *Findings*: Normocytic, normochromic anemia, without reticulocytes, positive IgG, and IgM serology for parvovirus; positive serum dot blot hybridization or PCR for parvovirus B19. The diagnosis is most likely with severe anemia (i.e., hemoglobin <8 g/dL, no reticulocytes and CD4 count <100 cells/mm^3) (JID 1997;176:269).
  - *Treatment*: May eradicate pathogen with ART (CID 2001;32: E122). Standard treatment with persistent parvovirus B19 and immunosuppression is IVIG 400 mg/kg/d × 5 days (Ann Intern Med 1990;113:926; CID 2013;56:968).
- *Nutritional deficiency*: Common in late-stage HIV, including vitamin B_{12} deficiency in 20% of AIDS patients (Eur J Haematol 1987;38:141) and folate deficiency due to folic acid malabsorption (J Intern Med 1991;230:227).
  - *Findings*: Megaloblastic anemia (MCV >100 not ascribed to AZT or d4T) ± hypersegmented polymorphonuclear cells, low reticulocyte count, low serum B_{12} (cobalamin) level (<125–200 pg/mL), elevated methylmalonic acid, and total homocysteine levels (NEJM 2013; 368:149, Semin Hematol 1999;36:75) or a serum folate level <2. *Note*: A single hospital meal may significantly increase the serum folate level.

- *Treatment*: Folate deficiency: Folic acid 1–5 mg/d × 1–4 mos. B_{12} deficiency: Cobalamin 1 mg IM qd × 7 days, then every week × 4 wks, then every month, or 1–2 mg po qd (Blood 1998;92:1191; Fam Pract 2006;23:279).
- *Iron deficiency*: Common causes include malnutrition, gastrointestinal losses from esophagitis, gastritis, peptic ulcer disease, helminth infections, angiodysplasia or malignancy, and menstrual losses in women (NEJM 2015;372:1832).
  - *Findings*: low Fe (normal range 10–30µg/dL), transferrin saturation >16% (normal >16%–<45%), and low ferritin. Ferritin (<30 ng/mL suggests iron deficiency and <10 ng/mL is 99% sensitive and 83% specific for iron deficiency anemia). In patients with anemia of chronic disease and iron deficiency: low Fe, low-normal transferrin saturation, and ferritin <100 ng/mL (J Gen Intern Med 1992;7:145; NEJM 2015;372:1832).
  - *Treatment*: Identify and treat the source of loss. Oral iron supplementation of 120 mg/d of elemental iron for 3 mo. (Am Fam Physician 2013;87:98; NEJM 2015;372:1832).
- *Drug-induced marrow suppression ± red cell aplasia*: ART (AZT); therapy for OIs (ganciclovir, valganciclovir, dapsone, amphotericin B, flucytosine, ribavirin, pyrimethamine, primaquine, TMP-SMX); chemotherapeutic agents; interferon.
  - *Findings*: Normocytic, normochromic anemia (macrocytic with AZT or d4T), low or normal reticulocyte count.
  - *Treatment*: Discontinue implicated agent ± EPO.
- *Drug-induced hemolytic anemia*: Most common with dapsone, primaquine, and ribavirin. Hemolytic anemia is also seen with thrombocytopenic purpura (TTP). The risk with dapsone and primaquine is dose-related and most common with G6PD deficiency.
  - *Findings*: Reticulocytosis, increased lactic acid dehydrogenase (LDH), increased indirect bilirubin, methemoglobinemia, and reduced haptoglobin. The combination of a haptoglobin <25 mg/dL + elevated LDH is 90% specific, and 92% sensitive for hemolytic anemia (JAMA

1980;243:1909). Peripheral smear may show keratocytes, "bite cells," "blister cells," and irregularly contracted cells (NEJM 2005; 353:498). *Note*: Coombs test may be positive in drug-related immune hemolysis.

- *Treatment*: Discontinuation of implicated drug, oxygen, and blood transfusion. Severe cases in absence of G6PD deficiency are treated with IV methylene blue (1–2 mg/kg) (JAIDS 1996;12:477; South Med J 2011;104:757).

DIAGNOSTIC EVALUATION: Laboratory tests: CBC, MCV, peripheral smear, reticulocyte count, bilirubin (total and direct), iron studies (ferritin, iron, transferrin, TIBC), vitamin B_{12}, folate, methylmalonic acid, and homocysteine levels; stool Hemoccult; consider bone marrow biopsy.

Suggested algorithm:

- Macrocytic anemia (MCV >100 fL):
  1. *Vitamin B_{12} deficiency*: Low vitamin B_{12}, high methylmalonic acid, high homocysteine.
  2. *Folate deficiency*: Low total folate, normal vitamin B_{12}, normal methylmalonic acid, high homocysteine.
  3. *Myelodysplastic syndrome*: Vitamin B_{12}/folate levels may be normal. Dysplastic cells and other cytopenias may be present.
  4. *Other causes*: Liver disease, hypothyroidism, drug-induced (AZT).
- *Normocytic anemia* (MCV 80–96 fL):
  1. Anemia of chronic disease
  2. Chronic kidney disease
  3. Acute blood loss
  4. Drug-induced marrow suppression
  5. Hemolytic anemia
- *Microcytic anemia* (MCV <80 fL):
  1. Iron deficiency anemia
  2. Sideroblastic anemia
  3. β- or α-thalassemia

Neutropenia

DEFINITION: Absolute neutrophil count <1500/μl (risk of infection increases below ANC of 1,000/μl).

CAUSE: Usually due to HIV or to drugs such as AZT, amphotericin B, ganciclovir, valganciclovir, foscarnet (less common), ribavirin, flucytosine, pyrimethamine, pentamidine (less common), sulfonamides, interferon-α, and cancer chemotherapy (Int Rev Immunol 2014;33:511). AZT remains a common cause in countries that still rely on this drug (PLoS One 2017;12:e0170753).

SYMPTOMS: Reported risk of bacterial infections is variable, but the largest review shows an increase in hospitalization with an ANC of <500/mm³ (Arch Intern Med 1997;157:1825). Other reviews show that few PLWH have excessive neutropenia-associated infections (CID 2001;32:469).

TREATMENT:

- *HIV-associated*:
  - With ART initiation, ANC increase with immune reconstitution is variable (CID 2000;30:504; JAIDS 2001;28:221). Severe and persistent neutropenia may respond to granulocyte colony stimulating factor (G-CSF) and granulocyte/macrophage colony stimulating factor (GM-CSF).
- *Drug-associated*:
  - Treatment is to discontinue the implicated drug.
  - *G-CSF*: Usual dose is 1–5 μg/kg/d SQ or 3×/wk. Dose can be titrated to lowest dose necessary to maintain ANC >1,000/mm³ (NEJM 1987;371:593; Br J Haematol 2015;171:695).

Thrombocytopenia

DEFINITION: Platelet count <100,000/mL.

CAUSES:

- *HIV-associated immune thrombocytopenic purpura (ITP)*: Ascribed to ineffective platelet production from HIV infection of multilineage hematopoietic progenitor cells in the marrow (NEJM 1992;327:1779; CID 2000;30:504), as well as platelet destruction from platelet-antibody complexes (BMC Res Notes 2015;8:595). Incidence has declined in the HAART era (BMC Res Notes. 2015;8:595).

- *Drug-induced*: Immune thrombocytopenia: Antibody mediated. Multiple medications have been implicated, including those used to treat infectious complications in PLWH: β-lactams, ethambutol, quinine, rifampin, sulfonamides, trimethoprim-sulfamethoxazole, vancomycin (Blood 2010;116:2127). HIV may increase risk for heparin-induced thrombocytopenia (CID 2007; 45:1393).

TREATMENT: See Table 8.9.

Thrombotic Microangiopathy (TMA) and Thrombotic Thrombocytopenic Purpura

DEFINITION: Characterized by microangiopathic hemolytic anemia, thrombocytopenia, renal failure, fever, and neurologic changes (CID 2006;42:1488; NEJM 2014; 371:654; Br J Haematol 2015;171:695).

CAUSE: HIV infection of vascular endothelial cells resulting in dysfunction, localized thrombin generation, and consumption of ADAMTS13, or von Willebrand factor cleaving protein (Br J Haematol 2015;171:695). HIV infection itself, AIDS-related disorders, or treatment-induced immune reconstitution may trigger episodes of TTP in susceptible patients (J Clin Apher 2018 Jan 26). Infection with HIV increases the risk of TMA. AIDS-related disorders may also mimic the clinical features of TTP, such as CMV infection, HHV-8 infection, disseminated malignancy, and HIV-associated nephropathy with malignant hypertension (CID 2009;48:1129).

DIAGNOSIS: (1) Anemia, (2) thrombocytopenia (platelet count <150,000/μL), (3) peripheral smear with fragmented red blood cells

TABLE 8.9 Treatment of HIV-associated ITP

Clinical Status	Treatment
Asymptomatic and platelet count >30,000/μl	Discontinue implicated drugs and monitor response (Median time to recovery with discontinuation of the implicated agent is 7 days (Ann Intern Med 1998;129:886).
	ART improves platelet counts (Korean J Hematol 2011;46:253, CID 2000;30:504; NEJM 1999;341:123; ClD.1998;26:207; Ann Intern Med 1988;109:718).
Bleeding symptoms or platelet count <30,000/μl	Discontinue implicated drugs.
	Antiretroviral therapy.
	Prednisone 1 mg/kg/day for 21 days and taper gradually over 4–8 wks. Initial response seen in 4–14 days, peak at 7–28 days.
	IVIG 1 g/kg for 1–2 days or 400 mg/day for 5 days. Initial response seen in 1–4 days, peak at 2–7 days.
	anti-D immune globulin 50–75 μg/kg for 1–2 doses. Initial response seen at 1–3 days, peak at 3–7 days.
	Splenectomy: experience is variable; some good (Arch Surg 1989;124:625), some bad (Lancet 1987;2:342).

From Blood 2011;117:4190; Adv Hematol 2012;2012:910954.

(RBCs) (schistocytes, helmet cells) ± nucleated cells, (4) increased creatinine, (5) evidence of hemolysis (increased reticulocytes, indirect bilirubin, and LDH plus low haptoglobin), and (6) normal coagulation parameters.

TREATMENT: The usual course is progressive with irreversible renal failure and death without treatment. Standard treatment is plasma exchange until platelet count is normal, and LDH is normal (NEJM 1991;325:393). With poor response, add prednisone 1 mg/kg qd, fresh frozen plasma transfusion, or rituximab. A review of 24 cases found prompt initiation of ART and plasma exchange ± steroids led to prompt remission. Rituximab was used in some refractory cases (Br J Haematol 2005;128:373; Brit J Haematol 2011;153:515).

Immune Reconstitution Inflammatory Syndrome (IRIS)

DEFINITION: A practical definition is a paradoxical worsening of a preexisting infection or the presentation of a previously undiagnosed condition in PLWH soon after commencement of ART (CID 2009; 48:101). Most cases occur in the first few weeks or months of ART. IRIS is highly heterogeneous, with manifestations differing depending on the pathogen, organ system involved, and the preexisting morbidity.

- *Paradoxical IRIS* applies to patients who have worsening of a previously treated infection after starting ART. In this case, the pathogens may not be cultivable at the time of IRIS.
- *Unmasking IRIS* refers to flare-up of an underlying, previously undiagnosed infection after starting ART (Curr Opin HIV AIDS 2010;5:504). Unmasking IRIS may be confused with a new OI in a patient with a low CD4 count (HIV AIDS [Auckl] 2015; 7:49).

"Official definitions":

1. M. A. French: Must have major criteria A and B, or major criteria A and any two minor criteria (AIDS 2004;18:1615).
   - Major criteria:
     A. Atypical presentation of opportunistic infection or tumors in patients responding to ART:
        - Localized disease (e.g., severe fever or painful lesion)
        - Exaggerated inflammatory response (e.g., severe fever or painful lesions)

- Atypical inflammatory response (e.g., necrosis, granulomas, suppuration, or perivascular lymphocytic inflammatory cell infiltrate)
- Progression of organ dysfunction or enlargement of preexisting lesion after definite clinical improvement with pathogen-specific therapy prior to ART and exclusion of treatment toxicity and new diagnoses

B. Decrease in VL >1 $\log_{10}$ copies/mL

- Minor criteria
  - Increased CD4 cell count
  - Increase in an immune response specific to the relevant pathogen (e.g., DTH response to mycobacterial antigens)
  - Spontaneous resolution of disease without specific antimicrobial therapy, or tumor chemotherapy with continuation of ART

Other authors have proposed definitions for IRIS that are slightly different from the preceding one. These include definitions by Shelburne (Medicine 2002; 81:213), Robertson (CID 2006, 42:11), and Grant (PLoS ONE 2010;5: e11416). Other definitions for TB-IRIS (Lancet Infect Dis 2008; 8:516), and cryptococcal IRIS (Lancet Infect Dis 2010; 10:791) have been created by the International Network for the Study of HIV-associated IRIS (INSHI) to be used in resource-limited settings.

Haddow et al. (CID 2009;49:9) suggested separate definitions for paradoxical and unmasking IRIS:

PARADOXICAL IRIS:

Clinical criteria:

1. Temporal relationship: ART initiation must precede clinical deterioration
2. One of the following:
   a. Worsening of an infectious or inflammatory condition that was recognized and ongoing at the time of ART initiation, following a clinical response to appropriate treatment

    b. Deterioration with atypical or exaggerated clinical, histological, or radiologic findings in terms of severity, character of inflammatory response, rapidity of onset, or localization

    c. Recurrence of an episodic infectious or inflammatory condition, worse than episode within 1 yr preceding ART in terms of frequency, severity, or response to therapy

Exclusion of other causes (worsening not explained by):

1. Expected clinical course of underlying condition, given current therapy and the susceptibility profile of the organism
2. Drug toxicity
3. Other infection or inflammatory condition
4. Withdrawal of previously effective therapy
5. Failure of antiretroviral treatment: presumptive, based on either nonadherence or resistance to ART, or confirmed, based on VL assay if available.

UNMASKING IRIS:

Clinical criteria:

1. *Temporal relationship*: ART initiation must precede clinical deterioration
2. New onset of symptoms of an infectious or inflammatory condition after initiation of ART
3. Consistent with presence of preexisting causative pathogen or antigen at the time of starting ART
4. Either one of the following:

    a. Onset within 3 mos after initiating ART

    b. Atypical or exaggerated clinical, histological, or radiological findings in terms of severity, character of inflammatory response, rapidity of onset, or localization

Exclusion of other causes (event not explained by):

1. Expected clinical course of another condition
2. Drug toxicity

3. Newly acquired infection, based on clinical history or other evidence

4. Failure of antiretroviral treatment: presumptive, based on either nonadherence or resistance to ART, or confirmed, based on VL assay if available

PATHOGENESIS: The presumed mechanism is severe CD4 lymphopenia and a dysregulated immune response, followed by qualitative and quantitative recovery of pathogen-specific cellular and humoral responses to opportunistic pathogens including primarily mycobacteria, fungi, and viruses (Science 1997;277:112; CID 2000;30:882; JID 2002;185:1813; Drugs 2008;68:191; Curr Opin HIV AIDS 2009;22:651; Clin Microbiol Rev 2009;22:651). IRIS may target viable or dead microbial pathogens, host antigens (with autoimmune disease), or tumor antigens. There is an increased incidence of IRIS in patients with more advanced immunosuppression and disseminated OIs, which suggests the higher antigen load/burden they provide might cause excessive inflammation as the immune system starts to recover.

The imbalance between the innate and acquired immunity to specific pathogens and their regulatory mechanisms is responsible for IRIS. While the exact molecular mechanisms are yet to be determined, elevated proinflammatory markers (C-reactive protein [CRP]) and cytokines (IL-6, IL-12, TNF-α) in various body fluids suggest a proinflammatory cascade along a pathway that is common to most forms of IRIS (HIV AIDS [Auckl] 2015;7:49).

EPIDEMIOLOGY: Variations in geographical incidence of infection, diagnostic criteria, study methodology, diagnostic capability, pathogen, organ involvement, baseline immunosuppression, and morbidity are some of the factors that affect the incidence of IRIS (Lancet Infect Dis 2010;10:251). The most frequently reported cases of IRIS are with TB, MAC, and cryptococcal meningitis. One retrospective review found rates of 30–34% for each of these three OIs (AIDS 2005; 19:399). Others report lower rates of 10–23% (CID 2006; 42:418; HIV Med 2005;6:140; AIDS 2006;20:2390; CID 2009;49:1424). A large meta-analysis

(Lancet Infect Dis 2010; 10:251) showed an overall incidence of 13%, varying from 6% for Kaposi sarcoma-related IRIS to 38% for CMV-IRIS; variations in IRIS rates due to specific infections were seen in different income settings. IRIS may be underrecognized and undertreated in resource-limited settings, thus explaining the lower incidence and higher mortality seen in retrospective reviews from these areas (HIV AIDS [Auckl] 2015;7:49). The rate in the United States in ACTG 5164 was 8%, but that may be deceptively low since Pneumocystis pneumonia (PCP) was the most common OI, and steroid treatment may have reduced rates in that subset (PLoS ONE 2009;4:e5575). Prospective studies have shown lower rates of IRIS than retrospective studies (PLoS ONE 2010;5: e11416).

Overall mortality rate varies from 0% to 15% (Lancet Infect Dis 2010; 10:251, AIDS 2013:27:1603) and varies based on baseline morbidity, degree of immunosuppression, geography, and associated OI (e.g., in patients with cryptococcal meningitis associated IRIS, mortality is as high as 20%; in CNS-TB-IRIS, mortality rates can be up to 75%) (HIV AIDS [Auckl] 2015;7:49).

CLINICAL FEATURES: Manifestations depend on the pathogen and affected organ, as well as systemic or local inflammation. CNS IRIS due to TB meningitis, cryptococcal meningitis, progressive multifocal leukoencephalopathy (PML), or other CNS infections is associated with worse outcomes due to accompanying edema and raised intracranial pressure from the inflammation (Nat Clin Pract Neurol 2006;2:557; Curr Infect Dis Rep 2013;15;583). The interval from ART to IRIS ranges from 3 to 658 days with 60% occurring within 60 days (Curr Opinion Infect Dis 2006; 19:20).

Risk factors for the development of IRIS include CD4 count <50–100/mL at initiation of ART, high VL at baseline, rapid fall in HIV VL, treatment-naïve at time of OI treatment, and short interval between ART and OI treatment (HIV Med 2000;1:107; AIDS 2005;19:399; CID 2006;42:418).

Genetic predisposition may play a role; the following have been implicated: HLA-A, -B44, -DR4 (associated with herpes virus IRIS); TNFA-308*1; and IL6-174*G (associated with mycobacterial IRIS).

PRINCIPLES FOR PREVENTION AND TREATMENT: Prevention refers to methods of managing OIs that are likely to cause IRIS when treating both the OI and HIV. Prophylaxis and screening for OIs prior to onset of ART is crucial to preventing IRIS (HIV AIDS [Auckl] 2015; 7:49). *IRIS can be completely prevented* by early HIV diagnosis and early ART, before the CD4 count falls into OI range.

- *When to start ART*: The 2018 DHHS guidelines identify multiple scenarios for initiating ART in HIV treatment-naïve patients who present with an OI:

  The OI has no specific therapy: ART should be given immediately. Improvement of immune function with ART might improve disease outcomes. Examples are cryptosporidiosis, microsporidiosis, HIV-associated dementia, and PML.

  The OI has specific therapy, but IRIS is uncommon: ART should be given immediately. Examples are histoplasmosis, coccidioidomycosis, and leishmaniasis.

  The OI has specific therapy and is known to have IRIS as a common feature, and a brief delay in ART is appropriate (usually ≤2 wks). Examples are disseminated MAC, PCP, CMV, and toxoplasmosis. ACTG 5164 randomized 282 patients in this category to "immediate ART" (within 14 days) or "deferred ART" (>28 days). Results favored "immediate treatment" in terms of rates of death/AIDS progression (14% vs. 24%; p = NS). There were no significant differences in grade 3 or 4 adverse events, adherence, hospitalizations, or risk of IRIS (PLoS ONE 2009;4: e5575). The median delay of ART in the "immediate" group was 12 days. On the basis of these data, the recommendation is to initiate ART rapidly with a delay of no more than 2 wks when immediate therapy risks IRIS, polypharmacy and adverse reactions, and drug interactions.
- Treatment of IRIS usually consists of continued treatment of the OI and HIV ART with use of NSAIDs and/or corticosteroids for symptomatic treatment of IRIS. NSAIDs are preferred, but systemic symptoms that are severe or cases with large

inflammatory masses usually require steroids: prednisone 1–2 mg/kg/d for 1–2 wks followed by tapering based on symptoms. Most patients show improvement within 3 days (Thorax 2004; 59:704; CID 2005; 41:1483). In some cases, it is necessary to give prolonged courses, surgically resect masses, drain abscesses, or even stop treatment of HIV and/or OI due to life-threatening IRIS. A case report of the use of maraviroc in PML-IRIS in patient with multiple sclerosis suggested the possible benefit of maraviroc in patient with HIV-IRIS (NEJM 2014; 370:486). The CADIRIS study comparing maraviroc with placebo in patients with IRIS showed no decrease in morbidity or mortality in patients treated with maraviroc. However, the study was not powered to detect a benefit in patients with forms of IRIS associated with worse outcomes such as cryptococcal meningitis or TB meningitis (Lancet HIV 2014;1: e60).

SPECIFIC IRIS FORMS:

- *TB-IRIS*:
  TB-IRIS is one of the most common forms of IRIS given how prevalent TB is worldwide. Paradoxical TB-IRIS was reported to occur in 15.7% of TB patients starting ART (Lancet Infect Dis 2010;10:251). Higher incidence rates are seen in countries where the TB burden is higher, such as India and South Africa, with rates between 47% and 54% (PLoS One. 2013; 8: e6354; CID 2013; 56:450).

  Clinical presentation: The most common presentations include fever, adenopathy, worsening pulmonary infiltrates, and/or pleural effusions (Lancet Inf Dis 2005;5:361). Extrapulmonary manifestations include expanding CNS lesions, meningitis, cord lesions, and cervical adenopathy. In the STRIDE study, only 7% of patients with TB-IRIS had CNS involvement (JAIDS 2014;65:423). Most cases occur within 8 wks of initiating ART; extrapulmonary TB often occurs later—often 5–10 mos later (CID 1994; 19:793; CID 1998; 26:1008).

Time of initiation of ART: The greatest concern is delayed ART in patients with late-stage HIV (CD4 <50/mL) resulting in early mortality, which is usually attributed to delayed ART and rarely to TB-IRIS (JAIDS 2007;44:229). The STRIDE (NEJM 2011; 16:1482), CAMELIA (NEJM 2011;16:1471), and SAPiT (NEJM 2011;16:1492) trials showed that for patients with CD4 of <50, ART initiated within 2 wks of TB therapy improved survival. As these studies all involved pulmonary TB, the findings may not apply to extrapulmonary TB or TB meningitis. The incidence of IRIS varied in each study but was consistently higher in patients with CD4 counts of <50 than those with CD4 >50. In these three studies the overall mortality in patients with CD4 of <50 was lower, suggesting that the benefits of early initiation of ART outweighed the risk of IRIS in these patients

TB Meningitis: In a study conducted in Vietnam, patients were randomized to immediate ART, or to ART deferred 2 mos after initiation of TB treatment. A significantly higher rate of severe (Grade 4) adverse events was seen in patients who received immediate ART than in those with deferred therapy (80.3% vs. 69.1% for early and deferred ART, respectively; $P = 0.04$).

One study showed that in patients with TB-IRIS (excluding TB-meningitis–IRIS), use of prednisone reduced morbidity but not mortality (AIDS 2010:24:2381). The recommended course of corticosteroids is variable, but often reported at 20–80 mg/d for 5–12 wks (AIDS Res Ther 2007;4:9).

- *MAC*: The most common presentation is pulmonary disease or lymphadenitis with abscess formation (Lancet 1998; 351:252; Lancet Inf Dis 2005; 5:361). This usually occurs at 1–3 wks after initiation of ART but can be up to 84 days (JAIDS 1999; 20:122). Large abscesses may require excision, drainage, or needle aspiration; postoperative healing is often poor (CID

2004; 38:461). Other presentations include pneumonitis, osteomyelitis, or septic arthritis.

CMV: IRIS after CMV retinitis with vitritis is reported in 18–63% of cases (JID 1999; 179:697; HIV Med 2000; 1:107; Ophthalmology 2006; 113:684). This can occur rapidly and cause blindness. The usual therapy is intraocular corticosteroids (Br J Ophth 1999;83:540; Retina 2003;23:495). Clinically significant CMV IRIS is lower at 0.04 per person/yr (Ophthalmology 2010;117:2152).

• *Cryptococcal meningitis*:

Paradoxical IRIS is reported to occur in 13%–45% of PLWH who start ART after treatment for cryptococcal meningitis. It occurs a median of 4–9 wks following ART initiation, but delayed cases have been reported up to a year. (PLoS Med 2010;7:e1000384).

Clinical presentation: C. neoformans IRIS meningitis is not dissimilar from AIDS-related cryptococcal meningitis (CID 2005;40:1049). The most common presentation is worsening meningitis symptoms (CID 2005;40:1049). Non-neurological presentations are less common, but include lymphadenitis, pneumonitis, and eye and soft tissue disease (Lancet ID 2010;10:791).

TIME OF INITIATION OF ART: All patients with CD4 counts of <100 should be screened with a serum cryptococcal antigen at diagnosis of HIV and prior to ART initiation. If serum crypto Ag is positive at HIV diagnosis, there is no need to repeat it prior to ART initiation. A study in Zimbabwe showed that starting ART at 72 hrs versus waiting 10 wks was associated with higher mortality at 3 yrs (88% vs. 54%). While overall mortality at 3 yrs was 73%, most deaths in both arms occurred in the first 2 wks after ART initiation (CID 2010; 50:1534). The Cryptococcal Optimal ART Timing (COAT) trial was an open label, randomized trail conducted in Uganda and South Africa. ART-naïve patients with cryptococcal meningitis were randomized to early ART initiation (7–14 days after starting amphotericin) or deferred (after 5 wks); the trial was stopped when significantly higher mortality was seen in the early ART arm. The higher mortality rate was more pronounced in patients with low CSF cell count. However, the incidence of IRIS was not significantly different between both groups (NEJM 2014; 370:2487). While the DHHS guidelines recommend waiting 2–10 wks before initiating ART, in high-income settings where complications of cryptococcal meningitis and IRIS can be managed more easily, waiting 4–6 wks before starting ART is probably optimal. Delay in ART is important in patients with low (<5 cells/μgL) CSF cell count and increased intracranial pressure.

Treatment of the IRIS meningitis form includes anticryptococcal agents, LPs to control intracranial pressure, and systemic corticosteroids (Int J STD AIDS 2002;13:724). Patients with persistent cryptococcal growth in CSF cultures at the time of ART initiation and who have less than expected rise in CD4 count with ART are more likely to have cryptococcal meningitis-related IRIS (AIDS 2013; 27:2089).

- *Hepatitis B or C*: Elevated transaminase is usually mild, but can cause liver decompensation with cirrhosis.
- *PML*: New or worsening CNS disease (CID 2002; 35:1250; J Neurovirol 2005;11 Suppl 2:16). A retrospective review of 54 patients with PML IRIS showed patients who had worsening of PML IRIS with ART initiation (paradoxical response) developed IRIS sooner and had higher burden of disease and worse survival than patients who developed IRIS and PML (unmasking response) simultaneously with ART initiation (Neurology 2009;72:1458). Patients with unmasked PML were shown to have longer survival than patients with paradoxical PML IRIS or PML that developed >6 mos after ART initiation (J Neuroimmunol 2010; 219:100). Initiation of ART >3 mos after diagnosis of PML has been shown to be associated with improved survival (J Neurovirol 2003; 9 Supp 1:73). Development of CD8+T-cell responses specific to JC virus is

associated with control of infection (Neurology 2013; 81:964) and survival (J Neurol Neurosurg Psychiatry 2010;81;1288 Neurology 2009; 73:1551). Maraviroc has been successfully used in PML-IRIS in a patient with MS on natalizumab therapy (NEJM 2014;370:486) and HIV (AIDS 2009;23:2545) but caused death in a patient with HIV-related PML (Case Rep Med 2014;2014:381480), suggesting that more research is necessary before MVC can be routinely recommended.

- *KS-Related IRIS*: Paradoxical KS-IRIS occurs in 7–31% cases when ART is initiated. Frequently presents with inflammation or enlargement of a prior lesion. In the most severe cases, it can cause acute airway obstruction or significant GI bleeding. Onset is usually in the first 12 wks post ART initiation. Treatment includes systemic chemotherapy and supportive measures. Liposomal anthracyclines (e.g., doxorubicin) are first-line. Corticosteroids may be harmful as there is an association with acute progression of KS lesions, possibly due to a permissive effect on HHV-8 viral replication. ART should be continued (HIV AIDS [Auckl] 2015; 7:49).

TABLE 8.10 IRIS

Pathogen/Condition	Clinical Expression
Infectious Diseases	
Aspergillosis	Pulmonary disease with mucous impaction (case report)
Bartonellosis	Lymphagangitis, splenic inflammation
Chlamydia trachomatis	Reiter syndrome
Herpes simplex	Erosive lesions
Histoplasmosis	Pulmonary disease; adenitis; skin lesions
HHV-8	Worsening of Kaposi sarcoma; Castleman disease
Human papillomavirus	Warts

(*continued*)

TABLE 8.10 Continued

Pathogen/Condition	Clinical Expression
JC virus	Inflammatory PML with enhancement on MRI
Leishmaniasis	Increased skin disease, visceral disease, uveitis
Molluscum contagiosum	Increased skin lesions
M. tuberculosis	Fever, lymphadenopathy (abdominal, mediastinal, cervical), pneumonitis, pleural effusions, lung abscesses, expanding CNS lesions
Other mycobacteria	Skin abscess, adenitis
BCG	Skin ulcerations, neuritis
M. leprae	Pneumonia
M. xenopi	Adenitis
M. genavense	Adenitis, parotitis
M. scrofulaceum	Pneumonia
M. kansasii	
P. jirovecii	Progressive pneumonia, ARDS, granulomatous pneumonia
Parvovirus B19	Encephalitis
Strongyloides stercoralis	Disseminated disease
Toxoplasmosis	Encephalitis
Noninfectious Diseases	
Autoimmune disorder	Hyperthyroidism; SLE, rheumatoid arthritis, Graves' disease
Malignancy	Kaposi sarcoma with inflammatory skin and mucosal lesions, pneumonitis, adenopathy
	Non-Hodgkin lymphoma—relapse
Miscellaneous	Guillain Barré syndrome, tattoo ink inflammatory response, interstitial lymphoid pneumonitis and sarcoidosis; parotid gland enlargement

Liver and Pancreatic Disease

In the era of effective ART, the survival of PLWH has improved significantly. Increased life expectancy has been accompanied by the advent of nonopportunistic diseases that affect those with HIV infection disproportionately compared to the general population (AIDS 2017;31;1633), including liver disease. Liver disease has become a leading cause of morbidity among PLWH (Lancet 2011;377:1198; AIDS 2017;31;1633) and is now the most common non–AIDS-associated disease cause of death in PLWH (AIDS 2017;31;1633), largely in part due to co-infection from viral hepatitis (an estimated 66% of liver-related deaths are from hepatitis C; Lancet 2011;377;1198).

HIV infection itself is associated with immune activation, development of hepatic fibrosis, and rates of hepatic decompensation that exceed those of HBV or HCV monoinfection (Hepatol Comm 2017;1:987). HIV may promote liver disease by infecting Kupffer cells, affecting overall total cell density, or by affecting translocation of gut microbes, thus altering liver disease pathogenesis (Hepatol Comm 2017;1:987). Other proposed mechanisms of liver injury include increased oxidative stress, mitochondrial injury, lipotoxicity due to increased free fatty acids, direct cytotoxicity on hepatocytes by triggering apoptosis, toxic metabolite accumulation, senescence, and nodular regenerative hyperplasia (BMJ Open Gastroenterol 2017;4). Other contributing factors of liver disease in PLWH are HBV co-infection, alcohol abuse, drug-induced hepatotoxicity, and, possibly, hepatic injury from ART agents (Lancet 2011;377:1198). With major advancements in effective antiviral therapy for both HBV and HCV in recent years, nonalcoholic fatty liver disease (NAFLD), nonalcoholic steatohepatitis (NASH), and hepatocellular carcinoma (HCC) are becoming more frequent causes of chronic liver disease in HIV patients, accounting for approximately 11% of deaths (World J Hepatol 2012;4:91). The following is a brief review of management issues dealing with liver disease in PLWH.

ART-Associated Liver Disease

- *Factors associated with increased risk of ART hepatotoxicity* (Clin Gastroenterol Hepatol 2010;8:1002):
  - Co-infection with HBV or HCV
  - Advanced fibrosis
  - Baseline transaminitis
  - Alcohol abuse
  - Older age
  - Female gender
  - First exposure to ART
  - Significant increase in CD4 count after ART initiation
  - Concomitant use of TB medications
  - Cocaine use
- *There are four primary mechanisms for ART-related liver damage* (Clin Gastroenterol Hepatol 2010;8:1002):
  1. Direct drug toxicity and/or drug metabolism
  2. Hypersensitivity reactions
  3. Mitochondrial toxicity
  4. IRIS (HBV may reactivate and HCV-associated fibrosis may rapidly progress to cirrhosis with IRIS)
- NRTIs, NNRTIs, and PIs are the classes of ART most commonly implicated with hepatotoxicity, which can range in severity from transient elevations in transaminases to hepatic failure and death (World J Hepatol 2012;4:91):
  - *NRTIs*: AZT, ddI, d4T (not commonly used in the United States), and ABC (may be part of hypersensitivity reaction) (Lancet 2011;377:1198).
  - *NNRTIs*: EFV, NVP, and ETR:
    - *NVP hepatitis*: May also note rash and other symptoms of a hypersensitivity reaction. Most common in females with baseline CD4 of >250/mL or in men with baseline CD4 of >400/mL.
    - *EFV hepatitis*: May be symptom of a hypersensitivity reaction (Lancet 2011;377:1198).
  - *PIs*: Tipranavir, darunavir, and ritonavir.

- *CCR5 inhibitor* (maraviroc): Hepatitis in hypersensitivity reaction.
- *Fusion inhibitor* (enfuvirtide): Hepatitis in hypersensitivity reaction.
- *PI/NNRTI transaminitis*: 15–30% rate is increased 2-fold with HCV coinfection (JAMA 2000;283:74; CID 2002;34:831; Hepatology 2002;35:182).
- Other risks for drug-related hepatotoxicity are renal failure and thrombocytopenia (JAIDS 2006;43:320).
- Noncirrhotic portal hypertension has been linked with ART, particularly ddI (Lancet 2011;377:1198).
- Benign increased indirect bilirubin due to ATV and IDV (Gilbert-like syndrome).

Cholangiopathy, AIDS

See Clin Gastroenterol Hepatol 2010;8:1002.
CAUSE: Infection-related strictures in the biliary tract causing biliary obstruction:

- *Cryptosporidium parvum* is the most commonly identified microbial cause. Other causes: microsporidia, CMV, MAC, histoplasma, and *Cyclospora*.

FREQUENCY: Relatively rare in ART era and seen primarily in late-stage AIDS.

PRESENTATION: Right upper quadrant pain, LFTs show cholestasis. Fever, nausea, vomiting, and diarrhea may also occur. Jaundice is uncommon. Late-stage HIV with CD4 count of <200 cells/mm^3.

DIAGNOSIS: Alkaline phosphatase levels are high, often >8× ULN. Level predicts prognosis. Usual method to establish the diagnosis is endoscopic retrograde cholangiopancreatography (ERCP) (gold standard); ultrasound is 75–95% specific.

TREATMENT: ART is the most important treatment. Treat pathogen when possible. Usual treatment is mechanical (i.e., sphincterotomy) and based on lesion. ERCP is used for both diagnosis and treatment.

Acalculous Cholecystitis

See Clin Gastroenterol Hepatol 2010;8:1002.

CAUSE: Usually associated with CMV or *Cryptosporidium*. Other causes include *Isospora* and microsporidia.

PRESENTATION: Right upper quadrant pain and fever. LFTs show cholestasis. Often there is no leukocytosis.

DIAGNOSIS: Ultrasound shows a thickened, distended acalculous gallbladder. HIDA scan shows nonfunctioning gallbladder.

TREATMENT: Cholecystectomy.

Hepatitis

- *Hepatitis A, B, and C.* Hepatitis E often has a self-limited acute increase in ALT (World J Hepatol 2012;4:91–98).
- *Alcohol toxicity* or other substance abuse (JAIDS 2001; 27:4426).
- *Excessive alcohol consumption* is an important risk factor for progressive liver disease and mortality, irrespective of viral hepatitis status (Lancet 2011;377;1198–1209).
- *Chronic nonviral*: Alcoholic, nonalcoholic steatohepatitis (see later discussion), autoimmune hepatitis, hemochromatosis, sarcoidosis.
- *Drug toxicity*: Acetaminophen (CID 2004;38:565), INH, statins, ART agents (see section on ART and Liver Disease).
- *Hypersensitivity*: Phenytoin, ABC, TMP-SMX, NVP
- *OIs*: Infections including MAC, TB, and CMV:
  - *Fungal infections* with hepatic involvement such as *Cryptococcus, Histoplasmosis, Coccidioides, Candida, Aspergillus*, extrapulmonary PJP.
  - *Bartonellosis* (bacillary peliosis hepatis).

- Disseminated HSV, HHV-6, VZV, EBV, adenovirus, toxoplasmosis, strongyloidiasis.
- *Hepatotropic infections* including schistosomiasis (can lead to portal hypertension), leishmaniasis, herpes viruses, liver abscess (World J Hepatol 2012;4:91).

NAFLD and NASH

Nonalcoholic fatty liver disease (NAFLD) can range from mild steatosis (fat deposition in hepatocyte) to nonalcoholic steatohepatitis (NASH), caused by necroinflammation, macrovascular steatosis, hepatocellular ballooning, Mallory's hyaline, and fibrosis (Lancet 2011;377;1198). NAFLD and NASH affect PLWH more than the general population of North America or Europe or even worldwide (AIDS 2017;31;1633). Estimated prevalence worldwide of NAFLD in PLWH is 35%, and 45% for NASH (Lancet 2011;377:1198; BMJ Open Gastroenterol 2017;4; AIDS 2017;31:1621), and NAFLD has been identified in up to 30% of HIV mono-infected Americans (World J Hepatol 2012;4:91). Metabolic factors, particularly elevated BMI, insulin resistance, diabetes mellitus, and dyslipidemia (World J Hepatol 2012;4:91; Lancet 2011;377:1198; AIDS 2017;31:1621) confer the greatest increased risk of NAFLD in HIV infection. CD4 cell count has also been associated with NAFLD, suggesting a role for immune recovery (AIDS 2017;31:1621). Though NRTIs have been implicated as a cause for NAFLD or NASH (Hepatol Commun 2017;1:987), a recent systematic review and meta-analysis did not demonstrate this association (AIDS 2017;31:1621); however, the contribution of ART class to liver disease has been understudied.

The diagnosis is suspected by elevated ALT and AST and metabolic risk factors, and is established by biopsy or with imaging by ultrasound (US), CT, or MRI. A major contemporary cause is HCV co-infection, which is associated with significant hepatic fibrosis (AIDS 2005;19:585; Hepatology 2008;47:1118; JID 2005;192:1943). A review of 28 patients with HIV/HCV co-infection that had sequential biopsies showed that 74% had significant regression of hepatic steatosis with ART and increased CD4 counts (Gastroenterology 2011;140:809). The authors recommended attention to prevention of the dominant comorbidities of obesity and alcohol intake.

Hepatocellular Carcinoma (HCC)

See Lancet 2011;377:1198; Hepatol Comm 2017;1:987.
Incidence and prevalence of HCC has increased due to HBV and HCV co-infection. PLWH diagnosed with HCC are younger, more frequently symptomatic, have multiple or invasive disease, and have advanced tumor stages compared with patients without HIV infection. Median survival in PLWH with HCC is poor (7 mos), although this statistic is affected by screening intervals and approach to therapy, which differs worldwide. In the United States, it is recommended to screen for HCC every 6 mos using liver ultrasound in PLWH with stage 3 fibrosis or cirrhosis. All standard treatments (radiofrequency ablation, transarterial chemoembolization, and liver transplantation) should be considered on an individual patient basis.

Viral Hepatitis

HEPATITIS B
See Hepatology 2009;50:661.

PREVALENCE: HBV is transmitted like HIV, by blood, sex, and childbirth. Primary HBV infection in adults is usually subclinical and self-limited, but about 6% develop chronic HBV infection defined by persistent HBsAg × 6 mos. The seroprevalence of HBsAg in US adults is about 0.2%; it is higher in MSM, intravenous drug users (IDUs), persons with multiple sex partners, and immigrants from areas where HBV is endemic (Africa, Southeast Asia, and Eastern Europe). The prevalence of HBsAg in PLWH in the US and Europe is 6–14%). Rates of co-infection are much higher in some countries where HBV is endemic (Af J Med Sci 2006;35:337; World J Gastroenterol 2014;20:17360; J Hepatol 2006;44:S6).

TABLE 8.11 Viral hepatitis (A–E)

Type	Prevalence and Transmission	Incubation Period	Diagnosis	Course
A	Cases in the US have decreased by more than 95% since the vaccine was made available in 1995. Fecal–oral or exposure to contaminated food or water. Populations at high risk: travelers to endemic countries, people who use drugs, MSM, household contacts.	Average of 28 days (range of 15–50 days)	Very high ALT/AST Acute: IgM Prior infection or vaccination: Total HAV antibody (IgG)	Fulminant and fatal in 0.6%; fulminant in 15% with HCV Self-limited in >99% No chronic form
B	Sex, blood (including injection drug use), and perinatal Seroprevalence of HbsAb: vaccinated <10 yrs previously 90%; general population 3–14%; IDU 60–80%; MSM 35–80% Seroprevalence of HbsAg (chronic HBV): general population 0.1–0.2%; MSM 6–17%; IDU 7–10%; immigrants from high-risk areas 13%; PLWH (US) 7–10%	Average of 90 days (range of 60–150 days)	Acute: HBsAg + anti-HBc IgM Chronic: HBsAg × 6 mos + anti-HBc IgG Vaccinated: HBsAb	Fulminant and fatal in 0.9%. Chronic hepatitis in 25% of those infected during childhood and 15% of those who were infected in adulthood. 8–10% I those with HIV.

(continued)

TABLE 8.11 Continued

Type	Prevalence and Transmission	Incubation Period	Diagnosis	Course
C	Blood (> sex and perinatal) 2.7–3.9 million in the US with chronic hepatitis C (70–90% are injection drug users) Populations at high risk: People who inject drugs, Recipients of blood transfusions before 1992, chronic hemodialysis patients, people with HIV, MSM	4–12 wks	Anti-HCV antibody (EIA or CIA), HCV RNA (qualitative or quantitative)	Chronic hepatitis after acute HCV in 75–85% Cirrhosis in 5–20% in 20 yrs but increased risk of progression with HIV coinfection or ETOH HCV has little or no effect on rate of HIV progression
D	"Delta hepatitis" Uncommon in the US; incomplete virus that requires the helper function of hepatitis B to replicate. Occurs only among those infected with hepatitis B.			
E	Rare in the US; most cases in developing world. Fecal–oral transmission; possible zoonotic transmission in developed countries. Populations at high risk: Pregnant women, solid transplant recipients on immunosuppressive therapy	40 days (range of 15–60 days)	Hepatitis E Ab or RNA but no serologic tests have been FDA approved in US for diagnosis.	Mostly self-limited; fatality rate during outbreaks is 1%. Chronic cases in hepatitis E genotype 3 in developed countries and in transplant recipients.

From Centers for Disease Control, 2015.

NATURAL HISTORY: The natural history of chronic HBV mono-infection is highly variable. About 25% have persistent active viral replication with HBeAg and high levels of HBV DNA in serum (usually >20,000 IU/mL) associated with progressive liver injury with cirrhosis and a risk of HCC. Others have spontaneous remission with a spontaneous decrease in HBV DNA levels and seroconversion from HBeAg positive to HBeAg negative, and anti-HBe. This transition occurs at a rate of about 10%/yr in monoinfected patients, but less often with HIV/HBV co-infection (Ann Intern Med 1981;94:744; Clin Gastroenterol Hepatol 2006;4:936). Levels of HBV DNA are lower in HBeAg negative patients, but some of these patients have progressive liver disease with HBV levels of >2,000 IU/mL, or there may be progressive severe HBeAg-negative liver disease. Uncommon extrahepatic complications of HBV infection include glomerulonephritis, polyarteritis nodosa, and vasculitis.

The impact of HIV on HBV infection is substantial (Hepatology 2009;49 Suppl 5:S138):

- HIV confers an increased risk of chronic HBV after acute infection (10–15%) especially with low CD4 count.
- Decreased HBeAg clearance.
- Decreased hepatic inflammatory response with lower ALT levels
- Higher levels of HBV DNA and rates of HBeAg positivity with the associated risks of HBV-associated liver disease and hepatocellular carcinoma (JAMA 2006;295:65; CID 2003;37:1678; Lancet 2002 360;1921: JAIDS 1991;4:416). This is the presumed explanation for the 19-fold increase in the risk of hepatic deaths associated with HIV co-infection in the MACS cohort (Lancet 2002;360:1921).
- Treatment of both infections is confounded by overlapping antiviral activities and risk of resistance with nucleos(t)ide analogues including 3TC, FTC, TDF, and ETV (entecavir).

LAB TESTING AND MONITORING:

- *HBV screening*: Hepatitis B surface antigen (HBsAg), antibody to hepatitis B surface antigen (HBsAb), antibody to hepatitis B core antigen (HBcAb) (see Table 8.12).
- *Negative HBsAb, HBsAg*: Vaccinate
- *Baseline testing (HBsAg-positive)*:
  - *HBV replication*: HBeAg, HBeAb, and HBV DNA (HBV DNA indicates active HBV infection)
  - *Liver function*: ALT, albumin, bilirubin, prothrombin time, CBC with platelet count
  - *Assess co-infection*: anti-HCV and anti-HAV
- *Note*: HBsAb may disappear with reappearance of HBsAg especially with low CD4 counts. May need to repeat screening test with otherwise unexplained increase in LFTs.
- *Isolated anti-HBc without HBsAg* is unclear, but may indicate occult HBV; screen for HBV DNA before vaccinating (JAIDS 2004;36:869; World J Gastroenterol 2014;20:17360).

TABLE 8.12 Diagnostic Tests for Hepatitis B

Status	HBs Ag	HBs Ab	HBc Ab	HBe Ag	HBe Ab	Viral Load
Incubation	+	−	−	+/−	−	Low
Acute HBV	+	−	+	+	−	High
Inactive	+	−	+	−	+	Low
Chronic	+	−	+	+/−	−	High/Low
Resolved	−	+	+	−	+	Negative
Vaccinated	−	+[a]	−	−	−	Negative
Occult HBV infection	−	−	+	−	−	High/Low

[a] Ab titer ≥10 IU/L required for immunity

MONITORING IN ABSENCE OF HBV TREATMENT:
LFTs every 6 mos including ALT, albumin, bilirubin, prothrombin time, and CBC with platelet count. For hepatocellular carcinoma risk, the American Association for the Study of Liver Diseases (AASLD) recommends ultrasound every 6 mos with or without AFP (Hepatology 2018;67:358). The NIH/CDC/IDSA Guidelines for Prevention and Treatment of Opportunistic Infections in HIV-Infected Adults and Adolescents (https://aidsinfo.nih.gov/guidelines/html/4/adult-and-adolescent-oi-prevention-and-treatment-guidelines/344/hbv) agree with the recommendation for imaging.

TERMS:
See Tables 8.13 and 8.14.

- *Chronic HBV infection*: HBsAg-positive 2× separated by 6 mos.
- *HBeAg-negative inactive chronic hepatitis B*: HBsAg-positive with negative HBeAg, low-level plasma HBV DNA (<2,000 IU/mL), and normal ALT. Prognosis is improved with respect to progression of liver fibrosis and the risk of HCC; however, the risk of HCC is not eliminated, and these individuals remain at risk of reactivation (J Med Virol 2005;77:173; Semin Liver Dis 2005;25:143; Hepatology 2002;35:1522).
- *HBeAg seroconversion*: Indicates loss of HBeAg and development of HBeAb. This occurs spontaneously at about 10% per year in mono- infected patients; data for co-infected patients are not available, but probably lower (Ann Intern Med 1981;94:744).
- *Reactivation or HBV flare*: This may occur spontaneously, with immunosuppression or with chemotherapy and is usually expressed with increased ALT and HBV DNA level. Can be exacerbated by withdrawal of ART or development of resistance to anti-HBV agents (see Table 8.13) (CID 1999;28:1032; JAMA 2000;283:2526; Hepatology 2000;32:635; J Infect 2000;41:192).

MANAGEMENT:
See also Tables 8.13 and 8.14.

- *Hepatitis B vaccination*: PLWH should be screened with HBsAg, anti-HBc, Patients with negative HBsAg and anti-HBs should receive HBV vaccine. There is no strong evidence to guide management of patients who are negative for HBsAg and anti-HBs but positive for anti-HBc only (termed "isolated anti-HBc"). For people with isolated anti-HBc, HBV vaccination can be considered in those with isolated anti-HBc and negative HBV DNA.

- Patients with chronic HBV co-infection should (1) be advised to avoid or limit alcohol consumption; (2) receive HAV vaccine, preferably when CD4 count is >200 cells/mm^3; (3) be evaluated for HBV treatment, (4) choose antiretroviral regimens for HIV based on anti-HBV activity of the nucleoside analog components; (5) be counseled on the risks of HBV transmission, including the need for barrier protection of sexual partners; and (6) be advised that contacts should be evaluated for HBV vaccine.

- *Treatment of HIV with HBV coinfection* (Table 8.14): Many of the reverse transcriptase inhibitors with activity against HBV also have activity against HIV. Therefore, among persons with HIV/HBV coinfection, HBV must be treated concurrently with a fully suppressive ART regimen for HIV. As such, all persons with HIV/HBV coinfection should be initiated on an ART regimen that includes tenofovir disoproxil (TDF) or tenofovir alafenamide (TAF). While emtricitabine and lamivudine have antiviral effect against HBV, use of an ART regimen with either of these agents as the sole anti-HBV component is not recommended due to the high risk of development of resistance (2017 NIH/CDC/IDSA Guidelines for Prevention and Treatment of Opportunistic Infections in HIV-Infected Adults and Adolescents https://aidsinfo.nih.gov/guidelines/html/4/adult-and-adolescent-oi-prevention-and-treatment-guidelines/344/hbv).

- Primary goal of HBV treatment is to prevent progression of HBV-related morbidity and mortality, such as development of liver failure and hepatocellular carcinoma.
- *Serologically*:
  - *Primary endpoint*: Sustained undetectable levels of HBV DNA combined with loss of HBsAg, with or without sero-conversion to HBsAb positivity.
  - *For individuals with HBeAg-positive disease, secondary end-point*: sustained suppression of HBV DNA combined with loss of HBeAg, with or without seroconversion to HBeAb positivity.
- *Monitoring response*: ALT and HBV DNA level every 3 mos initially. Detectable HBV DNA at 6 mos usually indicates treatment failure and the need to modify therapy (AIDS Rev 2007;9:40).

TABLE 8.13 Management of HBV with HIV co-infection

HBV Treatment	
Indication for HBV treatment	1. *Immune active disease*: • Elevated HBV DNA (>20,000 IU/mL if HBeAg+ or >2,000 IIU/mL if HBeAg−) plus ALT >2 times ULN[a]; OR at least moderated hepatic inflammation or fibrosis 2. *Cirrhosis* 3. *Extrahepatic manifestations of HBV present*[b] 4. *Pregnancy*
HIV/HBV Category	***Recommendations***
On ART for HIV	Fulminant liver failure • Avoid TDF and TAF until hepatic insult has resolved (if on TDF- or TAF-containing ART regimen, switch to 3TC-containing regimen.

(continued)

TABLE 8.13 Continued

HIV/HBV Category	Recommendations
	Creatinine clearance >60ml/min • Regimens containing TAF+FTC or TDF+FTC Creatinine clearance 30–59 mL/min • Regimens containing TAF+FTC (TDF not recommended) Creatinine clearance <30 • Add entecavir Duration: Indefinite[d]
No ART; HBV treatment only	Treatment of HBV without concurrent treatment of HIV is NOT recommended Peg-IFN 2a 180 mg SQ/wk × 48 wks can be considered in rare cases where treatment of HBV but not HIV is needed. Fulminant liver failure • Initiation of ART is not recommended until acute hepatic insult has resolved
HBV treatment failure	Defined as <1 log decline in HBV DNA level after 12 wks of anti-HBV therapy • Medication adherence counseling • HBV resistance testing and medication switch based on results

Disease and treatment monitoring

Test	Frequency
Hepatitis B serologies HBsAg HBsAb HBeAg HBeAb HBV DNA	Every 3–6 mos
Liver enzymes ALT AST	ALT above the upper limit of normal • Every 3 mos ALT within limits of normal • Every 3–6 mos

TABLE 8.13 Continued

Disease and treatment monitoring

Test	Frequency
Hepatocellular carcinoma screening Liver US with or without AFP, CT, or MRI abdomen	Every 6 mos

Based on 2018 NIH/CDC/IDSA/AASLD Guidelines, the HIV clinical guidelines program, and the American Association for the Study of Liver Diseases (AASLD) (https://aidsinfo.nih.gov/contentfiles/lvguidelines/adult_oi.pdf; https://www.hivguidelines.org/adult-hiv/coinfections/hbv-hiv-coinfection/;

https://www.aasld.org/sites/default/files/guideline_documents/hep28156.pdf)

[a] Upper limit of normal per AASLD: women 19 IU/mL, men 30 IU/mL

[b] Extrahepatic manifestations include: polyarteritis nodosa, glomerulonephritis, cryoglobulinemia

[c] Entecavir: only with complete HIV suppression since entecavir has low level activity against HIV with risk of 184V mutation (AIDS 2008;22:947; NEJM 2007;356:2614). If HBV strain is known to be resistant to 3TC, there is concern for the increased likelihood of entecavir resistance by HBV; increase entecavir dose to 1.0 mg/d and monitor HBV DNA levels q3mos.

[d] Discontinuation of anti-HBV therapy is not recommended due to risk of reactivation of HBV infection, and risk of hepatic failure.

Adefovir and telbivudine are no longer recommended for HBV treatment, and lamivudine as sole anti-HBV agent within a combination ART regimen is not recommended due to risk of on-treatment development of HBV resistance.

HEPATITIS C

EPIDEMIOLOGY: The estimated prevalence of HCV in the United States is 3.5 million (1%) (NHANES, 2014). This includes 2.7 million chronically infected in the general population and 800,000

TABLE 8.14 Medications for HBV/HIV co-infection

Drug Dose	Activity vs.		Comment
	HIV	*HBV*	
3TC 300 mg/d	++	++	YMDD mutants with HBV resistance emergence rate with monotherapy: 21% at 1 yr, 94% at 4 yrs (AIDS 2006;20:863; CID 2004:37:1678): Give with TDF
FTC 200 mg/d	++	++	Assumed to be nearly identical to 3TC except longer T½
TDF 300 mg/d	++	++	Good activity, especially when combined with 3TC or FTC vs. HBV (NEJM 2003:348:177)
TAF 25 mg/d	++	++	Approved by FDA for HBV in 2016. Very good activity. Combined with 3TC or FTC vs. HBV (Expert Rev Clin Pharmacol. 2017;10:707)
Peginterferon 5 MU/d or 10 MU 3x/wks 16-48 wks	+	+	No resistance issues. Only drug shown to cause HBsAg conversion (J Gen Intern Med 2011;26:326)—Disadvantage is toxicity and CD4 decrease with HIV
Entecavir 0.5–1.0 mg/d	+	++	Resistance requires 3 mutations: (AAC 2004;48:3498). Resistance more common with 3TC resistance—Weak HIV activity can lead to 184V mutation if HIV not fully suppressed (NEJM 2007;356:2614)

infected among the incarcerated, institutionalized, or homeless population. Globally, 71 million individuals were infected with HCV worldwide in 2015 (Ann Gastroenterol 2018;31:35). In the NHANES survey, chronic HCV infection is highly correlated with illicit drug use (IDU, representing 70–90% of cases), as well as age 40–59, male sex, black race, and lower socioeconomic status. Fifty-two percent of participants reported any lifetime injection drug use (Ann Intern Med 2014;160:293). Unfortunately, about 50% of those infected are unaware of their diagnosis. IDU is the most significant risk factor for acquiring HCV, accounting for at least 60% of acute infections in the United States. Healthcare exposures are also an important source of transmission, as well as the receipt of blood products before 1992, receipt of clotting factor concentrates before 1987, hemodialysis, needle-stick injuries among healthcare workers, and patient-to-patient transmission from poor infection control. Other risk factors include perinatal transmission, incarceration, or percutaneous or parental exposures in an unregulated setting (i.e., tattoos) (Epidemiol Infect 2004;132:409).

Since 2004, there has been a substantial increase in HCV rates in MSM in Europe, Australia, and the United States (Lancet 2011;377:1198; Curr Infect Dis Rep 2010;12:118; AIDS 2011;25:1083). Twenty-five percent of PLWH in the United States are co-infected with HCV (Lancet 2011;377:1198). Co-infection with HIV is common because both viruses are transmitted by the same mechanisms: contaminated blood, sex, and perinatal transmission (J Hepatol 2006;44:Suppl S6; AIDS 2005;19: 969; CID 2007;44:1123). However, the rates of transmission in these categories are very different, as summarized in Table 8.15.

NATURAL HISTORY: HCV can lead to chronic liver disease, cirrhosis, and HCC; it is the main cause of liver disease in developed and developing countries (Lancet 2011;377:1198; Ann Gastroenterol 2018;31:35). Acute HCV infection occurs 4–12 wks after HCV transmission with ALT levels usually 10–20× ULN at 2–8 wks, HCV-RNA at 1–2 wks, and anti-HCV at 6–8 wks (Am J Gastroenterol 2008;103:1283). About 20–30% develop symptoms, usually at 6–8 wks. Spontaneous resolution occurs in 18–34% and is associated

TABLE 8.15 Transmission rates of HIV and
HCV (in absence of treatment or prophylaxis)

	HIV	HCV
Needle stick injury	0.3%	3%
Discordant couples	13%/yr	3%/yr
Perinatal transmission	20–30%	2–5%

with several genetic factors, including *IL28B* inheritance (J Hepatol 2014;61:S58). If acute resolution occurs, there are no long-term sequelae.

HCV-RNA detected ≥6 mos after infection is defined as chronic HCV. The transition from acute to chronic HCV is usually subclinical, so the time course from acute to chronic HCV is difficult to specify. With chronic HCV mono-infection, the natural history remains incompletely defined but is characterized by persistent hepatic inflammation with progression to cirrhosis in 10–20% after 20–30 yrs of infection; however, there are varying progression rates to cirrhosis in the literature. After cirrhosis, the rate of progression to liver failure is 3–6%/yr, and to HCC is 1–5%/yr. The development of fibrosis is influenced by many factors including age at infection, male sex, alcohol consumption, obesity, insulin resistance, type 2 diabetes, co-infection with HBV or HIV, immunosuppressive therapy, and genetic factors. Treatment of chronic HCV with a sustained virologic response (SVR) is associated with a reduction in portal hypertension, hepatic decompensation, HCC, and liver-related mortality (J Hepatol 2014;61:S58).

HIV-HCV co-infection is common due to shared risk factors. Overall, about 30% of PLWH in the United States and Europe are co-infected with HCV (Clin Gastroenterol Hepatol 2010;8:1002). Coinfection with HIV is associated with an increased rate of progression of chronic HCV to cirrhosis. (Ann Gastroenterol 2018;31:35). HIV alters the natural HCV course: PLWH are less likely to clear HCV viremia, have higher HCV RNA levels, have an accelerated progression to fibrosis, have an increased risk of developing cirrhosis, and a have a higher risk of decompensated liver disease once cirrhotic. HIV/HCV co-infected patients have a 2-fold increased risk of cirrhosis and 5-fold increased risk of decompensated liver disease compared to HCV mono-infected (Lancet 2011;377:1198; Clin Gastroenterol Hepatol 2010;8:1002). Other factors associated with more rapid progression of HCV are detectable HIV viremia, male sex, alcohol use >50 g/d, age >25 yrs, and low CD4 count (Lancet 2011;377:1198). ART reduces the rate of hepatic fibrosis and hepatic decompensation with HCV (Hepatol Comm 2017;1:987; J Hepatol 2006;44:47; CID 2006;42:262; Antivir Ther 2006; 11:839; Lancet 2003;362:1708); however, some studies have shown that the ABC/3TC backbone, PIs, and NNRTIs are associated with increased progression of fibrosis (Hepatol Comm 2017;1:987). One report noted the 3-yr survival with HCV/HIV and cirrhosis is relatively good (87%) but is poor with hepatic decompensation (AIDS 2011;25:899). It was previously thought that HCV did not affect HIV disease; however, the Swiss HIV Cohort Study showed that those with HIV/HCV co-infection had a faster progression to AIDS and slower CD4 recovery than those with HIV infection alone (Lancet 2000;356:1800). There are limited data on the effect of achieving SVR on the HCC risk in PLWH; however, co-infection with HCV accounts for 93% of the cases of HCC occurring in patients with HIV. Ongoing tumor surveillance may be needed in this group after SVR regardless of pretreatment fibrosis stage (J Hepatol 2014;61:S58).

ART-ASSOCIATED HEPATOTOXICITY (WITH HEPATITIS C): Chronic HCV can be associated with a higher risk of ART-related hepatotoxicity; antiretroviral agents can induce severe changes in aminotransferase levels in HIV/HCV co-infected individuals (JAMA 2000;283:74; AIDS 2000;14:2895; JAIDS 2001;27:426). Patients on PIs have the highest risk of developing hepatotoxicity; however, one large cohort of co-infected patients found that these changes were often self-limited, even when the PI was continued, and there were no cases of irreversible liver failure (JAMA 2000;283:74). NNRTIs, especially NVP, are associated with hepatotoxicity, hypersensitivity reactions, and lipid disorders. Those on ritonavir have a greater than 2-fold increase in the risk of hepatotoxicity if co-infected with HCV.

There are no clear guidelines for modifying ART with co-infection, although a common recommendation is to discontinue these agents if patients are symptomatic, or have transaminase levels >5× ULN or >3.5× baseline levels. Most patients with grade 3/4 toxicity are asymptomatic (JID 2002;186:23). In these cases, there should be an investigation for other causes of liver disease (hepatitis A or B, OIs, alcohol, or other hepatotoxic medications). Consider a change in antiretroviral agents if no reversible cause can be found. If the ALT level does not change or if it increases, consider liver biopsy and HCV treatment. If the ALT decreases, resume ART with a new drug regimen and monitor ALT closely. NVP and TPV/r are antiretroviral agents that are often considered to be contraindicated with baseline hepatic disease including HCV coinfection, but there is no evidence that the hepatic necrosis seen with this drug has any association with HCV (Lancet 2004;363:1253; JAIDS 2004;36:772).

DIAGNOSIS: HCV testing should be performed in people who have the risk factors, as mentioned earlier. The CDC established risk-based HCV testing guidelines in 1998 that were then expanded in 2012, recommending all persons born between 1945 and 1965 to have one-time HCV testing without prior ascertainment of HCV risk factors.

In addition to testing in those who use injection drugs, one-time HCV testing should be done in those with HIV or who use intranasal drugs illicitly. Annual HCV testing is recommended for people who inject drugs and for HIV-infected MSM. Other conditions that warrant HCV testing include those who are sexually active and about to start pre-exposure prophylaxis (PreP) for HIV, those with unexplained chronic liver disease or transaminitis, and those who are solid organ donors.

Tests for HCV include (1) screening tests, with EIA or CIA for anti- HCV; (2) confirmatory test with quantitative HCV RNA; and (3) genotyping, because this guides selection of appropriate antiviral therapy. If seronegative HCV is suspected based on elevated transaminases or risk factors, then a test for HCV RNA should be performed (Clin Liver Dis 2003;7:179). False-negative screening serology is most common with CD4 of <100/mL. Unlike HIV, HCV VL does not correlate with progression.

MANAGEMENT:

- *All HCV/HIV co-infected patients should*: (1) Be advised to abstain from alcohol use or at least limit consumption to <20–50 g alcohol/wk (2–5 drinks); (2) avoid hepatotoxic drugs, including iron supplements in the absence of iron deficiency and acetaminophen in doses >2 g/d; (3) be informed about methods to prevent transmission of both infections (use condoms and avoid needle sharing); (4) receive vaccinations for HBV and HCV, if susceptible; (5) be evaluated for HCV disease severity and treatment; (6) consider ART for all HCV-infected patients with HIV regardless of CD4 count; and (7) consider evaluation for HCC by ultrasound or α-fetoprotein (AFP) every 6 mos.
- *If patients have signs or symptoms of decompensated cirrhosis*, refer to a liver transplant center before starting HCV therapy.
- *Indications to treat*: The goals of therapy are to eradicate HCV as indicated by an SVR, the elusive cure that cannot be achieved with HIV or HBV. The success of treatment (SVR rate) has historically been judged largely by the experience with genotype type 1, since this is the most refractory to therapy and the dominant genotype in the United States, Europe, and Japan. Initial studies with genotype 1 infection using interferon for 6 mos yielded a cure rate of 5%; the addition of ribavirin and prolongation to 48 wks increased the SVR to 25%. Pegylated interferon was associated with an SVR of 40% (Lancet 2001;359:958; NEJM 2002;347:975). The advent of multiple new agents (designated direct-acting antivirals [DAAs]) began in 2011 with testing and FDA approval of telaprevir and boceprevir, orally administered PIs, which, when combined with peginterferon/ribavirin (PEG-IFN/RBV), achieved cure rates of 55–75% (Lancet 2010;376:705; NEJM

2009;360:1827). In 2014, the FDA approved sofosbuvir/ ledipasvir (Harvoni), the first combination pill that does not require ribavirin or interferon. Since then, more DAAs have become available. The section below, summarizes treatment options and recommendations, as well as drug interactions with ARVs that should be avoided, as per the joint IDSA-AASLD guidelines in 2018 (hcvguidelines.org). Issues with cost and controversy regarding timing of therapy initiation still remain.

RECOMMENDATIONS FOR EVALUATION AND TREATMENT:
Pre-therapy: General evaluation:

- *Assess comorbidities*: Substance abuse, psychiatric disease, cardiopulmonary disease, renal disease. Perform pregnancy testing in women of childbearing age and assess contraceptive use, if using ribavirin.
- Assess if there has been any prior HCV treatment experience
- Counsel patient on benefits and risks, importance of adherence, and necessity for close supervision and blood tests during and after treatment
- Perform medication reconciliation to assess for drug–drug interactions
  - Consider modification of ART based on interactions with HCV therapy. See Table 8.18 for highlighted interactions and refer to PLoS ONE 2015;10:e0141164 or hcvguidelines. org for comprehensive interactions guide.
- Laboratory tests:
  - *Quantitative HCV RNA* by RT-PCR.
  - *HCV genotype*: This guides selection of treatment regimen.
  - *Hepatic transaminases*: Note that ALT and AST values fluctuate and may be normal with advanced liver disease (Gastroenterology 2003;124:97).
  - CBC, eGFR, ALT, AST, bilirubin, INR.
  - *Evaluate HIV status*: CD4 count, VL, active OIs.

- *Evaluate HBV status*: Hep B sAg, sAb, cAb. If Hep B sAg is positive, assess HBV DNA and start equally effective HIV and HBV regimen before HCV treatment (see Hepatitis B section).
- *HCV resistance testing* for RASs (resistance-associated substitutions), if use of elbasvir/grazoprevir is planned in a genotype 1a patient.
- Test to evaluate the fibrosis stage:
  - *Liver biopsy*: Invasive but considered the gold standard. The concern is sampling error (Am J Gastroenterol 2015;110:1169).
  - *FibroScan*: Uses ultrasound transient elastography to measure liver stiffness, but may not be applicable in the setting of obesity, ascites, or limited operator experience (Gastroenterology 2012;142:1293). Approved by FDA in 2013.
  - *Laboratory test formulas*: Readily available, but variable in sensitivity and specificity (Hepatology 2006;41:175; AIDS 2003;17:721; JAIDS 2005;40:538; JAIDS 2006;41:175; J Clin Gastroenterol 2008;42:827; Liver Int 2008;28:486; Clin Chim Acta 2007;381:119; Intervirology 2008;51 Suppl 1:11 and 27; J Hepatol 2008;48:835).
    - FIB-4: Predicts significant fibrosis based on age and three variables (AST, ALT, and platelet count). This was used to calculate the Ishak fibrosis score based on correlates with liver biopsies in 832 patents. The derived formula is based on this analysis: age (years) × AST (UI/L) × PLT (109/L) × ALT (IU/L). The corresponding scores were fibrosis class 1, <1.45; class 2, 1.46–3.25; and class 3, >3.25 (Hepatology 2006;43:1377).
    - APRI index: Based on the AST-to-platelet ratio: AST (with ULN 40 IU/L/platelet count (platelets × 109/L) × 100. The corresponding scores are APRI class 1, <0.5; class 2, 0.51–1.5; and class 3, >1.5 (JAIDS 2005;40:538). An advantage to these systems is the ability to avoid liver biopsy in many cases (CID 2011;52:1164).

- *Ultrasound* to assess for HCC if stage 3 or 4 (cirrhosis). If HCC is present, refer to oncology before starting HCV therapy.

THERAPY: In general, HIV/HCV-co-infected patients should be treated the same as people without HIV. The goal of therapy is SVR/virologic cure, which has been shown to be durable and improve liver disease and decrease risk of HCC, as well as reduce extrahepatic manifestations. Therefore, all patients should be offered therapy, except those with short life expectancies not expected to improve with treatment of HCV.

TABLE 8.16 AASLD/IDSA/IAS-USA Recommendations for treating HCV in treatment-naive patients with and without compensated cirrhosis

DAA Therapy Options	Genotype	Duration (wks)	Major Studies
Ledipasvir/ sofosbuvir (Harvoni)	1a, 1b, 4, 5, 6	12	ION-1, ION-3, SYNERGY
Paritaprevir/ ritonavir/ ombitasvir + dasabuvir (Viekira Pak)	1a, 1b, 4	12 (24 if cirrhosis[a]; add RBV for 1a)	SAPPHIRE-1, PEARL-1, PEARL-IV TURQOISE-I & -II, AGATE-1 & -2
Elbasvir + grazoprevir (Zepatier)	1a, 1b, 4	12 (if 1a & NS5A polymorphisms, add RBV, treat 16 wks)	C-EDGE, C-WORTHY
Sofosbuvir/ Velpatasvir (Epclusa)	1–6	12	ASTRAL-1, ASTRAL-2, ASTRAL-3, POLARIS-2, POLARIS-3

TABLE 8.16 Continued

DAA Therapy Options	Genotype	Duration (wks)	Major Studies
Sofosbuvir/ velpatasvir/ voxilaprevir (Vosevi)	3	12 (as an alternative)	POLARIS-3
Glecaprevir/ pibrentasvir (Mavyret)	1–6	8 (12 if cirrhosis)	SURVEYOR-1, SURVEYOR-2, ENDURANCE-1, ENDRANCE-3, ENDURANCE-4, EXPEDITION-1, EXPEDITION-2
Daclatasvir + sofosbuvir	1a, 1b, 2, 3	12 (16-24 if cirrhosis with or without RBV)	ALLY-2, ALLY-3, SAPPHIRE-I, PEARL-IV, TURQUOISE-II, ENDURANCE-3
Simeprevir + sofosbuvir	1a, 1b (avoid if Q80K mutation)	12 (24 if cirrhosis with or without RBV)	OPTIMIST-1, OPTIMIST-2

See also hcvguidelines.org for regularly updated information.

* There is a 2015 FDA warning against use of the Viekira Pak in advanced cirrhosis due to reports of serious liver injury (http://www.fda.gov/Drugs/DrugSafety/ucm468634.htm).

Zepatier is the only approved DAA for patients with renal impairment or on hemodialysis. There is very limited data on the use of the other DAAs in patients with creatinine clearance <30 mL/min.

Retreatment: Refer to the AASLD-IDSA guidelines for up-to-date recommendations (hcvguidelines.org).

TABLE 8.17 AASLD/IDSA/IAS-USA Recommendations for treating HCV in treatment-experienced patients with and without compensated cirrhosis

Prior HCV Treatment	Genotype	Cirrhosis Status	DAA Option	Duration (wks)	Major Studies
PEG-IFN/RBV	1a	None	Elbasvir/grazoprevir (add RBV if NS5A RASs)	12 (16 of NS5A RASs)	C-EDGE TE
			Glecaprevir/pibrentasvir	8	ENDURANCE-1
			Ledipasvir/sofosbuvir	12	ION-2
			Sofosbuvir/velpatasvir	12	ASTRAL-1
		Cirrhosis	Elbasvir/grazoprevir (add RBV if NS5A RASs)	12	C-EDGE TE
			Sofosbuvir/velpatasvir	12	ASTRAL-1
			Glecaprevir/pibrentasvir	12	EXPEDITION-1
	1b	None	Elbasvir/grazoprevir	12	C-EDGE TE
			Glecaprevir/pibrentasvir	8	ENDURANCE-1
			Ledipasvir/sofosbuvir	12	ION-2
			Sofosbuvir/velpatasvir	12	ASTRAL-1
		Cirrhosis	Elbasvir/grazoprevir	12	C-EDGE TE
			Sofosbuvir/velpatasvir	12	ASTRAL-1
			Glecaprevir/pibrentasvir	12	EXPEDITION-1
NS3 + PEG-IFN/RBV	1	None	Ledipasvir/sofosbuvir	12	ION-2
			Sofosbuvir/velpatasvir	12	ASTRAL-1
			Glecaprevir/pibrentasvir	12	MAGELLAN-1

	Prior treatment	Cirrhosis	Regimen	Duration (weeks)	Clinical trials
		Cirrhosis	Sofosbuvir/velpatasvir	12	ASTRAL-1
			Glecaprevir/pibrentasvir	12	MAGELLAN-1
1	Non-NS5A, SOF-containing regimen	With or without cirrhosis	Sofosbuvir/velpatasvir/voxilaprevir (1a)	12	POLARIS-4
			Sofosbuvir/velpatasvir/voxilaprevir (1b)	12	POLARIS-4
			Glecaprevir/pibrentasvir	12	ENDURANCE-1, EXPEDITION-1
1	NS5A	With or without cirrhosis	Sofosbuvir/velpatasvir/voxilaprevi	12	POLARIS-1
2	PEG-IFN/RBV OR SOF+RBV	With or without cirrhosis	Glecaprevir/pibrentasvir	8 (12 if cirrhosis)	SURVEYOR-II, EXPEDITION-1, ENDURANCE-2
			Sofosbuvir/velpatasvir	12	ASTRAL-2, POLARIS-2, POLARIS-4
3	PEG-IFN/RBV	None	Sofosbuvir/velpatasvir	12	ASTRAL-2, POLARIS-2
		Cirrhosis	Elbasvir/grazoprevir	12	C-ISLE
			Sofosbuvir/velpatasvir/voxilaprevir	12	POLARIS-3, ASTRAL-3

(continued)

TABLE 8.17 Continued

Prior HCV Treatment	Genotype	Cirrhosis Status	DAA Option	Duration (wks)	Major Studies
Any DAA	3	With or without cirrhosis	Sofosbuvir/velpatasvir/voxilaprevir (add RBV if prior NS5A used and cirrhosis)	12	POLARIS-1, POLARIS-4
PEG-IFN/RBV	4	With or without cirrhosis	Sofosbuvir/velpatasvir	12	ASTRAL-1
			Glecaprevir/pibrentasvir	8 (12 if cirrhosis)	SURVEYOR-II, EXPEDITION-1
			Elbasvir/grazoprevir + RBV	16	Integrated analysis
			Ledipasvir/sofosbuvir	12	SYNERGY
			Sofosbuvir/velpatasvir/voxilaprevir	12	POLARIS-1, POLARIS-4
Any DAA	4	With or without cirrhosis	Sofosbuvir/velpatasvir/voxilaprevir	12	POLARIS-1, POLARIS-4
PEG-IFN/RBV	5 or 6	With or without cirrhosis	Glecaprevir/pibrentasvir	8 (12 if cirrhosis)	Integrated analysis
			Ledipasvir/sofosbuvir	12	NCT01826981
			Sofosbuvir/velpatasvir	12	ASTRAL-1
Any DAA	5 or 6	With or without cirrhosis	Sofosbuvir/velpatasvir/voxilaprevir	12	POLARIS-1

See also: hcvguidelines.org for alternative regimens and regularly updated information.

TABLE 8.18 Recommendations of HCV medication interactions with HIV ART

DAA	HIV ART DDIs
Daclatasvir	Decrease daclatasvir dose to 30mg/d with ATV/r, ATV/c, EVG/r, EVG/c co-administration. Increase daclatasvir dose to 90 mg/d with EFV, ETR (and possibly NVP) co-administration.
Elbasvir/ grazoprevir	Use with ABC, FTC, ENF, 3TC, RAL, DTG, RPV, TDF, TAF Avoid with COBI, EFV, ETR, NVP, any protease inhibitors
Glecaprevir/ pibrentasvir	Use with ABC, FTC, ENF, 3TC, RAL, DTG, RPV, TDF; monitor for hepatic toxicity if used with EVG/COBI Avoid with ATV, EFV, ETR, any ritonavir-containing regimen
Ledipasvir/ sofosbuvir	Can increase tenofovir levels. Avoid TDF with CrCL <60ml/min. TAF can be considered with PI/r, PI/c, EVG/r, EVG/c co-administration.
Simeprevir	Use with ABC, FTC, ENF, 3TC, MVC, RAL, DTG, RPV, TDF Avoid COBI, EFV, ETR, NVP, any protease inhibitor
Sofosbuvir/ velpatasvir	Avoid with EFV, ETR, NVP, TPV/r; Can increase tenofovir levels. Avoid TDF with CrCL <60 mL/min. Consider TAF
Paritaprevir/ ritonavir/ ombitasvir/ dasaabuvir	Use with ATV (300 mg/d without ritonavir), DTG, FTC, ENF, 3TC, RAL, TDF, TAF Avoid with DRV, EFV, LPV/r, ETR, NVP, COBI, RPV, TPV/r
Sofosbuvir/ velpatasvir/ voxilaprevir	Use with DTG, FTC, ENF, 3TC, RPV, RAL; monitor for hepatic toxicity with DRV/r and EVG/COBI Avoid with ATV/r, EFV, ETR, NVP May increase tenofovir levels. Avoid TDF with CrCL <60 mL/min. Consider TAF

See hcvguidelines.org for more information.

MONITORING DURING THERAPY:

- CBC, CMP, quantitative HCV RNA after 4 wks of treatment:
  - >10-fold, persistent, asymptomatic increases in ALT or <10-fold, symptomatic increases in ALT should prompt discontinuation of therapy.
  - If HCV RNA is detectable after 4 wks of therapy, repeat after 2 additional weeks of treatment.
    - If 6-wk HCV RNA is increased by >10-fold, discontinue treatment.
  - If on elbasvir/grazoprevir, monitor LFTs at 8 wks of treatment (and again at 12 wks, if receiving 16 wks of treatment).
  - More frequent assessment (i.e., of CBC) may be needed if receiving ribavirin.
- HCV RNA 12 wks after the end of therapy:
  - SVR12 is considered a virologic cure (Hepatology 2015;61:41).
  - For Hep BsAg-positive patients who are not already on therapy, monitor HBV DNA level during and immediately after therapy.

RISK FOR HEPATITIS B REACTIVATION: Reactivation of HBV has been reported in patients starting DAA HCV therapy who are not on active HBV agents. For PLWH who have HBV infection, tenofovir-based HIV regiments are preferred since tenofovir also has activity against HBV. For patients who are only Hep BcAb positive, LFTs should be followed, and if there is an elevation in transaminases, HBV DNA testing should be pursued to assess for reactivation.

POST-TREATMENT FOLLOW-UP: For patients with advanced fibrosis (stage 3 or 4), CBC, CMP, INR, and imaging for HCC surveillance every 6 mos. Assess for recurrence with repeat quantitative HCV RNA, testing only if risk of reinfection or unexplained hepatic dysfunction develops. Refer patients with cirrhosis for endoscopic screening for esophageal varices. If treatment failed to achieve SVR, monitor disease progression every 6–12 mos with hepatic function panel, CBC, and INR.

DECOMPENSATED CIRRHOSIS: Refer to liver transplant center. For treatment, weight-based ribavirin may be used in combination with ledipasvir/sofosbuvir, sofosbuvir/velpatasvir, or daclatasvir/sofosbuvir for 12 wks. For patients who are ribavirin ineligible, the same fixed-dose combinations of DAAs may be used without ribavirin, for an extended period of 24 wks. Patients should be referred to a liver transplant center before starting HCV therapy.

LIVER TRANSPLANTATION WITH HIV INFECTION: Optimal control of HIV disease is required for all HIV patients undergoing liver transplantation. In patients with portal hypertension, splenic sequestration can decrease the CD4 count; a threshold of CD4 of >100 can be used in these patients. Initial case series of PLWH undergoing liver transplant demonstrated poor outcomes, but this was before the introduction of continuous ART regimens. Now, PLWH not co-infected with HCV have excellent outcomes following liver transplant, similar to HIV-negative patients. However, if liver transplantation is done in an HIV/HCV co-infected patient, fibrosis rates are accelerated with graft cirrhosis rates of 30% at 5 yrs (J Hepatol 2014;61:S58), predominantly due to HCV recurrence. A US-based prospective study of HIV/HCV co-infected patients undergoing liver transplantation showed 1- and 3-yr patient survival rates were 76% and 60%, respectively, in the HIV/HCV cohort compared to 92% and 79%, respectively, in the HCV mono-infected cohort ($P < 0.001$). Similar to previous reports, the graft loss was significantly higher in the co-infected cohort. Multivariate analysis identified HIV infection as the only baseline factor associated with an increased risk of death (Am J Transplant 2012;12:1866).

Pancreatitis

See Am J Med 1999;107:78.
INCIDENCE: Data from the early HAART era (2001–2006) found varying rates in different cohorts:

- *EuroSIDA*: 1.3 cases/1,000 person years (AIDS 2008;22:47) with individual case reviews.

- *Johns Hopkins cohort*: 2.6 cases/1,000 person years (AIDS Patient Care STDS 2008;22:113) using individual case reviews.
- *Kaiser Permanente*: Range from 5.1–8.0/1,000 person years (AIDS 2008;22:145), but cases defined simply by lipase >4× ULN.

MAJOR CAUSES:

- Drugs, especially ddI or ddI + d4T ± hydroxyurea. May be complication of lactic acidosis (NRTI-associated mitochondrial toxicity) or secondary to PI-associated hypertriglyceridemia with elevated triglyceride levels—usually >1,000 mg/dL. Less common drugs: d4T, 3TC (pediatrics), LPV/r, RTV, INH, rifampin, TMP-SMX, pentamidine, corticosteroids, sulfonamides, erythromycin, paromomycin. Rare case reports with currently used drugs (e.g., DTG) (AIDS 2015;29:390).
- *Opportunistic infections*: CMV. Less common: MAC, TB, cryptosporidium, toxoplasmosis, cryptococcus.
- *Conditions that cause pancreatitis in general population*, especially alcoholism. *Less common*: Gallstones, hypertriglyceridemia (average level is 4,500 mg/dL), post ERCP (3–5% of procedures), trauma. *Note*: Despite association between hypertriglyceridemia and PIs, other medications appear to account for >90% of cases (Pancreas 2003;27:E1).

DIAGNOSIS:

- Amylase >3× ULN; *p*-isoamylase is more specific but not usually measured (Mayo Clin Proc 1996;71:1138). Other causes of hyperamylasemia: other intraabdominal conditions, diseases of salivary gland, tumors (lung and ovary), and renal failure.
- Other tests:
  - *Lipase*: As sensitive as amylase, but more specific. Need for amylase plus lipase is arbitrary.

- *CT scan*: Best method to image (Radiology 1994;193:297). Used to (1) exclude other serious intraabdominal conditions, (2) stage pancreatitis, and (3) detect complications.

TREATMENT: Supportive care: IV fluids, pain control, and NPO.

PROGNOSIS: Best predictor of outcome is APACHE II score (Am J Gastroenterol 2003;98:1278).

Malignancies

EPIDEMIOLOGY: HIV infection is a well-established risk factor for the development of several tumors designated as AIDS-defining cancers (ADC). Compared to the general population, the incidence rates of Kaposi sarcoma (HHV-8), non-Hodgkin lymphoma (EBV), and cervical cancer (HPV) in PLWH is substantially magnified (JNCI 2011;103:753). The widespread availability of ART has led to a significant decrease in the frequency of the 3 ADCs. However, the incidence of non–AIDS-defining cancers (NADCs) including lung, liver, renal, anal, head and neck, skin, and Hodgkin lymphoma has increased, and these cancers now account for nearly two-thirds of all cancers in the post-HAART era. NADCs are now a leading cause of death among PLWH (JAIDS 2016;73:190; Cancer Epidemiol Biomarkers Prev 2017;26:1027).

There are several reasons for the increased rate of NADCs, including (1) HIV itself: the virus may contribute directly through activation of proto-oncogenes, alterations of cell cycle regulation, inhibition of tumor suppressor genes including p53, enhancement of tumor growth, and rendering of tissue more susceptible to the effect of environmental carcinogens; (2) chronic immunosuppression and immune activation; (3) high prevalence of co-infection with other oncogenic viruses (e.g., HBV, HCV, HPV, EBV, HHV8) (AIDS 2016;30:273); (4) high frequency of tobacco and alcohol use (CID 2012;55:1228; AIDS 2016;30:273); (5) aging of the HIV population; and (6) possibly ART itself (anal cancer may be associated with PIs) (AIDS 2012;26:2223).

TABLE 8.19 Crude cancer type-specific incidence rate and all-cause death rates, by HIV infection status, NA-ACCORD

	HIV Incidence Rate Per 100,000 PY	General Population Incidence Rate Per 100,000 PY
Kaposi sarcoma	130.4	0.2
Non-Hodgkin lymphoma	153.5	12.6
Lung cancer	129.3	45.4
Anal cancer	60.1	1.2
Colorectal cancer	36.4	27.7
Liver cancer	46.3	10.9
Hodgkin lymphoma	33.5	1.9
Melanoma	16.4	14.5
Oral cavity/pharyngeal cancer	34.3	18.4
Death	3686	833

Adapted from Ann Intern Med 2015;163:507.

PREVENTION:

Cancer prevention strategies include:

- *ART:* (reduces KS and NHL)
- *Smoking cessation*
- *Safe sex* and IDU rehabilitation to prevent oncogenic virus acquisition: HBV, HCV, HPV, and HHV8; condoms shown to reduce HPV transmission (only)
- *HCV and HBV therapy*
- *HPV vaccination* (Lancet 2011;377:2085)
- *Standard cancer screening* per general population guidance:
  - Colonoscopy
  - Mammogram
  - Cervical Pap smear
- *Anal Pap smear:* MSM; conflicting guidelines from authoritative sources

- *Cirrhosis*: Semi-annual α-fetoprotein (AFP) or ultrasound, but unclear cost-effectiveness

PROGNOSIS: Outcome is largely dictated by tumor type and stage at presentation. However, there is increasing evidence that patients with HIV have poorer cancer outcomes compared to the general population (CID 2010;51:1099; Cancer Epidemiol Biomarkers Prev 2015;24:1167; J Clin Oncol 2015;33:2376). However, the gap is decreasing (Int J Cancer 2015;137:2443) and is significantly improved with ART (AIDS 2013;27:1109).

Kaposi Sarcoma

CAUSE: HHV-8. Transmission of infection is thought to be by HHV-8 in saliva (JAIDS 2006;42:420; Sex Transm Infect 2006;82:229; Nat Rev Cancer 2010;10:707).

EPIDEMIOLOGY: Rate is up to 3,640-fold higher in PLWH compared with general population and 300-fold higher than other immuno-suppressed patients (Lancet 1990;335:123; JNCI 2002;94:1204). The postulated mechanism is HIV-induced upregulation of cytokines that regulate angiogenesis and lymphangiogenesis (Lancet 2004;364:740). The rate has decreased about 5- to 6-fold in the HAART era (JAMA 2002;287:221; JNCI 2010;103:753; JAMA 2011;305:1450).

PRESENTATION: Firm purple to brown-black macules, patches, nodules, or papules that are usually asymptomatic, neither pruritic nor painful, and usually on legs, face, oral cavity, and genitalia. Complications include lymphedema (especially legs, face, and genitalia) and visceral involvement (especially mouth, GI tract, and lungs). ART reduces the frequency of KS (JAIDS 2003;33:614), and, when it develops during ART, the course is typically less aggressive (Cancer 2003;98:2440).

DIFFERENTIAL: Bacillary angiomatosis (biopsy with silver stain to show organisms), hematoma, nevus, hemangioma, B-cell lymphoma, and pyogenic granuloma. Biopsy should be performed on at least one lesion to confirm the diagnosis. This is particularly important with rapidly growing lesions.

PROGNOSIS: CD4 count plus tumor burden staging (ACTG; J Clin Oncol 1989;7:201). TIS: Extent of Tumor (T), Immune status (I), Severity of systemic illness (S). TIS predicts survival (J Clin Oncol 1997; 15:385). Good prognosis: lesions confined to skin, CD4 count >150/mL, no "B" symptoms.

DIAGNOSIS:

NYS AIDS Institute Guidelines:

- *Skin and oral cavity*: Inspection plus biopsy of one typical lesion
- *Lung*: Suspect with cutaneous lesion plus unexplained dyspnea, wheezing, or hemoptysis. Evaluation: X-ray or CT scan shows bilateral perihilar/lower zone reticulonodular infiltrates. These are often flame-shaped (Ann Thorac Med 2010;5:201). *Diagnosis*: Bronchoscopy to detect typical red raised or flat lesions, usually at bronchial branch points. Diagnosis is established by inspection; biopsy is unnecessary and may cause bleeding.
- *GI*: Suspect with cutaneous lesion plus unexplained GI symptoms. Usually pain, bleeding, or obstruction. Diagnosis via upper and lower endoscopy to detect typical raised, red mucosal lesion.

TREATMENT:

- *ART*: Associated with lesion regression, decreased incidence, and prolonged survival (J Clin Oncol 2001;19:3848; J Med Virol 1999;57:140; AIDS 1997;11:261; Mayo Clin Proc 1998;73:439; AIDS 2000;14:987).
- *Antiviral therapy*: Foscarnet, cidofovir, and ganciclovir are active against HHV-8 (J Clin Invest 1997;99:2082), but these drugs do not appear to cause tumor regression (JAIDS 1999;20:34)

- *Chemotherapy*: Vinblastine injections, topical cis-retinoic acid gel (Panretin gel), imiquimod, liquid nitrogen, radiation (low dose), cryosurgery, or laser therapy.
- *Systemic therapy*:
  - Indications: (1) Pulmonary KS, (2) visceral KS, (3) extensive cutaneous lesions (arbitrarily >25 skin lesion), (4) rapidly progressive cutaneous KS, or (5) KS associated lymphedema.
  - Systemic treatment:
    Optimize ART management and OI prophylaxis first
    Agents: Liposomal anthracyclines: liposomal doxorubicin (Doxil), or liposomal daunorubicin (DaunoXome); paclitaxel (Taxol).

RESPONSE: KS cannot be cured; goals of therapy are to reduce symptoms and prevent progression. Complete remission is rare. ART is associated with reduced tumor burden. Antiviral drugs directed against HHV-8 have no established benefit (JAIDS 1999;20:34).

- *Local therapy*: Local injections of vinblastine cause reduced lesion size, but not elimination in most patients (Cancer 1993;71:1722).
- *Systemic therapy*: Liposomal anthracyclines usually show good results with few side effects. Paclitaxel is as effective but more toxic due to neutropenia and thrombocytopenia; side effects are dose-related; lower doses appear as effective with less marrow suppression.
  For refractory/relapsed therapy:
    Preferred regimen: Pomalidomide.
    Alternatives: Bevacizumab, etoposide, gemcitabine, imatinib, interferon alfa, nab-paclitaxel, thalidomide, vinorelbine.
- *Immune reconstitution KS*: In a review of 150 treatment-naïve patients with KS who started ART, 10 (6.6%) developed progressive KS (J Clin Oncol 2005;23:5224).

TABLE 8.20 Frequency, presentation, and diagnosis of Kaposi sarcoma

Site	Frequency*	Presentation	Diagnosis
Skin	>95%	Purple or black-brown nodular skin or oral lesions ± edema	Appearance and biopsy
Oral	30%	Usually palate or gums	Appearance and biopsy (skin biopsy preferred)
GI	40%	Pain, bleeding, or obstruction • Most are asymptomatic • Most have skin lesions • May occur at any level	Endoscopy to see hemorrhagic nodule; biopsy is often negative (Gastroenterology 1988;89:102). Assume diagnosis if skin biopsy is positive
Lung	20–50%	Dyspnea, cough, wheezing, and/or hemoptysis. May cause parenchymal or endobronchial lesions or pleural effusion. Pleural effusion: serosanguineous, cytology negative. X-ray: infiltrates diffuse or nodular.	CT scan and bronchoscopy. Endobronchial TB—red raised lesions—biopsy often negative.

Clinical presentation consists of worsening KS with lymphadenopathy, more skin lesions, skin lesions that are more violaceous, and associated with more edema (CID 2004; 39:1852).

HIV-Associated Lymphomas

Most are B-cell lymphomas. Histologic types include diffuse large B-cell lymphoma (DLBCL), HHV8-positive DLBCL, primary effusion lymphoma, plasmablastic lymphoma, primary CNS lymphoma (PCNSL), Burkitt lymphoma, and Hodgkin lymphoma. In an analysis of 6,788 NHL cases, 96 (1.4%) were T-cell lymphomas; the relative risk in AIDS patients versus the general population was 15. T-cell lymphomas include mycosis fungoides, peripheral lymphomas, cutaneous lymphomas, and adult T-cell lymphoma (JAIDS 2001;26:371). Most HIV-associated lymphomas increase in frequency with declining CD4 counts. Hodgkin lymphoma is an exception, which presumably explains the increasing rate of Hodgkin disease during the HAART era (Blood 2006;108:3788; JNCI 2011;103:753). A review of 187 HIV-associated cases of Hodgkin lymphoma found strong correlations with low CD4 count (50–100 cells/mm^3) and onset within 1–3 mos after starting ART, suggesting a form of immune reconstitution (Blood 2011;178:44; AIDS 2011;25:1395).

Non-Hodgkin Lymphoma (NHL)

CAUSE: Immunosuppression (CD4 count <100 cells/mm^3) and EBV (50–80%).

EPIDEMIOLOGY: NHL is 200–600 times more common among PLWH compared with the general population (Int J Cancer 1997;73:645; JAIDS 2004;36:978). The rate is about 3% for patients with AIDS (JAIDS 2002;29:418). Most (70–90%) are high-grade DLBCL or Burkitt-like lymphomas (Am J Med 2001; Brit J Haematol 2001;112:863). NHL incidence has decreased substantially during the HAART era (CID 2009;48:633). A recent review of 61 cases of NHL in AIDS patients in France showed the median age at diagnosis of NHL was 40 yrs. The median CD4 count was 237, and the major independent risks were time with CD4 of <350 mL and VL >500 c/

mL (CID 2009;49:1109). HIV viremia has also been associated with increased incidence of NHL (JID 2009;200:79; CID 2014;58:1599).

PRESENTATION: Compared with NHL in the general population, PLWH have higher rates of stage IV disease with "B" symptoms and frequent extranodal involvement. Common sites of infection and forms of clinical presentation are fever of unknown origin, hepatic dysfunction, marrow involvement, lung disease (effusions, multinodular infiltrates, consolidation, mass lesions, or local or diffuse interstitial infiltrates, hilar adenopathy), GI involvement (any level), and CNS involvement (aseptic meningitis, cranial nerve palsies, CNS mass lesions).

DIAGNOSIS: Lymph nodes that are >2 cm or progressively enlarging should be biopsied. Imaging of nodes is recommended for unexplained constitutional symptoms such as fever, weight loss, or night sweats ≥2 wks. Biopsy new, enlarged (>2 cm) or enlarging nodes. The diagnostic yield of fine-needle aspiration (FNA) in patients with HIV infection and adenopathy is reported at 65–75% (Internat J STD AIDS 2008;19:553; ACTA Cytol 2001;45:589; Acta Cytol 2000;44;960); an excisional biopsy is frequently required. The differential diagnosis includes infection and other metastatic malignancies.

EVALUATION: (1) Blood tests: CBC, liver function tests, creatinine, calcium, phosphorus, LDH; (2) marrow aspiration and biopsy; (3) contrast-enhanced brain MRI; (4) LP for cells, protein, and EBV RNA test. Positron emission tomography (PET)/CT scans are commonly used to help diagnose lymphomas, localize the tumor, and evaluate response to chemotherapy (Cancer 2005;104:1066), but there is still a need to confirm the diagnosis with biopsy and considerable clinical skill is required to interpret disseminated disease as well as response to treatment (Transfus Apher Sci 2011;44:167).

TREATMENT:

- *ART*: Patients receiving ART should continue it during chemotherapy. AZT, COBI, and RTV-boosted protease inhibitors should generally be avoided during chemotherapy.

Integrase inhibitors (RAL, DTG), MVC, RPV, TAF/FTC, ABC/3TC have been widely used in this setting due to the lack of drug–drug interactions with chemotherapy (Clin Microbiol Infect. 2014;20:O672).

- *OI prophylaxis*: Should be based on CD4 count. If >400/ml, use prophylaxis dictated by immunosuppression of the chemotherapy regimen.
- *Chemotherapy*: Full dose if possible:
  - EPOCH + rituximab (etoposide, prednisone, vincristine, cyclophosphamide, doxorubicin (Cancer 2012;118:3977; Blood 2010;115:3008).
  - CHOP + Rituximab (cyclophosphamide, doxorubicin vincristine and prednisone) (J Clin Oncol 2006;24:4123).
  - CDE (cyclophosphamide, doxorubicin and etoposide) + Rituximab (Blood 2005;105:1891).
  - *G-CSF* for all patients.
  - *Rituximab* may improve tumor response, but may increase risk of infectious death with CD4 <50/mL (Blood 2005;105:1891; Br J Haematol 2008;140:411; Cancer 2008;113;117).
  - If CD4 <50, maximize supportive care.
- *CNS prophylaxis*: Predicted by CSF EBV DNA (J Clin Oncol 2000;18:3325).
- *Peripheral stem cell transplant* in PLWH with lymphomas is feasible in the HAART era; about 100 cases have been reported with complete remission in 48–90% (Cell Transplant 2011;20:351).

RESPONSE: Initial response to chemotherapy rates are 50–60%, but relapse rates are high and the long-term prognosis is poor, with median survival <1 yr (AIDS 2013;27:1109; Leuk Lymphoma 2015;19:1). The usual cause of death is progressive lymphoma (AIDS 2013;27:1109). The prognosis is significantly better with ART; one report showed an 84% 1-yr survival with ART + chemotherapy (AIDS 2001;15:1483), and viremia during the 6 mos after diagnosis has been shown to predict mortality (AIDS 2013;27:2365). The prognosis with lymphoma plus HIV infection in the HAART era is significantly worse than for lymphoma alone. A review of 259 HIV-infected and 8,230 HIV-uninfected incident NHL patients showed a 2-yr mortality rate of 59% for the HIV-infected group compared to 30% in the HIV-uninfected group. Poor prognostic correlates were CD4 count of <200/mL, prior AIDS-defining diagnosis, or Burkitt subtype (AIDS 2010;24:1765). Nevertheless, one report found that patients who achieve complete remission with chemotherapy had a 3-yr survival (74%) comparable to that of HIV-negative patients with NHL (CID 2004;38:142). Another report found that ART is associated with reduced chemotherapy-related toxicity as well as improved survival (J Clin Oncol 2004;22:1491).

Burkitt Lymphoma

Standard therapy used in patients without HIV.

Plasmablastic Lymphoma

Reviewed in Lancet ID 2008;8:261. Use standard regimens (no successful regimens known).

Hodgkin Lymphoma

Classical Hodgkin lymphoma is associated with immunosuppression and includes three categories: HIV-associated, iatrogenic (chronic corticosteroids, etc.), and post-transplant. All forms are treated with ABVD: adriamycin, bleomycin, vinblastine, and dacarbazine (Am J Hematol 2011;86:170). Use of ART has enabled more aggressive treatment. Prognosis is significantly improved now, and survival approaches that seen in the general population (CID 2015;61:1469).

Primary Effusion Lymphoma (PEL)

CAUSE: HHV-8 and EBV (NEJM 1995;332:1186; Clin Microbiol Rev 2002;15:439; CID 2008;47:1209).

EPIDEMIOLOGY: Rare: tumor registries crossed with AIDS registries show a frequency of 0.004%, or 0.14% of NHL in patients with AIDS (JAIDS 2002;29:418).

PRESENTATION: Serous effusions (pleural, peritoneal, pericardial, joint spaces) with no masses (Hum Pathol 1997;28:801). Development of solid tissue lymphomas is rare (Acta Hematol 2010;123:237).

DIAGNOSIS: Effusions are serous, contain high-grade malignant lymphocytes and HHV-8.

TREATMENT:

- *ART* plus same regimen for non-Hodgkin lymphoma.

RESPONSE: This tumor usually does not extend beyond serosal surfaces, but prognosis is poor, with median survival of 2–6 mos (JAIDS 1996;13:215; J Clin Oncol 2003;21:3948; AIDS 2008;22:1685; AM J Hematol 2008;83:804). Most patients show temporary response to therapy with decrease in effusion size. The CD4 count is the most important predictor of progression (CID 2005;40:1022). A case report showed complete regression of PEL with ART (AIDS 2008;22:1236).

NEUROLOGIC COMPLICATIONS: CNS complications were frequent in the pre-HAART era, although the incidence of many of the following conditions is now substantially decreased, particularly the OIs. HIV-associated neurocognitive disorders (HAND) remain an important source of morbidity in PLWH. The most important factor when considering the differential diagnosis is the CD4 count.

TABLE 8.21 Features of selected CNS conditions in PLWH

Agent/Condition Frequency (All AIDS) Patients	Clinical Features	CT Scan/MRI	Cerebrospinal Fluid (CSF[a])	Other Diagnostic Tests
Toxoplasmosis (2–4%)	Fever, reduced alertness, headache, focal neurological deficits (80%), seizures (30%) Evolution: < 2 wks CD4 <100/mL	Location: Basal ganglia, gray-white junction Sites: Usually multiple Enhancement: prominent; Usually ring lesions (1–2 cm) Edema/mass effect: Usually not as great as lymphoma	Normal: 20–30% Protein: 10–50 mg/dL WBC: 0–40 (monos) Experimental: Toxo Ag (ELISA) or PCR	Toxoplasma serology (IgG) false-negative in <5% Response to empiric therapy: >85%; most respond by day 7 (NEJM 1993;329:995) MRI: Repeat at 2 wks Definitive diagnosis: Brain biopsy
Primary CNS lymphoma (2%)	Afebrile, headache, focal neurological findings; mental status change (60%), personality or behavioral; seizures (15%) Evolution: 2–8 wks CD4 <100/mL	Location: Periventricular, anywhere, 2–6 cm Sites: One or many Enhancement: Prominent; usually solid, irregular Edema/mass effect: Prominent	Normal: 30–50% Protein: 10–150 mg/dL WBC: 0–100 (monos) EBV PCR + in 50–80%	Suspect with negative toxoplasma IgG, single lesion, or failure to respond to empiric toxoplasmosis treatment (MRI and clinical evaluation at 2 wks) Thallium 201 SPECT scan (90% sensitive and specific)

Condition	Clinical features	Imaging	CSF/Laboratory	Diagnosis
Cryptococcal meningitis (8–10%)	Fever, headache, alert (75%); less common are visual changes, stiff neck, cranial nerve deficits, seizures (10%); no focal neurologic deficits. Evolution: <2 wks. CD4 <100/mL	Usually normal or shows increased intracranial pressure. Enhancement: Negative or meningeal enhancement. Edema mass effect: Ventricular enlargement/obstructive hydrocephalus	Protein: 30–150 mg/dL. WBC: 0–100 (monos). Culture +: 95–100%. India ink +: 60–80%. Cryptococcal Ag: >95% sensitive and specific	Cryptococcal Ag in serum – sensitivity 95%. Definitive diagnosis: CSF Crypto Ag sensitivity and specificity >99% and/or positive culture
CMV encephalitis (>0.5%)	Fever ±, delirium, lethargy, disorientation; headache; stiff neck, photophobia, cranial nerve deficits; no focal neurologic deficits. Evolution: <2 wks. CD4 <100/mL	Location: Periventricular, brainstem. Site: Confluent. Enhancement: Variable, prominent to none	CSF may be normal. Protein: 100–1,000 mg/dL. WBC: 10–1,000 (polys)/mL. Glucose usually decreased. CMV PCR + >80%. CSF cultures usually negative for CMV	Definitive diagnosis: Brain biopsy with histopathology and/or positive culture. Hyponatremia (reflects CMV adrenalitis). Retinal exam for CMV retinitis

(continued)

TABLE 8.21 Continued

Agent/condition frequency (all AIDS) patients)	Clinical features	CT scan/MRI	Cerebrospinal fluid (CSF[a])	Other diagnostic tests
HIV dementia (7%)	Afebrile; triad of cognitive, motor, and behavioral dysfunction Early: Decreased memory, concentration, attention, coordination; ataxia Late: Global dementia, paraplegia, mutism Evolution: Weeks to mos CD4 <200 cells/mm^3	Location: Diffuse, deep white matter hyperintensities Site: Diffuse, ill-defined Enhancement: Negative Atrophy: Prominent No mass effect	Normal: 30–50% Protein: Increased in 60% WBC: Increased in 5–10% (monos) β-2 micro- globulin elevated (>3 mg/L)	Neuropsychological tests show subcortical dementia HIV dementia scale for screening

| Neurosyphilis (0.5%) | Asymptomatic
Meningeal: Headache, fever, photophobia, meningismus
± seizures, focal findings, cranial nerve palsies
Tabes dorsalis: Sharp pains, paresthesias, decreased DTRs, loss of pupil response
General paresis: Memory loss, dementia, personality changes, loss of pupil response
Meningo-vascular: Strokes, myelitis
Ocular: Iritis, uveitis, optic neuritis
Any CD4 cell count | Aseptic meningitis: May show meningeal enhancement
General paresis: Cortical atrophy, sometimes with infarcts
Meningo-vascular syphilis: Strokes | Protein: 45-200 mg/dL
WBC: 5–100 (monos)
VDRL +: Sensitivity 65%, specificity 100%
Experimental: PCR for *T. pallidum* | Serum VDRL and FTA-ABS are clue in >90%; false-negative serum VDRL in 5–10% with tabes dorsalis or general paresis
Definitive diagnosis: Positive CSF VDRL (found in 60–70%)
Note: Most common forms in PLWH are ocular, meningeal, and meningo-vascular |

(continued)

TABLE 8.21 Continued

Agent/condition frequency (all AIDS) patients)	Clinical features	CT scan/MRI	Cerebrospinal fluid (CSF[a])	Other diagnostic tests
PML (1–2%)	No fever; no headache; impaired speech, vision, motor function, cranial nerves Evolution: Weeks to mos CD4 <100/mL; some >200/mL	Location: White matter, subcortical, multifocal Sites: Variable Enhancement: Negative No mass effect	Normal CSF PCR + for JC virus: Sensitivity 95% (Neurology 2013;80:1430)	Brain biopsy: Positive DFA stain for JC virus

Tuberculosis (0.5–1.0%)	Fever, reduced alertness, headache, meningismus, focal deficits (20%) CD4 <350/mL	Intracerebral lesions in 50–70% (NEJM 1992;326:668; Am J Med 1992;93:524)	Normal: 5–10% Protein: normal (40%) 100–500mg/dL WBC: 5–2000 (average is 60–70% monos) Glucose: CSF/serum <50% AFB smear +: 20% CSF PCR: Sensitivity 57% (Clin Microbiol Infect 2014;20:O600)	Chest x-ray: active TB in 50%; PPD positive: 20–30% Definitive diagnosis: positive CSF culture

[a]Normal values: Protein: 15–45 mg/dL; traumatic tap: 1 mg/1,000 RBCs; glucose: 40–80 mg/dL or CSF/blood glucose ratio >0.6; leukocyte counts: <5 mononuclear cells/mL, 5–10 is suspect; bloody tap: 1 WBC/700 RBC; opening pressure: 80–200 mm H_2O.
*CSF analysis in asymptomatic PLWH shows 40–50% have elevated protein and/or pleocytosis (>5 mononuclear cells/mL); the frequency of pleocytosis decreases with progressive disease.

Cytomegalovirus Encephalitis

CAUSE: CMV with CD4 <50/mL.

FREQUENCY: <0.5% of patients with AIDS.

PRESENTATION: Rapidly progressive delirium, cranial nerve deficits, nystagmus, ataxia, headache with fever ± CMV retinitis.

DIAGNOSIS: MRI shows periventricular confluent lesions with enhancement. CMV PCR in CSF is >80% sensitive and 90% specific, and cultures of CSF for CMV are usually negative.

TREATMENT:

> *Ganciclovir* 5 mg/kg IV q12h; foscarnet 90 mg/kg IV q12h *plus* ART.

RESPONSE: Pre-HAART trial of foscarnet plus ganciclovir showed a median survival of 94 days, compared with 42 days in historic controls (AIDS 2000;14:517).

HIV-Associated Neurocognitive Disorders (HAND)

HISTORICAL CONTEXT: The impact of HIV infection on cognitive function (which was profound) was recognized early in the epidemic and led to the term "AIDS dementia complex" (ADC). Two categories were proposed: (1) HIV-associated dementia and (2) a milder form with minor cognitive or motor impairment (Neurology 1991;41:778). More recently there was an alternative classification with three categories: (1) asymptomatic neurocognitive impairment (ANI), (2) HIV-associated mild neurocognitive disorder (MND), and HIV-associated dementia (HAD) (Neurology 2007;69:1789). Specific criteria for the 2007 definition (the Frascati Criteria) (Neurology 2007;69:1789) are:

- *HIV-associated ANI*:
  1. Acquired impairment in cognitive function that is >1 SD below a demographically corrected mean using neuropsychological testing that assesses seven cognitive areas.
  2. Cognitive loss does not impair daily function
  3. No evidence of delirium, dementia, or preexisting cause.
- *HIV-associated MND*:
  1. Acquired impairment of cognition.
  2. Cognitive impairment causes at least mild interference of mental acuity and inefficiency in work, homemaking, or social observation.
  3. No evidence of delirium or dementia.
- *HAD*:
  1. Acquired cognitive impairment of at least 2.0 SD below demographically corrected mean.
  2. Cognitive impairment causes substantial interference with work, homemaking, or social functioning.

The CHARTER study of 1,316 PLWH from six US HIV programs (Neurology 2010;75:2087) showed 53% were considered normal, 38% had ANI, 12% had MND, and 2.4% had HAD. This indicates a substantial decrease in the 10–15% prevalence of HAD in the pre-HAART era (Neurology 1992;42:472). A major risk factor for HAD was a nadir CD4 <200/mL. This analysis found no significant or favorable relationship between the use of drugs that have high CNS penetration scores, although others have found a correlation (Neurology 2011;76:693; Ann Neurol 2004;56:416).

CAUSE: Chronic encephalitis with progressive or static encephalopathy due to CNS HIV infection with prominent immune activation. Some work suggests that there is an up-regulation of endogenous antioxidant defenses in the brain. The failure of this neuroprotective mechanism causes accumulation of sphingomyelin and impairs cognitive function. Comorbidities that play a role are aging, HCV, and drug abuse (Int Rev Psychiatry 2008;20:25; Neurology2008;70:1753).

INCIDENCE: Prior reports suggested the incidence of HAD was 7% after AIDS in pre-HAART era, and 2–3% in the early HAART era (Neurology 2001;56:257). More recent work with sensitive neurocognitive testing and imaging indicates that about half of PLWH have neurocognitive defects (J Neurovirol 2009;15:187).

PRESENTATION: Prior studies showed high rates of subcortical dementia in late-stage HIV with CD4 of <200/mL. Early symptoms are apathy, memory loss, cognitive slowing, depression, and withdrawal. Motor defects include gait instability and reduced hand coordination. Late stages show global loss of cognition, severe psychomotor retardation, and mutism. There may be seizures, which are usually easily controlled. The rate of progression is highly variable, but the average from first symptoms to death in the pre-HAART era was 6 mos (Medicine 1987;66:407). Physical examination in early disease shows defective rapid eye and limb movement and generalized hyperreflexia. In late stages, there is tremor, clonus, and frontal release signs. The more recent studies just noted (J Neurovirol 2009;15:187) showed high rates of cognitive impairment even in early-stage HIV infection that correlated with central white matter damage demonstrated with diffusion tensor imaging. Changes were seen at all stages of HIV but were more widespread in patients with AIDS. Cognitive changes correlated with white matter injury in the internal capsule, corpus callosum, and superior longitudinal fasciculus.

DIAGNOSIS: History, physical examination, and screening with HIV Dementia Scale. Formal testing includes Trail Making B, Digital Symbol, Grooved Pegboard, and the HIV Dementia Scale. MRI shows cerebral atrophy (which can be present without symptoms), typically with rarefaction of white matter (J Neurol Neurosurg Psych 1997;62:346). CSF shows increased protein with 0–15 mononuclear cells; pleocytosis is absent in 65%. Main goal is to exclude alternative diagnosis because no test is specific for HAD.

TREATMENT: The HIV Dementia Scale can be used to follow response to ARV treatment. ART has reduced the frequency

TABLE 8.22 HIV Dementia Scale

Maximum Score	Test*
See below	Memory registration: Four words given (hat, dog, green, peach) and have the patient repeat them.
6	Psychomotor speed: Record the time, in seconds, that it takes the patient to write the alphabet. Score: <21 sec = 6; 21.1–24 sec = 5; 24.1–27 sec = 4; 27.1–30 sec = 3; 30.1–33 sec = 2; 33.1-36 sec = 1; >36 = 0
4	Memory recall: Ask for the four words from above. For words not remembered give semantic clue, e.g., "animal" (dog), "color" (green), etc. 1 point for each correct answer.
2	Construction: Copy a cube and record time. Score: <25 sec = 2; 25–35 sec = 1; >35 = 0

From AIDS Reader 2002;12:29.

≤7/12 is threshold for dementia but is nonspecific requiring additional neurologic evaluation.

TABLE 8.23 AIDS dementia complex staging

Stage	Description
Stage 0	Normal
Stage 0.5	Subclinical: Minimal—equivocal symptoms; no work impairment.
Stage 1.0	Mild: Minimal intellectual or motor impairment; able to do all, but more demanding work or ADL.
Stage 2.0	Moderate: Cannot work or perform demanding ADL; capable of self care.
Stage 3.0	Severe: Major intellectual disability; unable to walk unassisted.
Stage 4.0	End stage: near vegetative stage; paraplegia or quadriplegia.

of HAD, but there are limited data to show efficacy of ART for reversing established HAD (J Neurovirol 2002;8:136; J Neurol 2004;10:350). Some studies suggest that CNS penetration of antiretrovirals is an important correlate with neurologic improvement (Arch Neurol 2004;61:1699; J Neurovirol 2016;22:349), but others do not (AIDS 23;23:1359; J Neurovirol 2009;15:187). CNS penetration was studied in CHARTER, an analysis of 374 patients receiving ART who had simultaneous serum and CSF level measurements. Antiretroviral agents with the best CNS penetration based on CSF levels are AZT, ABC, NVP, LPV/r, and IDV/r (see Table 8.24) (HIV Med 2008;16:15; AIDS 2009;23:83; AIDS 2009;23:83). Some patients who have progressive dementia despite good virologic control by conventional monitoring have resistant virus in the CNS, suggesting that genotypic resistance tests of HIV isolated in CSF could facilitate regimen selection (J Virol 2004; 78:10133). However, there are no specific treatments for HIV dementia (Int Rev Psychiatry 2008;20:25), and a recent

TABLE 8.24 CNS penetration effectiveness rankings scoring system

Class	Ranking			
	1	*2*	*3*	*4*
NRTI	TDF	ddI 3TC d4T	FTC ABC	AZT
NNRTI		ETR	EFV RPV	
PI	NFV RTV SQV/r TPV/r	ATV ATV/r FPV	DRV/r FPV/r LPV/r	IDV/r
Integrase inhibitor		EVG/c	RAL	DTG

RCT compared use of CNS Penetration Effectiveness (CPE)-based CNS-targeted regimens to non–CNS-targeted regimens to compare effectiveness in treating HAD found no difference, although extensive limitations of the study were noted (CID 2014:58:1015).

RESPONSE: ART is associated with significant increases in survival (AIDS 2003;17:1539) and reduced incidence of HAD, but its role in treatment of HAD specifically is less clear (Brain Path 2003;13:104). Severe progressive dementia similar to the course seen in the pre-HAART era is infrequently seen. The issue of response of HAD to ART is obviously a key issue. This was addressed by the HIV Imaging Consortium, which did proton magnetic resonance spectroscopy in 124 patients with HIV dementia (AIDS 2011;25:625). Results showed that brain injury persists. There is also evidence that clinically stable patients may have progressive cognitive impairment (JAIDS 2005;38:3; AIDS 2010;24:983).

CNS PENETRATION EFFECTIVENESS RANKS 2011 SCORING SYSTEM: The CPE score is a method to estimate CNS penetration of antiretroviral drugs (Arch Neurol 2008;65:65) provided by the CNS HIV Anti-Retroviral Therapy Effects Research (CHARTER) study, a multicenter, prospective observational study cohort based in six North American locations. Penetration of ART drugs is estimated based on CSF pharmacology, chemical characteristics, and effectiveness in CNS infections. Validation was done by assessing antiviral effect with simultaneous measurement of CSF and plasma HIV viral load in 833 patients receiving these drugs (Arch Neurol 2008;65:65). The ranking is 1–4, with 4 indicating the best penetration and 1 indicating the least (Table 7.18). The metric used to analyze changes with standardized tests with periodic testing is the NPZ3 score: Neurocognitive Z (standardized T score) converted to Z by averaging three measurements. Several studies have demonstrated the relevance of the CPE score, including a multicenter analysis of 2,636 patients (median CD4 244 cells/

mm^3) who underwent standardized neurologic testing. Patients taking ART regimens with better CPE scores performed better with sequential neurocognitive testing (AIDS 2011;25:357). There are two points of concern in these analyses. First, analysis of 22,356 patients who initiated ART between 1996 and 2008 in the UK collaborative HIV Cohort (CHIC) Study found that the median CPE score (Table 7.18) increased from 7 in 1996–97 to 9 in 2000–01, but then declined to 6 in 2006–08 (Neurology 2011;76:693). Of note, this analysis also found a correlation between the CPE score and CNS complications. The second concern is the previously cited ACTG (ALLRT) cohort, which demonstrated the positive correlation between the CPE score and neurocognitive function (AIDS 2011;25:357), also found that more than three antiretrovirals may be required to treat HIV in the CNS. Several recent analyses evaluating pharmacokinetics and pharmacodynamics of ART and CNS penetration highlight the limitations of the CPE scoring system (Clin Pharmacokinet 2014;53:891; Clin Pharmacokinet 2015;54:581). This remains an active and controversial area of research.

Primary CNS Lymphoma (PCNSL)

CAUSE: Virtually all are EBV-associated (Lancet 1991;337:805).

FREQUENCY: The prevalence in the period 1985–90 was >1,000 times higher than in the general population (Lancet 1991;338:969). Incidence has declined in the HAART era, but not as much as with other HIV complications (JAIDS 2000;25:451). HIV infection now accounts for 27% of CNS lymphomas; rates have decreased about 10-fold during the HAART era, from 297/100,000 to 26/100,000 (JAMA 2011;305:1450).

PRESENTATION: A review of 248 cases of immunocompetent patients showed 43% had neuropsychiatric signs, 33% had increased intracranial pressure, 14% had seizures, and 4% had ocular symptoms (Arch Neurol 2010;67:291). "B" symptoms (fever, weight loss, night sweats) are rare. CD4 is usually <50/mL.

DIAGNOSIS: MRI with contrast usually shows a single enhancing lesion, but there may be multiple lesions, and MRI may show ring enhancement (Am J Neuroradiol 1997;18:563). These lesions usually involve the corpus callosum, periventricular area, or periependymal area; they are often >4 cm in diameter and usually show a mass effect (Neurology 1997;48:687; J Neurooncol 2005;72:169). The diagnosis is established with brain biopsy, positive CSF cytology, and possibly by EBV DNA in CSF (see later discussion). Major differential diagnosis is toxoplasmosis.

Factors favoring CNS lymphoma are (1) typical neuroimaging results (above), (2) negative anti-*Toxoplasma* IgG serology, (3) failure to respond to empiric treatment of toxoplasmosis within 1–2 wks, (4) lack of fever, and (5) thallium single proton emission CT (SPECT) scan with early thallium uptake. CSF EBV PCR is >94% specific and 50–80% sensitive (Lancet 1992;342:398; JNCI 1998;90:364; CID 2002;34:103). Others report much lower specificity of CSF EBV DNA and suggest quantitation with a 10,000 c/mL threshold (J Clin Virol 2008;42:433). Stereotactic brain biopsy is definitive and usually reserved for patients who fail to respond to toxoplasmosis treatment (AIDS 1995;9:1243; CID 2002;34:103). A review of nearly 500 AIDS patients undergoing stereotactic brain biopsy showed a 4% morbidity rate (CID 2002;34:103).

THERAPY:

- *Standard*: Radiation plus corticosteroids (J Neuro Sci 1999;163:32), or methotrexate (J Clin Oncol 2003;21:1044). A comparison of 41 patients with HIV-associated CNS lymphomas and 45 without HIV showed the latter group had a much better treatment response and survival (J Neurooncol 2011;101:257).
- *Chemotherapy*: May be combined with radiation plus corticosteroids. Usually reserved for patients with elevated CD4 counts. The benefit of methotrexate plus rituximab continues to be supported (Neurology 2014;83:235). A recent trial of methotrexate, temozolomide, and rituximab also shows promise (J Clin Oncol 2013;31;3061).

RESPONSE: Response rates to radiation therapy plus corticosteroids is 20–50%, but these results are temporary, and the average survival following symptom onset was only about 4 mos in the pre-HAART era (Crit Rev Oncol 1998;9:199; Semin Oncol 1998;25:492). Survival has improved marginally in the HAART era, but is still poor (AIDS 2011;25:691; AIDS 2014;28:397).

Toxoplasmosis

PERIPHERAL NERVOUS SYSTEM

HIV-Associated Neuromuscular Weakness Syndrome (HANWS)

CAUSE: Postulated to be caused by mitochondrial toxicity attributed to deoxy NRTIs, primarily d4T (NEJM 2002;346:811; CID 2003;15:131; AIDS 2004;18:1403).

CLINICAL FEATURES: A review of 19 probable cases showed a median lactic acid level of 4.9 mmol/L; 88% had taken d4T for a median duration of 10.5 mos (AIDS 2004;18:1403). The only treatment is withdrawal of d4T. Pathology studies and electromyography (EMG) showed involvement of peripheral nerves, muscles, or both. Clinical features include ascending paresis, areflexia, and cranial neuropathies. CPK levels are often elevated. Diagnosis is based on the finding of new onset limb weakness ± sensory involvement that is acute (1–2 wks), or subacute (>2 wks) involving legs or arms/legs and the absence of alternative confounding illnesses such as Guillain-Barré syndrome, myasthenia gravis, myelopathy, hypokalemia, stroke. This complication has nearly disappeared with phase-out of d4T, although it is still seen in some resource-limited countries where d4T is used (J Med Assoc Thai 2011;94:501).

Cytomegalovirus Radiculitis/Inflammatory Demyelinating Polyneuropathy

CAUSE: Unclear; immunopathogenic mechanism with inflammation and breakdown of peripheral nerve myelin is suspected.

FREQUENCY: Uncommon.

DIAGNOSIS: There are two forms:

- *Acute demyelinating neuropathy* (AIDP, Guillain-Barré syndrome) occurs early in the course of HIV.
- *Chronic inflammatory demyelinating polyneuropathy* (CIDP) is a more chronic relapsing motor weakness that usually occurs in late-stage HIV.

Both present with a progressive ascending paralysis with mild sensory involvement. CSF shows increased protein and mononuclear pleocytosis or normal white blood cell (WBC) count; EMG and nerve conduction studies are critical for diagnosis. Nerve biopsy may be needed; should show mononuclear, macrophage infiltrate, and internodal demyelination (Ann Neurol 1987;21:3240; JAMA Neurol 2015;72:1510).

TREATMENT:

- *AIDP*: Plasmapheresis: 5 exchanges with maintenance as needed; or, as alternative, IVIG 0.4 g/kg/d × 5 days (monitor renal function).
- *CIDP*: Oral prednisone (1 mg/kg/d) or intermittent plasmapheresis or IVIG: Each continued until there is a therapeutic response.

RESPONSE: Treatment usually halts progression; CIDP may require prolonged courses (Ann Neurol 1987;21:3240).

Peripheral Neuropathy and Sensory Peripheral Neuropathy

Peripheral neuropathy is defined as loss of vibratory sensation of both great toes or absent/hypoactive ankle reflexes bilaterally. This form is asymptomatic and detected by neurologic exam. Sensory peripheral neuropathy (SPN) includes two forms: HIV-associated distal sensory polyneuropathy (HIV-DSP) and ART toxic neuropathy (ATN). These sensory neuropathies resemble the neuropathies that occur with diabetes and alcoholism. Diagnosis is based on a history of numbness, paresthesias, or burning pain in the feet; exam shows reduced or absent ankle jerks.

A review of 2,141 patients in ACTG trials from 2000 to 2007 showed the frequency of peripheral neuropathy was 32%, and for SPN it was 9% (AIDS 2011;25:919). Drugs implicated in ATN are ddI and the thymidine analogues, primarily d4T >AZT. These are rarely used now except in resource-limited countries (Neurology 1988;38:794; Neurology 2006;66:1679). The major findings of the ACTG review were:

- The prevalence of asymptomatic PN was 23% and 4% for symptomatic PN.
- The findings persist regardless of HIV treatment and treatment response in terms of viral suppression and immune recovery.
- The frequency of symptomatic PN increased with increasing age, baseline CD4 <200/mL, high baseline VL, history of diabetes, and use of a statin (Neurology 2002;58:1333).
- Patients who stopped receiving neurotoxic ART drugs showed 54% had persistent symptoms, while 18% cleared the symptoms.

TABLE 8.25 Differential diagnosis of lower extremity symptoms in PLWH

Syndrome	Symptoms	Clinical Features	Ancillary Studies/Treatment
Distal sensory neuropathy (DSN)	Pain and numbness in toes and feet; ankles, calves, and fingers involved in more advanced cases CD4 count <200/mL, but can occur at higher CD4 levels	Reduced pinprick/ vibratory sensation Reduced or absent ankle jerks Contact allodynia (hypersensitivity) present in most cases	Skin biopsy shows epidermal denervation Electromyography/nerve conduction velocities (EMG/NCV) show a predominantly axonal neuropathy Quantitative sensory testing, or thermal thresholds may be helpful
Antiretroviral toxic neuropathy (ATN)	Same as DSN (above), but symptoms occur after initiation of ddI, d4T Any CD4 cell count More common in older patients and patients with diabetes	Same as DSN (above)	EMG/NCV show a predominantly axonal neuropathy Discontinuation of presumed neuro-toxic medication, if severe Symptoms may worsen for a few weeks (coasting) before improving *(continued)*

TABLE 8.25 Continued

Syndrome	Symptoms	Clinical Features	Ancillary Studies/Treatment
Tarsal tunnel syndrome	Pain and numbness predominantly in anterior portion of soles of feet	Reduced sensation over soles of feet Positive Tinel's sign at tarsal tunnel	Infiltration of local anesthetic in tarsal tunnel may provide symptomatic relief
HIV-associated neuromuscular weakness syndrome	Ascending paresis with areflexia ± cranial nerve, or sensory involvement Usually associated with prolonged d4T use	Lactate and CPK levels usually ↑ EMG/NCV – axonal neuropathy and myopathy	Discontinue NRTIs, especially d4T Prognosis for survival is poor
HIV-associated myopathy/AZT myopathy	Pain and aching in muscles, usually in thighs and shoulders Weakness with difficulty when rising from a chair, or reaching above shoulders Any CD4 cell count	Mild/moderate muscle tenderness Weakness, predominantly in proximal muscles (i.e., deltoids, hip flexors) Normal sensory exam/ normal reflexes	CPK ↑ EMG shows irritable myopathy Discontinue AZT and follow CPK every 2 wks. Symptoms/signs/CPK should improve within 1 mo

| Polyradiculitis | Rapidly evolving weakness and numbness in legs (both proximally and distally), with bowel/bladder incontinence
May occur at high or low CD4 cell count | Diffuse weakness in legs
Diffuse sensory abnormalities in legs and buttocks
Reduced/absent reflexes at knees and ankles | EMG/NCV show multilevel nerve root involvement
Spinal fluid helpful in determining CMV or HSV as cause
Treat CMV polyradiculopathy with ganciclovir or foscarnet |
| Vacuolar myelopathy | Stiffness and weakness in legs with leg numbness
Bowel/bladder incontinence in advanced cases
CD4 count <200 cells/mm^3 | Weakness and spasticity, mainly in hip, knee, and ankle flexors
Brisk knee jerks, upgoing toes
If sensory neuropathy coexists, then distal sensory loss and reduced/absent jerks | Spinal fluid may show elevated protein 0–10 cells/mm^3
Exclude B-12 deficiency and HTLV-1 co-infection
Thoracic spinal imaging normal
No established therapy, but physical therapy or methionine (3 g bid) and ART may be helpful (Neurology 1998;51:266) |

(continued)

TABLE 8.25 Continued

Syndrome	Symptoms	Clinical Features	Ancillary Studies/Treatment
Inflammatory demyelinating polyneuropathies	Predominantly weakness in arms and legs, with minor sensory symptoms CD4 count: may occur at any level	Diffuse weakness including facial musculature, asymmetric in early cases, with diffuse absent reflexes Minor sensory signs	EMG/NCV show a demyelinating polyneuropathy Spinal fluid shows a very high protein with mild to moderate lymphocytic pleocytosis, but all cultures are negative Treatment: Plasmapheresis, IVIG, and/or ART
Mononeuritis, or mononeuritis multiplex	Mix of motor and sensory defects Asymmetric Evolves over weeks CD4 count variable	EMG and NCV–asymmetric and multifocal defects R/O CMV (CSF or sural nerve biopsy), and HCV	CD4 count >200 cells/mm^3—possible steroids CD4 counts <50 cells/mm^3 and severe—treat for CMV

Distal Sensory Peripheral Neuropathy and Antiretroviral Toxic Neuropathy

See AIDS 2002;16:2105.

CAUSE: HIV infection per se, usually with CD4 <200/mL and/or dideoxy NRTIs: ddI and d4T (AIDS 2000;14:273). Distal sensory peripheral neuropathy (DSPN) and antiretroviral toxic neuropathy (ATN) are indistinguishable by clinical features or biopsy.

TREATMENT: Contributing drugs and conditions to address: ddI, d4T, metronidazole (long term), vitamin B_6 overdose, INH (but incidence only 0.07%) (AIDS 2010;24 Suppl 5:S29), elevated triglycerides (AIDS 2009;23:2317; AIDS 2011;25:F1), vincristine, thalidomide, B_{12} deficiency, alcoholism, diabetes, and uremia. HCV does not appear to play a role (Neurology 2009;73:309).

- *Pharmacologic treatment*:
  - *Gabapentin* (Neurontin) 300–1200 mg po tid. One placebo-controlled trial showed modest benefit (J Neurol 2004;251:1260).
  - *Lamotrigine* 25 mg bid increasing to 300 mg/d over 6 wks; one of the few treatments with confirmed benefit in clinical trials (Neurology 2000;54:2115), but results are inconsistent, and there is a high incidence of rash (Cochrane Database Syst Rev 2011;2:CD006044).
  - *Tricyclic antidepressants*: Nortriptyline 10 mg hs increased by 10 mg q5d to maximum 75 mg hs or 10–20 mg po tid; other tricyclics (amitriptyline, desipramine, or imipramine) are considered comparable (JAMA 1998;280:1590; Pain 2010;150:575). *Note*: PIs and cobicistat can increase TCA concentrations.
  - *Ibuprofen*: 600–800 mg tid.
  - *Gabapentin* 400 mg bid to ceiling 3,600 mg/d ± nortriptyline 10 mg bid to ceiling target of 100 mg/d (Lancet 2009;374:1252). Participants had diabetic or postherpetic neuralgia. At maximum tolerated doses, both drugs showed

significant reductions in pain scores but optimal results with the combination of both.

- *Capsaicin*: A high-concentration patch (8%) tested with a 30- or 60-minute application repeated every 90 days effectively reduced pain for up to 1 yr (Drugs 2010;70:1831), with most common adverse reaction being irritation at site of application. Pretreatment with topical lidocaine or oral tramadol was explored with no significant difference in tolerability of treatment between the two arms (Eur J Pain 2014;18:1240).
- *Lidocaine* 20–30% ointment (lidocaine gel) was not effective in a controlled trial (JAIDS 2004;37:1584).
- *Phenytoin* 200–400 mg/d. (*Note*: Drug–drug interactions with PIs, cobicistat, NNRTIs, TAF, RPV.)
- *Marijuana*: Smoked/medicinal marijuana has been shown to reduce pain (Neurology 2007; 68:515; J Opioid Manag 2009;5:257).
- *Severe pain*: Methadone, up to 20 mg qid. (*Note*: drug–drug interaction with EFV, NVP, and some PIs.)
- *Fentanyl patch* 25–100 μg/hr q72h or morphine. (*Note*: drug interactions between fentanyl and PIs and cobicistat.)
- *Acupuncture* failed in one reported trial (JAMA 1998;280;1590).
- *Miscellaneous*: Avoid tight footwear, limit walking, wear bridge at foot of the bed, use foot soaks.

RESPONSE: Sensory neuropathy due to NRTIs is usually reversible if the implicated agent is discontinued early (e.g., within 2 wks of the onset of symptoms). If continued, the pain eventually becomes irreversible and may be incapacitating. Response with drug discontinuation is often delayed for several weeks and then shows gradual improvement that may require up to 12 wks after discontinuing nucleosides (JAIDS 1992;5:60; Neurology 1996;46:999). Treatment of sensory neuropathy, beyond discontinuing implicated medications and addressing contributing conditions, is medication directed at pain control. Placebo-controlled trials have shown benefit with gabapentin, nortriptyline, topical capsaicin, cannabis, and lamotrigine.

Ophthalmic Complications

HISTORICAL PERSPECTIVE: CMV was the dominant ocular complication in the pre-HAART era, with a 30% lifetime risk (Arch Ophthalmol 1996;114:821; Arch Ophthalmol 1996;114:23). ART brought a dramatic decrease in this complication that exceeded that seen with all other OIs (Am J Ophthalmol 1997;124:227; AIDS 1998;12:1931). However, some late presenters still develop this complication, and some patients relapse despite high CD4 counts (CID 2001;32:815; Ann Intern Med 2002;137:239).

A retrospective study in Tokyo involving 1,515 HIV-positive patients from 2004 to 2013 evaluated role of routine ophthalmologic screening. Median CD4 count was 210/mL. Vast majority of cases (71% with CMV retinitis, 82% with any ocular disease) were asymptomatic. No patients with CMV retinitis had a CD4 of >200/mL. Authors recommend routine ophthalmologic screening for all PLWH with CD4 <200/mL (PLOS One 2015;10:e0136747). 2013 IDSA guidelines recommend dilated funduscopic exam every 6–12 mos for patients with CD4 <50/μL (CID 2014;58:e27).

With widespread use of ART, the focus should be on screening for ocular complications associated with noninfectious comorbidities, including diabetes mellitus, hyperlipidemia, and non–AIDS-defining malignancies (Clin Epi Research 2014;28:47).

CMV Retinitis

CLINICAL PRESENTATION: Patient presents with late0stage HIV infection (CD4 <50) complaining of variable visual problems depending on which part of the retina is affected; these include scotomas, decreasing visual acuity, peripheral and central visual field loss, floaters, and flashing lights. Of these, floaters and flashing lights are the most powerful predictors of CMV retinitis

TABLE 8.26 Frequency of ocular diseases among 1,515 screened patients

	All Patients, n = 1515	CD4 <50/µL, n = 308	CD4 <100/µL, n = 490	CD4 <200/µL, n = 731	CD4 ≥200/µL, n = 784
Any ocular diseases	204 (14)	81 (26)	130 (27)	162 (22)	42 (5.4)
CMV retinitis	24 (1.6)	14 (4.5)	20 (4.1)	24 (3.3)	0
HIV retinopathy	127 (8.4)	62 (20)	97 (20)	111 (15)	16 (2)
Cataract	31 (2)	2 (0.6)	9 (1.8)	15 (2.1)	16 (2)
Ocular syphilis	4 (0.3)	0	0	3 (0.4)	1 (0.1)

From PLoS One 2015;10:e0136747.

(Ophthalmology 2004;111:1326). Funduscopic exam typically shows perivascular yellow-white retinal infiltrates +/– intraretinal hemorrhage, sometimes referred to as "scrambled eggs and ketchup." Little to no inflammation is noted in the vitreous body. If left untreated, the disease progresses in 2–3 wks to blindness. The diagnosis is usually established on the basis of the combination of typical funduscopic changes in the patient with advanced HIV infection. CMV can be detected by PCR in vitreous and aqueous humor and is highly specific, but usually unnecessary.

OI DIFFERENTIAL DIAGNOSIS: Toxoplasmosis, HSV, VZV, syphilis, TB.

Cryptococcus Chorioretinitis

Cryptococcal lesions are usually located in the choroid and retina and appear as multiple, discrete yellowish spots of varying sizes. Difficult to eradicate. Treatment is with IV amphotericin plus 5-FC as in cryptococcal meningitis. Addition of intravitreal amphotericin B and vitrectomy may be indicated (Retina 1987;7:75)

Herpes Simplex Keratitis

Can cause painful, recurrent corneal ulcerations. Characteristic branching or dendritic pattern seen on slit lamp exam. Treatment is trifluorothymidine, cycloplegic drugs, debridement of the ulcer. Recurrent episodes are reduced with oral acyclovir 400 mg bid × 1 yr (NEJM 1998;339:300).

Immune Recovery Uveitis (Vitreitis)

First described in 1998 (Am J Ophthal 1998;125:292) as a consequence of rapid immune reconstitution (CD4 increase >100/μL) after starting ART in patients with prior CMV retinitis. Additional risk factors include extent of retinitis (>30% retinal area) and previous use of cidofovir. Findings on exam are similar to CMV retinitis, but anterior chamber involvement is much more extensive. Optic disc and macular edema may also be seen. Corticosteroids (systemic and local) are used for treatment (Expert Rev Ophthalmol 2012;7:555).

Kaposi Sarcoma

Diagnosis is made by inspection of lesions and confirmation by biopsy. Lesions respond similarly to treatment of systemic lesions. Immune reconstitution itself may result in resolution of lesions.

Microangiopathy

HIV microangiopathy may present with cotton wool spots, intraretinal hemorrhages, and/or microaneurysms. These are more common with low CD4 counts; they are inconsequential and require no treatment. Microaneurysms associated with anemia often respond to increased hematocrit. Other findings may respond to ART.

Microsporidial Keratoconjunctivitis

The cause is usually *Encephalitozoon hellem*. Diagnosis by ophthalmologist with slit lamp, plus conjunctival scrapings or biopsy. Treatment is fumagillin plus albendazole and ART.

Molluscum Contagiosum

Lesions can be asymptomatic or cause conjunctivitis. Diagnosis is made by exam. Treatment is surgical excision or cautery to ablate the lesions and ART.

Pneumocystis jirovecii Choroidopathy

Yellow or orange lesions at posterior pole of retina. Treatment is standard systemic PCP regimens.

Progressive Outer Retinal Necrosis

Necrotic retinitis caused by varicella zoster virus. Present as punctate white spots that quickly coalesce; typically dense vitritis is absent. Can result in permanent blindness in a few days and/or retinal detachment. Treatment should be in conjunction with ophthalmologist but is not always effective (J Clin Vir 2007;38:254).

Syphilis

Ocular forms include uveitis, optic neuritis, and chorioretinitis. Standard treatment is the same as for CNS syphilis using aqueous penicillin G 18–24 million units/d IV × 10–14 days.

Toxoplasma Retinitis

Diagnosis is based on multiple white or cream-colored retinal lesions without hemorrhages (as commonly seen with CMV) and without pigmented lesions (as seen with toxoplasmosis retinitis in immunocompetent hosts). Treatment is similar to regimens for CNS toxoplasmosis.

Zoster Ophthalmicus

Diagnosis is presumptive based on typical dermatomal rash in the distribution of the first branch of the trigeminal nerve (V1). Due to the high frequency of ocular involvement and potential complications, treatment should be in conjunction with an ophthalmologist.

Osteoporosis

Multiple studies show increased rates of bone disease in PLWH, with relative risk of 6.4 and 3.7 for decreased bone density and osteoporosis, respectively, compared to controls (AIDS 2006;20:2165). PLWH have elevated fracture risk (J Clin Endocrinol Metab 2008;93:3499; CID 2011;52:1061; JAIDS 2015;70:54; PLoS One 2011;6:e17217), with sociodemographic factors and comorbidities partially accounting for the increased risk. Osteoporosis does not account for all fractures as 12% of fractures occurred in nonosteoporotic patients (Osteoporos Int 2014;25:2263; HIV Med 2015;16:563).

CAUSE: The increased prevalence of low bone mineral density (BMD) in PLWH is multifactorial.

- Immune activation leading to increased bone turnover
- Use of cART (particularly TDF, but association appears independent of regimen used; BMD loss is most intense in first year after ART initiation, then gradually decreases)
- Premature aging associated with HIV infection
- Aging population of PLWH
- Comorbid osteoporosis risk factors in PLWH

Traditional causes of secondary osteoporosis are common in PLWH, including: frailty, hypogonadal states, adrenal insufficiency, thyrotoxicosis, hemophilia, sickle cell disease, emphysema, chronic metabolic acidosis, malabsorption, dietary calcium deficiency, vitamin D deficiency, chronic renal disease, alcohol use, tobacco use, methadone or opiate use, sedentary lifestyle, depression, chronic infection, and use of ART, glitazones, glucocorticoids, proton pump inhibitors, among others (CID 2010;51:939).

DIAGNOSIS: Dual-energy X-ray absorptiometry (DXA) scan is the gold-standard for diagnosis of low BMD; some guidelines also recommend use of the WHO Fracture Risk Assessment (FRAX) (http://www.shef.ac.uk/FRAX/), as a diagnostic tool. Note that HIV infection is not taken into account in FRAX, and FRAX risk assessment based on clinical risk factors (without BMD measurement) has been found to correlate poorly with BMD results (JID 2010;202:330; Arch Osteoporos 2014;9:181). Even counting HIV as a secondary cause of osteoporosis in a large VA study, FRAX still grossly underestimated risk of subsequent fracture (JAIDS 2016;72(5):513–20).

EVALUATION FOR SECONDARY CAUSES OF LOW BMD: PLWH diagnosed with osteopenia or osteoporosis were found to have an additional 3.8 risk factors for low BMD in addition to HIV (JIAPAC 2012;11:239). Testing for additional causes is warranted to identify potentially treatable conditions. All patients with low BMD should have a targeted history and physical exam and medication review, plus the following laboratory tests: CBC, CMP (with calcium), 25-OH vitamin D, PTH, TSH, free T4, total and free testosterone (men), SPEP, 24-hr urinary calcium, fractional excretion of phosphate if on TDF (urinary and serum phosphate, sodium, and creatinine), tryptase, and IgG/IgA to tissue transglutaminase (JID 2012;205:S391). Young, amenorrheic women should have estradiol, FSH, LH, and prolactin levels checked. Evaluation for less common causes can be pursued based on clinical suspicion (Eur J Endocrinol 2012;162:1009).

PREVENTION AND TREATMENT:

1. Address modifiable risk factors (e.g., smoking cessation, alcohol consumption).
2. Address risk factors for falls and encourage participation in a structured exercise program.
3. Assure adequate intake of calcium and vitamin D through diet or supplementation: calcium 800–1,200 mg/day + vitamin D 800 IU/day (Eur J Endocrinol 2010;162:1009). Titrate to normal calcium levels and 25-OH vitamin D >30 ng/mL. One study showed mitigation of BMD loss with ART initiation by routine calcium and vitamin D supplementation (Ann Intern Med 2015;162:715).
4. Treat any conditions that contribute to osteoporosis (e.g., hyperthyroidism, hypogonadism, vitamin D deficiency).
5. Discontinue contributing medications, as feasible (e.g., corticosteroids, PPIs). It is prudent to avoid or replace TDF with TAF, ABC, or NRTI-sparing regimens, as feasible in patients with osteoporosis, or high risk of fracture.
6. *Pharmacologic therapy*:
   - *Bisphosphonates*: A small early study of once-weekly alendronate showed reversal of osteoporosis at 96 wks in 73% vs. 4% in placebo (AIDS 2005;19:343). A 2014 meta-analysis of alendronate and zoledronic acid showed modest, but statistically significant increases in BMD over time with both bisphosphonates (AIDS Rev 2014;16:213). Alendronate (70 mg weekly or 10 mg/d) is recommended as first-line therapy for osteoporosis in the general population and is the most studied bisphosphonate in HIV. If adherence is a concern, annual IV zoledronic acid can be considered, but ~10% can have an acute-phase reaction with fever and body aches. A small phase IIb trial of prophylactic one-time zoledronic acid infusion on the day of ART (TDF/FTC/ATV/RTV) initiation showed blunting of ART-related bone resorption and BMD loss over the first 48 wks of ART (CID 2016;63(5):663–71).

- *Indications for bisphosphonates*: Men or postmenopausal women >50 yrs with (1) fragility fracture; (2) osteoporosis at hip, femoral neck, or lumbar spine; or (3) osteopenia with 10-yr risk of a fracture of the hip, shoulder, wrist, or spine of >20% (all 3 combined) or >3% (hip alone) based on FRAX (as noted earlier, however, FRAX may underestimate risk in HIV).
- The appropriate duration of bisphosphonate use in HIV has not been studied. Recommendations for the general population vary; most advise reassessing use of bisphosphonate after 3–5 yrs due to risk of adverse effects. Due to ongoing high-risk of fracture, some patients will benefit from continued use. There are no data to guide healthcare providers on reinitiation of bisphosphonate after discontinuation.
- *Use of estrogen replacement therapy* and selective estrogen receptor modulators is controversial given lack of supportive data and potential harms. Intranasal calcitonin, teriparatide, and denosumab can be considered.

MONITORING: There is no consensus among professional society guidelines on the appropriate interval for follow-up DXA for screening or for monitoring response to treatment. Intervals for screening should likely be based on degree of BMD abnormality seen on initial testing. Advice on obtaining monitoring DXA scans during the first 3–5 yrs of therapy is conflicting. Following initial treatment, patient can be monitored for BMD stability periodically.

FURTHER READING:

1. Curr Opin HIV AIDS 2016;11:351.
2. Curr Opin HIV AIDS 2016;11:261.
3. Osteoporos Int 2014;25:2359.
4. Enferm Infecc Microbiol Clin 2018;36:312.
5. Ann Intern Med 2017;166:818.
6. Endocr Pract. 2016;22:Suppl4;1–42.
7. CID 2015;60:1242.

Psychiatric Complications

Behavioral, mood, and psychiatric disorders are quite common among PLWH (Neurol Clin 2016;34:33). It is important to rule out underlying medical conditions that may present with behavioral/psychiatric manifestations.

DIFFERENTIAL: Nonpsychiatric conditions that are often mistaken as psychiatric include:

- Infection: HIV-associated dementia; neurosyphilis.
- Deficiencies: Vitamin B_6, B_{12} or A; thiamine; zinc.
- Endocrine disorders: thyroid disease, uncontrolled diabetes, adrenal insufficiency, or hypogonadism.
- Medication adverse reactions: EFV, DTG, corticosteroids, interferon:
  - DTG: Recent reports of increased neuropsychiatric side effects in some studies (AIDS 2016;30:2831; AIDS 2017;31:1201; HIV Med 2017; 18:56; J Antimicrob Chemother 2017;72:1752); however, others have not found increased rates compared to other agents (JAIDS 2017;74:423).
- Substance abuse or withdrawal
- Cardiopulmonary disease leading to hypoxia: sleep apnea, pulmonary hypertension, COPD.
- Metabolic disorders: Chronic renal or liver disease.
- Electrolyte abnormalities: Hyper-/hypocalcemia; hyper-/hyponatremia.

Bipolar Disorder (Manic Depression)

FREQUENCY: Seventeen percent of male PLWH and 4% of female PLWH in a large nationally representative sample of US adults had diagnosis of bipolar disorder (J Clin Psychiatry 2012; 73:384).

DIAGNOSIS: Manic episodes, depressive episodes, and mixed episodes. Differential includes familial bipolar disorder and HIV mania (no family history, no episodes prior to late stage HIV, comorbid cognitive impairment). Mania is defined as a period of abnormal mood that is elevated, expansive, or irritable with ≥3 of the following: (1) grandiosity, (2) decreased sleep (<3 hrs/d), (3) excessive talking, (4) psychomotor agitation, (5) racing thoughts, (6) distractibility, (7) excessive pleasurable activities, and/or (8) psychomotor agitation.

TREATMENT:

HIV mania: ART (acute management); newer atypical neuroleptics are favored given their improved side effect profile: olanzapine, quetiapine, aripiprazole, ziprasidone, risperidone. Valproic acid can also be used. Favored agents to control symptoms: valproic acid, gabapentin, and other anticonvulsants. Care should be directed by a psychiatrist.

Delirium

DIAGNOSIS: Impaired consciousness, inability to focus or sustain interest, cognitive changes, global derangement of brain function, acute onset, altered consciousness, or disorganized thinking. Reported frequency in hospitalized PLWH is 12–29% (Alzheimer Dis Assoc Disord 1987;1:221); however, very little is known about the prevalence of delirium in PLWH following the introduction of HAART (HIV/AIDS [Auckl] 2015;7:35).

TREATMENT: Focus should be on correcting the underlying condition first.

- *Agitation*: Neuroleptics such as haloperidol, chlorpromazine, or risperidone.
- *Agitation that puts others at risk*: Neuroleptics + low dose of lorazepam for sedation.

Major Depression

FREQUENCY: Twelve percent of male PLWH, and 6% of female PLWH in a large nationally representative sample of US adults had diagnosis of major depression (J Clin Psychiatry 2012; 73:384). Prevalence varied from 17% to 47% among PLWH in the United Kingdom (Int J STD AIDS 2018;29:704).

PRESENTATION: Depressed mood, loss of pleasure from activities (anhedonia), anorexia, morning insomnia or hypersomnia, difficulty concentrating, thoughts of suicide. Depression is a major contributor to medication nonadherence (J Gen Intern Med 2011;26:1175).

DIFFERENTIAL: Dementia, delirium, demoralization, intoxications or withdrawal, neurologic diseases.

DIAGNOSIS: Start with two-question screening test:

- Do you feel sad, depressed, or hopeless?
- Have you lost interest/pleasure in things that you usually enjoy?

If yes to both, recommend Patient Health Questionnaire PHQ-9 (found online at http://www.actiondepression.org/information/depression/depression-self-test).

TREATMENT: Antidepressants (Table 8.27 and 8.28) starting with low doses and titrating slowly ("start low and go slow") with appropriate attention to side effects and serum levels. Treatment of depression led to improvements in viral suppression rates in one study (AIDS 2017;31:2515).

RESPONSE: Response rates to antidepressants are 85%; cure rate 50–79% (Psychosomatic 1997;38:423; Int J STD AIDS 2015;26:998).

Commonly used agent by class:

- *SSRIs*: Citalopram sertraline, fluoxetine, paroxetine, escitalopram.
- *Tricyclics*: Nortriptyline, desipramine, doxepin, imipramine.
- *Novel antidepressants*: Bupropion, venlafaxine, mirtazapine.
- *Psychostimulants*: Methylphenidate, dextroamphetamine.

TABLE 8.27 Depression drug selection

Agent	Advantages	Disadvantages
SSRIs	Relatively safe and well tolerated Compared with tricyclics: Fewer drug interactions and side effects Safety with overdose	ADRs: Sexual dysfunction, substrate, and inhibitor of P450 enzymes Use with PI (DRV/r) or NNRTI (EFV) may decrease level of some SSRIs (sertraline, paroxetine)
Tricyclics	Equally effective compared with SSRIs Also useful for neuropathy, insomnia, and diarrhea	ADRs: Anticholinergic effects, dry mouth, blurred vision, orthostasis Use with PI may increase tricyclic level Refractory arrhythmia with overdose

Reviewed in Cochrane Database Syst Rev January 22, 2018.

Sleep Disturbance

The incidence of insomnia in PLWH ranges from 30% to 97% (Psychosom Med 2005;67:260; Sleep Med 2015;16:901; AIDS Behav 2016;20:339). Insomnia in PLWH may be multifactorial: direct effects of HIV infection, adverse effects of ART (e.g., EFV), comorbid neuropsychiatric disorders, and OIs.

DIAGNOSIS: Evaluate patient for cause (psychiatric: major depression, PTSD, substance abuse, mania, substance use disorder, demoralization; and nonpsychiatric: obstructive sleep apnea, restless leg syndrome, uncontrolled medical conditions, medication induced, etc.) and refer for appropriate treatment.

TABLE 8.28 Specific antidepressant recommendations

Drug Regimen	Comment
Paroxetine 10–40 mg/day	May sedate: If insomnia—give qhs; may cause sexual dysfunction, headache or nausea
Sertraline 50–100 mg/day	Use higher doses with PIs (DRV/r) and EFV due to drug interactions; may cause insomnia, agitation, sexual dysfunction, headache; note long half life
Fluoxetine 10–40 mg/day	Rarely sedating, not fatal with overdose, no anticholinergic effects, may cause insomnia agitation, sexual dysfunction; note long half life
Citalopram 10–60 mg/day	Fewer drug interactions compared to other SSRIs; may cause nausea and sedation
Venlafaxine XR 75–375 mg/day	Less drug interactions; may cause headache, nausea, sexual dysfunction
Mirtazapine 15–45 mg/day	Start with 15 mg qhs and then increase to 15 mg at 7 days; may cause weight gain & dry mouth

TREATMENT: Optimal therapy for insomnia in PLWH has not been studied in randomized controlled trials. First-line therapy for insomnia is improved sleep hygiene and cognitive behavior therapy (Psychol Res Behav Manag 2011;4:21). If symptoms remain following nonpharmacologic therapy and intervention is warranted, addition of pharmacologic therapy is indicated. Note that PIs can interact with most medications used to treat insomnia; such patients should be started at low doses and titrated for effect. Side-effect profile, interaction with other medications, type of sleep disturbance, and duration of comorbid conditions should be considered when choosing a particular agent (AIDS Rev 2014;16:3; J Clin Sleep

Med 2009;5:251; Psychosom Med 2005;67:260; J Assoc Nurses AIDS Care 2013; 24:S72).

Commonly used agents include:
- *Benzodiazepines*: High addictive potential; should be used for short course and with caution:
  - Temazepam, lorazepam, and alprazolam
- *Non-benzodiazepines*: Can be habit forming
  - Zolpidem (Ambien), zaleplon (Sonata), eszopiclone (Lunesta)
- *Antidepressants* (have low abuse potential):
  - Doxepin, mirtazapine, and trazodone
- *Antipsychotics* (low abuse potential, but PLWH are at increased risk of EPS, so use with caution):
  - Olanzapine and quetiapine

Substance Use Disorders

FREQUENCY: Substance use disorders were diagnosed in 38% of male and 20% of female PLWH in a large, nationally representative sample of US adults (J Clin Psychiatry 2012; 73:384). Substance abuse is associated with increased risk of acquisition and transmission of HIV (MMWR Surveill Summ 2014; 63:1; Front Microbiol 2015;6:690), reduced adherence to ART, and decreased rates of viral suppression (Expert Opin Drug Metab Toxicol 2015;11:343; Addiction 2008;103:1242). Enrollment in comprehensive substance abuse programs has been associated with increased adherence to ART in PLWH who have abused illicit substances (Addiction 2008;103:124).

DIAGNOSIS: Use of substances despite clear evidence of negative consequences.

Dependence is defined as persistent use or drug seeking behavior, withdrawal, tolerance, and physical dependence.

TREATMENT:
See J Manag Care Pharm 2010;16(1 Suppl B):S14.

- *Opioid dependency*:
  - *Methadone treatment*: Usually started with mandated visits 5–6 days/wk with gradual reduction to weekly attendance at 1 yr. Initial dose usually 30–40 mg/d with increases to maintenance doses of 80–120 mg/d. EFV and NVP can decrease methadone concentrations up to 51%.
  - *Buprenorphine treatment*: Provider requirements for prescribing: (1) 8-hr course, (2) registration with US Drug Enforcement Agency (DEA), and (3) limit to 30 patients/physician for the first year, then 100 patients/physician. Usual starting dose is 8 mg on day 1, then titrate based on withdrawal symptoms with a target dose of 16 mg/day (maximum 32 mg/d).
  - *Naltrexone*: Only if methadone or buprenorphine cannot be used.
- *Cocaine dependence*:
  - No drug is approved for cocaine dependency. Nonpharmacologic treatments include the 12-step program and acupuncture.
- *Benzodiazepines*:
  - Detoxification
- *Methamphetamine*:
  - Possible benefit from bupropion, modafinil, and baclofen.

TABLE 8.29 Detoxification

Agent	Treatment
Sedative/hypnotic, EtOH, benzodiazepines, and barbiturates	Long-acting benzodiazepines (chlordiazepoxide, diazepam
Alprazolam (Xanax)	Substitute clonazepam and taper
Cocaine	Suicidal symptoms common; may need brief hospitalization
Opioids	Clonidine for autonomic instability. Buprenorphine or methadone tapers; dicyclomine for GI distress

Suicide

PLWH commit suicide at rates several times higher than the general population, but observed suicide rate has decreased 40–60% following introduction of HAART. However, suicide still accounts for 4–6% of all deaths in PLWHH (AIDS 2010; 24:1537, Am J Psychiatry 2010;167:143, AIDS 2009;23:1743; HIV Med 2013; 4:195; Lancet. 2014;384:241). Suicide deaths in PLWH appear to be related to diagnosis of psychiatric illness including substance abuse, recent diagnosis of HIV, and low socioeconomic status; these were all factors associated with increased risk of suicidal death in PLWH (J Clin Psychiatry 2012;73:1315; Am J Psychiatry 2010; 167:143; PLoS One 2014;9:e89089), while CD4 counts of >500 were associated with decreased risk of suicide death (Am J Psychiatry 2010; 167:143). Among antiretrovirals, efavirenz has the strongest association with neuropsychiatric side effects. Several published reports including one cross-study analysis of four AIDS Clinical Trials Group studies found increased risk of suicide in PLWH taking EFV-based regimens (Ann Intern Med 2014;161:1).

Pulmonary Complications

Pulmonary diseases have been among the most common complications of HIV infection, but the spectrum of pulmonary complications, both infectious and noninfectious, has changed over the decades with the advent of ART, as well as the establishment of PCP prophylaxis and pneumococcal vaccination as standard of care (Am J Respir Crit Care Med 2001;164:2120; Proc Am Thorac Soc 2011:8:17).

In the early (pre-ART) years of the epidemic, pulmonary infections such as PCP, TB, and bacterial pneumonia were the most frequent complications. Currently, infectious diseases are less common although still prevalent, and diseases such as emphysema, pulmonary arterial hypertension (PAH), and lung cancer appear to be increasing; IRIS may also manifest as pulmonary disease (Proc Am Thorac Soc 2011:8:17).

The incidence rates of bacterial pneumonia, COPD, TB, pulmonary hypertension, and pulmonary fibrosis are all significantly increased with HIV infection, even after adjustment for confounders (PLoS ONE 2013;8:e58812). The risk for these pulmonary complications also correlates with age and smoking. A study of two large observational cohorts of PLWH and HIV-uninfected participants (Multicenter AIDS Cohort Study (MACS) and Women's Interagency HIV Study (WIHS), tracked the incidence of multiple infectious and noninfectious respiratory conditions over a 20-yr period, both prior to and during the HAART era. Compared to HIV-uninfected participants, PLWH had more incident respiratory infections both pre-HAART (MACS: aOR 2.4) and after HAART (MACS: aOR 1.5; WIHS: aOR 2.2). After HAART availability, noninfectious lung diseases were not significantly more common in PLWH in either cohort. However, PLWH in the HAART era with respiratory infections had an increased risk of death compared to those without HIV (MACS: aHR 1.5; WIHS: aHR 1.9).

COPD

Multiple studies have found HIV infection to be an independent risk factor for COPD independent of tobacco and IDU. In a study assessing pulmonary function tests in PLWH at a university hospital, the most prevalent abnormality was decreased diffusion capacity (DLCO 72.1% of predicted) at a rate of 65% of total population and in 50% of nonsmokers. The average forced expiratory volume (FEV$_1$) was 92.8% of predicted and the use of ART was noted to be an independent risk factor for lower FEV$_1$ (Am J Respir Crit Care Med 2010;182:790). Elevated diffusing capacity of lungs (DLCO) may be attributable to early emphysema (Am J Respir Crit

Care Med 1999;160:272). Pathophysiology is unclear but possible theories include:

- *Malnourishment,* as BMI was an independent risk factor with malnourishment linked to elastase induced lung injury (Am J Respir Crit Care Med. 1999;160:272).
- *Pulmonary hypertension*
- *Elevated metalloproteases* due to direct infection by virus in alveolar macrophages with resultant release and also upregulation of matrix metalloproteases in uninfected neighboring cells (Diagn Mol Pathol 2005;14:48).
- *ART:* It is unclear exactly how ART may be associated with obstruction. Possible explanations include decreased expression of peroxisome-proliferator-activated receptor, which is involved in cytokine metabolism and provides antiinflammatory effects in lungs and airways. Other potential explanations include abnormal immune restoration which may result from occult infection or colonization in lower respiratory tract leading to airway obstruction (PLoS ONE 2009;4:e6328).

Lung Cancer

HIV infection is associated with an increased risk for lung cancer independent of smoking, even in the current ART era (CID 2007;45:103; J Clin Oncol 2006;24:1383). Lung cancer is the most frequent non–AIDS-defining cancer in PLWH and is the leading cause of cancer-related death among PLWH in a large US population-based registry (CID 2010:51:957). Average age at diagnosis of lung cancer in PLWH is consistently younger than in general population (Ann Intern Med 2010;153:452). Most diagnoses are made with advanced stage disease (III or IV). Two meta-analyses estimated that the risk of lung cancer in PLWH was more than 2-fold higher than in the general population (Lancet 2007:370:59; JAIDS 2009:52:611), and the risk is relevant for all main lung cancer subtypes (squamous cell carcinoma, adenocarcinoma, and small cell carcinoma). PLWH who also smoked or used injection drugs are at particularly higher risk, although the risk remains increased even after adjusting for smoking (AIDS 2012;26:1017). PLWH are less likely to be treated for lung cancer and suffer higher mortality than HIV-negative patients with lung cancer (AIDS 2013;27:459).

Pneumonia

CAUSE: With the introduction of combination ART, the incidence of PCP and TB has decreased (AIDS 2007:21:2093). Invasive pneumococcal disease has also decreased in PLWH after the introduction of the pneumococcal vaccine (Ann Intern Med 2006:144:1), but remains higher than that of the general population (BMC ID 2011;11:314). Community-acquired methicillin resistant *Staphylococcus aureus* (MRSA), and *P. aeruginosa* are more frequent in PLWH than in HIV-uninfected individuals (Ann Intern Med 2008:148:249; AIDS 2002:16:85).

The single major prospective study of pulmonary complications of HIV was in the pre-HAART era (before 1995) (Am J Respir Crit Care Med 1997;155:72). Most common infections then were PCP 45%, common bacteria 42%, TB 5%, CMV 4%, *Aspergillus* 2%, and cryptococcosis 1%. A more recent large comprehensive review was the VA Aging Virtual Cohort Study consisting of 33,420 HIV-infected veterans and 66,840 matched controls (1999–2007) (Am J Resp Crit Care Med 2011;183:388). The rate of bacterial pneumonia was 5-fold greater in the HIV group compared to veterans without HIV. The most common bacterial pathogen was *S. pneumoniae*; other bacteria disproportionately represented were *S. aureus* and *P. aeruginosa* (NEJM 1995;333:845; Ann Intern Med 1986;104:38; Crit Care Med 2001;29:548; J Intensive Care Med 2011;26:151; Eur Respir J 2014;43:708; PLoS ONE 2013;8:e58812).

A prospective observational study of 331 consecutive adult community-acquired pneumonia (CAP) cases in PLWH from January 2007 and July 2012 in a hospital in Barcelona, Spain,

TABLE 8.30 Microbial etiology of CAP in PLWH

Microorganisms	Total Population (n = 331)
Unknown etiology	31%
Streptococcus pneumoniae	30%
Pneumocystis jirovecii	13%
Mixed etiology	12%
Respiratory viruses	5%
Haemophilus influenzae	2%
Staphylococcus aureus	2%
Pseudomonas aeruginosa	1%
Legionella pneumophila	1%
Escherichia coli	0.3%
Klebsiella pneumoniae	0.3%
Mycoplasma pneumoniae	0.3%
Other	2%

From Eur Respir J 2014:43:6:708.

found that *S. pneumoniae* was the most frequent microorganism in the group with CD4 of ≥200/mL; *P. jirovecii* was the most frequent microorganism in the group with CD4 of <200/mL. Also, WBC ≤4×10^{12}/L (OR 3.7), lactate dehydrogenase (LDH) level ≥598 U/L (OR 12.9), and multilobar infiltration (OR 5.8) were predictors of *P. jirovecii* (Eur Respir J 2014:43:6:708).

- *Bacteria*: The most common bacterial causes of pneumonia are, in rank order: *S. pneumoniae, H. influenzae, P. aeruginosa,* and *S. aureus* (CID 2006;43:90; CID 1996;23:107; Am J Respir Crit Care Med 1995;152:1309; NEJM 1995;333:845; JID 2001;184: 268; AIDS 2002;16:2361; JAIDS 1994;7:823; AIDS 2003;17:2109). The risk of pneumococcal bacteremia is increased 25-fold with HIV (CID 2014:59:1168). *H. influenzae* pneumonia usually involves nontypeable strains (JAMA 1992;268:3350). *P. aeruginosa* is a cause of pneumonia in late-stage HIV infection and often causes bacteremia and relapses (JAIDS 1994;7:823; NEJM 2010;362:812).

- *Atypical*: Pneumonia due to *M. pneumoniae, C. pneumoniae*, and *Legionella* appear to be relatively uncommon in patients with HIV infection (Eur J Clin Microbiol Infect Dis 1997;16:720; NEJM 1997;337:682; NEJM 1995;333:845; Am J Resp Crit Care Med 1995;152:1309; CID 1996;23:107; Am J Resp Crit Care Med 2000;162:2063; CID 2004;40[suppl 3]:S150); AIDS Patient Care STDS 2008;22:473).
- *Influenza* does not appear to be unusually common or severe in PLWH. A combination of reported case series in the 2009 H1N1 epidemic showed one death among 88 hospitalized PLWH (JAIDS 2011;56:e111). Data from California showed that PLWH accounted for 22 of 1,088 (3%) hospitalized patients and 4 of 110 (4%) deaths (JAMA 2009;302:1896).

PRESENTATION: Cough, dyspnea, and fever ± sputum production.

- *Differential diagnosis* depends on CD4 count (see Table 8.31).
- *Time course*: Pyogenic infections and influenza evolve rapidly. PCP develops slowly in PLWH, with an average duration of symptoms of 3 wks prior to presentation.

TABLE 8.31 Etiology correlated with CD4 count

CD4 Cell Count	Etiology
>500 cells/mm^3	Bacterial pneumonia, primary MTB, NHL, bronchogenic cancer
<500 cells/mm^3	Recurrent bacterial pneumonia
<200 cells/mm^3	Pneumocystis pneumonia, cryptococcal pneumonia, disseminated TB, non-Hodgkin lymphoma
<100 cells/mm^3	Toxoplasmosis pneumonitis, *Nocardia, Staphylococcus*, and *Pseudomonas* pulmonary Kaposi sarcoma
	Talaromycosis—if in appropriate endemic location
<50 cells/mm^3	Coccidiosis, histoplasmosis, MAC (all usually disseminated) CMV Aspergillus

DIAGNOSTIC TESTING:

- *Expectorated sputum*: Controversial, due in part to poor technique in collecting, transporting, and processing specimens. Expectorated sputum for *M. tuberculosis* (MTB): the yield with three specimens is 50–60% for AFB stain (Am J Respir Crit Care Med 2001;164:2020).

- Xpert MTB/RIF: New tool for diagnosing TB and is now in use in many regions. It consists of an automated, cartridge-based real-time PCR system that detects MTB in sputum samples within 2 hrs with minimal need for technical expertise. Xpert MTB/RIF detects RIF resistance by targeting the MTB rpoB gene. The presence of RIF resistance is thought to be a good marker for MDR-TB (Ann Glob Health 2014;80:476).

  - A 2014 Cochrane review calculated pooled sensitivity for Xpert MTB/RIF test of 79% in PLWH (Cochrane Database Syst Rev 2014;1:CD009593). Most of the molecular tools now available, such as Xpert MTB/RIF, suffer from decreased accuracy in PLWH due to multiple challenges associated with HIV-TB co-infection, including (1) higher rate of smear-negative disease, (2) less frequent "typical" symptoms of TB, (3) higher likelihood of extrapulmonary TB (Am J Respir Crit Care Med 2011;184:132). Table 8.32 shows the diagnostic accuracy of Xpert MTB/RIF in HIV-positive and HIV-negative patients, from five studies that evaluated molecular test for TB, three of these studies in PLWH.

- *Induced sputum*: Recommended as an alternative to expectorated sputum for detection of MTB in patients who cannot produce an expectorated sample and as an alternative to bronchoscopy for detection of PCP. Sensitivity for detection of TB by AFB smear is about the same as it is for expectorated sputum; for PCP, sensitivity averages 56% (Eur Resp J 2002;20:982). PCR methods are sensitive, but asymptomatic carriage of *P. jirovecii* limits specificity (Proc Am Thorac Soc 2011;8:17; JCM 2011;49:1872).

TABLE 8.32 Diagnostic accuracy of Xpert MTB/RIF in patients with and without HIV

HIV-negative		HIV-positive		Smear Positive	Smear Negative	Overall
Sensitivity	Specificity	Sensitivity	Specificity	Sensitivity	Sensitivity	Specificity
83–98%	96–100%	70–94%	92–96%	95–99%	47–78%	94–100%

From Ann Glob Health 2014;80:476.

- *Bronchoscopy*: The yield for PCP is 95% or comparable to open-lung biopsy (JAMA 2001;286:2450). For MTB, sensitivity is similar to that for expectorated sputum (above). For other bacteria, bronchoscopy is no better than expectorated sputum.
- *Miscellaneous*: Tests to consider in atypical or nonresponsive pulmonary infections include *Legionella* urinary antigen, *Histoplasma* serum and urinary antigen, serum cryptococcal antigen, 1-3 β-D-glucan, CT scan, and bronchoscopy with biopsy.

IMAGING:

- Chest x-ray is adequate for most pulmonary complications of HIV. One blinded trial of PLWH showed accurate detection in 64% of bacterial pneumonias, 75% of PCP cases, and 84% of TB cases (Thor Imaging 1997;12:47). High-resolution CT scan is more expensive, sensitive, and accurate, including accurate detection for 90% of KS and 94% of PCP and a 93% negative predictive value for excluding active pulmonary disease (Ann Thor Med 2010;5:201).
- *Specific conditions*:
  - *Bacterial pneumonia*: Same as changes in immunocompetent hosts, especially lobar or segmental consolidation and rapid progression.
  - *PCP*: X-rays often lag clinical symptoms. *Classic changes*: bi-lateral symmetric perihilar or diffuse infiltrates appearing

as reticular or ground glass infiltrates. Cysts and pneumothoraces are common. Normal chest x-rays in 10% (CID 2010;30:S5).

- *Influenza*: Typical changes are bilateral with multiple lobe involvement, predominance in perihilar and peripheral areas with ground-glass, consolidation, or nodular opacities (Radiology 2010;255:252).
- *TB*: with CD4 count of >200/mL, the changes with TB are typical for an immunocompetent host with reactivation with upper lobe cavitary disease. However, with lower CD4 counts, there is often lower lobe involvement, patchy consolidation, effusions, adenopathy, cavities, and/or nodules. About 15% are normal on the chest x-ray, but high resolution CT will show abnormalities with adenopathy and "tree-in-bud" pattern, which is asymmetric (NEJM 1999;340:367; J Thorac Imaging 2002;17:28).
- *KS*: Bilateral, perihilar, and lower zone reticulonodular infiltrates; sometimes with the classical flame-shaped nodules. Pulmonary effusions are common (J Comput Assist Tomogr 1993;17:60; Ann Intern Med 1985;102:471).
- *Lymphoma*: Well-defined single or multiple nodules that are often large and peripheral (unlike KS) (Chest 1996;110:729).

PROPHYLAXIS: TMP-SMX effectively reduces incidence of PCP and bacterial pneumonia, including cases involving *S. pneumoniae*, *Legionella*, *H. influenzae*, and *S. aureus*. Influenza vaccine appears to decrease the risk of influenza (Arch Intern Med 2001;161:441). Pneumovax shows variable results (Br Med J 2002; 325:292), and a systematic review of 15 reports concluded "moderate support" and the need for more data (HIV Med 2011;12:323). INH substantially reduces the risk of TB (JAMA 2005; 293:2719).

TABLE 8.33 Correlation of chest x-ray changes and etiology of pneumonia

Change	Common	Uncommon
Consolidation	Pyogenic bacteria, Kaposi sarcoma, cryptococcosis	*Nocardia*, *M. tuberculosis*, *M. kansasii*, *Legionella*, *B. bronchiseptica*
Reticulonodular infiltrates	*P. jirovecii*, *M. tuberculosis*, histoplasmosis, coccidioidomycosis	Kaposi sarcoma, toxoplasmosis, CMV, Leishmania, lymphoid interstitial pneumonitis
Nodules	*M. tuberculosis*, cryptococcosis	Kaposi sarcoma, *Nocardia*, PCP
Cavity	*M. tuberculosis*, *Nocardia*, *P. aeruginosa*, cryptococcosis, coccidioidomycosis, histoplasmosis, aspergillosis, anaerobes, Staphylococcus, Klebsiella	*M. kansasii*, MAC, *Legionella*, *P. jirovecii*, lymphoma, *Rhodococcus equi*
Hilar nodes	*M. tuberculosis*, histoplasmosis, coccidioidomycosis, lymphoma, Kaposi sarcoma	*M. kansasii*, MAC
Pleural effusion	Pyogenic bacteria, Kaposi sarcoma, *M. tuberculosis* (congestive heart failure, hypoalbuminemia	Cryptococcosis, MAC, histoplasmosis, coccidioidomycosis, aspergillosis, anaerobes, *Nocardia*, lymphoma, toxoplasmosis, primary effusion lymphoma
Adenopathy	*M. tuberculosis*	*Cryptococcus*, cancer

From Ann Thorac Med 2010;5:201.

EMPIRIC TREATMENT FOR BACTERIAL PNEUMONIA IN PLWH
See AIDS Guidelines 2017:H-5-7; 2007 IDSA/ATS Guidelines.

- *Outpatient*: Oral β-lactam plus an oral macrolide (AII), or an oral respiratory fluoroquinolone (AII). Preferred β-lactams are high-dose amoxicillin (3 g/d) or amoxicillin-clavulanate (2 g q12h); alternatives are cefpodoxime or cefuroxime. Preferred macrolides are azithromycin or clarithromycin. Doxycycline is an alternative to the macrolide (CIII). Preferred oral respiratory fluoroquinolones are moxifloxacin or levofloxacin.
- *Hospitalized patient*: Respiratory fluoroquinolone (moxifloxacin of levofloxacin) or a combination of a β-lactam (cefotaxime or ceftriaxone or ampicillin-sulbactam) plus a macrolide (usually azithromycin) (AII).
- *ICU admission*: β-lactam plus either a macrolide or β-lactam + respiratory fluoroquinolone. MRSA coverage should be considered based on epidemiological risk.
- *Empiric P. aeruginosa treatment*: If risk factors for *Pseudomonas* infection are present, an anti-pneumococcal, anti-pseudomonal β-lactam plus either ciprofloxacin or levofloxacin (750 mg dose) should be used (BIII). Preferred β-lactams are piperacillin-tazobactam, cefepime, imipenem, or meropenem. Alternatives are an anti-pneumococcal, anti-pseudomonal β-lactam, plus an aminoglycoside and azithromycin (BIII), or an anti-pneumococcal, anti-pseudomonal β-lactam plus an aminoglycoside and an anti-pneumococcal fluoroquinolone (BIII).
- *Empiric S. aureus treatment*: In patients who have risk factors for *S. aureus* infection, including community-acquired MRSA, vancomycin or linezolid should be added to the antibiotic regimen (BIII). This should be considered in all patients who are in septic shock or intubated who require ICU level of care. Although not routinely recommended, the addition of clindamycin (to vancomycin, but not to linezolid) may be considered if severe necrotizing pneumonia is present to minimize bacterial toxin production (CIII).

- Transition to po therapy should occur in patients who have improved clinically, can take po, and have normal GI function. This should be considered in patients who have oral temp of <37.8°C, heart rate <100 bpm, respiratory rate <24 breaths/min, blood pressure >90 mm Hg, and on room air with spO_2 >90%.

PREVENTING PNEUMONIA IN PLWH
See AIDS Guidelines 2017:H8.

- PLWH, both adults and adolescents, who have never received any pneumococcal vaccine should receive a single dose of PCV13, regardless of CD4 count (AI).
- Patients with CD4 ≥200/mL should then receive a dose of 23-valent PPV (PPV23) at least 8 wks later (AII).
- PLWH with CD4 <200/mL can be offered PPV23 at least 8 wks after receiving PCV13 (CIII); however, it may be preferable to defer PPV23 until after the CD4 count increases to >200/mL on ART (BIII).
- Clinical evidence supporting use of PPV23 in persons with CD4 <200/mL appears strongest in patients who also have HIV RNA <100,000 copies/mL; evidence also suggests benefit for those who start ART before receiving PPV.
- Duration of the protective effect of PPV23 is unknown; a single revaccination with PPV is recommended if ≥5 yrs have elapsed since the first dose of PPV23 was given (BIII).
- A third dose of PPV23 should be given at age 65 yrs or later, as long as 5 yrs have elapsed since the most recent dose and it was given before age 65 yrs (BIII).
- PCV13 should also be given in PLWH who have already received PPV23 (AII). However, such patients should wait at least 1 yr after their most recent dose of PPV23 before receiving a single dose of PCV13 (BIII).
- Subsequent doses of PPV23 should be given according to the schedule outlined above (i.e., at least 5 yrs between doses of PPV23 with no more than 3 lifetime doses).

- High-dose inactivated influenza vaccine should be administered annually during influenza season to all PLWH (AIII).
- This recommendation is pertinent to prevention of bacterial pneumonia, which can occur as a complication of influenza. Use of live attenuated influenza vaccine is contraindicated and is not recommended in PLWH (AIII).
- The incidence of *H. influenzae* type b infection in PLWH adults is low. Therefore, *H. influenzae* type B vaccine is not usually recommended for adult use (BIII) unless a patient also has anatomic or functional asplenia.

Pulmonary Hypertension

See Adv Cardiol 2003;40:197; Am J Resp Crit Care Med 2008;177:108; Arch Broncopneumol 2012:48:4:126.

CAUSE: Unclear but likely multifactorial; there is an association with HLA II DR52/DR6 (Am J Respir Crit Care Med 1996;153:1299). gp120 stimulates secretion of endothelin I (J Immunol 1993;150:4601). Nef+ viruses induce plexiform lesions typical of PAH. TAT is a known downregulater of BMPR2, a protein which functions to be anti-proliferative and pro-apoptotic to pulmonary artery smooth muscle cells. (J Leukoc Biol 2006;79:192).

FREQUENCY: Infrequent (0.5%), but risk is 2,500-fold higher with HIV based on low rates in the general population (Expert Rev Respir Med 2011;5:257; Chest 1991;100:1268). A review of the Veterans Cohort Study with 33,420 US veterans found that the rate of pulmonary hypertension was 1.2/1,000 PY compared to 0.8/1,000 age-matched controls (Am Respir Crit Care Med 2011;183:388). The rate of pulmonary hypertension in this and other reports does not correlate with CD4 (Clin Microbiol Infect 2011;17:25). Prevalence of PAH in PLWH is 0.5% even in the modern era of HAART, suggesting it may be independent of ART (Am J Respir Crit Care Med 2008;177:108).

SYMPTOMS: Major symptom is dyspnea. In a review of 154 case reports, the average CD4 at diagnosis was 352/mL, average duration of known HIV infection was 4.3 yrs, mean age was 35 yrs, and main symptoms were dyspnea (93%), pedal edema (18%), syncope (13%), and fatigue (11%) (HIV Med 2010;11:620).

DIAGNOSIS: X-ray shows enlarged pulmonary trunk or central pulmonary vessels (early), massive right ventricular and right atrial enlargement (late). TTE shows dilated right atrium and ventricle ± tricuspid insufficiency. Doppler echocardiogram shows pulmonary arterial systolic blood pressure>30 mm Hg. Sleep study should be normal. The best test is right-sided cardiac catheterization to demonstrate increased pulmonary artery pressure (>25 mm Hg), increased right atrial pressure, and normal pulmonary capillary pressure. Lung scan and pulmonary function tests are normal.

TREATMENT:
See HIV Med 2010;11:620; Clin Microbiol Infect 2011;17:25; Circulation 2015:131:1361.

- *ART*: There are dual (opposing) effects of ART on pulmonary arterial remodeling, and each drug may differentially affect pulmonary hypertension in patients (Circulation 2015:131:1361). In some studies ART decreased mortality from PAH and prevented worsening of functional status versus no HAART or NRTI (Clin Infect Dis 2004;38:1178).
- *PAH therapy* has also advanced in recent years, with the availability of targeted therapies; four classes of drugs are currently approved as "specific therapy" for PAH. However, evidence to support best management of HIV-PAH is still lacking. Patients are generally treated like other patients in Group I PAH. Exception is that vasoreactivity tests are not done, as they are almost always negative. See Table 8.35.

PROGNOSIS: Mortality improved now compared to previous era. In the early 2000s, mortality ranged from 27% to 66%. A newer study

TABLE 8.34 Important immunizations targeting respiratory pneumonia pathogens

Vaccine Type	Recommendation
Pneumococcal	• Recommended for all • If CD4 count is <200 cells/μL, may be less effective; consider revaccination when CD4 count increases in response to ART • Two types of pneumococcal vaccine; both should be given, as follows
Pneumococcal (polysaccharide) (PPV23)	• 1 dose as soon as possible after HIV diagnosis (or PCV13 may be given first, see below); revaccinate 5 yrs after initial vaccination • For those who received 1–2 doses of PPV23 before age 65, repeat at age ≥65 if ≥5 yrs since their previous dose • PPV23 should not be given <8 wks after PPV13 (see below)
Pneumococcal 13-valent conjugate (PPV13)	• 1 dose recommended for all adult PLWH; timing varies according to whether PPV23 has been given • No previous pneumococcal vaccination • 1 dose PCV13 followed by PPV23 ≥8 wks after PCV13 (If CD4 <200 cells/μL, PPV23 can be offered ≥8 wks after PCV13 or can await increase of CD4 to >200 cells/μL.) • Previous PPV23 vaccination: 1 dose of PCV13, given ≥1 yr after last receipt of PPV23
Influenza (inactivated vaccine)	Recommended (yearly) • Vaccination is most effective among persons with CD4 counts of >100 cells/μL and HIV RNA of <30,000 copies/mL • In patients with advanced disease and low CD4 cell counts, inactivated vaccine may not produce protective antibodies. A second dose of vaccine does not improve response in these patients

TABLE 8.34 Continued

Vaccine Type	Recommendation
	• Live, attenuated cold-adapted vaccine (LAIV, FluMist) is not recommended for use in patients with HIV infection as the efficacy of the vaccine in this population has not been evaluated. It is no longer recommended in the US for any patient population as of 2016
	• Close contacts of severely immunocompromised persons (including household members and healthcare personnel) should not receive live, attenuated influenza vaccine

From AIDS Guidelines 2017:H-5-7;2007 H-8.

found 1- and 3-yr survival rates of 88% and 72%, respectively (AIDS 2010;24:67).

Smoking Cessation

Tobacco smoking remains a prevalent behavior in PLWH, with estimates ranging between 40% and 75% in comparison to the current general US smoking rate of 19%. Smoking is associated with impaired immune functioning, increased cardiovascular risk, and decreased response to ART (Am J Public Health 2010;100:1896). Smoking is the most important modifiable risk factor for cardiovascular disease, and, given the high prevalence of cigarette smoking in HIV patients, smoking cessation should be a top priority for all HIV care providers (J Assoc Nurses AIDS Care 2014;25:32; Curr HIV/AIDS Rep 2015;12:413). A recent modeling study showed that PLWH entering HIV care at 40 yrs who continued to smoke, lost >6 yrs of life expectancy compared with never smokers; those who quit smoking upon entering care regained almost 5 yrs of life expectancy (JID 2016;214:1672).

TABLE 8.35 HIV-PAH therapy

PAH targeted therapies
Prostacyclin analogues

• Epoprostenol IV	Several studies suggest that these
• Treprostinil SC	agents improve exercise tolerance,
• Iloprost INH	hemodynamics, 6 min walk distance, and
• Beraprost po	symptoms in HIV-PAH which all were
	maintained >17 mos on two of the studies

Endothelin receptor antagonists

• Bosentan po	Bosentan and Ambrisentan, selective
• Ambrisentan po	endothelin receptor antagonists, are
• Macitentan po	considered an appropriate oral selective
	pulmonary vasodilator in patients
	with HIV-related PAH. Several studies
	confirm the long-term benefits of
	bosentan therapy in HIV-PAH with
	improvement in symptoms, 6 min walk
	distance and hemodynamics and with
	favorable overall survival. Several studies
	showed good tolerance and long term
	clinical improvement observed following
	ambrisentan treatment, including a post
	hoc meta-analysis. In one trial, Macitentan
	was used in 10 patients
	Significant drug-drug interaction between
	bosentan, all PIs, and most NNRITs.
	Co-administer low dose bosentan (62.5mg
	q24–48h) with PIs only at steady-state
	(after 10 days of continuous PI dosing)
	EFV, NVP, and ETR may decrease bosentan
	concentrations. Bosentan dose may need
	to be increased
	No data with cobicistat. Avoid or use with
	caution
	PI/r or PI/cobi may significantly increase
	concentrations of ambrisentan and
	macitentan. Avoid or use with caution

TABLE 8.35 Continued

Phosphodiesterase type 5 inhibitor
- Sildenafil po   Some reports suggest the beneficial effects
- Tadalafil po   of sildenafil in patient with HIV-PAH,
                           but data on its long-term benefit are still
                           lacking
                         Little data available on the use of tadalafil,
                           with only a case series with eighteen HIV-
                           PAH subjects, three of which were treated
                           with tadalafil
                         *D-D interaction with all PIs and cobicistat
                         High dose sildenafil not recommended with
                           PIs and cobicistat
                         With PI/r (once at steady-state after
                           7 days): use tadalafil 20 mg/d (max 40 mg/
                           d) EFV, NVP, ETR may decrease sildenafil
                           and tadalafil concentrations. Dose may
                           need to be increased after 10–14 days of
                           co-administration

Soluble guanylate cyclase stimulator
- Riociguat po   No HIV-PAH patients were enrolled in recent
                          trial, where the efficacy of riociguat, a
                          soluble guanylate cyclase stimulator, has
                          been assessed

From Am J Respir Crit Care Med 2003;167:1433; Eur Repir J 2004;23:321; Eur J Clin Invest 2015:45:5:515; AIDS 2001;15:1747; AIDS 2002;16:1568; NEJM 2000;343:1342; Am J Respir Crit Care Med 2000;162:1846.

A systematic review on smoking cessation interventions studies for HIV patients between 1989 and 2012 found the highest likelihood of smoking cessation in two RCTs using cell phone technology interventions. Another intervention that significantly reduced smoking-cessation rates was the utilization of interviewing techniques (J Assoc Nurses AIDS Care 2014;25:32). Brief smoking cessation interventions delivered by clinicians can significantly increase abstinence rates of current smokers (HIV Med. 2015;16:201). The US Surgeon General has developed guidelines for clinicians to use during clinic visits to help patients who are interested in smoking cessation. These include use of the Five A's model, which provides a brief and structured framework for addressing smoking cessation in clinical settings (see Table 8.36) (HRSA Guidelines for HIV/AIDS Clinical Care 2014:190).

In addition to counseling, the use of pharmacologic interventions such as nicotine replacement therapy and other adjuvant therapies should be considered. These therapies were developed for the general population, but current clinical guidelines suggest that they should be efficacious for HIV-infected smokers (see Table 8.36; HRSA Guidelines for HIV/AIDS clinical care 2014:190).

TABLE 8.36 Five A's model for addressing smoking cessation in clinical settings

Component	Action	Example
ASK every patient about tobacco use	Identify and document tobacco use at every visit	Incorporate questions about tobacco use when obtaining vital signs, or when reviewing a patient's history • "Do you currently use tobacco?" • "Do you currently smoke cigarettes?"
ADVISE to quit	Using a clear, strong, and personalized message, urge every tobacco user to quit	• "It is important for you to quit smoking now." • "Quitting is the most important thing you can do to protect your health." • "I can help you quit." Also link smoking with something specific to the patient, such as secondhand exposure to children or partners, his/her own lung, cardiovascular, or cancer risk, or the expense of cigarettes.

TABLE 8.36 Continued

Component	Action	Example
ASSESS readiness to make a quit attempt	Determine whether the tobacco user is willing, and ready to make a quit attempt within 30 days	• "Are you willing to give quitting cigarettes a try?"
ASSIST in the quit attempt	For the patient willing to quit, assist in developing a quit plan. Provide practical counseling, support, and supplementary materials	• Have patient set a quit date and enlist the support of his/her family and friends • Offer pharmacotherapy, as appropriate, including nicotine replacement • Provide counseling that includes problem solving and skill building
ARRANGE for follow-up	Arrange for follow-up contacts beginning within the first week after the quit date	• Contact patient via telephone or in person soon after the quit date. This can be done by the primary clinician or other trained staff members. • During the follow-up encounter, assess, and identify any problems, review medication use and side effects, provide reminders about additional resources. • Congratulate patients on their successes. • Help those with relapses assess problems with and barriers to quitting, and offer additional or different assistance. • For patients who report a relapse, help them identify the circumstances that led to the relapse, and assist them with recommitting to smoking abstinence.

TABLE 8.37 Pharmacologic options for smoking cessation

Drug Recommended	Dosing	Common Side Effects	Comments
Nicotine formulations			
Nicotine patch (available OTC) Dosage varies by brand: Nicoderm or Habitrol: • 21 mg/24 hrs • 14 mg/24 hrs • 7 mg/24 hrs Nicotrol: • 15 mg/24 hrs • 10 mg/24 hrs • 5 mg/24 hrs	Dosing recommendations vary based on the number of cigarettes smoked. Individualize treatment Sample treatment recommendation for smokers who smoke ≥10 cigarettes per day: • High-dose patch for 4-6 wks, then • Medium-dose patch for 2 wks, then • Low-dose patch for 2 wks For smokers who smoke <10 cigarettes per day or <45kg: • Medium-dose patch for 6-8 wks, then • Low-dose patch for 2 wks • Consider combination with lozenges or gum in heavy smokers, which has shown to decrease >6 mos abstinence rates than patch alone	Local skin reaction can take 1% Hydrocortisone cream as needed; insomnia, or vivid dreams	• Apply before sleeping • Place patch on a relatively hairless location, rotating sites to avoid irritation. • If experiencing sleep disturbance, remove patch prior to bedtime, or use the 16-hr patch.

Nicotine lozenge (available OTC) • 2 mg and 4 mg	• For patients who smoke their first cigarette >30 minutes after waking, start with 2 mg dose. • For patients who smoke their first cigarette within the first 30 minutes after waking, start with 4 mg. • Allow lozenges to dissolve, do not chew or swallow. Most individuals use 9 lozenges per day; maximum is 20 per day. • Most patients should use 1 lozenge q1–2h with max five every 6 hrs. • Lozenges should be used for up to 12 wks. Gradually reduce number of lozenges per day over decreasing dosing from 1 lozenge q1–2h for the first 6 wks; to 1 lozenge q2–4h during wks 7–9; and 1 lozenge q4–8h during wks 9–12.	Nausea, hiccups, heartburn, headache, cough	• Do not eat or drink anything except water for 15 minutes before using a lozenge.

(continued)

TABLE 8.37 Continued

Drug recommended	Dosing	Common side effects	Comments
Nicotine inhaler (prescription only) • 4 mg per inhalation • 10 mg cartridge	Recommended dosage: 6–16 cartridges per day for first 6–12 wks then taper in the next 6–12 wks.	Local irritation in the mouth and throat, cough, rhinitis; may cause bronchospasm (<1%)	• Use caution in persons with severe reactive airway disease.
Nicotine Nasal Spray (prescription only) • 0.5 mg per spray	• Patient should use 1–2 sprays each nostril per hour (total 1–2 mg per hour); increasing as needed for symptom relief. • Minimum recommended treatment is 16 sprays (8 mg) per day, with a maximum limit of 80 sprays per day (10 sprays per hour). • Recommended duration of therapy: 3–6 mos. • Do not sniff, swallow, or inhale through the nose while administering doses. Tilt head slightly back when dosing.	Nasal irritation, transient changes in sense of smell and taste; may cause bronchospasm (<1%)	• Use caution in persons with severe reactive airway disease. • Nicotine nasal spray has highest dependence potential of the nicotine

Non-Nicotine Medications, First Line

Bupropion SR
• 150 mg

Begin 1–2 wks before quit date.

• Start at 150 mg daily for 3 days, then increase to 150 mg BID for 7–12 wks. Can decrease to once a day if having side effects. Similar efficacy.

• May consider longer-term therapy.

Insomnia, dry mouth, agitation, headache

• May lower seizure threshold in certain patients.

• Levels increased in patients on P450 3A4 inhibitors. (ritonavir and other PIs).

• EFV and TPV may decrease levels by 40–50%

• Use with caution in patients with history of seizures or eating disorders, and those who have used a monoamine oxidase (MAO) inhibitor in the past 14 days

(continued)

TABLE 8.37 Continued

Drug recommended	Dosing	Common side effects	Comments
Varenicline • 0.5 mg and 1 mg	• Begin 1 week before quit date. • Start with 0.5 mg daily for 3 days, increase to 0.5 mg BID for 4 days, then 1 mg BID for duration of therapy. • Typical duration: 12 wks. • Patients may benefit from additional 12 week prolongation of varenicline, if tolerating medication as this has been observed to show increased rates of abstinence (JAMA 2006;296(1):64). • Varenicline is approved for maintenance therapy for up to 6 mos.	nausea; flatulence; headache; sleep disturbance; abnormal, vivid, or strange dreams; depression; agitation; hostility	• After randomized control trials including a meta-analysis showed no increased risk of neuropsychiatric effects even in patients with underlying mental illness compared to placebo. FDA removed Black box warning in 2016 (BMJ 2015;350: h1109.) • Dosage reduction recommended for patients who have creatinine clearance (CrCl) of <30 mL/min, or are on dialysis. • To reduce nausea, should be taken with food. To reduce insomnia, second pill can be taken at dinner rather than at bedtime. • Dosage may be reduced for patients with adverse effects.

From HRSA Guidelines for HIV/AIDS Clinical Care 2014:190.

Renal Complications

- *Screening for renal disease risk*: Race, family history, CD4 count, HIV VL, nephrotoxic drugs (current and prior use), comorbidities (hypertension, diabetes, hepatitis C).
- *Recommendations for routine serum creatinine* (with basic chemistry) at entry to care, every 6–12 mos before ART, at ART baseline, at 2–8 wks and then every 6–12 mos while on ART; plus urinalysis at entry to care, at ART initiation, and then every 6 mos if receiving TDF or every 12 mos if not (2017 DHHS Guidelines, CID 2014;59:e96). Importance of screening is increased in those with a risk for HIVAN or other renal disease.
  - *Annual screening* if high risk (African American, CD4 <200 cells/mm^3, HIV RNA >4,000 copies/mL), high-risk comorbidity (diabetes, hypertension, HCV), or receiving TDF (CID 2014;59:e96).
  - *Proteinuria >1+ by dipstick*: Quantitate proteinuria with "spot" urine protein:creatinine ratio. A protein:creatinine ratio ≤0.2 is normal; a ratio of 1 equates to 1 g protein/day; and a ratio of 2–3 indicates nephrosis and presumed glomerular disease.
  - *Chronic kidney disease* is defined as renal disease >3 mos.
  - CKD Epidemiology Collaboration (CKD-EPI) creatinine equation has been shown to be more accurate than Modification of Diet in Renal Disease (MDRD) or Cockcroft-Gault equation in PLWH (serum creatinine measured in mg/dL) (Kidney Int Suppl 2013;3:1; CID 2014;59:e96); however, the FDA continues to recommend the use of MDRD or Cockcroft-Gault equation for drug dosing in patients with decreased renal function:
  - *Females*:
    - If serum Cr ≤0.7: glomerular filtration rate (GFR) = 144 (SCr/0.7) – 0.329 × 0.993^{Age} (×1.159 if black)

- If serum Cr >0.7: GFR = 144 (SCr/0.7) – 1.209 × 0.993^{Age} (×1.159 if black)
- *Males*:
  - If serum Cr ≤0.9: GFR = 144 (SCr/0.9) – 0.411 × 0.993^{Age} (×1.159 if black)
  - If serum Cr >0.9: GFR = 144 (SCr/0.9) – 1.209 × 0.993^{Age} (×1.159 if black)
- *Chronic kidney disease*: Ultrasound to detect stones and assess renal size.
  - *Small* (<9 cm): Often severe kidney disease, heroin nephropathy (HAN)
  - *Large* (≥12 cm): HIVAN (but nonspecific, increased echogenicity more characteristic of HIVAN) (J Ultrasound Med 2004;23:603)
- *Other studies*: HBV, HCV, complement, ANA, cryoglobulins, quantitative immunoglobulins, blood glucose, protein electrophoresis.

Acute Kidney Injury (AKI)

DEFINITION: An increase in serum creatinine by 0.3 mg/dL within 48 hrs, or decrease in urine output to <0.5/mL/kg/hr for 6 hrs. Incidence is reported at 6 cases per 100 patient-years (Kidney Int 2005;67:1526).

CAUSE: Most common HIV-associated causes are HIVAN, HCV cryoglobulinemia, and drug-related (CID 2006;42:1488). Predictors include concurrent diabetes, chronic renal or liver disease, and hepatitis (AIDS 2006;20:561). One review of 2,274 patients found that the risk is much higher with CD4 counts of <100 cells/mm^3 (OR 7) and decreases by >10-fold with HIV treatment >3 mos (CID 2008;47:242). Drugs most likely to cause AKI in this population are aminoglycosides, amphotericin, cidofovir, foscarnet, pentamidine, TMP-SMX, and high-dose acyclovir. Antiretroviral drugs implicated are IDV and ATV with crystalluria (JAIDS 2003;32:135;

CID 2012;55:1262) and TDF with acute tubular necrosis (CID 2006;42:283). More recent reports of AKI in outpatients found that causes were diverse, including prerenal azotemia (38%), acute tubular necrosis (20%), or drug-related (15%) (HIV Ther 2010;4:589; Kidney Int 2010;78:478). An observational study of PLWH with AKI on admission to a hospital in Malawi showed that sepsis and nephrotoxins were the main causes (BMC Nephrol 2017;18(1):21). A review of 29 patients with AKI who had acute interstitial nephritis found that most had drug toxicity due to NSAIDs or TMP-SMX (Clin J Am Soc Nephrol 2010;5:798). ARV agents were implicated in only 3, and none had the classic triad of fever, rash, and pyuria (Clin J Am Soc Nephrol 2010;5:798).

Chronic Kidney Disease (CKD)

DEFINITION: Chronic renal disease defined as a GFR of <60/mL/min/1.7 mm^3 (Ann Intern Med 2003; 139:137) is relatively common in PLWH, with an incidence rate of 11 cases/1,000 person years in one report (JID 2008;197:1548). HIV infection leads to greater decline in renal function over time versus in uninfected individuals (JID 2017;216:622). Proteinuria is detected in 5% of PLWH (AIDS 2007;21:1003), and 2–10% have reduced eGFR.

CAUSE: In black patients, HIVAN is a common cause. In non-blacks, a common cause is immune complex-mediated kidney disease (HIVICK) (Kidney Int 1993;44:1327); other common causes include diabetes, hypertension, and HCV (Int J Nephrol Renovasc Dis 2016;9:223).

RISK FACTORS:

- Risk score for prediction of CKD in PLWH has been developed and externally validated (PLoS Med 2015;12:e1001809).
- Risk factors for progression to end-stage renal disease (ESRD) include HIVAN, African American descent, family history of ESRD, proteinuria, and advanced immunosuppression (Am J Kidney Dis 1999;34:254; AIDS 2007;21:2435;

JID 2008;197:1548; Am J Nephrol 2008;28:478; AIDS 2010;24:1877; AIDS 2008;22:841; CID 2014;59:e96).

- *HIV medication-associated renal injury*: Most common and important is TDF, which can cause AKI or CKD (CID 2010;51:496). IDV may cause AKI due to IDV crystallization and interstitial nephritis (AIDS 1998;12:2433; Ann Pharmacother 1998;32:843). ATV has also been associated with renal crystallization and interstitial nephritis (AIDS 2010;24:2239; Antivir Ther 2011;16:119). In a EuroSIDA cohort study with 6,843 patients, CKD was associated with use of TDF, IDV, ATV, and LPV/r; each additional year of use increased the rate of CKD by 16% for TDF and 22% for ATV; when ATV and TDF were combined, the increase in CKD was 41%/yr (AIDS 2010;24:1667). The prodrug TAF has lower tenofovir plasma levels and is associated with less nephrotoxic effects including improvement in proteinuria, albuminuria, and proximal renal tubule function compared to TDF (JAIDS 2017;75:226; Lancet ID 2016;16:43).

- *Racial differences*: Once chronic renal disease develops, risk of progression to ESRD is far greater in blacks with a hazard ratio of 17.7 and a GFR decline that is 6-fold more rapid (JID 2008;197:1548). This racial disparity appears to be independent of underlying etiology, although HIVAN appears to be nearly exclusively seen in patients of African descent (see later discussion). The association of black race with ESRD in patients with AIDS was noted early in the epidemic (NEJM 1984;310:669) and in the US Veterans Affairs Medical System (J Am Soc Nephrol 2007;18:2968). ESRD is relatively rare in European whites (AIDS 2007;21:1119; JID 2008;197:1490). A report from Zimbabwe on 3,316 African patients given ART found that 52 (1.6%) developed a GFR of <30 mL/min/1.7 m^2 by week 96 (CID 2008;46:1271). There was no significant association with any ART regimen, although 74% received TDF.

- *CVD*: CKD and CVD share common risk factors as well as strong association among PLWH. An analysis of the D:A:D study showed that individuals at high risk for CKD had a 1.31 times increase in CVD events, while persons at high risk for CVD had a 5.63 times increase in CKD events (PLOS Med 2017;14(11):e1002424).

Hepatitis C Coinfection

See J Am Soc Nephrol 1999;10:1566.

CAUSE: Mixed cryoglobulinemia, membranoproliferative glomerulonephritis. There is increased risk of renal disease among HIV-HCV co-infected patients compared to PLWH (BMC Inf Dis 2017;17(1):246).

SYMPTOMS: Palpable purpura, decreased complement, and renal disease with hematuria and proteinuria; may present with acute renal failure and/or nephrotic syndrome (J Hepatol 2008;49:613).

DIAGNOSIS: (1) evidence of hepatitis C (positive EIA and HCV RNA), (2) renal disease (hematuria and proteinuria) that may be in the nephrotic range, (3) low complement levels, (4) renal biopsy evidence of HCV-immune complexes, and (5) circulating cryoglobulins ± skin biopsy of purpuric lesion.

TREATMENT: Therapy is targeted against HCV as well as underlying renal manifestations. Historically, antiviral treatment included pegylated interferon and ribavirin-based regimens (Clinic Rev Allerg Immunol 2014;47:299). However, novel HCV DAAs are currently available and are better tolerated. Potential drug interactions between DAA and ART must be evaluated prior to initiating therapy (AASLD and IDSA HCV Guidelines 2017). In severe cryoglobulinemia, some recommend high-dose corticosteroids and plasmapheresis (Clinic Rev Allerg Immunol 2014;47:299). With progressive renal failure and/or nephrotic range proteinuria, some recommend cyclophosphamide or rituximab as means of immunosuppressive therapy (Kidney Int 2006;69:436; Kidney Int 2009;76:818).

Heroin Nephropathy (HAN) (CID 2005;40:1559)

CAUSE: Unknown, possibly glomerular epithelial cell injury from toxin contaminant (Am J Kidney Dis 1995;25:689).

FREQUENCY: Unknown, but decreased with increasing purity of street heroin. Frequency is increased in African Americans, who account for 94% of renal failure cases in one series of 98 patients (JAMA 1983;250:2935). HAN among blacks is more commonly associated with focal segmental glomerulosclerosis (FSGS), while membranoproliferative glomerulonephritis (MPGN) is more frequently associated with Caucasian heroin users (Clin J Am Soc Nephrol 2006;1:655; Forensic Sci Int 1998;95:109).

DIFFERENTIAL: Main differential is HIVAN. Characteristics of HAN: (1) hypertension, (2) small kidneys by ultrasound, (3) less rapid progression to ESRD (20–40 mos vs. 1–4 mos), (4) less proteinuria, and (5) differences on renal biopsy (Semin Nephrol 2003;23:117).

HIV-Associated Nephropathy (HIVAN)

CAUSE: Unknown, but most likely HIV infection of glomerular endothelial and mesangial cells (NEJM 2001;344:1979; Nat Med 2002;8:522). HIVAN is found almost exclusively in patients of African descent (Am Kidney Dis 2000;35:884; Kidney Int 2004;66:1145; JID 2008;197:1548). One proposed genetic mechanism is via apolipoprotein L1 (APOL1) gene on chromosome 22q13.1 with variants that predispose patients to kidney disease. Interestingly, these variants are found more often in African American patients (Kidney Int 2014;86:266; Front Microbiol 2015;6:571).

FREQUENCY: An analysis of 3,976 PLWH in Baltimore (78% African American) found an incidence rate for ESRD due to HIVAN in African Americans to be about 1/1,000 patient-years (JID 2008;197:1548); a review in the UK showed an incidence rate of 0.6/1,000 patient years for black patients (CID 2008:46:1288). A review of PLWH with reduced baseline GFR found that 100/284 (35%) progressed to ESRD, of whom 99 were African American. Renal biopsies in 73 showed HIVAN in 37 (37%). Risk factors for HIVAN in African Americans include AIDS and a VL of >100,000 copies/mL, male sex, family history of renal disease (Am J Kidney Dis 1999;34:254; Am J Kidney Dis 2000;35:884; CID 2006;42:1488), and injection drug use (NEJM 1987;316:1062; Kidney Int 1987;31:1678; Kidney Int 1990;37:1325). ART has a protective effect, with a 60% reduction in incidence in one large study (AIDS 2004;18:541). However, another review of 61 cases showed that viral suppression with ART had a survival benefit but no benefit with respect to renal outcome (CID 2008;46:1282) (see later discussion). The incidence of HIVAN has significantly decreased with time in the HAART era (Am J Nephrol. 2008;28(3):478).

DIAGNOSIS: Baseline proteinuria is a sensitive predictor of chronic renal disease (JAIDS 2003;32:2003; Clin Nephrol 2004;61:1). Characteristic features are (1) nearly all patients are of African descent, (2) there is a rapid rise in creatinine, (3) nephrotic range proteinuria (>3 g/d), and (4) detectable HIV VL (Topics HIV Med 2007;14:164). Other common features are normal blood pressure, large echogenic kidneys, lack of peripheral edema despite hypoalbuminemia, late-stage HIV infection, and rapid progression to ESRD in 1–4 mos (NEJM 1987;316:1062; Kidney Int 1995;48:311; Am J Roentgenol 1998;171:713; Semin Dialy 2003;16:233). Thus, typical clinical features are GFR <60 mL/min for >3 mo, proteinuria >1.5 g/24 hr, typical echogenic kidneys, and absence of alternative causes (CID 2008;46:1282). *Definitive diagnosis requires renal biopsy.* Renal biopsy shows a collapsing focal glomerulosclerosis with tubulointerstitial injury. Renal biopsy is recommended to establish this diagnosis according to an NIH review of HIV-associated renal disease (Ann Intern Med 2003;139:214). A review of 55 PLWH with >3 g/d proteinuria, plus renal biopsy found that only 29 (53%) had HIVAN, emphasizing the need for renal biopsy (Am J Med 2006;118: 1288). Collapsing glomerulopathy, the hallmark of HIVAN, has now been described in patients with autoimmune diseases without HIV (Lupus 2011;20:866).

TREATMENT:

- *ART*: All patients should be treated with ART regardless of CD4 count. ART also appears to protect against HIVAN (2017 DHHS Guidelines). A 12-yr study found HIVAN in 7% of African Americans with AIDS who were receiving ART and 26% in those who were not treated (AIDS 2004;18:541). Initial data based on biopsy results indicate benefit with ART (Lancet 1998;352:783; Clin Nephrol 2002;57:335; NEJM 2001;344:1979). Some show dramatic improvement (NEJM 2001;344:1979), but this may be only temporary (AIDS Patient Care STD 2000;14:657), as another report found that, once HIVAN is established, the use of ART has little impact on progression to ESRD (CID 2008;46:1282).
- *Dialysis* (Am J Kidney Dis 1997;29:549): One report found that one-third of HIVAN patients required dialysis within 1 mo of the diagnosis (Nephrol Dial Transplant 2006;21:2809).
- *ACE inhibitors and ARBs*: Treatment with captopril (6.25–25 mg po tid) and other ACE inhibitors has beneficial results and should be used in patients who do not respond to ART (J Am Soc Nephrol 1997;8:1140; Am J Kidney Dis 1996;28:202; Kidney Int 2003;64:1462).
- *Corticosteroids*: Prednisone (60 mg/d × 2–11 wks, followed by 2–26 wk taper) shows variable results in terms of renal function and proteinuria (Am J Med 1994;97:145; Kidney Int 2000;58:1253; Semin Nephrol 1998;18:446). Supporting data are limited (Clin Nephrol 2002;57:336).
- *Renal transplantation*: Cohort of 11 patients with biopsy-proven HIVAN were retrospectively reviewed (PLoS ONE 2015;10:e0129702):
  - *Graft survival*: 1 yr, 100%; 3 yrs, 81%.
  - *Rejection incidence*: 1 yr, 18%; 3 yrs, 27%.

HIV-Associated Immune-Complex Kidney Disease (HIVICK)

DEFINITION: Includes postinfectious glomerulonephritis, membranous nephritis, IgA nephritis, fibrillary glomerulonephritis, immunotactoid glomerulopathy, and membranoproliferative glomerulonephritis (Nephrol Dial Transplant 1993;8:11; Ann Intern Med 2003;139:214; Kidney Int 2005;67:1381; CID 2006;42:1488).

FREQUENCY: Estimated at 15–80% in PLWH with chronic renal disease (CID 2006;42:1488). A cohort of 751 PLWH in Baltimore revealed that HIVICK was predominant in patients of African America descent; however, ESRD incidence was decreased compared to HIVAN (Clin J Am Soc Nephrol 2013;8:1524). Similar results were observed in the UK CHIC cohort study (Nephrol Dial Transplant 2016;31:2099).

TREATMENT: ART, ACE inhibitors, and/or corticosteroids (Nephrol Dial Transplant 1997;12:2796; Clin Nephrol 2003;60:187).

Nephrotoxic drugs: COBI, DTG, and RPV have been associated with increases in serum creatinine due to inhibition of tubular creatinine secretion. These are not associated with reduced GFR as outlined below (CID 2014;59:e96):
- *Cobicistat*: Uptake by renal organic cation transporter (OCT2) leads to inhibition of multidrug and toxin extrusion transporter (MATE1), which decreases urinary creatinine secretion (Kidney Int 2014;86:350).
- *Dolutegravir*: Inhibits OCT2 causing decreased urinary creatinine secretion; leads to small elevations in serum creatinine (by 0.1–0.2 mg/dL) in treatment-naïve adults but is not associated with change in eGFR as confirmed in phase I studies (CID 2014;59:265).
- *Rilpivirine*: Also inhibits OCT2 (AIDS Rev 2014;16:199).

Thrombotic Thrombocytopenia Purpura, HIV-Associated Thrombotic Microangiopathy

Kidney Transplantation

Kidney transplant has been shown to be a viable option in PLWH. A consortium of 19 US transplant centers reported outcomes for patients with HIV (2003-2009) (NEJM 2010;363:2004).

- *Criteria*: (1) CD4 count >200 cells/mm^3; (2) HIV VL suppressed to <50 c/mL or <75 c/mL while receiving stable ART ≥16 wks prior to transplant; (3) no history of PML, cryptosporidiosis, CNS lymphoma, or visceral KS; and (4) if HBV or HCV, a liver biopsy that excludes cirrhosis.
- *Baseline data for 150 patients*: Median age 46 yrs, median CD4 534 cells/mm^3, HCV 19%, HBV 3%; cause of renal failure: HTN 25%, HIVAN 24%, diabetes 9%, other/unknown 36%.
- *Results*:
  - *Patient survival*: 1 yr, 94%; 3 yrs, 88%.
  - *Graft survival*: 1 yr, 90%; 3 yrs, 74%.
  - *Rejection incidence*: 31%.
  - *Progression of HIV*: Five AIDS-defining complications.
- *Conclusions*: Renal transplantation is "highly feasible" in this population. Rates of patient and graft survival were intermediate between transplant recipients without HIV and recipients >65 yrs. There was an unexpectedly high rate of rejection (by a factor of 2–3). Outcomes among HIV/HCV co-infected patients are worse. Data from the Scientific Registry of Transplant Recipients matching 510 PLWH 1:10 to HIV-negative controls (J Am Soc Nephrol 2015;26:2222):
  - *HIV-negative graft survival*: 5 yrs, 75.3%; 10 yrs, 54.4%.
  - *HIV-positive graft survival*: 5 yrs, 69.2%; 10 yrs, 49.8%.
  - *HIV/HCV co-infected graft survival*: 5 yrs, 52%; 10 yrs, 27%.
- *International experience*: Similar studies conducted in France, United Kingdom, Spain, and Brazil had similar outcomes

with patient survival, graft survival, and rejection incidence (up to 44%) (Am J Transplant 2010;10:2263; Nephrol Dial Transplant 2011;26:1401; Int J STD AIDS 2014;25:57; Transpl Infect Dis 2017;19(4):e12724).

- *HIV patients as donors*: A cohort of 27 PLWH in South Africa received kidney transplants from HIV-infected, deceased donors (only 1 donor had been receiving ART) (NEJM 2015;372:613).
  - *Results*:
    - *Patient survival*: 1 yr, 84%; 3 yrs, 84%; 5 yrs, 74%.
    - *Graft survival*: 1 yr, 93%; 3 yrs, 84%; 5 yrs, 84%.
    - *Rejection incidence*: 1 yr, 8%; 3 yrs, 22%.
    - *Progression of HIV*: Multiple non-HIV infections in most (30%) patients, 3 patients with infectious complications that led to death.
- In 2013, the US passed the HIV Organ Policy Equity (HOPE) Act to allow PLWH to donate organs to other PLWH. Research guidelines were published in 2015 in preparation for transplants (Final HIV Organ Policy Equity [HOPE] Act Safeguards and Research Criteria for Transplantation or Organs Infected with HIV, 2015). The first HIV-to-HIV kidney transplantation in the US was performed in 2016. There were 23 kidney transplants performed at US centers under approved research protocols by the end of 2017. Due to the relatively low number of transplants to date, additional studies are needed to evaluate the efficacy of HIV-to-HIV transplantation.

Index

Tables and figures are indicated by an italic *t* and *f*, respectively, following the page number.